# ELECTROACUPUNCTURE

## A PRACTICAL MANUAL AND RESOURCE

# ELECTROACUPUNCTURE
## A PRACTICAL MANUAL AND RESOURCE

Edited by

## DAVID F MAYOR, MA BAc MBAcC
**Practising Acupuncturist, Welwyn Garden City, UK**

Forewords by

Angela and John Hicks
Joint Prinicipals of the College of Integrated Chinese Medicine, Reading, UK

Zang-Hee Cho
Professor, Radiological Sciences and Psychiatry and Human Behavior,
Director, Functional Imaging and Acupuncture Research,
University of California, Irvine, California, USA

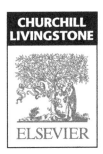

Edinburgh London New York Oxford Philadelphia St Louis Sydney Toronto 2007

**CHURCHILL**
**LIVINGSTONE**
ELSEVIER

Churchill Livingstone is a registered trackemark of Elsevier Limited

First published 2007
 Reprinted 2007

ISBN 13: 978 0 443 06369 5
ISBN 10: 0 443 0 6369 9

**British Library Cataloguing in Publication Data**
A catalogue record for this book is available from the British Library

**Library of Congress Cataloging in Publication Data**
A catalog record for this book is available from the Library of Congress

**Notice**
Knowledge and best practice in this field are constantly changing. As new research and experience broaden our knowledge, changes in practice, treatment and drug therapy may become necessary or appropriate. Readers are advised to check the most current information provided (i) on procedures featured or (ii) by the manufacturer of each product to be administered, to verify the recommended dose or formula, the method and duration of administration, and contraindications. It is the responsibility of the practitioner, relying on their own experience and knowledge of the patient, to make diagnoses, to determine dosages and the best treatment for each individual patient, and to take all appropriate safety precautions. To the fullest extent of the law, neither the Publisher nor the Editors assumes any liability for any injury and/or damage to persons or property arising out or related to any use of the material contained in this book.

**The Publisher**

For Churchill Livingstone:
Publishing Manager: *Karen Morley*
Project Development Manager: *Kerry McGechie, Louise Allsop*
Project Manager: *Cheryl Brant*
Design Direction: *Stewart Larking*

Printed in Spain

# Contents

# Foreword

We first saw electroacupuncture being used effectively over twenty-five years ago. The electroacupuncture machine was less sophisticated than those in current use and the practitioner possibly less skilled – but it worked! The patient felt no pain as her tooth was removed. It seemed – and was – miraculous. Since that time we have seen its increasing use in the treatment of many conditions – especially for painful conditions, for treatment in childbirth and for addictions.

Seen in the context of acupuncture's 2000+ -year history, electroacupuncture is still a relatively 'young' technique. Much of its potential is still being explored and its newness invariably throws up both new and exciting information as well as some conflicts and questions. David deals with this in the style of the oldest Chinese medicine traditions. He gives us the information and allows us to hold many truths simultaneously. He makes no secret of the conflicting research and protocols that can be found, but at the same time answers some of our most pressing questions such as: How is electroacupuncture used? What is it used for? What is the theory behind it? Is it thoroughly researched?

Some practitioners will wish to know about the practicalities of electroacupuncture. For them there are clear instructions about how to choose and use electroacupuncture machines as well as treatment protocols for a vast number of conditions. These include the treatment of pain, obstetrics and gynaecology, psychological and nervous conditions, stroke and cerebrovascular diseases and a huge array of other diseases. Accompanying many of these are case studies to illustrate the effects of the treatments and there are many contributions – at least twenty – by experts in their individual fields.

Other practitioners may wish to understand more about the theory of electroacupuncture. For them David has provided a meticulously researched, in-depth exploration into this subject. He has written chapters on electroacupuncture's historic roots and research into how it works. Best of all, he has provided a research database of over 8000 accessible studies on his accompanying CD-rom.

In *Electroacupuncture* David Mayor, together with his contributors, has given us not only a textbook, but also an encyclopaedia. It covers every aspect of the practice of this treatment mode. There is unlikely to be any other textbook on the subject of electroacupuncture to surpass this book in completeness of content and depth and breadth of research. As such it is likely to become a classic and will stay on our shelves as a reference book for countless years to come.

*Angela Hicks*
*John Hicks*
*Joint Principals*
*College of Integrated Chinese Medicine,*
*Reading, UK*

# Foreword

I am very pleased to have been asked to write this foreword by my friend David Mayor. Few people can be as knowledgeable as he is on the subject of electroacupuncture, with its roots in both Western science and Eastern tradition.

This unique and much needed book, based on many years of study, practice and teaching, is the most wide-ranging overview of modern times on acupuncture, and electroacupuncture in particular. It is the first description of acupuncture to integrate traditional concepts and modern science to such an extent.

The investigation of acupuncture, as defined by this book, is a complex interdisciplinary process, which we believe has to be based predominantly on modern neuroscience. It embraces complexities and uncertainties which no one person or group can possibly solve alone, although each investigator can contribute to understanding based on their own intellectual and scientific backgrounds.

Acupuncture research is still in its infancy and we do not know exactly how it works. We can hazard many guesses but have neither the definitive experimental results nor clear hypotheses to support particular theories. However, we do now have several established explanations derived from neuroscience, based on neurohumoral responses and autonomic nervous system reflexes. We even have some, albeit preliminary, neuroscientific results from neuroimaging research on the cortical activation that accompanies acupuncture stimulation. These can begin to explain some of acupuncture's main functions, such as its analgesic effects.

To fully understand acupuncture, however, we need a great deal more scientific exploration, with evidence to support its neurochemical, neurophysiological and neuroimmunological aspects. What seems important at this stage of development is unbiased and statistically well supported scientific experimental study as a foundation for progress towards better understanding. With sufficient basic data and proper scientific hypotheses, we can proceed further. In this connection, I am delighted to see this book, in my opinion possibly the most comprehensive acupuncture science publication ever attempted in its depth and breadth, covering the whole field from a classical acupuncture background to modern physics and electrical theory. I am sure there will be subsequent revisions and additions to this book by the author himself as well as others. With its associated database, it will certainly remain one of the most scientific and comprehensive resources for future acupuncture research.

But this is not a book just about physiological experiments, impersonal technology, theories and scientific evidence. It is also about human values and the application of knowledge in therapy, and offers a rich source of clinical information, remaining respectful of both scientific and traditional approaches.

As a scientist involved in acupuncture research, I can recommend this invaluable book without reservation, both for practising and student acupuncturists who would like to understand the basics of acupuncture in a modern scientific context and as a wonderful reference book for those in the field of acupuncture research.

*Zang-Hee Cho,*
*Professor, Radiological Sciences and Psychiatry and Human Behavior*
*Director, Functional Imaging and Acupuncture Research*
*Universtiy of California, Irvine, California, USA*

# Preface

There are many varieties of acupuncture, from highly traditional to outrageously avantgarde, although most practitioners are aware only of a few. This book was always intended to expand this awareness, and has been designed with acupuncture students, researchers and practitioners in mind, whether nonmedical acupuncturists, physical therapists or doctors.

It began as an attempt to organise electroacupuncture teaching materials into something more widely useful, after I had been exploring the method in practice for eight years or so, and reading the literature for a lot longer than that. I also did not want just to repeat what I had been taught or found for myself, but to pass on what was supported by more objective research. Inta Ozols of Churchill Livingstone, who had been looking for someone to write a book on electroacupuncture, expressed interest. Research and gestation began, the book started to grow ... and grow.

While the publishers wanted a thoroughgoing practical introduction to the subject, I had always stubbornly wanted to write more of a research resource, for people to dig into and discover for themselves the richness of nontraditional acupuncture. Over the years since it was first discussed in 1996, the project has developed into something which I think satisfies both the need for a textbook of reasonable length and, at a time when research is very much a focus for anyone involved in acupuncture, for a comprehensive research tool. The result should enable better practice, enhance understanding and increase knowledge.

Readers who want the basics will find their needs met in the book. Those who want more detail can find it in the longer chapter versions on the CD-Rom. And if you need to find out what has actually been done in clinical studies, the flexible CD-Rom database of more than 8000 studies on electroacupuncture and other acupuncture-related modalities should provide ample information. This also available on the Web, at www.electroacupunctureknowledge.com. For innovative content, an innovative structure seemed appropriate. Further information on the structure of this publication and how to use it can be found in the Introduction.

In life, completeness is unattainable, particularly in a large and rapidly changing field. Despite the resources of the Needham Research Institute and the British Library, and much hard work by translators, large chunks of the world acupuncture literature have remained inaccessible to me. And, given its current momentum, it will no doubt always outpace even the most diligent researcher. However, if readers do find mistakes or omissions that they can rectify, assistance would be warmly welcomed. It goes without saying that any such mistakes or omissions remain my responsibility.

On the other hand, as I am discovering, understanding does not mean having to know everything. A little mystery seasons the salad and, to quote Anaïs Nin, 'the most important of all achievements is to be a human being'.[1]

Writing this book has been a huge challenge. I am grateful for the opportunity it has given me to learn and grow and to practise acupuncture more effectively for my patients. I hope it will help others to do the same.

*DFM*
*Welwyn Garden City*

Note

1 Nin A 1970 The Journals of Anais Nin, 1939–1944 (ed G Stuhlmann). Peter Owen, London

# Endorsements

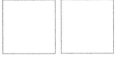

*Electroacupuncture: A Practical Manual and Resource* is timely, insightful and valuable. Unlike most medical authors, David F. Mayor recognizes that individual physicians build understanding and mastery in individual ways. Instead of providing a sterile tome of information to digest, Mayor provides a core resource of basic information that links readily to an in-depth coverage of key issues, an evidence base, a glossary of terms, references, and a website resource. The reader seeking to enhance his or her unique understanding finds a wide range of resources available, and it is possible to follow a particular thread of interest to multiple deeper levels. Unlike a standard medical text, this is a resource that engages the reader and invites exploration.

C Richard Chapman
*Professor and Director, Pain Research Center, Department of Anesthesiology, University of Utah School of Medicine*

With 22 special contributors, 85 illustrations, and over 8000 clinical references David F Mayor's research based Electroacupuncture book plus CD-Rom is a truly stunning achievement. The reader is taken through the techniques of applying EA to the beneficial application of EA across the complete range of clinical specialities. This, in itself, constitutes a valuable review of a wide range of disorders, for which carefully administered EA offers symptomatic and often causal relief. From the neurological pathways and neuropsychological effects of EA to a review of the theories and evidence for body bioelectricity, bioelectric circuitries, currents of injury and biophysical microresonances the author explores the informational dynamics of frequency interaction within the living matrix and its implications for therapeutic EA intervention. This book and its accompanying CD-Rom should be on the bookshelf of every acupuncturist, every NHS and GP service providing acupuncture, and in the library of every university faculty that offers courses in acupuncture and CAM therapies.

Robert A Charman
*Former lecturer in physiotherapy, University of Wales College of Medicine. Founder chairman, Association of Chartered Physiotherapists in Energy Medicine Editor,* Complementary Therapies for Physical Therapists (2000)

Most acupuncturists have no more than a passing knowledge of the practice of electroacupuncture and a comprehensive text on the subject has been sorely needed for some time, particularly in view of the accumulation of recent electroacupuncture research. Who better to compile such a book than David Mayor, whose long-standing absorption in the subject is reflected in this substantial work. For anyone who wants to expand and refine their range of treatment options, this is an essential text.

Peter Deadman
*Editor of the* Journal of Chinese Medicine *and co-author of* A Manual of Acupuncture. *Hove, England*

This comprehensive compilation of clinical *and* research information on electroacupuncture provides an outstanding resource to further the important dialogue between two key stake holders in the acupuncture community. Researchers can learn how to design protocols that best reflect clinical practice while acupuncturists can learn of numerous studies that are contributing to the evidence base for their traditional health care system.

Richard Hammerschlag
*Research Director, Oregon College of Oriental Medicine, Adjunct Professor of Neurology, Oregon Health and Science University, Past-president, Society for Acupuncture Research*

Electroacupuncture (EA) is a very important modality of acupuncture in its broadest sense. Compared to manual needling it has the benefit of stronger therapeutic effect and is more cost-effective for the patient. However, the proper application of EA requires knowledge not only of traditional acupuncture, but also of biophysics and other relevant disciplines that may not be familiar to most practitioners. One can hardly imagine that a single book could fulfil the requirements of clinicians on the one side and those oriented to research on the other. Moreover, the interests of acupuncturists who are traditionarily trained and those with a Western medical training will also be very different. However, by their innovative approach the author and publisher have successfully solved the problem by editing this publication in two parts, one classical book for a clear outline presentation and a CD-Rom for more detailed material and a huge updateable database. I am quite sure that the publication of this book will greatly foster the more general use of EA in clinical practice and help improve its therapeutic effect. One can predict that in the long run it will also stimulate research into the mechanisms of EA.

Han Jisheng
*Founder and professor, Neuroscience Research Centre, Beijing University, founder of the Chinese Association for the Study of Pain, member of the Chinese Academy of Sciences, author of* The Neurochemical Basis of Pain Relief by Acupuncture vols 1 and 2 (Beijing 1987, Wuhan 1988)

This book has been some time in preparation but the waiting has been worthwhile. David Mayor has covered his field most comprehensively; he has read very widely and considered many relatively unusual sources together with mainstream research papers. He has also remained true to his roots and the ideas of TCM are not absent, but quietly in the background. All efforts to integrate science and TCM in a meaningful way are to be applauded.

Physiotherapists using acupuncture as one of their professional skills have always been drawn to electroacupuncture. Electricity is just another "physical modality" and has been used by the profession to relax tissues and re-educate muscle for decades. When not dealing with pain in its myriad variations, physiotherapists are frequently concerned with the functioning of the nervous system. Electroacupuncture has often seemed like a key to both doors.

Val Hopwood
*Author of Acupuncture in Physiotherapy (2004), Leader, MSc Acupuncture course, Coventry University, England. Education Adviser, Acupuncture Association of Chartered Physiotherapists*

David Mayor has given us one of the most wanted books in acupuncture - The Book about electroacupuncture.

He has approached each chapter with an almost radical sense of compassion, as if all that any of us could do were to stumble ahead with the new knowledge we´re given. The result is a book crammed with wisdoms both from a scientific and clinical perspective. I don´t usually like books about acupuncture but if they were all like David Mayor´s - I´d read them by the truckload.

Thomas Lundeberg
*Professor in integrative physiology and senior consultant in rehabilitation medicine and algology, Stockholm, Sweden*

David Mayor has provided us with an outstanding compilation of information and research on electroacupuncture. With scholarship and attention to detail, he explores what he calls this "rich seam of knowledge". Undoubtedly this book will be the bible on electroacupuncture for many years to come.

Hugh MacPherson
*Senior Research Fellow, Department of Health Sciences, University of York, England. Co-editor of Acupuncture in Practice (1997)*

This book is an excellent resource for both practitioner and academic and is a valuable addition to the acupuncture literature. The novel approach, using written and computer media, has ensured the publication is user-friendly and allows a reader to target areas of individual interest. David Mayor has brought together a distinguished group of contributors, assuring readers of the highest quality of both clinical and research knowledge in this field. In this era of evidence-based practice, in-depth knowledge of the evidence underpinning practice is crucial; hence a resource containing such a vast number of clinical studies and numerous other references will be of immense value to practising clinicians as well as academics, researchers and teachers of acupuncture. The author gracefully integrates Traditional Chinese and western scientific principles underpinning electroacupuncture without conflict, in my belief, a hugely positive step for the practice of acupuncture itself.

Lynley Roberts
*Senior Lecturer, Faculty of Health & Sport Science, Eastern Institute of Technology, New Zealand*

This work is a masterpiece, an amazing achievement. It is the deepest and most critical assessment of the international literature to date. It is a labour of love that took nine years of painstaking research to compile.

Overall, because of its vast breath and depth of coverage, this is a difficult work to assimilate. It will take many readings but is a work destined to become the standard reference on electroacupuncture for many years to come. Hearty congratulations to its author and his team of expert contributers!

Phil Rogers
*Acupuncturist and student of Traditional Chinese Medicine, Dublin, Ireland*
http://homepage.tinet.ie/~progers

This is the most thorough text I have seen on the practice of electroacupuncture, covering every conceivable aspect of the field in an extremely user friendly, yet scientific manner. It will be used regularly by all practitioners and should be in the library of every acupuncturist, whether in practice, research or academia. Have this text in your library, read it and your patients will benefit.

Allen M Schoen
*Editor of Veterinary Acupuncture, Ancient Art to Modern Medicine (2nd edition, St Louis 2001) and co-editor, Complementary and Alternative Veterinary Medicine (St Louis 1998). Assistant Clinical Professor, Tufts University School of Veterinary Medicine, N Grafton, MA*

This book is dedicated

To the memory of four remarkable men, my mentors and friends:

Teddy Potter, who showed me the beauty of physics;

Herbert Weaver, who revealed for me the magical world of the dowser;

Roger Rose, who generously shared his enthusiasm for electroacupuncture in all its forms;

and Ken Chitty, whose tongue-in-cheek belief in the placebo value of electrical gadgetry
was always an inspiration and delight;

and to the many thousands of animals whose lives have been scarred or sacrificed
in the cause of acupuncture research.

# Contributors

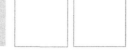

**Ken Andrews**
Modern acupuncturist, osteomyologist and biological terrain practitioner in private practice, Leigh, Lancashire, UK. Teaches auricular acupuncture and EAV internationally. Chairman, Auricular Association (GB).

**Steven KH Aung**
Family physician, Edmonton, Alberta, Canada. Assistant professor, University of Alberta, where he founded Certificate Program in Medical Acupuncture. Founder and President, World Natural Medicine Foundation. Author of books and articles on TCM.

**Mark Bovey**
Acupuncturist, Oxford. Coordinator, Acupuncture Research Resource Centre, Thames Valley University, West London. Faculty member, College of Integrated Chinese Medicine, Reading, UK.

**Ann Brownbill**
Naturopath specialising in acupuncture, Welwyn Garden City, UK. Also works in London at a clinic providing acupuncture to those with drug-misuse-related problems. Has a background in nursing.

**Sarah Budd**
Acupuncturist midwife, Maternity Unit, Derriford Hospital, Plymouth, UK. Has worked as a research assistant in the Acupuncture Research Resource Centre. Coauthored a report for Department of Health on the Regulation of Complementary Medicine in the UK.

**Josephine Cerqua**
Acupuncturist in both private and NHS practice, London. Clinic assistant, University of Westminster Polyclinic, London, UK.

**Jennifer Chu**
Associate Professor and Director, Electrodiagnosis Laboratory, Department of Rehabilitation Medicine, University of Pennsylvania, USA. Has pioneered automated and electrical twitch-obtaining intramuscular stimulation.

**Mike Cummings**
Medical Director, British Medical Acupuncture Society. Also works privately as a lecturer, medical acupuncturist and musculoskeletal physician in London, UK. Formerly a Medical Officer in the Royal Air Force.

**Stuart Ferraris**
Holistic dentist in private practice, Beaumaris, Wales, UK. Formerly a Dental Officer in the South African navy. Lectures nationally and internationally.

**Michael Flowerdew**
Electroacupuncture practitioner, Beccles, Suffolk, UK. Has coauthored a Cochrane review and instruction manuals and courses on modern approaches to acupuncture.

**J Gordon Gadsby**
Retired from private full-time electroacupuncture practice, Leicester, UK. Coauthor of a Cochrane review. Former nurse practitioner and lecturer, with a PhD on electroanalgesia.

**Goto Kamiya**
Ryodoraku practitioner in private practice, Yokohama, Japan. Standing Director, Japanese Society of Ryodoraku Medicine; author of Society's official basic ryodoraku textbook.

## Maureen Lovesey

Physiotherapist and acupuncturist in private practice, Berkhamsted, UK. Founder member and first Chairman, Acupuncture Association of Physical Therapists. Has lectured and published on various aspects of practice.

## Juliette Lowe

Practises acupuncture and Chinese herbal medicine in Ardross and Inverness, Scotland. Previously worked in London, UK, both privately and within the NHS.

## David F Mayor

Acupuncturist in private practice, Welwyn Garden City, UK. Lectures on electroacupuncture at a number of acupuncture colleges.

## Pekka J Pöntinen

Associate Professor of Anaesthesiology, Kuopio and Tampere Universities, Finland. President, Laser Therapy Institute, Zug, Switzerland. Editor in Chief, *Scandinavian Journal of Acupuncture and Electrotherapy*, 1986–1992. Author of over 200 articles and five books. Lecturer on acupuncture and laser therapy worldwide since the 1970s.

## Rodney S Robinson

Faculty administrator, Society of Biophysical Medicine, Liverpool, UK, where he also works with CIC – Drug Services and is closely involved with research and development of new electrostimulation and measurement approaches. Has a background in nursing, biomedical sciences and homeopathy.

## Lynnae Schwartz

Senior research fellow, National Institute of Neurological Disorders and Stroke, National Institutes of Health, and consultant for complex chronic pain in children through the Children's National Medical Center, Washington, DC, USA.

## Ron Sharp

Physiotherapist and acupuncturist at Stoke Mandeville Hospital. Teaches acupuncture for the Acupuncture Association of Chartered Physiotherapists and runs a private sports injury clinic.

## John L Stump

Practises at a private integrative medicine centre in Fairhope, AL, USA. Has doctorates in sports medicine, chiropractic and oriental medicine. Teaches for the International Academy of Medical Acupuncture. Author of several books and articles.

## Lyndsey Taylor (now Isaacs)

Acupuncturist in private practice, Rickmansworth, UK; also works at a clinic specialising in the use of electroacupuncture in the treatment of infertility. Has worked as a nurse in the UK, Australia, New Zealand and the USA.

## Adrian R White

Runs a small private acupuncture clinic in Saltash, Cornwall, UK; Editor in Chief, *Acupuncture in Medicine*; Past Chairman and Treasurer, British Medical Acupuncture Society; formerly Senior Lecturer, Department of Complementary Medicine, Exeter University. Has published systematic reviews, RCTs and other primary research on acupuncture.

## Jacqueline Young

Clinical psychologist and oriental medical practitioner, with a practice in central London, UK. Author of several books on natural medicine and a regular contributor to health publications and websites.

Further biographical details can be found in the CD-ROM ⊙ resource.

# Acknowledgements

This publication, so long in its maturing, would not have been possible without the help, support and patience of very many people.

In the first place, I would like to thank my respected teachers John and Angela Hicks of the College of Integrated Chinese Medicine (CICM), who encouraged me in my own aspiration to teach electroacupuncture, and also Bennie (Man Fong) Mei of AcuMedic, who first suggested I consider publishing my teaching notes in some form. Inta Ozols, who initially commissioned the book for Churchill Livingstone, was very generous in her trust, despite my wildly ambitious ideas, and that support has been continued by her successor as Elsevier's commissioning editor for complementary and integrative medicine, Karen Morley, and by Kerry McGechie and Louise Allsop, development editors. The production and marketing staff at Elsevier, and Richard Cook at Keyword, have been most helpful. I have particularly appreciated the calm support of my copy editor, Christine Wyard, and the indexing skills of Nigel d'Auvergne.

Those who have waited longest have been the many practitioners who contributed case studies early on for the book. I appreciate their patience, and hope that their work is presented as they would like it. Other contributors, who rescued the ship when I realised I could no longer row with only one oar, generously provided whole chapters, or chunks of chapters, and good humouredly put up with my bullying as time seemed to stretch inexorably past all deadlines. All these are named in the Table of Contents. I am also honoured that Zang-Hee Cho, and Angela and John Hicks, have written forewords for the publication.

Without editing, this book would have been totally unreadable. Those who have helped here include Rebecca Avern (Ch. 9.15), Clare Dobie (Chs 9.2 and 9.7), Mick Flowerdew (Ch. 9.14), Diana Griffin (Ch. 9.5), Susie Parkinson (Ch. 3), Karen Proudfoot (Ch. 9.8), Will Richardson (Ch. 9.4) and Billie Wray (Ch. 9.1). I am most grateful for their help, particularly Billie, who suggested that John Wheeler might be a good person to complete the job. Which he did, at immense speed, ploughing through all the chapters in the book with scalpels flailing, yet with great courtesy and understanding. I've no idea how he did it, in addition to the huge amount of work he was putting in for the British Acupuncture Council at the same time. Thank you, John.

Literature research to deal with many of the queries arising before the chapters could be finalised was carried out by Josephine Cerqua, Alex Griffin and Pekka Pöntinen.

At an earlier stage, before the chapters were edited, I was fortunate in that several people managed to read some of them through, in whole or in part. For this, I am grateful to Steven Aung, Panos Barlas, Ifor Capel, Dick Chapman, Bob Charman, Riccardo Cuminetti, Helen Dorrell, Gordon Gadsby, Alison Gould, Kuratani Kyomi, Jim Oschman (to whom I also apologise for some rather outspoken comments I have made publicly on his own books), Susie Parkinson, Jackie Young and particularly Richard Hammerschlag, who ploughed through chapter 7 in a rather noisy London pub with me one illuminating evening when things were looking especially difficult. I appreciate their helpful suggestions, although I have to say I happily ignored most of them, being a stubborn sort of animal. I did pay some attention, though, to the anonymous Churchill Livingstone reviewers who were helpful in shaping this book in its very earliest stages, although they may not think so now.

The text is only one part of this publication. Illustrations help where further words might only confuse, but this was one part of the process that I found most difficult and frustrating. Without Melissa Maudling's ability to interpret my scribblings as precise line drawings, Riccardo Cuminetti's skills with digital photography, and the facility and patience of Graeme

Chambers in preparing the final versions, I would truly have been lost. Thanks too to all those who provided other material (as indicated in figure captions throughout).

In addition, there is the database. Like the book, this grew from a small seed of an idea into something too large for any one person to handle. I have to thank all who have endured the tedium of entering clinical studies, from those at the beginning, when it was all unfamiliar territory, such as Karen Adams, Jane Curtis, Elke Hockings and Susannah Turner, to later stalwarts like Josephine Cerqua and Paul Smithson. Gordon Gadsby did a particularly useful job on the TENS studies. Translation work was also involved, and here I would have been totally out of my depth without Josephine Cerqua (French, Italian, Spanish), Natasha Gromak, Anna Nerukh and Irina Szmelskyj (Russian, Ukrainian), Ajna Matthey de l'Etang (French, German), Irmi Hochbein, Homayoun Pakzamir, Diana Schneidewind, Sabine Schnelle and Petra Werth (German), Cinzia Scorzon (Italian) and Ye Jing Huang (Chinese). Jing, in particular, has been a star, working her way with gusto through thousands of studies, in English as well as Chinese, despite her other commitments.

Others who have helped with translation queries include Park Jongbae, Giovanni Maciocia, Peter Offord and Hilary Smith (who worked on some of the Chinese experimental studies).

Without libraries, there would have been no studies to translate. I am indebted to Val Cooper and Wendy Roberts of Cambridge University Medical Library for their help in providing material and searching online databases, to John Moffett of the Needham Research Institute for his generosity in allowing Jing Huang and myself to work there whenever we wished, to Kath Boydell and others in my local library for putting up with my hundreds of requests for interlibrary loans, to Lynn Saliba at the British Library for her unfailing good humour and kindness. Other libraries consulted include those at the College of Integrated Chinese Medicine, the Northern College of Acupuncture, the Renshu College of Chinese Medicine and the New York Academy of Medicine, as well as several Cambridge libraries and libraries associated with University College, London.

A particularly tedious task has been formatting the thousands of references in both the text and the database. Here I would like first to acknowledge the help of my son Seth, who then handed on the baton to Alex and Alison Griffin of the Bishops Stortford Griffinery. Diana Griffin nobly wrestled with the intricacies of Excel to help format the database itself. Finally Cepha Imaging in Bangalore, genially mediated by Colin McEwan at Elsevier in Edinburgh, managed to shape it into something useful and manageable.

Subjecting myself and a succession of computers to a gruelling schedule over the past few years has taken its toll, I have to say. Without the help of my acupuncturists Helen Thomas and Xie Ming, osteopaths Sharon Winkler and Caroline Penn, and wonderful regular massage from Melissa Maudling, I know I would not have been able to continue. This publication owes a lot to them, as well as to Steve Ford, Keith Malpass and Chris Stocken, who have managed to calm me and my computers at times of electronic disaster.

Writing is only possible if you can spare the time to do it. I owe a great deal to my family for their financial support over the years, and realise that otherwise it would not have been possible to devote myself to this project as fully as I have. I am also indebted to the following, who have helped to fund the database and other work involved in this publication:

The Acupuncture Association of Chartered Physiotherapists
The British Acupuncture Council
Body Clock Health Care, London
Harmony Medical, London
Nidd Valley Medical, Knaresborough, N Yorkshire
Noma (Complex Homoeopathy), Southampton
Scarboroughs, Crewkerne, Somerset
Daniela Matal, Brentwood, Essex.

Finally, I am immensely and always grateful to Susan, my wife, whose unstinting hard work, quiet support and incisive intuitions have made everything possible, and to Seth, my son, for showing me that I do not have to be afraid of life 'beyond the book'.

Many others have helped with advice, discussion and support, dealt uncomplainingly with my endless questions, loaned equipment, allowed me to teach and learn from their students, taught me themselves, or helped with research. A fuller list of many of these people can be found in the CD-Rom resource. I am truly sorry there is not room to thank them here.

# Abbreviations and Icons

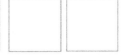

### List of abbreviations and icons

List of abbreviations used in this book (an expanded version of those used in the CD-ROM ⊙ resource can be found there).

| | |
|---|---|
| ~ | Approximately |
| < | Less than |
| > | More than |
| A | Ampère |
| Aβ | A-beta |
| Aδ | A-delta |
| Aγ | A-gamma |
| AA | Acupuncture analgesia |
| AC | Alternating current |
| ACE | Angiotensin-converting enzyme |
| ACh | Acetylcholine |
| AChE | Acetylcholinesterase |
| ACI | Acute cerebral ischaemia |
| AcP | Acupoint |
| ACR | Auriculocardiac reflex |
| ACTH | Adrenocorticotrophin |
| ADD | Attention deficit disorder |
| Adr | Adrenaline |
| AK | Applied kinesiology |
| ALS | Amyotrophic lateral sclerosis/acupuncture-like stimulation (low-frequency, high intensity) |
| ALTEAS | Acupuncture-like TEAS |
| ALTENS | Acupuncture-like TENS |
| AMED | Allied and Complementary Medicine Database |
| AMI | Apparatus for measuring the function of the meridians and the corresponding internal organs |
| AMPA | α-amino-3-hydroxy-5-methyl-4-isoxalone propionic acid |
| ANS | Autonomic nervous system |
| AP | Action potential/after polarisation |
| APS | Action potential simulation therapy |
| ATOIMS | Automated twitch-obtaining intramuscular stimulation |
| ATP | Adenosine triphosphate |
| βEP | Beta-endorphin |
| BDORT | Bidigital O-ring test |
| BFD | Bioelectronic function diagnosis |
| BP | Blood pressure/before polarisation |
| BPH | Benign prostatic hypertrophy |
| BSI | British Standards Institution |
| Ca²⁺ | Calcium ion |
| cAMP | Cyclic adenosine 3,5'-monophosphate |

| | |
|---|---|
| CCK | Cholecystokinin |
| CDC | Centers for Disease Control and Prevention |
| CEA | Conventional electroacupuncture |
| CEDS | Computerised electrodermal screening |
| CES | Cranial electrotherapy stimulation |
| CFF | Critical fusion frequency |
| CFS | Chronic fatigue syndrome |
| CGRP | Calcitonin gene-related peptide |
| CHD | Coronary heart disease |
| CINV | Chemotherapy-induced nausea and vomiting |
| CISCOM | Centralised Information Service for Complementary Medicine |
| Cl | Chlorine |
| CMP | Control measurement point |
| CNS | Central nervous system |
| CO₂ | Carbon dioxide |
| COPD | Chronic obstructive pulmonary disease |
| CRH | Corticotrophin-releasing hormone |
| CRPD | Complex/chronic regional pain disorder |
| CSF | Cerebrospinal fluid |
| CT | Computed tomography |
| CTD | Cumulative trauma disorder |
| CTEAS | Conventional TEAS |
| CTENS | Conventional TENS |
| CTS | Carpal tunnel syndrome |
| CVA | Cerebrovascular accident |
| CW | Continuous wave/current |
| DA | Dopamine |
| DC | Direct current |
| DD | Dense-disperse |
| DFM | Diagnostic system for functional medicine |
| DHEA | Dehydroepiandrosterone |
| DIP | Distal interphalangeal |
| DNIC | Diffuse noxious inhibitory control |
| DOMS | Delayed onset muscle soreness |
| DPA | D-phenylalanine |
| Dyn | Dynorphin |
| E | Energy |
| E₂ | Oestradiol |
| EA | Electroacupuncture |
| EAA | Electroacupuncture analgesia |
| EAP | Electroacupressure |
| EAV | Electroacupuncture according to Voll |
| ECG | Electrocardiogram |
| ECIWO | Embryo containing the information of the whole organism |
| ECMD | Electromagnetic compatibility directive |

| | | | |
|---|---|---|---|
| ECT | Electrochemical therapy | LASER | Light amplification by the stimulated emission of radiation |
| ED | Erectile dysfunction | | |
| EEG | Electroencephalogram | LBP | Low back pain |
| EGG | Electrogastrogram | LDL | Low-density lipoprotein |
| EHF | Extremely high frequency | LE | Leu-enkephalin |
| ELF | Extremely low frequency | LED | Light-emitting diode |
| EM | Electromagnetic | LEET | Low-energy emission therapy |
| EMBASE | Excerpta Medica database | LF | Low frequency |
| EMF | Electromotive force | LH | Luteinising hormone |
| EMG | Electromyogram | LHRH | Luteinising-hormone-releasing hormone |
| EMI | Electromeridian imaging | LILT | Low-intensity laser (or light) therapy |
| EMS | Electrical muscle stimulation | LISTEN | Life Information System Ten |
| Enk | Enkephalin | LSIP | Low skin impedance point |
| ENT | Ear, nose and throat | LTD | Long-term depression |
| EP | Evoked potential | LTP | Long-term potentiation |
| ES | Electrostimulation | $M\Omega$ | Megohm |
| EST | Electrostimulation treatment | $\mu A$ | Microampère |
| ESWL | Extracorporeal shockwave lithotripsy | mA | Milliampère |
| ESWT | Extracorporeal shockwave therapy | MA | Manual acupuncture |
| ETOIMS | Electrical twitch-obtaining intramuscular stimulation | MAA | Manual acupuncture analgesia |
| EU | European Union | MAOI | Monoamine oxidase inhibitor |
| F1, F2, | Spleen, Liver, Bladder and Stomach meridians | MAP | Mean arterial pressure |
| F4, F6 | in ryodoraku, respectively | MARF | Medical Acupuncture Research Foundation |
| FFR | Frequency following response | MCP | Metacarpophalangeal |
| 5HT | Serotonin | MDA | Medical Devices Agency |
| 5HTP | 5-hydroxytryptophan | MDD | Medical Devices Directive |
| fMRI | Functional magnetic resonance imaging | ME | Met-enkephalin |
| FMS | Fibromyalgia syndrome | MENS | Microcurrent electrical nerve or neuromuscular stimulation, or minimal electrical non-invasive stimulation |
| FSH | Follicle-stimulating hormone | | |
| G | Gauss | | |
| Ga(Al)As | Gallium (aluminium) arsenide | MEPZ | Motor end-plate zone |
| GABA | Gamma-amino butyric acid | MET | Modulation electrotherapy |
| GCSF | Granulocyte-colony-stimulating factor | MHRA | Medicines and Healthcare products Regulatory Agency |
| GH | Growth hormone | | |
| GHz | Gigahertz | MHz | Megahertz |
| GnRH | Gonadotrophin-releasing hormone | MP | Motor point |
| H4, H6 | Small Intestine and Large Intestine meridians | MRT | Microwave resonance therapy |
| | in ryodoraku, respectively | MS | Multiple sclerosis |
| HDL | High-density lipoprotein | MSG | Monosodium glutamate |
| HeNe | Helium neon | mT | Millitesla |
| HF | High frequency | MT | Magnet therapy |
| HIV | Human immunodeficiency virus | MTrP | Myofascial trigger point |
| HR | Heart rate | mW | Milliwatt |
| HVPG | High-voltage pulsed galvanic | mV | Millivolt |
| Hz | Hertz | MYMOP | Measure yourself medical outcome profile |
| IC | Interstitial cystitis | N | North pole |
| ID | Indicator drop | Na | Sodium |
| IFS | Individual frequency storage | NA | Noradrenaline |
| I(F)T | Interferential therapy | NaCl | Sodium chloride, common salt |
| IgE | Immunoglobulin E | NADA | National Acupuncture Detoxification Association |
| IgG | Immunoglobulin G | | |
| IMS | Intramuscular stimulation | NEAP | Neuroelectric acupuncture |
| IQ | Integrated charge | NK | Natural killer (cell) |
| IR | Infrared | nm | Nanometre |
| kHz | Kilohertz | NMDA | N-methyl-D-aspartate |
| $k\Omega$ | Kilohm | NRS | Numerical rating scale |
| $\lambda$ | Wavelength | NSAID | Non-steroidal anti-inflammatory drug |
| L-dopa | Laevodopa | OA | Osteoarthritis |
| LA | Laser acupuncture | $\Omega$ | Ohm |

| | |
|---|---|
| OP | Opioid peptide |
| PBP | Pseudobulbar paralysis |
| pd | Penetration depth |
| PD | Potential difference/Parkinson's disease |
| PEMF | Pulsed electromagnetic field |
| PENS | Percutaneous electrical nerve stimulation |
| PHN | Postherpetic neuralgia |
| PIP | Proximal interphalangeal |
| PL | Polarised light |
| PONV | Postoperative nausea and vomiting |
| PRR | Pulse repetition rate |
| PSM | Propagated sensation along the meridian |
| PT | Pain threshold/physical therapy |
| pTENS | Probe, point or punctate TENS |
| PVWM | Periventricular white matter |
| Q | Charge |
| QGM | *Qi Gong* machine |
| R | Resistance |
| RA | Rheumatoid arthritis |
| RCT | Randomised controlled trial |
| REPP | Reactive electropermeable points |
| RMD | Repetitive motion disorder |
| RMP | Representative measuring point |
| ROM | Range of motion |
| ROS | Review of symptoms |
| RRM | Resonant recognition model |
| RSD | Reflux sympathetic dystrophy |
| RSI | Repetitive strain injury |
| S | South pole |
| SBM | Society of Biophysical Medicine |
| SC | Skin conductance |
| SCI | Science Citation Index/spinal cord injury |
| SCN | Superior clunial nerve |
| SCS | Spinal cord stimulation |
| SD | Strength-duration |
| SEG | Segmentalelectrogram |
| SEP | Somatosensory evoked potentials |
| SLE | Systemic lupus erythematosus |
| SMP | Summation measurement point |
| SP | Skin potential |
| SPES | Subperception electrical stimulation |
| SR | Skin resistance |
| SSP | Silver spike point |
| T | Tesla |
| TCET | Transcranial electrotherapy |
| TCHM | Traditional Chinese herbal medicine |
| TCM | Traditional Chinese medicine |
| TDP | Type of far-infrared lamp |
| TEAS | Transcutaneous electrical acupoint stimulation |
| TENS | Transcutaneous electrical nerve stimulation |
| TES, TNS | Variants of TENS |
| TG | Thermography |
| TIA | Transient ischaemic attack |
| TLEA | TENS-like electroacupuncture |
| TLS | TENS-like stimulation |
| TMJ | Temporomandibular joint |
| TN | Trigeminal neuralgia |
| TOIMS | Twitch-obtaining intramuscular stimulation |

| | |
|---|---|
| TrP | Trigger point |
| TSE | Transcutaneous spinal electroanalgesia |
| UHF | Ultra-high frequency |
| ULF | Ultra-low frequency |
| URI | Upper respiratory tract infection |
| UV | Ultraviolet |
| UVB | Ultraviolet-B |
| V | Volt |
| V1 or OB | First or ophthalmic branch of the trigeminal nerve |
| V2 or MxB | Second or maxillary branch of the trigeminal nerve |
| V3 or MnB | Third or mandibular branch of the trigeminal nerve |
| VAS | Visual analogue scale |
| VHF | Very high frequency |
| VIP | Vasoactive intestinal polypeptide |
| VLF | Very low frequency |
| W | Watt |
| WHO | World Health Organization |
| WM | Western medicine |
| WMA | World Medical Association |
| YNSA | Yamamoto's new scalp acupuncture |

**Acupoint nomenclature**

Acupoints are listed using the standard alphanumeric method rather than Chinese point names, with the following abbreviations:

| | |
|---|---|
| LU | Lung |
| LI | Large Intestine |
| ST | Stomach |
| SP | Spleen |
| HE | Heart |
| SI | Small Intestine |
| BL | Bladder |
| KI | Kidney |
| P | Pericardium |
| SJ | *Sanjiao* (Triple Burner) |
| GB | Gall Bladder |
| LIV | Liver |
| Ren | Conception Vessel (*renmai*) |
| Du | Governor Vessel (*dumai*) |

Points on the Bladder meridian are numbered according to the convention:

| | |
|---|---|
| BL-36 | *chengfu* |
| BL-37 | *yinmen* |
| ... | |
| BL-40 | *weizhong* |
| ... | |
| BL-54 | *zhibian* |

Points on the Stomach meridian are numbered according to the convention:

| | |
|---|---|
| ST-5 | *daying* |
| ST-6 | *jiache* |
| ST-7 | *xiaguan* |
| ST-8 | *touwei* |

Extra points are labelled according to the system used in *Acupuncture: A comprehensive text*, and *A Manual of Acupuncture*.

Icons used in this publication, particularly for navigation in the CD-ROM resource.

 CD-ROM resource

 pTENS

 DATABASE

 CES

 CAUTION

 LA

 MA

 LILT

 EA

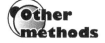 Other methods

 TEAS

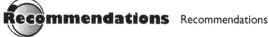 Recommendations

 TENS

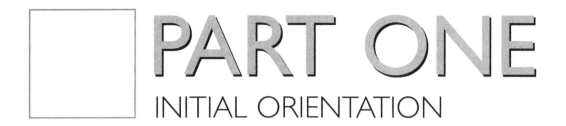

# PART ONE
## INITIAL ORIENTATION

## INTRODUCTION

Before starting any journey, it is useful to consult a map. The introductory chapter should help you navigate the rich oceans of knowledge on electroacupuncture (EA) presented in this book. You may want to keep your journey through the book simple and straightforward or, if more technically minded, you may enjoy the challenge of hidden reefs and complicated currents. **Chapter 1** includes basic definitions of acupuncture and electroacupuncture (a full list of technical terms used in the book is contained in the Glossary and on the CD-ROM),

and details the purpose of the book and its structure. Guides on to how to use the publication (book and CD-ROM) are presented, both for the practitioner who only wants minimum information before setting out to apply the practical techniques described, and for the reader who is more interested in the finer details of neurophysiology or research methodology.

**Chapter 2** is presented in the form of a timeline table, summarising the cycles and connections of EA, manual acupuncture and electrotherapy in East and West. A much fuller description of the history and context of EA is to be found in the CD-ROM ⊙ Resource.

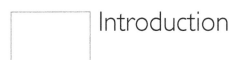

# Introduction

## ACUPUNCTURE – DEFINITIONS

This book is about the practice of electroacupuncture (EA) and other non-traditional approaches to acupuncture treatment. It is intended for those who are already qualified, or are training to become, acupuncture practitioners, and for other therapists who may wish to add non-invasive acupuncture-based methods to their therapeutic repertoire. It is also a resource for those who wish to understand and research this large subject, who may or may not be practitioners themselves.

Acupuncture, from the Latin words *acus* and *pungere*, has been defined as the insertion of needles into the body at specific points, together with the treatment of such points using non-invasive techniques that include electrostimulation and laser. There are many styles of acupuncture, some based on neurophysiological models, but most on traditional concepts of energy flow and balance. The latter I have loosely grouped together under the non-prescriptive banner of traditional Chinese medicine (TCM). There is no conflict between either of these approaches and the use of adjunctive devices for acupoint stimulation. Indeed, electricity, magnetism and light are used in some of the most subtle of Japanese acupuncture systems.

Electroacupuncture has been *broadly* defined as a comprehensive term for all procedures based on measurements or therapy derived from Chinese acupuncture but using modern electronics. It encompasses many different forms of treatment. With roots in eighteenth-century Japan and nineteenth-century France, it was rediscovered in China and France in the 1930s and 1950s, and in Germany and Japan in the 1950s, flourishing in both West and East in the 1970s. It has since played an important role in experimental neurophysiology, has much to contribute to clinical practice, and is still in a very creative phase.

Electroacupuncture is cosmopolitan, a place where therapists of many persuasions can meet. It is not the exclusive preserve of any one body of practitioners, nor a place for takeover bids. However, different groups may understand the term 'electroacupuncture' in different ways, depending on their training and inclination, and indeed may stimulate different points on the body (trigger or reflex points, or traditional meridian points, for example).

Some consider EA in a *narrow* sense, as electrical stimulation of acupoints exclusively through needles. Other terms have also been coined for this, such as 'percutaneous electrical nerve stimulation', with non-invasive stimulation being called 'neuroelectric acupuncture' or 'meridian therapy', for example.

In this book, EA will in most cases refer to needle stimulation. Other frequently used abbreviations are listed at the front of the book.

## WHY USE ELECTRO-ACUPUNCTURE?

Why should anyone turn to EA if they already have a grounding in acupuncture using simple needling (manual acupuncture, or MA) and moxibustion? There are many reasons:

- EA is more effective than MA in some situations, and often potentiates the effects of traditional methods (when treating pain, for instance).
- EA can be less time-consuming and less demanding of the practitioner than MA, in both training and practice.
- Results may in some cases be more rapid, and longer lasting.
- EA may have specific effects on pain, relaxation, circulation and muscle that are different from those of MA.
- EA is more readily controlled, standardised and objectively measurable than MA.
- EA allows stronger, more continuous stimulation than MA, and with less tissue damage.
- Non-invasive methods of electrostimulation may be more acceptable to:
  —children
  —needle phobics

—those with poor immune function or bleeding disorders
—those practitioners who are not acupuncturists.

- Non-invasive methods can be cost effective for home treatments, perhaps between sessions with a practitioner, although some forms of treatment will require supervision.
- As with EA, non-invasive methods may have specific effects that differ greatly from those of needling.
- Some of the more advanced equipment facilitates treatment planning, as well as treatment itself.
- The search for new pastures.

## TECHNOLOGY – LURE OR SUSPICION?

Technology can be exciting, but is certainly not the answer to every problem and will not remedy all of our deficiencies as practitioners.

Technology is also not the work of the devil, although for the technophobe it may seem quite frightening and impossible to master. There are no ghosts, gremlins or gods in machines unless we put them there. However, some traditionalists may not see the need for more equipment in a world already overdependent on electricity and power, and may not feel as comfortable with it as conventionally trained doctors. For some doctors, in turn, although the incorporation of electronics has made acupuncture more attractive, the languages of TCM may seem just as unreasonable.

In the end, therapeutic tools are just that and no more, even if, in skilled hands, they may appear powerful, even magical. Ecology need not be violated. Power can in fact be given back to the patient with many forms of EA (in its broad sense). It is certainly not in itself another agent of 'medical paternalism'.

## THE PURPOSE OF THIS BOOK – WHAT IT IS AND WHAT IT IS NOT

The primary purpose of this book is to enable better practice and greater understanding of EA. It is offered as both a practical guide and a research resource. Evidence is presented for how and whether EA works so that those who use EA, whether non-medical acupuncturists, physical therapists or doctors, can then make more informed decisions when it comes to their clinical practice, and better explain to others (or, if needs be, themselves) how what they do is useful.

A subsidiary purpose has been to introduce biomedical language and research to those who have trained in traditional acupuncture, as I myself did. It is important for us as TCM practitioners to become familiar with the language of mainstream Western medicine and also to be able to communicate something about what we do in terms that conventional medics can at least understand without too much unease. Otherwise we may well find ourselves marginalised, even in the world of acupuncture.

Although some of us may have turned to acupuncture as an alternative to mainstream medicine, as a 'flight from science', this book will, I hope, re-empower traditional acupuncturists who feel at sea with scientific language and foster dialogue and cross-fertilisation between practitioners from different backgrounds. Both biomedical and TCM language can seem impossibly dreary and obscure to the uninitiated. They need not be. As I have found while writing this book, learning the language of biomedicine can be quite a challenge for someone without conventional medical training, but is nevertheless quite possible, if not everyone's cup of tea. We should not be put off by linguistic barriers.

Nor must we be put off by research. Although it is becoming increasingly important, reading research is not the only avenue to understanding. Indeed, dependence on 'evidence' has been accused of discouraging practitioners from relying on their own practical experience, or even fostering a trend of 'perpetrating other people's mistakes instead of your own'. I hope that I have given enough space for those who learn in different ways to feel at home somewhere in this book and to be able to use the aspects of it that are right for them.

There are several things this book is not. It is not a stand-alone manual that will enable you to practise EA or the various modalities of electrotherapy without proper training. Nor is it an introduction to acupuncture. A basic knowledge and understanding of this is assumed. Although knowledge is power (if not measured in watts), alone it is not enough. This book provides a foundation. To use it, you need clinical experience under supervision. This book is not a substitute.

Many acupuncture books reiterate the same material that has been taught and retaught over generations. The intention here is, rather, to allow the material, the experimental and clinical research that has been carried out, as well as individual case studies by experts in the field, to speak for itself, and not to straitjacket it into a 'system' of standard treatments or hide the resulting contradictions and puzzles. Inevitably, this may be interpreted as favouring a Westernised or 'scientised' version of EA. This has not been my intention. If TCM theory is not discussed in detail, this is not to deny its necessary and ever-pervading presence in any discussion of acupuncture, but rather reflects the dearth of writing on EA and its TCM roots.

## THE STRUCTURE OF THIS PUBLICATION, AND HOW TO USE IT

This publication is divided into two parts: the book itself and the accompanying CD-ROM. The latter is referred to in the book as the 'CD-ROM resource,' or with the icon ⊙. In addition, some of the material on the CD-ROM is accessible in updatable form via the Internet at www.electroacupunctureknowledge.com.

Although the book can be read cover to cover, or consulted as a reference work, and provides quite enough information to permit safe and effective treatment of many conditions, it can also be used as a portal to the CD-ROM resource, which is designed more as a research resource for dipping into, with considerably more information on most topics. If you cannot find what you need in the book, the full version of each chapter can be browsed on the CD-ROM, using the 'Search' function and words or phrases from the printed chapters, or your own search terms. A unique component of the CD-ROM resource is the electronic database summary of more than 8000 clinical studies.

Full versions of all chapters in this publication may be found in the CD-ROM resource. For reasons of space, the book contains the abridged versions only. These function as stand-alone introductions to the subjects covered, with introductory and summary sections. Most chapters on clinical treatment contain information on points and stimulation parameters that can be used, and summary charts on the relevant sections of the database to consult.

The research-minded reader may initially be disappointed that the book does not contain references as such. However, all the necessary references, over 15 000 in total, are available on the CD-ROM resource. Many of them are not from English language publications, but most have been consulted in the original by the authors, or by collaborators with linguistic skills and acupuncture knowledge. In the book, instead of references, each chapter is followed by an annotated list of recommended titles, mostly in English, that are likely to be relatively accessible without having to consult specialist libraries.

To some readers, many words and abbreviations will be unfamiliar. When such technical words are used for the first time in the book, they are italicised and defined, while abbreviations are reintroduced in each chapter. There is a glossary and list of abbreviations in the book itself, with longer versions in the CD-ROM resource. The index can also be used to locate unusual terms.

**Part I** of the book contains this Introduction and a brief look at the historical context of EA.

**Part II**, Scientific and Clinical Foundations, is about EA research and its clinical application. Its main aim is to present the evidence for how and whether EA works. Its contents are as follows:

- Introduction, a discussion of EA research issues and methodology and an account of how research was carried out for this project.
- Chapter 3, some 'nuts and bolts' knowledge of electricity for those unfamiliar with it.
- Chapter 4, a brief guide to relevant aspects of the physics of electrotherapy and an outline of how it works.
- Chapter 5, introducing the neuroscience needed to understand the experimental EA research, with an exploration of the neurophysiology and electrical characteristics of the acupoints and meridians.
- Chapter 6, an in-depth description of the experimental findings on EA.
- Chapter 7, a summary of some of the main theories of how EA works.

- Chapter 8, a brief evaluation of controlled clinical trials on EA.
- Chapter 9, the longest section of the book, in which the clinical research on EA is explored, together with summaries on the acupoints and stimulation parameters likely to be most useful, and illustrative case histories from experienced practitioners.

**Part III** is more practical, focusing on the technology involved and its application in clinical practice:

- Chapter 10 offers an overview of the different families of electrotherapeutic and other equipment.
- Chapter 11 briefly outlines factors to consider when deciding what equipment might be appropriate for practice, followed by a description of design, safety, legal and marketing issues to be aware of; the second half of the chapter comprises an annotated listing of some commonly used devices.
- Chapter 12 covers the practical aspects of basic EA and other non-traditional acupuncture methods, and in the second half of the chapter the necessary precautions and contraindications to treatment.
- Chapter 13, on the integration of EA in clinical practice, is again in two sections; in the first, intention and an awareness of treatment levels are emphasised, and examples are then given of various possible simple strategies and treatment combinations.
- Chapter 14, the short final chapter in the book, draws together various themes woven into the fabric of the work and ends with a look at what the future may hold.

Appendices on useful resources and legislation are also included in the book. Further appendices, on drug interactions with electroacupuncture, a survey on the teaching of electroacupuncture in North America, and acupoint innervation and terminology, can be found on the ⊚. Unattributed chapters and appendices are by David Mayor.

There are a number of pathways through this book. For a quick start, the more practical reader may wish to start with an overview of EA applications (the summaries and case histories in Ch. 9), precautions and practicalities (Ch.12), followed by suggestions on integrating EA into existing practice (Ch. 13), and an overview of different devices and their current availability (Chs 10, 11). The other chapters (2–8) may then be used for reference.

The research-oriented practitioner, on the other hand, may want to plough through the material culled from published experimental and clinical studies (Chs 5–9) before embarking on the more practical side, while those who feel at sea with technical jargon from physics or physiology would be advised to familiarise themselves with this (Chs 3, 5) before proceeding further. Chapter 4, on the effects of physical agents such as electricity, magnetism and ultrasound, may only need a cursory glance from the experienced physical therapist, but for others provides useful background to their use in the context of acupuncture practice.

CD ROM

## Navigating the CD-ROM

Both the text and the database  on the CD-ROM are fully searchable.

You may:

- get to a chapter or section from the Contents pages
- bring up a figure, table or reference by clicking on the appropriate reference number
- navigate to treatments of the same modality using icons
- click on an abbreviation or technical term to bring up the appropriate entry in the list of abbreviations or glossary
- click on a cross-reference in the text to take you to where you want to go
- click on the summary chart at the end of each chapter to get to the relevant section of the electronic database.

In addition:

- Text material may be cut and pasted into word processor files for your own personal study and reference needs. However, if you wish to quote material from the book, please ensure you have read the full version on the CD-ROM before doing so. Further, be advised that the usual copyright restrictions apply.
- Similarly, images may be viewed independently of the text, and exported for use in presentations.
- Database material can also be exported and analysed.

Please refer to the CD-ROM for further instructions. Particularly in the CD-ROM resource, random dipping may enable you to make your own connections between seemingly unrelated topics. Creativity is yours.

## The website

The centrepiece of the website at www.electroacupunctureknowledge.com is the clinical studies database, which is also available on the CD-ROM resource, but with downloadable updates. In addition, sample material from the book is offered. A further appendix on the nomenclature and neuroanatomy of acupoints (Appendix 5 on the CD-ROM) is also available.

## Conventions used

Chinese terms are usually in *pinyin* rather than Wade-Giles form. In general, Chinese, Japanese and Korean family names are given first, and forenames second, except where the person referred to is resident in the West and prefers to conform to Western usage.

# Electroacupuncture East and West: the historical context

This chapter is presented in the form of a timeline table (Table 2.1). Patterns emerge, not only of how early methods, discoveries and ideas are repeated, but also of how waves of influence, interdependence and contradiction perform their dialectical *yin–yang* dance through time.

## ELECTROACUPUNCTURE, ITS CYCLES AND CONNECTIONS

*There is no new thing under the sun.*

*Ecclesiastes* (Ch. 1 verse 9)

History can be considered in terms of harmony with nature (*tianren heyi*), or conquest of the world about us (*ren ding shengitan*).

There is a curious difference between East and West in the origins of electrotherapy. Electric fish were used therapeutically in Fifth Dynasty Egypt, and their presence was a powerful impetus to later progress in understanding electricity. In China, however, although amber was known and used, it is highly unlikely that its electrical properties, far less dramatic than those of electric fish, informed treatment. In China electricity appears to have been a foreign import in the eighteenth century, the start of a process that would lead inexorably to the Maoist–scientific emphasis on *ren ding shengitan*.

Although a synthesis of acupuncture and electrotherapy occurred in France in the early nineteenth century, it was not until the mid 1930s that work on electroacupuncture (EA) was published in China. Indeed, in the late eighteenth and early nineteenth centuries, the West probably borrowed more from Oriental medicine than the other way about, as part of a fashion for 'romantic science' (1760–1830). Thus, as acupuncture became moribund in China in the early nineteenth century, it became relatively widely known

in the West. Here interest waned in the latter part of the century, and EA was almost forgotten, on one level because of technical difficulties with thick needles and crude, not always reliable, instrumentation. However, from the 1920s, the tide began slowly to turn again.

Acupuncture's resurgence under Chairman Mao in China, which emphasised 'union' or 'integration' with Western medicine, was paralleled by the creation of extraordinary hybrid forms of EA in France, Germany and Japan, as postwar scientific optimism gripped the industrialised nations. Electrical acupoint measurements were investigated in several such hybrid systems, explicitly in most cases to make acupuncture more scientific. Yet while 'traditional' Chinese medicine (TCM) was modernised and standardised, becoming yet more systematised and 'scientised' by the turn of the twenty-first century, a countertrend towards more traditional approaches became evident in North America and Europe, a balance to the engulfing world of technology. Within China itself, a greater openness to practices such as *qigong* in the 1970s and 1980s can be seen as a natural counterbalance to the rush to science.

An interesting pattern is also evident in the development of 'acupuncture analgesia' (AA), employing acupuncture (usually EA) intraoperatively to reduce pain and the need for drugs. 'Electroanaesthesia' was not uncommon in the USA of the late nineteenth century. In the early 1900s, France became the centre of this activity, but by 1925 this work was no longer included in major textbooks on anaesthesia, and it was not until the 1940s and 1950s that research was under way again, first in Russia and then once more in France. The methods generally used are known as transcranial electrotherapy (TCET), or cranial electrotherapy stimulation (CES), a gentler variant.

However, it was in China in 1958 that AA proper really had its genesis, first as manual acupuncture analgesia (MAA) in Shanghai, with EA analgesia (EAA) introduced shortly afterwards in Xian. There may have been some influence from Soviet TCET research at a time of rapprochement between the USSR and the People's Republic, but most writers are adamant that AA flowered because of Chairman Mao's dicta, such as:

> *Chinese medicine and pharmacology are a great treasure-house; efforts should be made to explore them and raise them to a higher level.*

> *We cannot just take the beaten track traversed by other countries in the development of technology and trail behind them at a snail's pace.*

> *Make the past serve the present and foreign things serve China.*

> *Unity and cooperation between the Chinese traditional doctors and Western-trained doctors.*

The development of AA was, then, as much political as medical in its inspiration. Here, as elsewhere, the history of acupuncture cannot be divorced from that of the cultures in which it has taken root. In French postwar acupuncture, for example, a need to assert the primacy of French discoveries after the ravages of war is very evident, while in Japan ryodoraku and other scientific reassessments of acupuncture were undertaken to preserve it against the wishes of the occupying American forces.

TENS (transcutaneous electrical nerve stimulation) is another modality where cross-currents of influence are evident. The 1965 publication of the gate theory of pain by Ronald Melzack and Patrick Wall led to a resurgence of interest in electrotherapy. This was further fuelled by the rediscovery of acupuncture by the West in the early 1970s, and by research into the neuropharmacological basis of pain modulation. Even if, on the surface, Western scientists distrusted Chinese research, much of the Chinese work on acupuncture neuroscience flowed easily into the mainstream of TENS research. EA has developed into a sophisticated neurophysiological research tool, as well as a therapeutic modality. TENS is commonly used at acupoints as an alternative to needles (as transcutaneous electrical acupoint stimulation, TEAS).

The scientisation of acupuncture continues. The challenge for the future is to rebuild a harmony between a medicine based on pharmacology and methods that can stimulate the bodymind's own self-balancing in ways that are respectful both of the patient and of the nuances of traditional theory. A pessimist may well fear that traditional core values will be eroded in the process, and that diversity of practice will be destroyed by the emphasis on proving efficacy and reducing risks. A more optimistic view is that with the subtlety of traditional acupuncture, possibilities for self-regulatory feedback between stimulation and measurement, and a refinement in the parameters of stimulation used based upon greater knowledge of bioelectrical processes, the *yin–yang* dance of electrotherapy and acupuncture looks set to evolve still further.

## ABOUT THE TIMELINE TABLE

The table on pages 9–19 includes information on key points in the history of acupuncture and electrotherapy that helps reveal the connections between them. It is an abridged version of a much fuller table in the CD-ROM resource ⊚, where other related treatment modalities, relevant scientific and medical discoveries, developments in technology and significant cultural, political and historical occurrences are also included, to provide a wider context.

(Note: 'BCE' is used instead of 'BC' for years before our current era, and 'CE' rather than 'AD'.)

## Additional Material in the CD-ROM resource

A longer version of this chapter, exploring its themes more fully, can be found in the CD-ROM resource.

## RECOMMENDED READING

*Standard histories of electrotherapy:*
Colwell HA 1922 An Essay on the History of Electrotherapy and Diagnosis. William Heinemann (Medical Books), London
Licht S 1967 History of electrodiagnosis. In: Licht S (ed) Electrodiagnosis and Electromyography. Elizabeth Licht, New Haven CT (2nd edn), 1–23

*On specific aspects of electrotherapy:*
Kellaway P The part played by electric fish in the early history of bioelectricity and electrotherapy. Bulletin of the History of Medicine. 1946 July; 20(2): 112–37
Turrell WJ Three electrotherapists of the eighteenth century: John Wesley, Jean Paul Marat and James Graham. Annals of Medical History. 1921 Winter; 3(4): 361–7

*On China:*
Lampton DM 1977 The Politics of Medicine in China: The policy process, 1949–1977. Westview special studies on China and East Asia. William Dawson, Folkestone, Kent
Chang J 1993 Wild Swans: Three daughters of China. Flamingo (HarperCollins), London

*On acupuncture:*
Feucht G 1977 Die Geschichte der Akupunktur in Europa. Karl F Haug Verlag, Heidelberg
Hsu E Outline of the history of acupuncture in Europe. Journal of Chinese Medicine (Hove, England). 1989 Jan; (29): 28–30
Lu GD, Needham J 1980 Celestial Lancets: A history and rationale of acupuncture and moxa. Cambridge University Press, Cambridge, UK

*On electroacupuncture:*
Macdonald AJR A brief review of the history of electrotherapy and its union with acupuncture. Acupuncture in Medicine. 1993 Nov; 11(2): 66–75

*Two general knowledge books that have fascinated me:*
Rosner L 2002 (ed) The Hutchinson Chronology of Science. Helicon, Oxford
Teeple JB 2002 Timelines of World History. Dorling Kindersley, London

**Table 2.1** Timeline Table

| Year | Electrotherapy | Manual acupuncture (MA) | Electroacupuncture (EA) |
|------|----------------|-------------------------|-------------------------|
| 2750 BCE | oldest known stone carvings showing use of electric fish (Nile catfish, *malopterurus electricus*) for painful conditions (Sakkara, Egypt) | | |
| 16th century BCE | | bronze needles in use in China | |
| 403 BCE | | *The Yellow Emperor's Classic of Internal Medicine* (*Huangdi Neijing*) written during Warring States Period | |
| 1683 | | *De Acupunctura*, by Wilhelm Ten Rhijne (Rhyne) (1647–1700), in which word 'acupunctura' is 1st used, published in London | |
| 1744 | Christian Gottlieb Kratzenstein (1723–1795): 1st recorded treatment using static electricity, on paralysed pnts | | |
| 1745 | Kratzenstein's book *Abhandlung von dem Nutzen der Electricität in der Arzneywissenschaft* appears; he notes that electrical treatment benefits circulation and relaxation, and considers electricity very much in terms of fire | | |
| 1749 | Jean-Étienne Deshais publishes *De Hemiplegia per Electricitatem Curanda* (Montpelier), 1st mainland European work on medical electricity | | |
| 1752 | Benjamin Franklin (1706–1790) treats 24-yr old woman for convulsive fits with 4 'shocks' morning and evening | | |
| 1756 | Richard Lovett (1692–1780) publishes *The Subtil Medium Prov'd*, 1st English language book on medical electricity; John Wesley starts to use electrotherapy in his free dispensaries for the poor | | |
| 1757 | | in China, Xu Dachun already writes of acupuncture as a 'lost art'; thus, at the very time acupuncture becomes available to Westerners, it is in a state of advanced decay | |
| 1759 | John Wesley (1703–1791, England) publishes popular book including many applications of electrotherapy; he believes that the 'subtile fluid' of electricity in some sense is | | |

*(Continued)*

**Table 2.1** Timeline Table—cont'd

| Year | Electrotherapy | Manual acupuncture (MA) | Electroacupuncture (EA) |
|---|---|---|---|
| | 'Soul of the Universe', or spirit of God made manifest, and (following Benjamin Franklin) writes about it as 'electrical fire' | | |
| 1764 | | | Gennai Hiraga (1728–1779) uses static electricity to treat muscle spasm and paralysis, Edo (Tokyo) |
| 1768 | 1st electrical apparatus installed in a London hospital | | |
| 1774 | 1st known case of resuscitation using electricity, in London; Jean Paul Marat (1743–1793, France) advises caution in using electrical treatment in presence of malignant tumours, and deplores its use for treating epilepsy; he understands it is of no benefit in cases of irreversible tissue pathology (cirrhosis, ankylosis) | François Dujardin (1738–1775, France) publishes his influential *Histoire de la Chirurgie*, with considerable coverage of acupuncture, concluding that its *modus operandi* is probably humoral | |
| 1801 | Christian Heinrich Ernst Bischoff (1781–1861, Germany) claims to treat hysterical paralysis using direct currents ('galvanism'); Friedrich Ludwig Augustin (1776–1854, Germany) refers to galvanism as sedative and sleep-improving; Hallé (France) notes that galvanic current, but not a static spark, makes a muscle contract in a pnt with facial palsy | | |
| 1802 | Thomas Gale (USA) publishes *Electricity, or Ethereal Fire, Considered*, stating enthusiastically: 'It is absolutely anti-febrile to all intents and purposes'; Giovanni Aldini (1762–1834, Italy), Galvani's nephew, treats severe depression with galvanic shocks | 1st serious mention of acupuncture in English medical press | |
| 1810 | | 1st known European trial of acupuncture, by Louis Berlioz (1776–1848, France), father of Hector Berlioz, composer; he treats a 24-year old woman suffering from 'nervous fever' and gastralgia | |
| 1812 | John Birch (St Thomas's Hospital, London) used electric shocks to treat nonunion of tibial fracture | | |

**Table 2.1** Timeline Table—cont'd

| Year | Electrotherapy | Manual acupuncture (MA) | Electroacupuncture (EA) |
|---|---|---|---|
| 1816 | | Louis Berlioz (France) writes: 'the introduction of several needles does not seem to me more efficacious than that of a single one. Further, ... it is never more successful than in cases where the procedure involves little or no pain' | Berlioz proposes that effects of MA may be enhanced by 'galvanic shocks produced by Volta's apparatus', and that its effects are due to stimulating nerves to replenish something they had lost; Jules Cloquet (1790–1883) argues that needles force a release of electricity in organs and arouse activity in nervous fluid |
| 1820 | François Magendie (1783–1855, France) employs galvanic current to treat neuralgia, cardialgia and epilepsy | 1st Italian book on acupuncture, by Bozetti | |
| 1821 | | James Morss Churchill (England), a surgeon, publishes 1st significant English language publication on acupuncture, *A Treatise on Acupuncturation*, emphasising technique rather than theory | |
| 1823 | | 1st issue of *Lancet* includes report of treatment of dropsy with acupuncture | Jean-Baptiste Sarlandière (1787–1838, France) starts to use EA, which he terms 'electropuncture', via mainly gold and silver needles; in one case of lead colic, needling was through the umbilicus (this was not painful; on the contrary, it was so 'delicious' 'he begged me to continue for ever' - suggesting possible endorphin release); Sarlandière used both static electicity ('franklinism') and galvanism, proposing initially that 'all lesions of motion should be treated by Franklinism and all those of sensation should be treated by Galvanism'; he considers electropuncture 'the most proper method' of treating rheumatism, nervous afflictions and gout; he treats asthma, migraine and various forms of paralysis |

*(Continued)*

**Table 2.1** Timeline Table—cont'd

| Year | Electrotherapy | Manual acupuncture (MA) | Electroacupuncture (EA) |
|------|----------------|--------------------------|--------------------------|
| 1824 | Charles Bew, surgeon-dentist to George IV, publishes an account of treating trigeminal neuralgia with 'a few slight shocks of electricity' | Churchill's book on acupuncture translated into German | |
| 1825 | | Churchill's book on acupuncture translated into French; Franklin Bache (1792–1864, USA), great-grandson of Benjamin Franklin, translates a book by S Morand (France), one of Jules Cloquet's students; Cloquet and Morand hold that pain is caused by accumulation of electrical fluid in nerves, which can be drained by inserting needles; they would sometimes leave these in for days | Sarlandière publishes on 'galvanopuncture'; several English medical journals publish accounts of French experiments on 'electro-magnetic' or 'galvanic' phenomena related to acupuncture; Sarlandière considers that needling draws electricity from the body, and 'électro-puncture' 'saturates' it and is more effective; he adds that the effects of electricity are well known, while those of simple acupuncture are often met with disbelief |
| 1826 | | *Lancet* starts to publish further articles in support of acupuncture; Franklin Bache (USA) publishes account of treating prisoners in Philadelphia State Penitentiary with acupuncture, for conditions such as muscular rheumatism, neuralgia and ophthalmia, retaining needles for up to 24 hrs | François Magendie, founder of discipline of pharmacology, anti-vitalist and one of 1st protagonists of animal experimentation, electrically needles nerves using steel or platinum needles; method was too painful to remain popular |
| 1827 | | John Elliotson (1791–1868, England) reports on 42 cases of chronic rheumatism; he concludes that acupuncture is not indicated for acutely inflamed, hot rheumatic joints | Gustav Landgren on a case of gout: 'after the release of 5 to 6 sparks that were clearly felt in the buttocks at the needle edge, pain was completely gone, and a profuse sweating covered his body. As this mode of application carried some difficulties, acupuncture was then used alone' |
| 1831 | with the discovery of induction by Michael Faraday (1791–1867, England) and 'the belief that at last the true medical electricity had been discovered', came a new era, with | by early 1830s, initial interest in acupuncture in England begins to wane, and continues to do so for several decades, partly because of a | Magendie continues to use galvanopuncture |

**Table 2.1** Timeline Table—cont'd

| Year | Electrotherapy | Manual acupuncture (MA) | Electroacupuncture (EA) |
|---|---|---|---|
| | the steady abandonment of galvanism in favour of the new machines | lack of understanding of its *modus operandi*, possibly also because of infection due to lack of aseptic techniques, although there is little evidence of this | |
| 1833 | | | Guillaume Duchenne de Boulogne (1806–1875, France), founder of modern electrotherapy, begins using EA (later he found comparable results possible without piercing skin if stronger stimulation is used, and switched to surface electrodes, or 'localised electrisation' as less painful - needles were thick, and electrical stimulation difficult to control) |
| 1834 | | | Francesco S da Camino (1786–1864, Venice, Italy) reproduces Sarlandière's EA work and publishes his first book on EA |
| 1844 | | | E Hermel (France) uses 'electro-puncture' for sciatica and lumbosacral neuralgia, with positive needle over site of pain |
| 1849 | Duchenne describes his treatment of paralysis, including hysterical paralysis, with 'faradic' (induction) currents; by this year, Bucknill (England) is treating melancholia with galvanic electricity | | |
| 1853 | | | Dr Holl (York County Hospital, Pennsylvania, USA) uses DC through acupuncture needles to treat longstanding nonunion of tibial fracture; Bacchetti uses 'electro-puncture' for extrauterine pregnancy |
| 1854 | *Die Electricität in ihrer Anwendung auf praktische Medicin*, by Moritz Meyer (1821–1893) is published in Germany | | |

**Table 2.1** Timeline Table—cont'd

| Year | Electrotherapy | Manual acupuncture (MA) | Electroacupuncture (EA) |
|------|----------------|-------------------------|-------------------------|
| 1859 | 1st edition of *A Treatise on Medical Electricity* by Julius Althaus (1833–1900, Germany/England) published in London, ending era of a purely empiricist approach to electrotherapy | | |
| 1868 | *Untersuchungen und Beobachtungen auf dem Gebiete der Elektrotherapie* by Rudolf Brenner (1821–1884) is published in Leipzig; he considers cathode stimulation as 'stimulating', and anode as 'calming' | | |
| 1871 | Duchenne reports effects on spasticity of activating antagonists to spastic muscles; George M Beard (1839–1883, USA) and Alphonso D Rockwell (1840–1925, USA) describe 'general faradisation', one electrode on feet, other moved systematically over definite pts of back, chest, abdomen, extremities, neck and head; they recommend this for neurasthenia, depression, sleep disturbance and alcoholism | Thomas Pridgin Teale (1831–1923, England) considers that acupuncture works by improving blood supply | |
| 1873 | A Newth uses generalised galvanism, with hands or feet in acidulated water, together with one electrode (usually cathode), other electrode being applied to head, neck or spine | | |
| 1878 | Rudolf Arndt (1835–1900, Germany) concludes that paralysis and depression should be treated with 'ascending' currents (cathode cephalad, anode caudad), mania with 'descending' currents (anode cephalad, cathode caudad); faradic currents are for those who need strong stimulation (stuporous conditions, long chronic illnesses, hysterical symptoms) | | |
| 1880 | | work of Amédée Dumontpallier (1827–1899) on contralateral needling for neuralgia, acute articular rheumatism and sciatica is published in England | |
| 1886 | F Heyden writes that faradic current is suitable for treatment of depression, as more stimulating, while galvanic current is more 'calming' or 'catalytic' | | J Brindley James (London) publishes an account of his 'percusso-punctator', a five-needle device which could also be electrified |

**Table 2.1** Timeline Table—cont'd

| Year | Electrotherapy | Manual acupuncture (MA) | Electroacupuncture (EA) |
|------|----------------|------------------------|-------------------------|
| 1889 | John MacWilliam (1857–1937) performs 1st experiments that later lead to development of cardiac pacemakers | | |
| 1890 | Jansen B Mattison (b 1845, USA) uses galvanism ('our most trusted ally') to replace opium and other drugs in habitués suffering from neuralgia | | |
| 1892 | | in his *Principles and Practice of Medicine,* William Osler (1849–1919, Canada) recommends *locus dolendi* acupuncture for lumbago (5–10 mins using 3–4 inch sterilised needles, even hat pins), as taught him by physiologist Sydney Ringer (1835–1910, England) | |
| 1893 | | 1st recognisably modern medical study on acupuncture (for 100 consecutive cases of sciatica) published by E Valentine Gibson in *Lancet* | |
| 1900 | by now most US doctors have at least one electrical machine in their office | | |
| 1909 | textbook *Électrothérapie* by Thomas Nogier (father of Paul Nogier) published | | |
| 1910 | decline of electrotherapy starts with publication of Flexner Report | | |
| 1915 | | | publication by Welshman Naunton Davies on 'galvanic acupuncture' for sciatica |
| 1921 | | | EA Goulden's publication on EA (2 mA, 10 mins, just below level of discomfort) for sciatica |
| 1925 | | George Soulié de Morant (1878–1955, France) starts to teach acupuncture in hospitals | Dimier (France) investigates EA with George Soulié de Morant; he considers that *qi* is either entirely electrical, or is carried by measurable electrical waves; Soulié de Morant states that 'the instruments prove, by their measures, the existence of the 'force vitale'; he applies both faradic and galvanic currents via needles, as well as HF electromassage on pts |

*(Continued)*

**Table 2.1** Timeline Table—cont'd

| Year | Electrotherapy | Manual acupuncture (MA) | Electroacupuncture (EA) |
|------|----------------|-------------------------|-------------------------|
| 1928 | Erwin Schliephake (1894–1994, Germany) introduces era of shortwave diathermy | P Charukosky reportedly applies acupuncture for 1st time in 20th century Russia | |
| 1932 | Albert Hyman (1893–1972, USA) 1st to carry out cardiac pacing through inserted needles | at about this time, George Soulié de Morant (France) starts to consider acupuncture in terms of autonomic function | |
| 1934 | | George Soulié de Morant (France) publishes précis on foundations of Chinese medicine, dedicated in large part to acupuncture | Tong Shi-chin's book *Investigation of Electroacupuncture* is published, 1st evidence of Chinese use of EA; EA equipment produced in China; Roger de la Fuye (1890–1961, France) recommends use of DC with needles |
| 1935 | | | Roger de la Fuye starts to use 'électropuncture', replacing needles by mild 'punctures électriques', or applying currents from his 'diathermopuncteur' to needles (10 kHz to 30 MHz, 0.125–2 secs/pt); he uses high frequencies to ensure deeper and painless penetration, and considers this method capable of reinforcing effects of homoeopathic medicaments, or indeed replacing them; white (steel) electrodes or platinum needles sedate, with a weak current, red or yellow (copper, gold) electrodes or gold needles tonify, with a stronger current; he considers both traditional and EA as 'above all … a remarkable preventive treatment' |
| 1939 | | George Soulié de Morant publishes vol 1 of his comprehensive textbook on acupuncture and Chinese medicine; he translates *qi* as 'energy' | |
| 1946 | | both in China and Japan, traditional medicine starts to become 'scientised' (standardised, adapted to classroom training); 'traditional medical practice was saved, but the *qi* paradigm was its ransom' | American occupying forces in Japan want to eradicate acupuncture and moxibustion as non-scientific, but permit study of acupuncture from a modern viewpoint, particularly at Kyoto University Faculty of Medicine, where Nakatani Yoshio studies acupuncture from viewpoint of autonomic |

**Table 2.1** Timeline Table—cont'd

| Year | Electrotherapy | Manual acupuncture (MA) | Electroacupuncture (EA) |
|------|----------------|-------------------------|--------------------------|
| | | | function; as Hyodo Masayoshi writes later: much Oriental medicine 'has become part of a new and rational physiotherapy' |
| 1947 | internationally, 13.66 MHz, 27.12 MHz and 40.98 MHz are set aside for shortwave medical applications | | Roger de la Fuye publishes his *Traité d'Acupuncture*, in which he states that whether applied to acupts directly or via needles, electrostimulation can tonify or sedate, and gives stronger effects than traditional needling; he warns against 'fantastical' acupuncture (a jibe at those followers of Soulié de Morant who were more interested in traditional theories than his own more pragmatic approach) |
| 1952 | Paul M Zoll pioneers cardiac pacing with surface electrodes on chest | effects of acupuncture on EEG are reported by RS Wei (China) | Roger de la Fuye's *Traité d'Acupuncture* translated into German, co-authored with Heribert Schmidt as *Die Moderne Akupunktur* |
| 1953 | | | Jacques Lavier (France) starts to experiment with EA on domestic animals, and then himself; together with Fritz Werner, Reinhold Voll (1909–1989, Germany) develops his 'Electropuncteur' device, but after protests from Roger de la Fuye, who seems to have considered he had a monopoly on the term 'electro-acupuncture', device was renamed rather clumsily 'K+F-Diatherapuncteur'; Zhu Longyu initiates animal research on EA in China; he notes its sedative effect in himself, followed by alertness |
| 1955 | | VG Vogralik (Russia) starts to use acupuncture for smoking cessation | Zhu Longyu (Shaanxi Province) uses both DC and AC, with needles in both traditional acupts and nerves, to treat pnts with psychiatric disorders; he publishes *Electroacupuncture in China*; Reinhold Voll (Germany) introduces facility for 1–10 Hz LF stimulation in his system |

*(Continued)*

**Table 2.1** Timeline Table—cont'd

| Year | Electrotherapy | Manual acupuncture (MA) | Electroacupuncture (EA) |
|------|---------------|------------------------|------------------------|
| 1956 | | new stage in successful development of acupuncture started in Russia, led by VG Vogralik and II Rusetzky | |
| 1958 | | | 1st operations using EA analgesia (EAA) |
| 1959 | | Fukushima Kodo (1910–1995?, Japan), blinded in the Sino-Japanese War in 1932, develops Toyohari method, originally for blind acupuncturists; in France, F Thoret experiments with Weihe's Tabacum pt (Ren14) for smoking withdrawal | Reinhold Voll states his working hypothesis that 'jede krankhafte Störung ihre eigene Wellenfrequenz hat' |
| 1960s | | | EA introduced into more general clinical practice in China, after several years of use for surgical anaesthesia; EA 1st used to induce ovulation in anovulatory women; EA convulsive therapy investigated in China as an alternative to ECT |
| 1962 | Carey and Lepley pioneer experimental use of DC for wound healing | | |
| 1965 | Gate theory of pain published by Ronald Melzack (b 1929, Canada) and Patrick Wall (1925–2001, England), rekindling interest in electrical control of pain | 1st controlled clinical trial of acupuncture in Japan | Hyodo Masayoshi, in his work at Department of Anaesthesiology, Osaka Medical College, begins to combine EA with nerve block; Han Jisheng 1st aware of acupuncture analgesia (AA) as a field for research |
| 1967 | Patrick Wall and William Sweet (1911–2001, USA) report use of HF peripheral nerve stimulation via needles for relief of chronic neurogenic pain; C Norman Shealy (b 1932, USA) and colleagues report experimental use of spinal cord stimulation for pain | | EA textbook published in Hong Kong |
| 1968 | William Sweet and James Wepsic publish study on treating chronic pain with peripheral nerve stimulation (implanted electrodes); 1st application of low-intensity DC for wound (chronic ulcer) healing in humans, by Dennis Assimacopoulos | | Hyodo Masayoshi (Japan) publishes account of treating whiplash injury with EA; Tokki LF EA device (Japan) developed |

**Table 2.1** Timeline Table—cont'd

| Year | Electrotherapy | Manual acupuncture (MA) | Electroacupuncture (EA) |
|------|---------------|------------------------|------------------------|
| 1971 | 1st research on bone healing since mid-19th century | | electrical plum blossom needling introduced (as a treatment for myopia); 1st popular publications on AA in China; 1st use of AA in West |
| 1972 | | George Soulié de Morant (France) publishes complete edition of his major work on acupuncture and Chinese medicine | huge upsurge of interest in EAA after President Nixon's visit to China; Wen Hsiang-lai (Hong Kong) visits China to study EAA; on return, he and his colleagues discover that auricular EA relieves drug withdrawal symptoms |
| 1973 | | | Michael O Smith, Yoshiaki Omura and Mario Wexu start to use Wen's protocol for drug withdrawal in New York |
| 1975 | | | MA starts to replace EA for drug withdrawal treatment at Lincoln Hospital, Bronx, New York |
| 1981 | | | ryodoraku now common in Japan |
| 1990s | 'electro-aesthetic' market burgeons; several modalities that were never popular in mainstream electrotherapy, or that have fallen from favour, are taken up by beauty therapists | acupuncture is used more and more in hospitals in Japan and the West | many Chinese clinics use EA; in some clinics almost every patient is treated with EA, in others much fewer |

Abbreviations: acupt = acupoint; AC = alternating current; DC = direct current; EA = electroacupuncture; ECT = electrochemical therapy; HF = high frequency; LF = low frequency; MA = manual acupuncture; pnt = patient; pt = point.

# PART TWO
## SCIENTIFIC AND CLINICAL FOUNDATIONS

# INTRODUCTION

This part of the book is about electroacupuncture research and its clinical application. Its main aim is to present the evidence for how and whether electroacupuncture (EA) works, so that readers can then make more informed decisions in clinical practice. The full versions of the chapters that follow are included on the accompanying CD-ROM, together with a longer version of this introduction that outlines some of the issues involved in experimental, theoretical and clinical research.

EA is not only a form of acupuncture, but also of electrotherapy. Some familiarity with the language of electricity is thus a prerequisite to understanding how it is used in practice and research. This is provided in **Chapter 3**. The following chapter provides a brief guide to relevant aspects of the physics of electrotherapy and an outline of how it works. For many practising acupuncturists, this will be unfamiliar territory, and it is presented as simply as possible consistent with the need for safety in use. The subsequent chapter introduces the neuroscience necessary for an understanding of the experimental EA research. Indeed, most experimental EA research is neuroscience based, and EA is sometimes used simply as an investigative tool without regard for its wider clinical applications. The chapter, therefore, developed as a resource for those, like myself, without a background or particular interest in the technicalities of neurophysiology and neurochemistry. In the second half of the chapter, acupuncture itself comes into view, with an exploration of the neurophysiology and electrical characteristics of the acupoints and meridians for non-technically minded readers.

Chapter **6** contains a lengthy in-depth description of the experimental findings on EA, best dipped into rather than read in one go. It suggests many possible avenues both for research and for improving the effectiveness of clinical application. The following chapter summarises some of the main theories of how EA works, starting with the better-known models based on neuroscience, with a foray into more speculative areas involving chaos theory, concepts of neurotransmitter frequency coding and brain resonance, biophysics and molecular resonance.

Chapter **8** begins with a brief evaluation of controlled clinical trials on EA. This is followed by **Chapter 9**, the longest section of the book, in which the clinical evidence for whether EA works is explored, together with recommendations for clinical application and illustrative case histories from experts in particular fields. Conditions are identified according to their Western rather than TCM classifications, in line with current practice in China. The summary sections in this chapter also draw on some of the clinically applicable findings from **Chapters 4–7**, particularly on the acupoints and stimulation parameters likely to be most useful.

It is as always important to remember, however, that in acupuncture there is often more than one way to approach a problem. Information given on points and parameters in **Chapter 9** should always be considered within the overall context of the patient–practitioner interaction, the patient as a unique individual with needs beyond simply relief of symptoms, and the practitioner's acupuncture experience and training. For those who just want to press on with using EA, it may be enough to read the summaries, together with **Chapter 3**, and to leave **Chapters 4–7** for later.

# ELECTROACUPUNCTURE RESEARCH – ISSUES AND METHODOLOGY

Much past acupuncture research, as in most fields of medicine, is of poor quality. Acupuncture itself has developed out of a different worldview to that of Western science, and there are fundamental difficulties when trying to apply scientific research methods to it. Indeed, the scientific method does not necessarily provide immutable and precise truths, and as scientific investigation becomes more complex and thorough what we seek becomes ever more elusive, even in the best-designed clinical trials. There may also be fundamental flaws in the methods of statistical analysis that are used in clinical research.

For a variety of reasons Chinese, Japanese and Russian studies tend to produce more positive results than those published in the West. Cultural and nationalistic biases exist in both the reporting and reviewing of acupuncture research. Since Chinese acupuncture research, in spite of its variety in scope and quality, tends to be lumped together as a homogenous entity, there is a risk that all non-Western acupuncture research becomes labelled as inadequate.

It is also worth remembering that acupuncture clinical trials have been carried out over a mere three decades, a miniscule period by comparison with the centuries in which acupuncture has been practised as a fully developed system, and not one on which to base conclusive judgements.

In the CD-ROM resource, a range of specific issues in electroacupuncture research is examined in detail. Amongst these are the following:

## Issues in experimental research

A measurable and repeatable stimulus such as EA is more useful in research than the inherently variable and irregular stimulus provided by manual acupuncture (MA). Thus there are many more experimental acupuncture studies using EA than MA. Experimental studies also tend to be of higher quality and better controlled than clinical ones.

In China, experimental EA research has inevitably been at the forefront of the movement to integrate Western science and TCM, with many new techniques developed to explore its complexities. However, the complicated science involved inevitably generates more factors to confound results. Another key issue is how relevant experimental EA research on animals is to actual clinical practice. There are important differences between species, and between experimental and clinical settings. Nevertheless, animals generally respond the same to EA as do humans, and the animal research that has taught us much about how EA may work cannot just be discarded wholesale. Furthermore, there may be ethical dilemmas involved in carrying out animal research. A considered and balanced view of these difficult issues is essential.

## Issues of mechanism and theory

Much effort has been put into creating a theoretical framework for acupuncture, and EA in particular, that is congruent with biomedical thinking. Indeed, more has probably been published on the neurophysiology of acupuncture than on the mechanisms of any other form of physical therapy. However, so far there is little evidence that any particular theoretical approach provides clinically superior results.

## Issues in clinical research

Clinical research on acupuncture, and EA in particular, has its own special problems. Studies are often inconclusive, not so much because acupuncture itself is at fault, but because problems have not been adequately addressed in their design. Some of the topics that need to be explored are *inclusion criteria*, the use of appropriate *controls*, *sample size* and attrition, *randomisation*, *bias*, *blinding*, the quality of acupuncture administered, point location, time and *crossover* effects, *endpoint measures* and *outcome*.

In the CD-ROM resource these are considered with particular reference to EA and associated methods, along with how research is reported and the extraordinary inaccuracies frequently found in study conclusions and abstracts. It is important to remember that just because acupuncture is used for a particular condition this does not necessarily mean it is effective.

# REVIEWING THE EXPERIMENTAL AND CLINICAL RESEARCH

The vast amount of research material that exists on electroacupuncture has to be reviewed in some way to make it accessible. Possible research methods range from informal narrative accounts based on one person's viewpoint, through consensus by acknowledged authorities in the field, to rigorous *systematic review* and *meta-analysis* by experts.

In reviewing the experimental and theoretical work on EA, I have chosen to carry out a narrative yet not uncritical review, presenting the results of studies, drawing together threads of evidence, and identifying shortcomings. The material is already highly technical and further rigorous analysis would probably exclude many of the more interesting findings. With the clinical research, the decision has been more difficult, and a two-level approach has been adopted, resulting in both critical and descriptive reviews.

## The clinical material critically reviewed

Adrian White has carried out a rigorous evaluation of EA controlled trials, on the basis of an extensive literature search up to the end of 2000. The result of his critical review of EA, presented here as Chapter 8, is that there is insufficient evidence of its therapeutic value in clinical practice. This may be disappointing, but is predictable given the number and quality of the studies reviewed and the review methodology employed. After all, the outcome of a systematic review depends on the quality of studies available, and there are clearly not enough good quality EA clinical trials to review. Thus, this evaluation is by no means a condemnation of EA as an ineffective treatment, and highlights the real need for larger, more carefully conducted studies.

## The clinical material descriptively reviewed

The descriptive review of clinical studies, including many uncontrolled ones, that forms the bulk of Chapter 9 has been carried out to look at what conditions are treated with EA and other non-traditional forms of acupuncture, and to find out what acupoints and treatment parameters are used. It also explores some similarities and differences between EA and other forms of electrotherapy. The clinical data on which this review is based can be found in the CD-ROM resource database 💿.

This informal overview of how EA is applied does not necessarily indicate best practice, but may prove a useful counterbalance to the purist rigour of Adrian White's approach. These two reviews also differ in that this one includes studies not just of EA defined as the application of electrical stimulation to acupoints through needles, but also of other non-traditional forms of stimulation at acupoints, such as transcutaneous electrical nerve stimulation (TENS), low intensity light therapy (LILT), ultrasound and so forth. However, research on specific forms of acupuncture may not be generalisable to other forms, so these studies are clearly distinguished from those dealing explicitly with EA.

## Finding the material

Finding material presents several problems, especially since building an EA research library has not been a high priority for any of the major UK acupuncture organisations. To create one's own database, logically the larger medical databases should be consulted first, abstracts read, and then copies of the relevant papers obtained. In reality, I already had a collection of textbooks and articles put together haphazardly over 20 years, from which references to further literature were extracted. Consulting the medical databases and trying to organise the material came later, along with writing to authors for further papers that might be of use, or for clarification on studies, abstracts or citations already in my collection.

The major databases consulted were MEDLINE (from 1964), and EMBASE (the Excerpta Medica database) and SCI, the Science Citation Index (both only available from 1980), all three until the end of 1998 (courtesy of Wendy Roberts at the University Medical Library in Cambridge). Also used were CISCOM 1973–1998 (the Centralised Information Service for Complementary Medicine, from the Research Council for Complementary Medicine, London) and AMED 1983–1998 (the British Library Allied and Complementary Medicine Database, courtesy of Mark Bovey at the Acupuncture Research and Resources Centre, then at Exeter University). Other electronic sources used have included the now defunct China a2z Acupuncture Progress, Alt-HealthWatch, and the useful monthly *Acubriefs* newsletter from MARF, the Medical Acupuncture Research Foundation in the USA. The latter has been the main source of references since 1998.

## Searching the material

A comprehensive search strategy was developed, using search terms derived from the titles and contents of papers already held. A simplified version was used with CISCOM. References and abstracts (where available) were retrieved in text format from the various databases consulted, and the references then entered in separate Idealist database bibliographies (4780 Medline records, 3080 for EMBASE, 3030 for the SCI, 1175 for AMED and 275 for CISCOM). The Cochrane Controlled Trials Register and the database of the Cochrane Field for Complementary Medicine were not available at this stage.

Many journals, of course, do not meet Medline's standards, and are not listed there at all. Some good quality journals, even with extensive English abstracts, may not be included either. Others, such as the *World Journal of Acupuncture-Moxibustion* or the *Liaoning Journal of TCM* (*Liaoning Zhongyi Zazhi*) are not included in any of the main academic databases used. Furthermore, journals are not added to Medline retrospectively so, although one may be listed now, not all past issues will have been indexed. Journals are also sometimes listed under different titles, such as the very informative *Acupuncture Research*. Until 1996 this was referenced as *Chen Tzu Yen Chiu*. Now this has been altered (retrospectively as well) to *Zhenci Yanjiu*, while issues from 1999 onwards are not listed at all! Worse, in AMED this journal is sometimes confused with *Acupuncture and Electro-therapeutics Research*.

Acupuncture studies are also published in many different journals. This problem of information 'scatter' is a serious one for any researcher. There is a very real need for a central register of acupuncture trials, freely accessible via the internet for both registration of trials and accessing data on those registered. The Cochrane Library is only really useful for sourcing the better quality studies that exist.

Searching for acupuncture studies on any database can be frustrating. Study titles and author names are not always listed as in the original papers, and not all authors may be listed if there are more than three. The type of acupuncture used is frequently not defined in the title, keywords or MeSH (medical subject heading) terms, or even the abstract. Thus many studies on 'acupuncture' may turn out to be on EA or laser acupuncture (LA), and articles on 'acupuncture analgesia' may be on manual acupuncture analgesia (MAA) or electroacupuncture analgesia (EAA). There are also some Western authors who would prefer that what they do is not seen as acupuncture, and refer to EA as 'sensory stimulation' to overcome publication bias, or hide behind the acronym

'PENS' (for 'percutaneous electrical nerve stimulation'). Mike Cummings has written an incisive review of the latter, showing how it is but EA under another name.

At the opposite extreme other authors keep publishing variants of the same study in different journals. Substantial parts of anthologies may thus be based on earlier publications (as with Zhang Xiangtong's 1986 *Research on Acupuncture, Moxibustion, and Acupuncture Anaesthesia* and the 1979 Beijing Symposium). Chinese authors especially may produce duplicate studies, the more polished versions for export to English language publications.

Sorting the material presents challenges. One grey area has been veterinary trials, which might be considered clinical by a veterinarian but experimental by a practitioner of human acupuncture. Another has been studies where results are primarily presented in terms of blood or physiological parameters. These have been variously discussed in the context of either experimental or clinical EA research, and sometimes both.

Visits to various libraries in Cambridge, particularly the Medical Library and that of the Needham Research Institute, together with the libraries associated with University College, London, and the British Library, have made it possible to obtain actual copies of most of the published material, and to carry out hand searches through complete runs of some key journals. In addition, full use was made of both national and international interlibrary loans, although this is an expensive way to obtain what are often quite short articles.

## Translating the material

Since most acupuncture research has been carried out in the Far East, Russia and some Eastern European states, much of the English language acupuncture literature depends on secondary sources. English abstracts are useful, but often give little precise data. Clearly, if we in the West cannot read original articles, much useful research will remain unknown. Therefore, one aim in preparing material for this book has been to present translated data from studies in languages such as Chinese and Russian that most Westerners cannot read.

Looking at the number of journals in which EA and associated studies detected by Medline were published in different years can be very revealing (Table P2.1).

**Table P2.1** Journals in which EA and associated studies detected by Medline have been published

| | 1991 | 1998 |
|---|---|---|
| British, North American, Australian and South African | 70 | 75 |
| Other European (or European language) journals | 19 | 13 |
| Chinese | 51 | 1 |
| Russian or other Eastern European | 60 | 14 |
| Japanese | 7 | 5 |

**Table P2.2** Journals in which EA and associated studies detected by EMBASE have been published

| | 1991 | 1998 |
|---|---|---|
| British, North American, Australian and South African | 107 | 118 |
| Other European (or European language) journals | 25 | 40 |
| Chinese | 10 | 3 |
| Russian or other Eastern European | 10 | 0 |
| Japanese | 4 | 5 |

On the surface it seems that something rather drastic happened to Russian and Chinese acupuncture research between 1991 and 1998. However, on scanning through my own holdings of similar journal articles from 1998, 39 were from Chinese journals previously listed on Medline but recently removed. Thus there appears to be, for whatever reason, bias against making the majority of the world's EA research available through Medline. This is also true of other electronic sources: Stephen Birch found that eight major databases did not list most Chinese, Japanese or Korean journals.

Comparable figures for EMBASE and the SCI are given in Tables P2.2 and P2.3.

## A small translation project – how detailed are Chinese experimental EA studies?

Given the paucity of information on acupoints and treatment parameters in journal abstracts in general, it was not surprising to find numerous Chinese studies with rather unhelpful abstracts. Thanks to a small grant from the

**Table P2.3** Journals in which EA and associated studies detected by the SCI have been published

| | 1991 | 1998 |
|---|---|---|
| British, North American, Australian and South African | 152 | 194 |
| Other European (or European language) journals | 16 | 22 |
| Chinese | 1 | 5 |
| Russian or other Eastern European | 28 | 3 |
| Japanese | 0 | 3 |
| Indian | 2 | 2 |

British Acupuncture Council, and with the help of John Moffett, librarian at the Needham Research Institute in Cambridge, I was able to enlist the skills of Hilary Smith, then a postgraduate student at the university, who very efficiently translated relevant sections from a sample of some 94 articles.

These were from three different journals:

A. 80 from *Acupuncture Research* (*Zhenci Yanjiu*)
B. 10 from *Chinese Acupuncture and Moxibustion* (*Zhongguo Zhenjiu*)
C. 4 from the *Chinese Journal of Integrated Traditional and Western Medicine* (*Zhongguo Zhongxiyi Jiehe Zazhi*).

The results can be summarised as follows:

- Requested details of points and parameters that were missing from the abstracts were found in the full articles in 50 (62.5%) of A, 1 (10%) of B, and 1 (25%) of C.
- These details were missing from the full articles in 7 (8.8%) of A, 1 (10%) of B, and 1 (25%) of C.
- They were partially present in 7 (8.8%) of A, 2 (20%) of B, and 1 (25%) of C.

They had not been requested for the remaining articles.

Chinese experimental studies usually give some indication of stimulation intensity, but do tend to report voltage rather than current or, failing that, the degree of motor activity elicited. They tend to give details of frequency, but commonly not of pulse duration or waveform. The amount of information given is probably little inferior to that in many studies published in Western journals of the same period (1985–1998). As for details of acupoints, the Chinese studies may be superior to comparable Western ones, at least at the beginning of the period considered.

Further specific details requested were found in 17 of 18 studies from A, 4 studies from B and 2 from C. In virtually all cases where it was not clear from the abstract whether EA or MA was used, this was clear in the full article, in 8 (10%) of A, 3 (30%) of B, and 1 (10%) of C. Some obvious mistranslations appeared in the abstracts, such as 'ankle' for 'back limb,' and *rong* for *ying* (Spring) points.

Furthermore, all authors' names were listed in all but one of the *Acupuncture Research* abstracts, and in this particular instance only the initial author's name was given in the full paper as well. Abstracts from *Chinese Acupuncture and Moxibustion* often did not list all the authors of an article, but these names were given in all of 38 full papers checked.

On the basis of this exercise, it seems that important treatment details omitted from abstracts of experimental studies published in some Chinese journals are in fact included in the full studies. A similar project to examine clinical trials is under way at the time of writing.

## SUMMARY

Some issues to note in this introduction are:

- the paradoxes involved in applying scientific methods to procedures developed or applied according to different paradigms
- the dangers of cultural bias
- technical issues in experimental research, together with the ethics of animal experimentation
- the relevance of laboratory work to clinical practice
- the need for high-quality research and reporting
- the importance of translation, with some data illustrating bias in standard electronic databases such as MEDLINE.

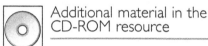 Additional material in the CD-ROM resource

A fuller version of this introductory chapter is available in the CD-ROM resource. The summary sections presented here are intended both for guiding readers to the fuller electronic versions and also to indicate the constraints and conditions under which much of the material for the CD-ROM was gathered. For those who mainly intend to use the book as their primary reference, it is important to be clear about the provenance of the material presented.

## RECOMMENDED READING

*There is now a wealth of material published on the methodology of acupuncture research. Several general textbooks with relevant contributions are listed in subsequent chapters. Another, which includes several chapters with a research perspective, is:*

Cassidy CM 2002 (ed) Contemporary Chinese Medicine and Acupuncture. Churchill Livingstone, Philadelphia, PA

*Other useful articles and books include:*

Sims J The mechanism of acupuncture analgesia: a review. Complementary Therapies in Medicine. 1997 June; 5(2): 102–11

Ewer T Methodological challenges of research into traditional, complementary and alternative medicine. Journal of the Acupuncture Association of Chartered Physiotherapists. 2001 Feb; 36–42

Felt RL Readers' rights: peer review in Chinese medical publication. Chinese Acupuncture and Oriental Medicine. 2001; 2(1): 9–16

Lewith G Acupuncture trial methodology. Acupuncture in Medicine. 1994 May; 12(1): 41–4

Vincent C, Furnham A, with Richardson P 1997 Complementary medicine. A research perspective. John Wiley, Chichester

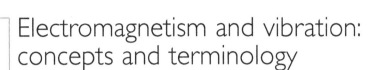
Electromagnetism and vibration:
concepts and terminology

This chapter introduces the language and ideas needed for basic understanding of the physics of EA and related techniques. This is necessary if equipment is to be used safely and effectively.

## PARTICLES AND WAVES

According to one view, physical matter is made up of atoms in different combinations and states. Elements (such as sodium, given the chemical symbol Na, or chlorine, Cl) consist of atoms of the same sort. Compounds (such as salt, NaCl) consist of combinations of atoms – molecules – of different sorts. An atom can be visualised as a miniature solar system, a nucleus surrounded by orbiting *electrons*. Each electron carries an identical negative electric *charge*, while the nucleus contains *protons*, each with a corresponding positive charge. A fundamental law is that such charges of opposite *polarity* attract, whereas similar ones repel. It is the electrostatic attractive force between the protons and electrons that holds the atom together.

An electric *field* is present in the space through which this force acts. The attraction can be imagined as acting along 'lines of force' between the particles; the field is these lines of force. If there are equal numbers of protons and electrons in the atom, the atom will be electrically neutral, with its electric field more or less contained.

However, atoms can also be affected by forces that are not simply electrical. For instance, *electromagnetic (EM) radiation*, made up of other particles, uncharged *photons*, may strike an atom and give an electron enough energy to escape from the atom, and perhaps even attach itself to another atom. The first atom then ends up positively charged, and the second negatively charged. Each has its own electric field, and if they are close enough they attract each other. Such non-neutral, charged atoms are called *ions*, and radiation

that can transform a neutral atom into an ion is called *ionising radiation*.

A complementary view is that neither atoms nor particles are fundamental, but waves. Energy moves as waves through space. In quantum physics, electrons and photons are not hard nuggets of matter, but clouds of vibrating energy that only appear to condense into particles when we try to locate or define them. Fields of force are not attractions between pre-existing particles; particles are condensations within fields.

## ELECTRIC FIELDS AND CURRENTS

Particles, waves, and fields are all useful concepts. For instance, in a force field produced by a charged particle (A), another such particle (B) will move towards or away from it, depending on its polarity. For oppositely charged particles, if they are far apart very little force is exerted on B, but as it moves closer to A more force is exerted. As a result, it will move faster and faster along the line of force between them. If the two are close together initially, B cannot pick up speed to the same extent. Thus A has more *potential energy* (the capacity to expend energy) the further apart the two particles are. It may be easiest to visualise this as follows: a stone on flat ground has less gravitational potential energy than a stone at the top of a mountain; a stone halfway up the mountain has an intermediate potential energy (Fig. 3.1).

*Energy* is the capacity for doing work, and *work* done is the product of force and distance moved. In other words, a stone rolling from the top of the mountain can do more work than one rolling only halfway. There is a difference between the amount of work needed to move the stone back to the ground from two different points on the mountain (electrically, this is called the *potential difference* (PD) between them). There is a potential gradient between the top and bottom of the mountain. So two stones at the same level are at the same potential – there is no potential gradient between them.

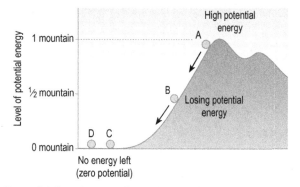

**Figure 3.1** Potential energy. Potential energy of a stone on a mountain is highest at the top of the mountain and lowest at its foot. The potential difference between A and C is greater than between B and C. There is no potential difference between C and D.

## Energy, charge and current

The electric *potential* at a point in the field is defined as the potential energy per unit charge of a positively charged particle placed at that point. Potential and potential difference are both measured in volts (V). One thousandth of a volt is a millivolt (mV). The potential energy a battery provides, its electromotive force (EMF), is also measured in volts. Energy (E) is measured in joules. The voltage V of a battery is the number of joules supplied to each unit of charge as it passes through the battery. Charge (Q) is measured in coulombs (C).

On flat ground, a stone will not move very far: its potential energy is not apparent. Without a source of consistent external power to supply the necessary energy or potential gradient, ions and electrons will also only mill around randomly. In electrical terms, such a power source could be a battery. The more work the battery can do (the higher it raises the top of the mountain), the more volts it can supply. One terminal of the battery will be positive, the other negative, so that there is a PD between them. Negatively charged particles will be attracted to one, repelled by the other. Now it becomes possible to move them in a consistent direction, down the hill towards the positive pole of the battery (Fig. 3.2). Such a consistent movement of charge is called an electric *current*. More particles will mean more current. Current is measured in ampères (or amps). An amp (1 A) is quite a lot of current. In electroacupuncture (EA) much smaller amounts of current are used, measured in milliamps (mA) and microamps (μA). As with volts, 1 A = 1000 mA or 1000 000 μA.

It is important to remember that a hill has a top and a bottom, and that both terminals of the battery need to be connected for a current to flow through a circuit. If this is broken (by a switch, or if a wire breaks), nothing will happen. Furthermore, as more and more stones roll down the hill, the hill itself slowly loses height: the battery gradually discharges.

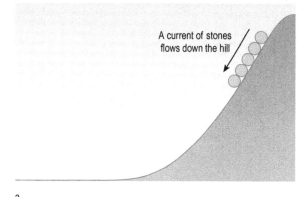

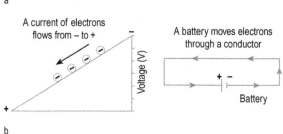

**Figure 3.2** Potential and current flow. (a) A 'current' of stones: gravity moves stones consistently down a mountain. (b) A current of electrons: a battery's electromotive force moves electrons through a conductor.

Once the battery goes (literally) flat, a battery charger may be able to increase the height of the mountain again.

## Resistance and power

A mountain can be smooth or rough, affecting the descent of the stones. Similarly, materials can be more or less electrically conductive. Some will present more *resistance* to a flow of current, and others less (Fig. 3.3). Put the other way around, a conductor will exhibit more *conductance* and an insulator less. In an insulator, the atoms and molecules are fixed; no charged particles are free to move. In a conductor, on the other hand, more ions are mobile, able to carry or conduct charge; there may also be electrons unattached to atoms, which are free to move. In metal conductors, only free electrons can carry charge; the ions are held in position in a lattice structure. Because like charges repel, electrons will tend to congregate on the surface of a conductor, in particular where its surface is most curved (e.g. at the tip of a needle). In a conductive liquid (an *electrolyte*), it is predominantly ions that carry charge. *Semiconductors* are substances such as silicon or germanium whose conductivity is intermediate between that of a conductor and an insulator. The human body consists of electrolytes and semiconductors rather than simple conductors.

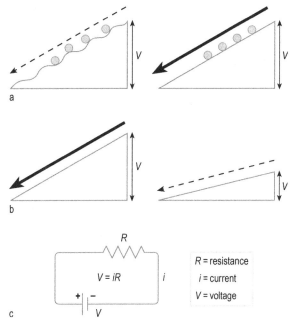

**Figure 3.3** Ohm's law: $V = iR$. (a) The greater the resistance, the less current flows, if voltage is constant. (b) The greater the voltage, the more current flows, if resistance is constant. (c) $R$, $i$ and $V$ in a circuit.

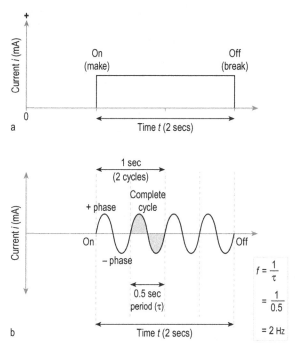

**Figure 3.4** Direct and alternating current. (a) A direct current (DC). (b) A sine wave alternating current (AC); frequency = number of cycles per second: $f = 1/\tau$.

Resistance $R$ is measured in ohms ($\Omega$), and conductance in mhos. In EA, the resistances concerned are generally larger, so are measured in kilohms (k$\Omega$) or megohms (M$\Omega$).

*Power* is defined as the rate at which work can be done: the more power, the more work can be done in a given time. Power is measured in watts or milliwatts (mW).

## Direct and alternating currents

The current supplied by a battery is *direct current* (DC): it always flows through a circuit in the same direction (Fig. 3.4a). Such a current is also known as *galvanic*. However, the battery can be replaced by a source of *alternating current* (AC), so that the polarity across the circuit alternates, and ions or electrons will flow first one way and then the other, in repeating identical *cycles*. The transition between the two is not abrupt: the ions slow down, stop, and then gather momentum in the opposite direction (Fig. 3.4b). AC is a sinusoidal current, its *waveform* a 'sine wave'. Each cycle has equal positive and negative *phases*, and is by definition *biphasic*: the current first flows in the direction conventionally considered as positive, then in the opposite direction. The duration of a cycle is its *period*; the number of cycles or direction changes per second is the *frequency* of the waveform. Frequency may be relatively low (LF) or high (HF).

Biphasic currents are not always sinusoidal. Rather than smooth cycles they may consist of *pulses*, which can be square or rectangular, sawtooth, triangular or trapezoidal, spike, exponential and so on. Each of these has different *rise time* and decay time characteristics. The pulses consist of bipolar phases that may follow each other without a break, or be separated by a short interval. In both cases, for rectangular pulses the total time for a complete pulse is called the *pulse duration* (each phase having its own phase duration), and the time between each pulse is the *interpulse interval*. For non-rectangular waveforms, pulse duration is defined rather arbitrarily as the duration at 50% of the maximum amplitude (Fig. 3.5). Pulsed DC is often termed *monophasic* current (in this case, the phase and pulse are identical). Continuous DC has zero frequency. The longer the pulse duration, the more charge is contained in the pulse (Fig. 3.6).

## Duty cycle, frequency and amplitude

The *duty cycle* of a waveform is defined as the ratio of 'on' time (pulse duration) to the total of 'on' and 'off' time before the next pulse starts (pulse duration plus interpulse interval) (Fig. 3.6).

Frequency is measured in units called hertz (Hz), or cycles per second. In the context of EA, a low frequency is a frequency of less than 10 cycles per second (<10 Hz), and a

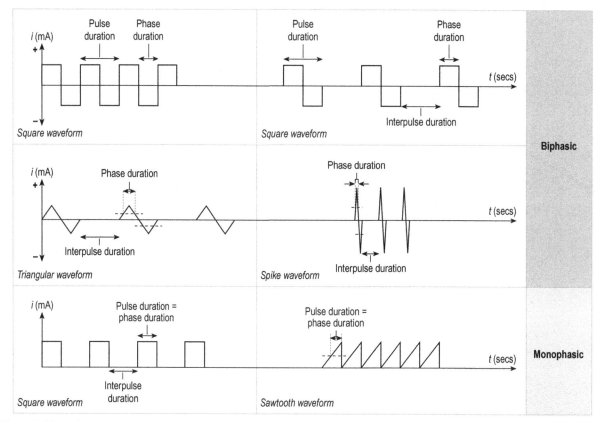

**Figure 3.5** Waveforms and pulse duration. Variants of continuous biphasic and monophasic wave forms, showing continuous pulses and pulses separated by an interpulse interval.

high frequency is around 50–200 Hz. However, conventions vary: in Western electrotherapy as a whole LF is taken as < 1 kHz, medium frequency as 1–10 kHz, and HF as more than 10 kHz (> 10 kHz), whereas in China the medium range is extended to 100 kHz.

The effect of two currents flowing in the same space is the same as the effect of the two currents added together. If they are of opposite polarity, they may cancel each other out. If they are biphasic, with the same frequency, whether their effects add or cancel depends on the *phase difference* (or phase angle) between them. They may be in phase, 180° out of phase, or somewhere between. In phase, their addition is called constructive *interference*, and in general two waves with identical parameters of frequency and amplitude that are also in phase are said to be *coherent*. Destructive interference occurs when they cancel each other out. If they have different frequencies, their interference will produce a *beat frequency* equal to the *difference* between their frequencies (Fig. 3.7).

Strictly speaking, only sine waves should be described as having simply 'frequency.' For other waveforms, it is more accurate to use the term *pulse repetition rate* (PRR) or pulse repetition frequency. The term *pulse frequency* will generally be used in this book, however, in place of the more cumbersome PRR, and will generally be abbreviated to 'frequency' unless the context demands otherwise.

Use of the word *amplitude* can also be confusing. Whereas this is straightforward for DC, when the current is biphasic it can be defined in different ways (Fig. 3.8). The *peak amplitude* of DC is the difference between its greatest value and zero, whereas the *peak-to-peak amplitude* of a biphasic current is measured between its greatest positive and negative values. The *average* value of a rectangularly pulsed DC is the product of the duty cycle and peak value. Clearly, for long interpulse intervals, there can be considerable differences between peak and average values: a high peak output does not guarantee a stronger stimulation.

## Variants of simple waveforms

Biphasic waveforms, as well as being *symmetrical*, with identical positive and negative phases, can also be *asymmetrical*. In this case, if the two phases have the same area, then the waveform is *charge balanced* (Fig. 3.9).

Currents used in the examples above are shown as *continuous current* (or *continuous wave*, CW), with constant amplitude, duration, and frequency. Currents may also be *pulse modulated* (Fig. 3.10): if the pulse frequency changes, they are frequency modulated, if the amplitude changes, they are amplitude modulated, and so on. Such modulation may be itself at a regular frequency, or not. A particular form of

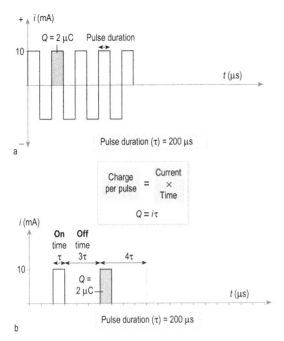

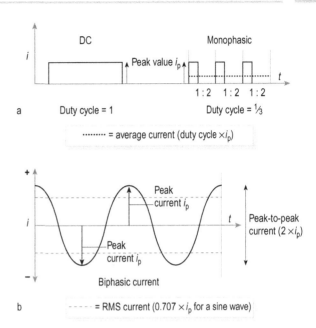

Figure. 3.8 The meaning of amplitude. (a) Peak and average values of DC and a monophasic pulse, showing average current = duty cycle × peak current. (b) Peak, peak-to-peak, and root-mean-square (RMS) current values for a sine wave, showing RMS = 0.707 × peak, with sine wave and monophasic pulse superimposed.

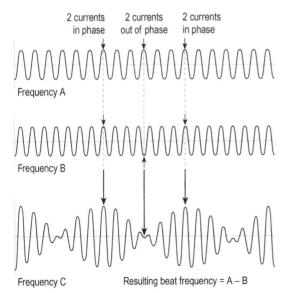

**Figure 3.6** Duty cycle. Continuous square wave currents with the same amplitude (10 mA) and pulse duration (200 μs), but different duty cycles. (a) Continuous biphasic pulses with no interpulse interval. Duty cycle is 1:1 or 100%. (b) Continuous monophasic pulses, with an interpulse interval of 600 μs. Duty cycle in this example is 1:4 or 25%.

frequency modulation is when trains of two different frequencies alternate (generally LF, and HF, or more or less than about 30 Hz). In the Chinese literature, this is often called the *dense-disperse* (DD) mode.

**Figure 3.7** Interference between two currents of different frequencies (A and B), to produce C.

Currents may also be *current modulated*, with changes to the overall pattern rather than the individual pulses. Most simply, they can be *interrupted* (burst, pulsed), whether they are AC or DC. Sometimes the distinction is made between bursts at short, millisecond intervals, and interrupted current with intervals of 1 second or more. With *burst current* or interrupted current, each burst or *train* of current pulses is followed by an *interburst interval*. In this case two different frequencies are involved: the frequency of the pulses themselves, and the slower frequency of the trains or bursts (Fig. 3.11).

With interrupted and DD currents, changes between the pulse trains are abrupt. Current amplitude and frequency can also be *ramped* to soften these changes.

## THE EFFECTS OF ELECTRICITY

### Electrolysis

In an electrolyte, there will be negative and positive ions. A current may be applied to the electrolyte through *electrodes* (Fig. 3.12). The negative electrode is the *cathode*, the positive the *anode*. Positive ions in the electrolyte will be attracted to the cathode (and so are called *cations*), negative ions to the anode (*anions*), a process called *electrolysis*. In salt water, acid will form at the anode and corrode it. With balanced biphasic current, it is assumed that the chemical products of electrolysis are neutralised with each

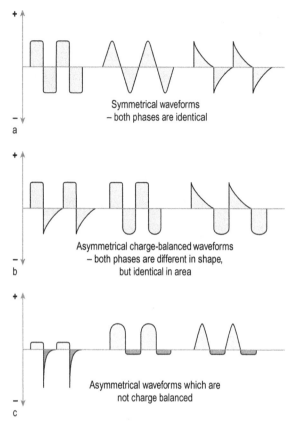

**Figure 3.9** Symmetry and charge balance. (a) Symmetrical waveforms. (b) Asymmetrical charge-balanced waveforms, made up of components from (a). (c) Asymmetrical waveforms that are not charge balanced.

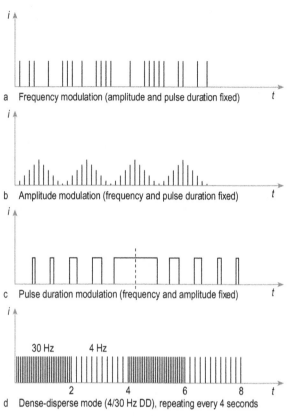

**Figure 3.10** Types of modulation. (a) Frequency modulation (FM). (b) Amplitude modulation (AM) at a regular frequency. (c) Pulse duration modulation. (d) A dense-disperse current of 4 Hz and 30 Hz.

polarity reversal. However, this may not be the case at low frequencies, or if the pulse duration or interphase interval is long.

## Magnetism

A moving electric charge produces a magnetic *field* at right angles to its direction of motion. Electrons spinning around randomly oriented atoms will produce random magnetic fields that tend to cancel each other out. In magnetic materials, on the other hand, atoms and molecules can be organised so that the magnetic fields add together. Using this principle, *permanent magnets* can be made, producing a constant (static) magnetic field. Electrons flowing in a wire create a magnetic field around the wire (the stronger the current, the stronger the field). A constant current produces a static magnetic field, and a changing one a changing magnetic field. In a wonderful symmetry, a changing magnetic field will create an electric potential difference along a conductor aligned with the field, and a current will result (this is called electromagnetic induction). Pulsed electromagnetic fields

(PEMF), with both electric and magnetic components, are used therapeutically.

Magnetism, like electricity, has polarity: north (N) and south (S) poles attract, while similar ones repel. Conventionally, the lines of force in a magnetic field emerge from the north pole and enter the south. The more densely these lines are packed together, the stronger is the magnetic field. Thus the field strength corresponds to the number of such lines passing through a unit area, the magnetic *flux density*, which is measured in gauss (G), or tesla (T). A magnet suspended with its N/S axis horizontal will align itself so that its north pole points roughly towards geographic north.

## Electromagnetic radiation

If moving electrons generate a magnetic field, *changes* in the movement of electrons produce EM radiation. Electrons flowing in a conductor collide with the lattice structure of its atoms and molecules and transfer their energy to other electrons in the miniature solar systems of the atoms, while

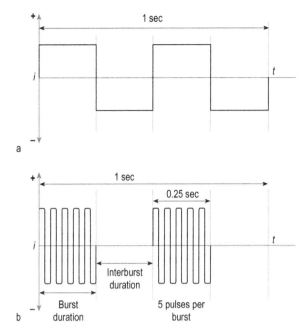

**Figure 3.11** Current modulation. (a) 2 Hz continuous wave (CW), unmodulated. (b) 2 Hz 'bursts' of current, with an internal frequency of 20 Hz and duty cycle 50% (burst and interburst duration identical).

not necessarily dislodging them altogether. The excited atomic electrons soon return to their original state, releasing energy in the form of photons.

In a conductor, the photon energy released manifests as heat or, at high enough temperatures, as light (as in the ordinary lightbulb). Heat and light are both forms of electromagnetic radiation, which can be described either as photons or as waves. The frequency of radiation emitted is proportional to its energy. In the visible spectrum, red has a lower frequency than blue or violet light. *Infrared* (IR) (radiated heat)

has a still lower frequency, and *ultraviolet* (UV) a higher one than any of the visible colours. White light is made up of radiation with many different frequencies. Light of only one frequency is termed *monochromatic*.

The more vigorously electrons collide with atoms, the higher is the energy of the photons emitted. In a gas-filled tube or in a vacuum, electrons can accelerate more easily than in a solid conductor, so higher-frequency radiation is produced (UV or X-rays, for example). Using different methods, a whole spectrum of different frequencies can be produced, from ELF and ULF (extremely and ultra low frequencies), through radio waves (e.g. VHF, very high frequencies), microwaves, far infrared, visible light and ultraviolet, to ionising X-rays and high-energy gamma rays (Fig. 3.13).

## POLARISATION AND WAVELENGTH

So far, waves have been described in terms of frequency and time. However, EM waves also travel through space, like waves travelling down a rope when you flick one end. If the rope passes through a wall with a vertical slit in it, it can only move up or down, so the waves occur in the plane of the slit, at right angles to the rope, not in any other direction. They are vertically *polarised*. Otherwise, they can move in many different planes, still at right angles to the rope, and are non-polarised. EM waves can also be polarised or non-polarised. Because they oscillate at right angles to the direction they move in, they are called transverse waves.

The *wavelength* (λ) of the radiation is the distance between successive wave crests; its speed is how far these travel in a given time. In a vacuum, all EM radiation travels at the same speed. Sometimes it is more convenient to describe radiation in terms of wavelength rather than frequency. Thus EHF (extremely high frequency) radiation with a frequency of 60 GHz may be easier to grasp as a wavelength of 5 mm. On the other hand, it makes more sense to consider a frequency of 100 Hz than a wavelength of 3000 km!

Box 3.1 details some properties of EM radiation.

## VIBRATION, SOUND AND ULTRASOUND

Whereas EM radiation is made up of *transverse waves*, the oscillations of mechanical vibration are *longitudinal*: regions of compression and rarefaction in the direction the waves are travelling through a medium. Sound and ultrasound are forms of vibration defined in relation to human hearing: sound can be heard between about 20 Hz and 20 kHz, at *infrasonic* frequencies (below about 20 Hz) vibration is experienced rather than sound, and *ultrasound* consists of frequencies above about 20 kHz. Like electric current, ultrasound can be CW or pulsed; ultrasound power density (sometimes termed intensity) is measured in $W/cm^2$. Just as with EM radiation, the energy of vibration can heat a substance.

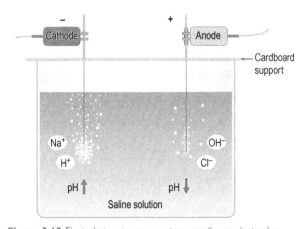

**Figure 3.12** Electrolysis, using acupuncture needles as electrodes.

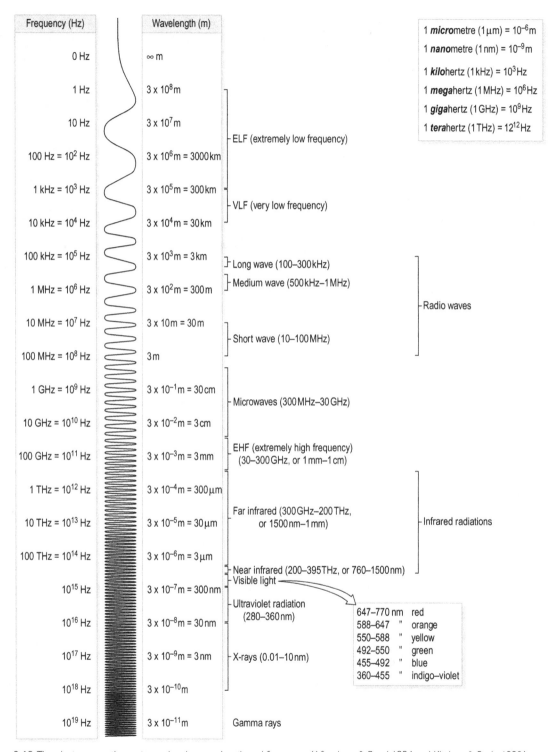

**Figure 3.13** The electromagnetic spectrum, showing wavelength and frequency. (After Low & Reed 1994 and Kitchen & Bazin 1998.)

All forms of EM radiation travel in straight lines, and can be reflected from the surface of physical matter or penetrate through it. More radiation will penetrate if it meets the surface at right angles. Inside matter, radiation may be refracted or scattered, transmitted or absorbed. Radiation that is completely transmitted without attenuation has no effect on matter. To do so, it must be absorbed, and its energy transferred (often resulting in heat). The more it is absorbed, the shorter the distance it will penetrate. Penetration is generally proportional to wavelength: as this increases, absorption will occur further from the surface. *Penetration depth* (pd) is the depth by which some 63% of radiant energy has been absorbed. At pd × 2, over 87% is absorbed. Some authors use the term 'half-depth,' the depth at which 50% of the initial energy is still present.

The energy and power of radiation are measured in joules and watts respectively, as with electricity. Another useful term is *energy density* (or radiant exposure), a measure of how much energy is applied over a given area in $J/cm^2$. Correspondingly, *power density* (irradiance) is measured in $W/cm^2$, as with ultrasound.

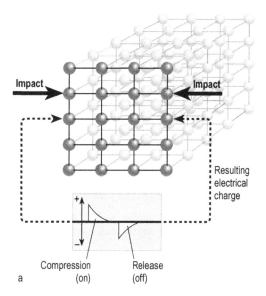

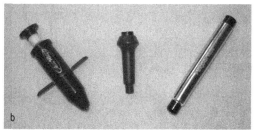

**Figure 3.14** The piezoelectric stimulator. (Photo by Riccardo Cuminetti.) (a) The principle: when some types of crystal are compressed and then released, an electrical pulse results. (b) Three piezoelectric stimulators.

## Resonance and standing waves

All objects with semirigid boundaries have a frequency at which they vibrate naturally, whether solid or hollow. Resonance occurs when external vibration is applied at this *resonant frequency*. Its amplitude is amplified, as when singing in the bathroom: certain notes sound louder, more sonorous, as the bathroom 'sings back' to you. The resonant frequency depends on the dimensions of the object. As sound waves reflect off the walls of the bathroom cavity, interference occurs between them. If two waves of the same frequency travelling in opposite directions interfere constructively then a *standing wave* results.

# STIMULATION DEVICES

To produce electric currents, EM fields and radiation, infra- and ultrasound for therapeutic application, electric circuits made up of different components are used. A battery or AC source of power is always necessary. Other components may be resistors, capacitors, inductances, switches, diodes and transistors, indicator meters (analogue or digital) and lamps, nowadays generally light-emitting diodes (LEDs).

Ultrasound is produced by a special transducer using the *piezoelectric effect*. Piezoelectric crystals change shape in an electric field, expanding or contracting in response to changes in voltage. This is used to generate the longitudinal

oscillations of ultrasound. Conversely, if pressure is put on such a crystal an electrical pulse is produced, with one in the opposite direction when the pressure is released (Fig. 3.14).

Microwaves are generally produced from resonant cavities of different shapes and sizes, although spark discharges are used in *microwave resonance therapy* (MRT) to generate EHF millimetre waves, which are then applied via a waveguide.

*LASER* light is produced by a quantum process called 'Light Amplification by the Stimulated Emission of Radiation', making use of standing waves in a crystal or gas-filled tube. Laser light is monochromatic, both spatially and temporally coherent, and *collimated* (does not diverge over distance).

## Electrodes

For most practitioners, what happens inside a stimulator is unimportant, provided it works. A standardised stimulator

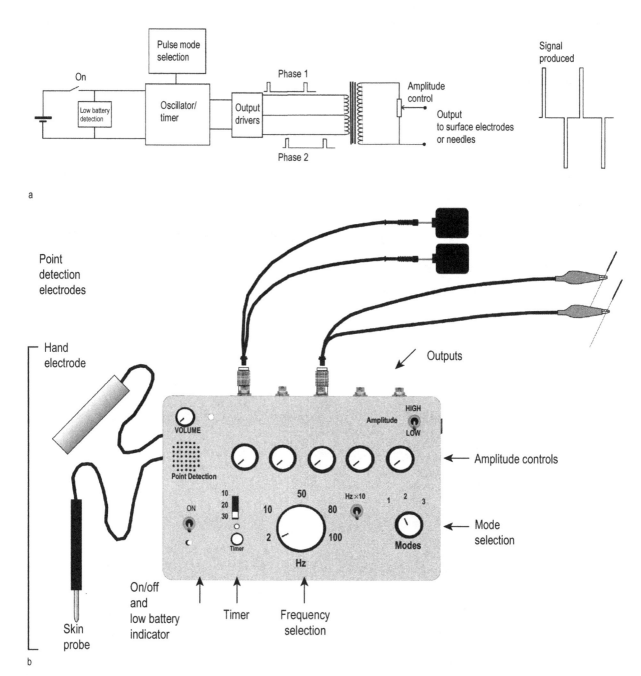

**Figure 3.15** A typical electroacupuncture stimulator. (Courtesy of Riccardo Cuminetti.) (a) Block diagram for a biphasic output stimulator. (b) A typical stimulator unit.

for EA is illustrated in Fig. 3.15. The current produced inside the device is applied to the body using electrodes. *Transcutaneous* electrodes transfer charge to the surface or skin of the body via the output lead(s), and are generally pads of various types, although small-diameter *probes* are also used. *Percutaneous* electrodes (such as acupuncture needles) are used to stimulate intramuscularly, beneath the skin.

The main difference between EA and *transcutaneous electrical nerve stimulation* (TENS, sometimes known as TNS or TES) is really one of usage. TENS by definition uses surface stimulation, and is nowadays primarily a home (outpatient) treatment, sometimes for extended periods. EA by definition uses needles, but practitioners may also use various forms of surface electrode. It is thus primarily a clinical treatment.

## Output type and current density

A stimulator supplies *constant current* or *constant voltage* depending on whether the current or the voltage remains the same when impedance varies at the interface between the patient's body and the electrode (*impedance* is the term for resistance when AC is used). The output type is determined by its internal circuitry: the output impedance of the former tends to be high (>100 k$\Omega$) and the amplitude control regulates the current, while the output impedance of the latter is low (< 500 $\Omega$), the output control regulating voltage.

For a given output current, the smaller the electrode area in contact with the body, the higher is the *current density* (in mA/cm$^2$).

## Additional material in the CD-ROM resource

In the electronic version of this chapter, additional material, mathematical detail and illustrations can be found on the following topics:
- Current and charge
- Ohm's law
- Electrolysis
- Magnetic polarity
- Electric circuits.

## RECOMMENDED READING

*For those who wish to explore the fundamentals of electro-therapy in more depth, some excellent textbooks are available. These include:*

Kitchen S, Bazin S 1998 (eds) Clayton's Electrotherapy. WB Saunders, Philadelphia, PA (10th edn)

Low J, Reed A 1994 Electrotherapy Explained: Principles and practice. Butterworth-Heinemann, London (2nd edn)

Nelson RM, Currier DP 1991 (eds) Clinical Electrotherapy. Appleton and Lange, Norwalk, CT

*Material specifically relevant to EA and laser can be found in:*

Filshie J, White A 1998 (eds) Medical Acupuncture: A western scientific approach. Churchill Livingstone, Edinburgh

*A very enjoyable introduction to physics, despite being over 40 years old, is:*

Feynman RB, Leighton RB, Sands M 1963 The Feynman Lectures on Physics 1. Mainly mechanics, radiation and heat. Addison-Wesley, Reading, MA

## SUMMARY

The most important things to remember from this chapter are:
- the different waveform patterns (Figs 3.9–3.11)
- electrolysis (Fig. 3.12)
- the different features of the EA stimulator (Fig. 3.15).

## Electroacupuncture in context:
## the effects of electrotherapy

This chapter offers a brief guided tour to the effects of electric currents, heat and cold, non-thermal radiation, magnetic fields, vibration, sound and ultrasound, together with an afterword on our relationship with the energetic world around us. The threads drawn together here will assist understanding of how the modalities of electrotherapy can be applied in the context of acupuncture practice.

# ELECTRIC CURRENTS

Electric currents have three effects: chemical, physical (or stimulatory) and thermal. These can influence the body at different levels: cellular, tissue, segmental and systemic.

## Direct current (DC) stimulation

Much electrotherapy depends on stimulating nerves to elicit the '*action potentials*' described in detail in Chapter 5 of the CD-ROM ⊙ resource. It is easier to activate the nerve action potential (AP) using negative rather than positive current. The negative electrode (cathode) is sometimes termed the 'active' electrode, and can provide more comfortable effective stimulation than the positive electrode (anode).

DC increases blood flow locally, with a resultant increase in temperature. It can also enhance tissue healing, for which researchers have usually adopted a protocol that involves negative stimulation initially, sometimes followed by positive currents, or even reversing polarity over several days. Pulsed DC has also been used. Cathodal high-voltage pulsed galvanic stimulation reduces acute oedema following injury, for example.

DC fields enhance bone and nerve repair if a field is applied in the same direction as the body's own electrical field. Nerves tend to grow towards the cathode. Although very low intensity DC can enhance growth and repair, stronger currents have a destructive effect. This has been utilised in treating tumours or aneurysms, in what has sometimes been called 'electropuncture,' or even 'electric moxa'.

The difference between weak and strong current effects is an example of a universal biological principle, the *Arndt–Schulz law*. This states roughly that above a certain threshold a weak stimulus enhances activity whereas a strong one inhibits it, and if strong enough can be destructive. For this reason, DC currents in electrotherapy are usually employed at relatively low intensities.

DC also has systemic effects. If it is applied in the same direction as the natural field of the body (forehead or vertex negative, occiput or leg positive), drowsiness and a sense of withdrawal may follow; there is alertness and mood elevation if current is applied in the opposite direction. Clearly, these findings could be taken into account when designing acupuncture treatments involving electrical stimulation.

## Low-frequency (LF) stimulation

Most electrotherapy devices apply current transcutaneously, but electroacupuncture (EA) utilises percutaneous rather than transcutaneous stimulation ('through' rather than 'across' the skin). The effects of both transcutaneous electrical nerve stimulation (TENS) and EA occur mainly at the cellular level, leading to tissue and segmental level effects. Thermal, electrolytic and other chemical effects are minimal.

The firing threshold for a nerve fibre depends on the amount of charge in the applied pulse, that is, on both its amplitude and duration. The exact relationship between these two factors can be illustrated in the strength–duration (SD) curve (Fig. 4.1). At short pulse durations, current has to be strong for an AP to result. The longer the pulse duration, the less current is needed, until at pulse durations greater than about 0.5 ms (for motor and sensory fibres) a minimal current is reached. For nerve stimulation, longer pulse durations are therefore unnecessary. Once the threshold is reached, the fibre fires. With more stimulation, more fibres are recruited.

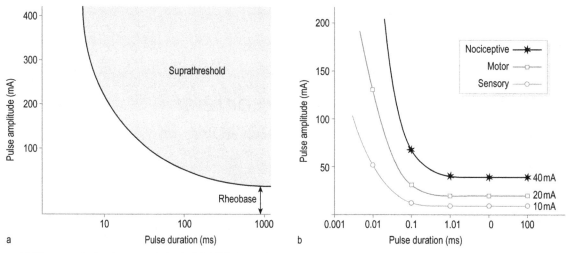

**Figure 4.1** The strength–duration curve. (After Walsh 1997, Low & Read 1994.) (a) Strength–duration (SD) curve. Note minimum current (rheobase) needed to trigger an action potential at long pulse durations. (b) Strength–duration curves for sensory (Aβ) fibre, motor (α) fibre, and nociceptive (Aδ or C) fibre. Note the increased separation between the three curves at shorter pulse durations.

The curves for the different sorts of fibres are more widely separated at shorter pulse durations making it simpler to activate them selectively, with *sensory level*, *motor level*, or *noxious level* stimulation. Thus very short pulses (~10 μs) or spikes are unlikely to activate motor fibres. However, when using HF (~100 Hz) TENS, cutaneous (more superficial) C fibres may in fact reach their threshold well before the deeper muscle afferents. Furthermore, thresholds differ in different parts of the body. Thus, to avoid exciting nociceptive C fibres inadvertently, it may be important to position electrodes as close as possible to the target tissue.

Using needles may have several advantages:

- The applied waveform is less distorted by the skin.
- Less current is needed to achieve motor stimulation.
- Deeper muscle afferents can be stimulated without pain from cutaneous C fibres.

The effect of trains of pulses is cumulative, so that less charge is required to stimulate the nerve, and stimulation feels more comfortable than with more widely spaced single pulses. Even a succession of subthreshold impulses may eventually trigger a nerve impulse.

Not only are pulse duration and amplitude important, but also the rise time and shape of the pulse. A rapid rise time, as with rectangular and spike waveforms, is needed to stimulate normal nerve. For sine waves, whose rise time depends on frequency, firing threshold is lowest at around 100 Hz.

Nerve fibres exhibit a *frequency following response* (FFR), with each stimulation pulse triggering the nerve to fire. Thinner fibres, with long '*refractory periods*', cannot follow high frequencies, but only low-frequency stimulation of high amplitude and long pulse duration. Thus pain-transmitting C fibres may fatigue even at 5 Hz, and will generally not fire at more than around 10 Hz. Thicker nerves may have a FFR up to ~1 kHz (1000 Hz). At higher frequencies still, around 4 kHz, nerve and muscle fibres no longer respond to stimulation.

Frequencies above 50 Hz may produce a short term 'block' of both Aδ and C nerve fibres (for more on fibre types, see Ch. 5).

Negative currents lower the threshold to further stimulation. Even with charge-balanced biphasic waveforms, especially asymmetric ones, this can mean that the two phases may not have identical effects.

## Muscle stimulation

Motor level electrical stimulation activates motor as well as sensory neurons, leading to muscle contraction. For normally innervated muscle, electrical stimulation always occurs via the motoneuron. However, in denervated muscle, where the nerve supply is interrupted, the muscle fibre itself is activated. Much greater currents and longer pulse durations are required to stimulate the latter, but rapid rise times and stronger currents are not necessary.

The FFR of normal muscle means that at low frequencies each incoming pulse produces a contraction. At around 10 Hz (the frequency of physiological tremor), this becomes a tremor. Above the *critical fusion frequency* (CFF), a smooth continuous (tetanic) contraction results. For most large muscles, tetanic stimulation is best applied between 30 and 50 Hz.

Interrupted currents, trains of pulses with relatively long intervals between them (see Fig. 3.11 on page 33), are frequently used in muscle stimulation, for muscle re-education, enhancing blood circulation and improving joint range of motion. Brief pulses and shorter trains are more comfortable than longer ones, while ramping stimulation up and down over several seconds gives a muscle action that feels more natural than simple bursts of stimulation.

Frequencies lower than 10 Hz are experienced as tapping or pulsating; those above 400 Hz are felt as vibrating or tickling, and are less likely to be uncomfortable than those around 100 Hz when using TENS. A frequency of 50 Hz may also be better tolerated.

## MUSCLE STRENGTHENING
*Electrical muscle stimulation* (EMS) cannot substitute for exercise in normal muscle, but can be useful if a muscle is weak or voluntary movement is restricted. Treatment has to be carried out several times a week for several weeks.

## FACILITATING MUSCLE CONTROL
Motor level stimulation can encourage patients to (re)gain control over voluntary muscle.

## REDUCING SPASTICITY
Stimulation can be helpful for various forms of spasticity, the effect lasting longer with more sustained treatment. The spastic muscles themselves, their antagonists, or both may be activated. If direct stimulation of spastic muscle leads to temporary aggravation, extrasegmental stimulation may decrease reflex excitability.

## AFFECTING CIRCULATION AND TISSUE REPAIR
Muscle movement exerts a pumping action on the blood and lymph, enhancing oxygenation and tissue nutrition, as well as removing lactic acid and other metabolic byproducts. If used consistently, stimulation (~10 Hz) increases muscular fatigue resistance, and after about 3 months even muscle structure is permanently altered. Interrupted stimulation, as with muscle strengthening, tends to increase effectiveness.

Effects on chronic oedema are sometimes disappointing, but biphasic LF stimulation can be very helpful for tissue repair, with electrodes positioned close to the wound.

## TREATING DENERVATED MUSCLE
Compression injury to a nerve results in *neurapraxia*, a conduction block that recovers relatively quickly (within days or weeks) or, if more severe, to *axonotmesis*, degeneration of the nerve beyond the injury, with subsequent slow regrowth of the nerve (1–2 mm daily). Complete severance of a nerve, *neurotmesis*, may mean the nerve never grows back to its target tissue. In neurapraxia (partial denervation), it is still possible to excite muscle via the motor nerve, but not in the case of complete denervation, when the muscle is paralysed. Without its usual electrical and neurochemical input, muscle soon atrophies, with increasing degeneration and fibrosis, a process beginning within 1–2 weeks after the initial lesion and complete (and probably irreversible) by about 3 years.

EMS can benefit muscle by maintaining nourishment to the tissue and aiding repair, thus delaying atrophy and fibrosis.

It also fosters a return to normal voluntary use once reinnervation occurs. However, since vigorous movement may actually damage muscle and increase fibrosis, low-intensity LF stimulation with short pulse durations and long interruptions between contractions may be more appropriate. One key factor is that the muscle be kept under tension (i.e. using isometric contractions) during treatment. It is important to start treatment as soon as possible after the initial lesion, and to maintain it consistently, since it may take up to 2 years for normal innervation to be re-established.

> **A cautionary aside on surface electrodes**
> High current densities can lead to thermal damage and breakdown of the outer layers of skin with some electrodes, particularly if the skin is dry or if a small-diameter handheld probe (pTENS) is used.

# HEAT AND COLD

Heat accelerates cellular metabolism and increases blood flow and vasodilation. It relieves pain and spasm, and increases joint and tendon mobility. Applied locally, heat encourages healing and inhibits surface infections. In combination with elevation and exercise, it is helpful for some oedema, and can also enhance visceral circulation.

Cold, locally applied, generally slows down cellular metabolism and causes an initial decrease in blood flow, followed by slowly alternating vasodilation and constriction. It can relieve pain and spasm, and may increase or decrease muscle strength. Cold may slow healing, but is used in the treatment of recent injury, chronic inflammation and oedema.

In the body, heat lowers the threshold to electrical stimulation and increases conduction, with cold having opposite effects. At frequencies higher than around 10 kHz, the energy of an applied current is absorbed and transformed into heat. Diathermy makes use of this principle. It may be longwave (~1 MHz), or shortwave (27.12 MHz).

Infrared and microwave can both be used for heating. Different wavelengths of infrared penetrate to different depths within the body. Neither penetrates as far as shortwave.

# NON-THERMAL EFFECTS OF RADIATION

## Microwaves (ultra high frequency, UHF)

Low-level microwave radiation, when not strong enough to cause heating, can enhance tissue repair. When modulated (pulsed) at extremely low frequencies (ELF), it has many more effects on living systems, including the heart and brain. These effects appear to occur at particular frequency or amplitude 'windows', such as 15 Hz or 16 Hz. Microwaves pulsed at this frequency alter calcium ion outflow from nerve cells, as well as some enzyme activity.

## Millimetre waves (extremely high frequency, EHF)

Millimetre waves (30–300 GHz, or $30–300 \times 10^9$ Hz), between microwaves and far infrared in the electromagnetic (EM) spectrum, exhibit non-thermal frequency window effects without modulation. At very low intensities, different frequencies will have different, even opposite, effects on bacterial growth, for example. These have been explained in terms of resonance, perhaps at the cell membrane level, or even of the amino acid constituents of deoxyribonucleic acid (DNA).

Athermal EHF accelerates nerve conduction and regrowth, and enhances the immune response and wound healing (particularly of peptic ulcer). Unlike microwave radiation, EHF does not appear to encourage mutation, and may indeed reduce bone marrow damage from subsequent radio- or chemotherapy.

As with acupuncture, EHF may have a *regulatory effect*, with little influence on an organism already in equilibrium. When used clinically, patients often exhibit a generalised 'sensor reaction' as soon as the most appropriate resonant EHF frequency is selected.

## Low-intensity lasers and polarised light

Low-intensity laser (or light) therapy (LILT) is the therapeutic application of low-output power (< 500 mW) lasers and monochromatic 'superluminous' diodes at athermal levels. LILT obeys the Arndt–Schulz law for dosage. As with microwave and EHF, there are windows of effective wavelengths, determined in part by the absorption characteristics of different biomolecules and cell components.

Helium neon (HeNe) and some gallium aluminium arsenide (GaAlAs) lasers produce red light. Other GaAlAs and carbon dioxide ($CO_2$) lasers produce infrared. Different lasers and superluminous diodes are often grouped together in a multiwavelength cluster array (for treating larger areas). The light from lasers and light-emitting diodes (LEDs) may be pulsed, or continuous (CW).

Once it enters the body, laser light is scattered, so in this context lasers have little advantage over other monochromatic light sources. Red light is useful to stimulate superficial structures directly; infrared may penetrate slightly further. However, the indirect effects of LILT go much deeper. They include changes in cellular proliferation and various enzyme processes, vasodilation, enhanced vascularisation and collagen synthesis, as well as other changes central to tissue repair, especially in its early stages. LILT can also enhance immune function. Like EHF, its influence on both tissue repair and immune function comes into play only when cells are already in an abnormal (or disease) state.

LILT has been used for nerve regeneration (retarding atrophy of denervated muscle), and cartilage, tendon and bone repair, as well as to enhance soft tissue healing.

More controversial than the use of LILT in tissue repair is its use for treating pain. Results in experimental studies are contradictory, and the mechanisms involved are not as well understood as those underlying LILT's role in tissue repair. However, LILT does appear to alter brain levels of various neurotransmitters, and may influence the EEG (electroencephalogram) as well. Thus there are claims that it can have contralateral, even systemic effects.

Polarised light, like LILT, can enhance immune activity, even if not monochromatic. Irradiation of only 400 cm² of skin (and the underlying subepidermal capillary network) can improve the circulatory and immunological characteristics of all the blood in the body, and hence of the whole body itself. Like LILT, polarised light appears to have a regulatory effect, stimulating or inhibiting to maintain homeostatic (or 'homeodynamic') balance. It also follows the Arndt–Schulz law.

# LOW-INTENSITY ELECTROMAGNETIC FIELDS

## Variable fields

Low-frequency pulsed electromagnetic fields (PEMF) have effects in some ways quite similar to those of high-frequency (VHF or microwave) radiation pulsed at the same low frequencies. As with all the low-intensity methods of stimulation, total energy transfer is less important than making use of certain intensity and frequency windows (15 Hz and 16 Hz again figure strongly). The Arndt–Schulz law plays its part, and initial state (at cell, tissue or whole organism level) determines the outcome of stimulation: a system in equilibrium (at rest) or fully activated does not respond, but PEMF can influence the rate of events between these two extremes, with more actively proliferating cells being most responsive.

PEMF have particular effects on some immune processes, on muscle spasm, circulation (e.g. vasodilation, atherosclerosis) and oxygenation, oedema, inflammation and arthritic states. PEMF also has marked effects on repair and regeneration, whether of nerve, tendon, ligament, bone, soft tissue, or even liver cells. As with pulsed microwave, it is likely that many of these effects are mediated by calcium ion transfer at the cell membrane. PEMF may also affect pain perception, although results are not so clear cut as in tissue repair, in part because the effects of low-intensity fields are subtle and often difficult to measure.

Waveform and frequency are important factors. Pulsed fields are more effective than sinusoidally modulated ones, and intermittent fields more effective than continuous ones. There are some interesting results on 10 Hz PEMF for ligament and bone repair, and on 2 Hz and 15 Hz for nerve repair; 2 Hz PEMF enhanced functional recovery even after nerve transection. However, there is also evidence that frequency responses may be specific to the individual. Varying treatment parameters, rather than keeping them fixed, has been found effective in some studies.

## Static fields

Static magnetic fields are produced by permanent magnets. Stronger fields penetrate the body more deeply, and in general results may be more consistent if fields stronger than about 500 G (50 mT) are used. Static fields influence cellular respiration, with dose-dependent (Arndt–Schulz) effects on blood chemistry, circulation, heart rate, thrombocytic activity, oedema, tissue healing, and even beneficial effects on tumours (in animal studies, with fields greater than about 4000 G). Static fields may also be *protective* against X-ray-induced mutagenesis, although this will depend on whether exposure to the magnetic field precedes or follows irradiation. As with DC electric fields, low-intensity static magnetic fields applied to the head will alter the EEG.

Although there are similarities between the biological effects of pulsed and static fields, in general the former seem to be stronger, and there is less convincing evidence for those of low-intensity static fields.

# VIBRATION, SOUND AND ULTRASOUND

Longitudinal oscillation in the form of mechanical vibration and sound can affect the body as much as EM stimulation. Cutaneous sensitivity is greatest at around 30–40 Hz, and that of deeper tissue at 250 and 125 Hz. Vibration is sensed at between 13–18 Hz and 2.6 kHz (large-diameter sensory neurons can 'follow' the applied frequency as far as this upper limit). Motoneurons also respond to vibration, but in a different way.

Various frequencies of vibration can relieve pain, although vibration also facilitates some muscular (flexor) reflexes to pain. It has contralateral as well as local effects. Usefully, 100 Hz vibration and 100 Hz TENS appear to alleviate pain synergistically. Vibration may also enhance bone mass, and affects the EEG (predominantly at around 10–15 Hz). Not surprisingly, however, sustained high-intensity vibration can cause lasting damage.

Ultrasound therapy is very widely used, with frequencies of 0.75–3 MHz and intensities up to 1.5 W/cm². At such high frequencies (and power), incident energy is predominantly converted into heat. Pulsed ultrasound, on the other hand, at not more than 0.5 W/cm², has minimal thermal effect, and also avoids the risks of high-intensity stimulation. Levels as low as 0.1 W/cm² have important effects for tissue repair.

Ultrasound penetrates deeper into the body at 1 MHz than at 3 MHz, and in any case considerably further than

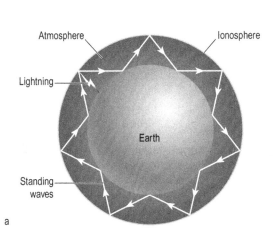

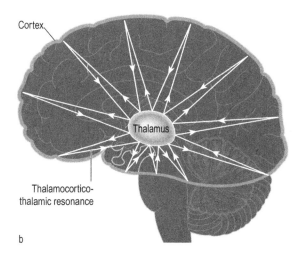

**Figure 4.2** Bioresonance: the earth and the brain. (a) Resonance in the cavity between earth and ionosphere. (After Oschman 2000.) (b) Resonance in the brain, between thalamus and cortex (see also Ch. 5).

---

**BOX 4.1**

**Living in the world – an afterword on bioresonance and the brain**

On our planet, we have developed surrounded and interpenetrated by a pulsating web of electromagnetic fields and radiation – our very existence depends on them.

In the 'cavity' between the earth's surface and the ionosphere, lightning discharges create standing waves at *Schumann resonance* frequencies (Fig. 4.2). The fundamental Schumann frequency is about 7.8 Hz. '*Sferics*' at very low frequencies (VLF) are also generated, again pulsed at extremely low frequencies (ELF). Over distance, these become damped, leaving a signal of around 10 kHz in fine weather. In the day, ELF predominates, at night the VLF sferics. The major power density of naturally occurring ELF is thus at around 10 Hz, and that of VLF at 10 kHz.

These same frequencies are echoed within our own bodies. For example, 10 Hz is the primary EEG frequency in all animals, while 7.8 Hz is a constituent of the ECG signal. Windows of particular biological sensitivity are defined accordingly. At much higher frequencies the atmosphere is particularly transparent to 60 GHz EHF. When it comes to visible light, is it just coincidence that the predominant wavelength of the Arctic daylight is the same as that found so useful for tissue healing, about 632 nanometres?

Changes in atmospheric ELF electric fields accompany shifts in the weather, and affect how we feel. So indeed do artificial fields: 3–6 Hz electric fields, for example, may lead to uncomfortable symptoms of headache and fatigue, while reaction times may be slower at 5 Hz than at 10 Hz. EEG patterns are in fact modified in accordance with these external changes, especially in those who are more sensitive to how the weather affects them. Even very-low-intensity ELF magnetic fields have powerful effects on the brain, leading to altered states of consciousness or sensations of vibration moving through the body. Research with very weak fields that mimic those occurring naturally in the brain itself, with frequencies in the theta range, or at around 16 Hz or 40 Hz, suggests that with both magnetic fields and electric currents it is the *information content* that is presented to brain tissue that is relevant, not intensity.

In the modern world, we are surrounded by an 'electromagnetic smog' of artificial fields and radiation that affects us. Ordinary household devices have been shown to affect the EEG, for example. Furthermore, we are often affected by the distortion of the natural EM fields around us caused by the construction of the buildings in which we live, by the acres of asphalt and concrete that isolate us from the earth, and by changes in surface water distribution.

It is thus possible that the drastically altered electromagnetic environment we have helped to create may adversely affect our long-term physical and mental health. Various protective countermeasures have been proposed, examples of which include ELF incoherent 'noise' and carefully positioned magnets or absorbent ceramic materials to mitigate the biological effects of exposure to temporally coherent LF fields or microwaves. However, a clear distinction has to be drawn between long-term EM exposure and short-term electrotherapy. Even long-term treatment has not been shown to have major adverse effects, and if any are found following electrical treatment it may well be that they are less significant than those of magnetic stimulation.

---

LILT (quite far enough to inactivate muscular trigger points, for example). As with several of the interventions described above, ultrasound pulsed at 16 Hz may have particular effects on calcium ion transfer.

Box 4.1 describes the phenomenon of bioresonance and the brain.

- frequency windows (resonance at invariant endogenous rhythms ~10 Hz or 16 Hz, 10 kHz, or even 60 GHz)
- regulatory (homeodynamic) interactions
- the importance of the initial state of the organism treated
- possible effects on the EEG.

## SUMMARY

EM and vibratory stimulation:

- have effects at various levels (cellular, tissue, systemic)
- are gross (neurostimulatory or thermal) or subtle (involving ionic currents rather than action potentials, or athermal).

Common themes that emerge are:

- cellular membrane ($Ca^{2+}$) and immune effects
- the Arndt–Schulz law

### Additional material in the CD-ROM resource

In the electronic version of this chapter, additional material and illustrations can be found on the following topics:

- Direct current (DC) stimulation, particularly for tissue repair
- Low-frequency (LF) stimulation
- Muscle stimulation, particularly for tissue repair and denervated muscle
- Technical information on differences between constant current and constant voltage stimulators, on electrodes and the distortion of electrical signals as they travel into the body

- Heat and cold
- Infrared and microwave methods of heating
- Non-thermal effects of radiation, particularly EHF and LILT
- Pulsed EM fields and permanent magnets
- Vibration and ultrasound
- Bioresonance and the brain.

## RECOMMENDED READING

*In addition to the standard electrotherapy texts recommended in Chapter 3, I cannot resist mentioning one interesting nineteenth-century textbook, much of which is still relevant today:*

Althaus J 1873 A Treatise on Medical Electricity, theoretical and practical, and its usage in the treatment of paralysis, neuralgia, and other diseases. Longmans, Green and Company, London (3rd edn)

*Standard textbooks on TENS and LILT, full of useful information, include:*

Walsh DM 1997 TENS: Clinical applications and related theory. Churchill Livingstone, Edinburgh

Baxter GD, with Diamantopoulos C, O'Kane S, Shields TD 1994 Therapeutic Lasers: Theory and practice. Churchill Livingstone, Edinburgh

*There are many books on the scientific basis of electrotherapy. Some of my favourites are:*

Blank M 1995 (ed) Electromagnetic Fields: Biological interactions and mechanisms. Advances in Chemistry 250. American Chemical Society, Washington, DC

Polk C, Postow E 1996 (eds) Handbook of Biological Effects of Electromagnetic Fields. CRC Press, Boca Raton, FL (2nd edn)

Reilly JP, with Antoni H, Chilbert MA, Skuggevig W, Sweeney JD 1992 Electrical Stimulation and Electropathology. Cambridge University Press, Cambridge

*A useful overview of wound healing is provided by:*

Vodovnik L, Karba R Treatment of chronic wounds by means of electric and electromagnetic fields. Medical and Biological Engineering and Computing. 1992 May; 30(3): 257–66

*A thought-provoking collection of papers on EHF stimulation is:*

Sitko SP, Andreyev EA, Binyashevski EV, Zhukovsky VD, Losimovich ED, Litvinov GS, Popovichenko NV, Talko JJ 1989 Microwave Resonance Therapy. The fundamental aspects of the application of mm range electromagnetic radiation in medicine. Provisional Collective "Otklik", Kiev

*A fascinating and readable book on the role of electromagnetic signalling, and much else, in development and wound repair:*

Becker RO, Selden G 1985 The Body Electric: Electromagnetism and the foundation of life. William Morrow, New York

# Neurophysiology, acupoints and meridians: Western and Eastern perspectives

This chapter touches on some of the endogenous electrical processes at the heart of life, seen from both a Western and an Eastern perspective. The electrophysiology of cells, nerves and muscle is described first, as well as some details of nerve transmission and the biochemistry of sensation and pain. These are necessary to understand the experimental studies of electroacupuncture (EA), as well as how best to apply EA in clinical practice. There then follows an account of the acupuncture points and meridians in both neurophysiological and bioelectrical terms.

at different frequencies. There are relationships between muscle force or motor control and frequency. The intrinsic frequencies of smooth muscle, in blood vessels or the gastrointestinal tract, tend to be lower than those of striated muscle.

Nerve fibres are classified by their diameter. Motoneurons tend to be thicker than many sensory neurons. From the skin, thicker sensory Aβ and Aγ fibres transmit signals from the mechanical receptors, Aδ fibres from cold and pain receptors (nociceptors), and C fibres from heat receptors

## ELECTRICITY AND LIFE – A WESTERN VIEW

The membrane of the living cell maintains different concentrations of positive ions inside and outside the cell, so that in effect each cell acts like a tiny battery (Fig. 5.1). Both the intracellular structures and the cell itself have their own resonant frequencies.

Information is transmitted around the body along neurons in the form of electrical signals, and across gaps (*synapses*) between neurons in the form of *neurotransmitter* chemicals (Fig. 5.2). *Efferent* nerves carry signals from the *central nervous system* (CNS) to the periphery, *afferent* ones in the opposite direction. The motor nerve, its end plates and the muscle fibres that it activates form the motor unit. The neurotransmitter at the neuromuscular junction is *acetylcholine* (ACh). Action potentials in muscle fibres result in muscle twitching. If frequent, these twitches eventually fuse, leading to a smooth contraction. There are various inherent striated muscle frequencies, those around 10 Hz being the most important when it is healthy. Smooth contraction of '*slow*' and '*fast*' muscle fibres can be elicited by stimulation

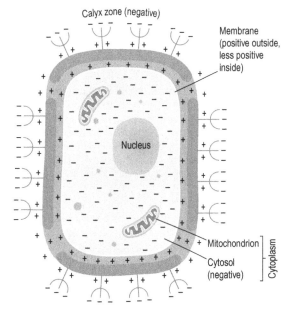

**Figure 5.1** The electrical zones and basic structures of the cell: a schematic view. (After Kitchen & Bazin 1996.)

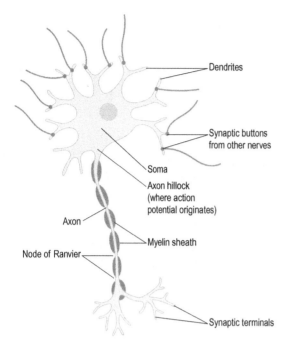

**Figure 5.2** The nerve cell: a typical neuron, showing cell body (soma), axon with myelin sheath and nodes of Ranvier. Note axon hillock (where action potential originates), and synaptic buttons from other nerves. (After Walsh 1997.)

and nociceptors. The sensation experienced depends on (but is not the same as) stimulus intensity, which affects both how many fibres fire and the frequencies at which they do so. Muscle afferents carry signals about the contractile state of the muscle itself.

Regular stimuli result in habituation ('bored' neurons). Neurons may also become sensitised or overreactive in certain circumstances. Most natural signals within the body are irregular: too little or too much variability may both reflect dysfunctional states.

The information in Box 5.1 outlines the additional detail available in the accompanying CD-ROM ⊚ resource, and details the chemical messengers and pathways involved in pain.

## Electricity and the brain

In the brain, electrical activity never ceases. It can be monitored locally, via implanted electrodes, or globally, using several scalp electrodes, to produce an electroencephalogram (EEG). The global picture, the EEG, is divided conventionally into frequency bands, known as delta (0.5–3 Hz), theta (3–7 Hz), alpha (7–12 Hz), beta (12–30 Hz), gamma (30–60 Hz) and so on. Lower frequencies are more prevalent the more relaxed a person is (Table 5.1). The *thalamus* is generally considered to be the brain's principal pacemaker (6 Hz and 10 Hz are its two main rhythms),

---

**BOX 5.1**

**Neuropharmacology in the CD-ROM ⊚ resource**

Although a grasp of the complex neurochemistry of the nervous system is not an absolute requirement for the safe and effective use of electroacupuncture, a basic understanding is helpful.

**The autonomic nervous system (ANS)**

The *autonomic nervous system* controls the functioning of glands and smooth muscle in the body, its efferent neurons grouped in ganglia either side of the spine. In simple terms, it has two functional divisions: the *sympathetic*, which prepares the body for 'fight or flight', and the *parasympathetic*, which in some respects has opposite properties, many of them mediated through branches of the *vagus nerve*. The ANS neurotransmitters are acetylcholine (ACh), *adrenaline* (Adr, epinephrine) and *noradrenaline* (NA, norepinephrine). NA acts more on α receptors, stimulating vasoconstriction and muscle contraction, adrenaline more on β receptors, stimulating vasodilation and relaxation of smooth muscle.

**The labyrinth of the CNS**

It is probably impossible for anyone to understand the CNS and its complex interconnections completely. However, some knowledge of its workings is needed to be able to follow the EA literature. In the CD-ROM resource the anatomy of the spinal cord is introduced first, with its various ascending and descending pathways (Fig. 5.3). The hindbrain, midbrain and forebrain, and the major centres within them, come next (Fig. 5.4), and some of the functions of these are briefly described, together with their interrelationships.

The different families of *neurotransmitters* and *neuromodulators* that play a part in EA are then listed, first the *peptides* (opioid, pituitary, circulatory, gut and so on), then the *monoamines* such as NA, dopamine (DA) and histamine, followed by the now familiar ACh, some amino acids, purines and the gases (the protean *nitric oxide*, for example). The opioid *peptides*, particularly important for EA, are described in some detail, together with their main locations in brain and spinal cord. The *endorphins*, like

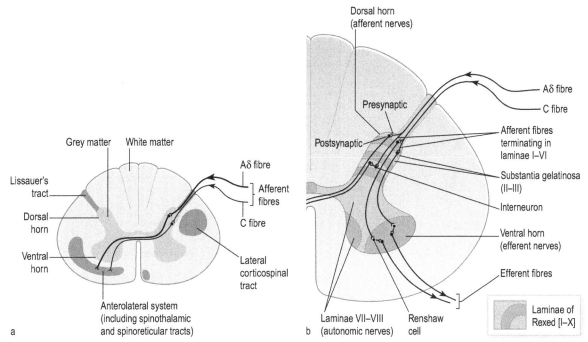

**Figure 5.3** The spinal cord. (a) A simplified cross-section of the spinal cord, showing the dorsal and ventral horns, some afferent and efferent nerve fibres, and some of the major ascending and descending tracts. Note how some fibres cross over to the opposite side, before ascending in the anterolateral system. (After Burt 1993.) (b) The laminae in the grey matter of the spinal cord, showing afferents, efferents and interneurons. (After Berne 2000.)

morphine, attach preferentially to μ ('mu') receptors, the *enkephalins* to δ ('delta') receptors, and the *dynorphins* to κ ('kappa') receptors. Naloxone is the major opioid antagonist used experimentally. Other peptides include adrenocorticotrophin (ACTH) from the pituitary, which induces cortisol release from the adrenal cortex, and the gut peptides vasoactive intestinal polypeptide (VIP), cholecystokinin (CCK) and substance P.

The functions and locations of the catecholamines Adr, NA and DA and their respective receptors are outlined briefly, as are those of another monoamine, histamine. *Serotonin* (5HT), one of the most researched neurotransmitters, is described in more detail. The roles of ACh and its receptors, and of the amino acid neurotransmitters and neuromodulators, are also described, as are those of the purines adenosine triphosphate (ATP) and adenosine. The second messengers cAMP and calcium ($Ca^{2+}$) are mentioned.

### The example of pain

*Nociceptive* and *neurogenic pain* are defined, one stemming from activation of nociceptors, the other from damage to neurons (although sustained by changes in the CNS). The peripheral, spinal, supraspinal and cortical elements involved in pain are described. Peripherally, peptides such as bradykinin and SP, as well as some *prostaglandins*, are associated with nociception. Neurogenic inflammation involves yet more biochemical processes. Pain, whether due to nociceptor activation or to neurogenic inflammation, triggers action potentials in afferent primary neurons, which then transmit to the *dorsal horn*. Some of the spinal reflexes that can aggravate pain are mentioned, as well as the receptors implicated in acute and chronic pain (AMPA and NMDA, respectively).
In neurogenic pain, further processes such as 'wind-up' within the spinal cord involve NMDA receptors and a number of other neurotransmitters.

Fast and slow pain signals ascend the spinal cord to the thalamus along different pathways. The first pain to arrive warns of possible tissue damage, the second, more likely to cause actual damage, has greater emotional and autonomic repercussions. Several other pathways transmit nociceptive information up the spinal cord. In response to pain, descending neurons from the brain release NA and 5HT from their terminations in the dorsal horn. 5HT boosts enkephalin levels, and these in turn inhibit substance P release in the afferent pathway. NA also inhibits pain-associated afferent activity. The result is reduced nociceptive transmission at spinal cord level.

*Continued*

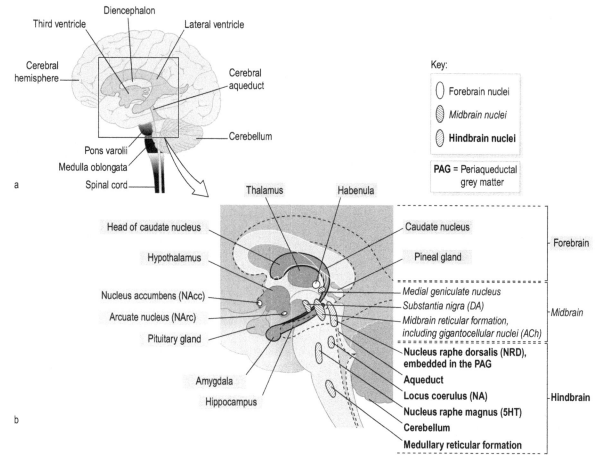

**Figure 5.4** Side views of the brain. (a) The divisions of the brain and some of the major nuclei. (After Williams et al. 1999.) (b) The periventricular nuclei, showing hippocampus, caudate nucleus, amygdala, nucleus accumbens (NAcc) and periaqueductal grey matter (PAG). (After Haines 2002.)

**Table 5.1** Brainwave frequencies and the associated spectrum of states of mind

| Frequency range | Associated state of mind |
| --- | --- |
| 0.5–3 Hz ('delta', δ) | Characteristic of deep sleep |
| 3–7 Hz ('theta', θ) | Present when in a state of reverie, or falling asleep – parietotemporal region |
| 7–12 Hz ('alpha', α) | Present when in a relaxed waking state, or during conscious physical relaxation – posterior occipital cortex |
| 12–30 Hz ('beta', β) | Present when awake and carrying out ordinary daily activities; associated with thinking, enhanced by anxiety |
| 30–60 Hz ('gamma', γ) | Present when particularly tense or alert (40 Hz may well be associated with creativity) |
| 60–120 Hz ('lambda', λ) | Has no specific associated state |

but other areas such as the *hippocampus* are also important, with its memory and learning functions.

There are locations where particular '*resonance modes*' seem to be concentrated, and such modes appear to have particular functional correlates. For example:

- Delta may be associated with 'dystrophy, degeneration and damage'. It normally occurs at the midbrain–pons junction, in the spinal cord, and possibly in the somatosensory cortex.
- Theta may be associated with consolidation of personally meaningful experience ('scanning for pleasure'). It is a major operating rhythm in the frontal cortex and limbic system, and is also found in the brainstem.
- Different alpha rhythms are generated in many different parts of the brain. In general, evoked alpha responses appear to be associated with sensory processing ('scanning for pattern'). Synchronised 10 Hz activity may indicate sympathetic overactivity (the images that can herald migraine tend to flicker at about this frequency).
- 40 Hz (gamma) has been found as a preferred frequency mode in the spinal cord, and is a marker for some aspects of higher sensory processing.

Despite the existence of resonance modes, signals in the healthy brain are continually changing, even chaotic. Limited variability may be associated with temporary habituation, or may be part of a disease process: it is characteristic of the EEG in epilepsy, for example, and is also found in degenerative brain conditions such as Alzheimer's and Creutzfeld–Jakob disease. Reduced variability also occurs in the thalamus and spinal cord with some forms of chronic pain.

Some correlations also exist between electrical activity in the brain and neurotransmitter activity. For example, noradrenaline (NA) is associated with HF activity and alertness, *serotonin* (5HT) with LF activity and decreased arousal, while *dopamine* (DA) and *GABA* may share control of gamma (40 Hz) oscillations. Many correlations (resonances) also occur between the different rhythmic systems of our bodies: EEG, ECG, EMG (electromyogram, whether of smooth or skeletal muscle) and respiration.

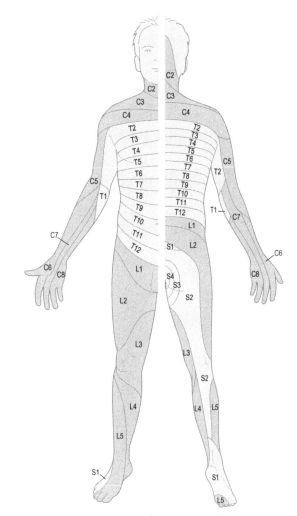

**Figure 5.5** Dermatomes on the front and back of the body. (After Walsh 1997.)

# PATTERNS AND POINTS – AN EASTERN PANORAMA

The body *segment*, with its interrelationship between *dermatome*, *myotome*, *sclerotome* and *viscerotome* (Figs 5.5–5.8), provides a useful conceptual framework to precede a description of *trigger points* (TrPs), *motor points* (MPs) and *acupoints* (AcPs), with their similarities and differences (Fig. 5.9). There is a possible association of acupoints with nerve, vascular and lymphatic structures (the '*neurovascular bundle*').

The electrical nature of the skin itself is a linking strand in this discussion. The skin is a battery, its outer surface around 40–80 mV more electrically negative than its deepest layers. This skin potential (SP) has its own rhythms, from the circadian to the vasomotor (~0.1 Hz). If the skin is punctured, a *current of injury* starts to flow, and is intimately associated with the healing process (Fig. 5.10). Measuring such currents, and other electrical skin characteristics, is surprisingly complex, but has been explored within the context of Oriental medicine.

## The electrical properties of acupuncture meridians and points

Locating painful points according to their electrical characteristics has been a method used for nearly a century. In the

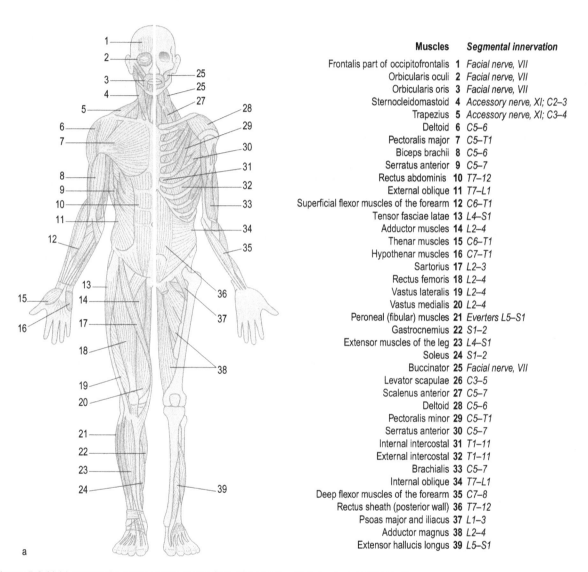

| Muscles | | Segmental innervation |
|---|---|---|
| Frontalis part of occipitofrontalis | 1 | Facial nerve, VII |
| Orbicularis oculi | 2 | Facial nerve, VII |
| Orbicularis oris | 3 | Facial nerve, VII |
| Sternocleidomastoid | 4 | Accessory nerve, XI; C2–3 |
| Trapezius | 5 | Accessory nerve, XI; C3–4 |
| Deltoid | 6 | C5–6 |
| Pectoralis major | 7 | C5–T1 |
| Biceps brachii | 8 | C5–6 |
| Serratus anterior | 9 | C5–7 |
| Rectus abdominis | 10 | T7–12 |
| External oblique | 11 | T7–L1 |
| Superficial flexor muscles of the forearm | 12 | C6–T1 |
| Tensor fasciae latae | 13 | L4–S1 |
| Adductor muscles | 14 | L2–4 |
| Thenar muscles | 15 | C6–T1 |
| Hypothenar muscles | 16 | C7–T1 |
| Sartorius | 17 | L2–3 |
| Rectus femoris | 18 | L2–4 |
| Vastus lateralis | 19 | L2–4 |
| Vastus medialis | 20 | L2–4 |
| Peroneal (fibular) muscles | 21 | Everters L5–S1 |
| Gastrocnemius | 22 | S1–2 |
| Extensor muscles of the leg | 23 | L4–S1 |
| Soleus | 24 | S1–2 |
| Buccinator | 25 | Facial nerve, VII |
| Levator scapulae | 26 | C3–5 |
| Scalenus anterior | 27 | C5–7 |
| Deltoid | 28 | C5–6 |
| Pectoralis minor | 29 | C5–T1 |
| Serratus anterior | 30 | C5–7 |
| Internal intercostal | 31 | T1–11 |
| External intercostal | 32 | T1–11 |
| Brachialis | 33 | C5–7 |
| Internal oblique | 34 | T7–L1 |
| Deep flexor muscles of the forearm | 35 | C7–8 |
| Rectus sheath (posterior wall) | 36 | T7–12 |
| Psoas major and iliacus | 37 | L1–3 |
| Adductor magnus | 38 | L2–4 |
| Extensor hallucis longus | 39 | L5–S1 |

**Figure 5.6** (a) Myotomes: the major muscles on the front of the body, with their segmental innervation.

(Continued)

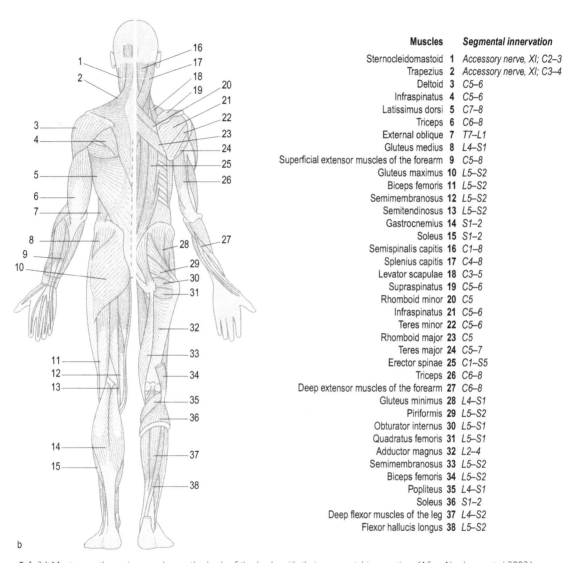

| Muscles | | Segmental innervation |
|---|---|---|
| Sternocleidomastoid | 1 | Accessory nerve, XI; C2–3 |
| Trapezius | 2 | Accessory nerve, XI; C3–4 |
| Deltoid | 3 | C5–6 |
| Infraspinatus | 4 | C5–6 |
| Latissimus dorsi | 5 | C7–8 |
| Triceps | 6 | C6–8 |
| External oblique | 7 | T7–L1 |
| Gluteus medius | 8 | L4–S1 |
| Superficial extensor muscles of the forearm | 9 | C5–8 |
| Gluteus maximus | 10 | L5–S2 |
| Biceps femoris | 11 | L5–S2 |
| Semimembranosus | 12 | L5–S2 |
| Semitendinosus | 13 | L5–S2 |
| Gastrocnemius | 14 | S1–2 |
| Soleus | 15 | S1–2 |
| Semispinalis capitis | 16 | C1–8 |
| Splenius capitis | 17 | C4–8 |
| Levator scapulae | 18 | C3–5 |
| Supraspinatus | 19 | C5–6 |
| Rhomboid minor | 20 | C5 |
| Infraspinatus | 21 | C5–6 |
| Teres minor | 22 | C5–6 |
| Rhomboid major | 23 | C5 |
| Teres major | 24 | C5–7 |
| Erector spinae | 25 | C1–S5 |
| Triceps | 26 | C6–8 |
| Deep extensor muscles of the forearm | 27 | C6–8 |
| Gluteus minimus | 28 | L4–S1 |
| Piriformis | 29 | L5–S2 |
| Obturator internus | 30 | L5–S1 |
| Quadratus femoris | 31 | L5–S1 |
| Adductor magnus | 32 | L2–4 |
| Semimembranosus | 33 | L5–S2 |
| Biceps femoris | 34 | L5–S2 |
| Popliteus | 35 | L4–S1 |
| Soleus | 36 | S1–2 |
| Deep flexor muscles of the leg | 37 | L4–S2 |
| Flexor hallucis longus | 38 | L5–S2 |

b

**Figure 5.6** (b) Myotomes: the major muscles on the back of the body, with their segmental innervation. (After Abrahams et al 2003.)

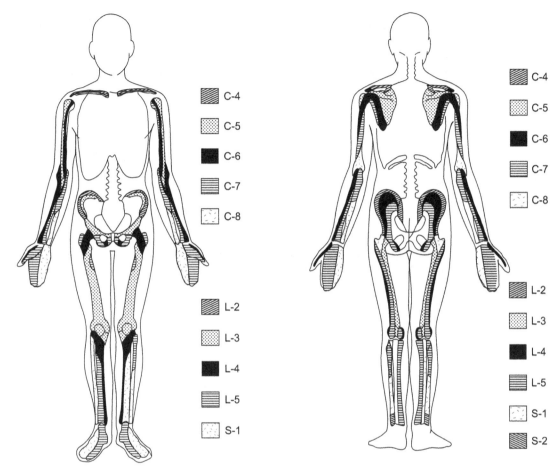

**Figure 5.7** Sclerotomes on the front and back of the body (thorax omitted). (From Chusid J 1982, with permission.)

1950s, Jean Niboyet in France and Nakatani Yoshio in Japan both independently explored the possibility that electrical skin resistance (SR) might be low at acupoints. Another key figure, Richard Croon in Germany, used weak, low-frequency currents to locate three families of electrically reactive points, some fixed, and others that appeared only in the presence of underlying pathology.

More influential was Reinhold Voll, whose system, EAV ('Electroacupuncture according to Voll'), made use of DC measurements of skin conductance and its decrease over time (the '*indicator drop*', ID). He interpreted these readings in terms of organ irritation or degeneration. Voll also proposed that other meridians than the traditionally accepted ones could exist, associated with different processes of degeneration (Fig. 5.11).

In France, Niboyet carried out very detailed research on SR measurements, using both DC and AC devices, even performing some measurements on cadavers. Like Voll, he advocated separating the tasks of point detection and measurement. Unlike Voll, although he found that 90% of the points he found appeared to coincide with the traditional meridian points of acupuncture, he did not attempt to erect a diagnostic system on the basis of his work. Georges Cantoni and Jacques Pontigny, focusing on SP rather than SR measurement, found that SP at AcPs tends to be positive with respect to the surrounding skin in healthy subjects. Using ideas developed by the American Robert Becker, they went on to interpret their findings in *yin–yang* terms.

In Japan, Nakatani explored the correlations between meridians and the 'ryodoraku' (lines of good electrical conductivity) when using DC measurements, although at higher voltages than Voll or Niboyet. He found points that became more reactive in disease, and developed a

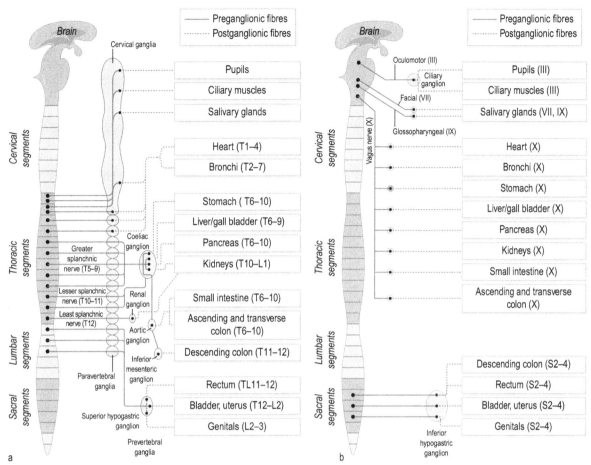

**Figure 5.8** Viscerotomes: autonomic innervation of the internal organs. (From Bibliographisches Institut 1979.) (a) The sympathetic innervation of the viscera. (b) The parasympathetic innervation of the viscera, showing the importance of the vagus nerve.

diagnostic system that could be used as a basis for treatment decisions. Twenty years later, another Japanese researcher, Motoyama Hiroshi, developed a very different method of SP measurements. In terms of basic science, this is the most conceptually complex system to date (Fig. 5.12), and also one of the most intriguing. Some of Motoyama's findings, for instance, are better explained in terms of meridian theory rather than those of neurophysiology.

Currents and potentials between different parts of the body have long been known, shifts in the latter accompanying other changes in the body, such as variations in temperature, ovulation and physical or mental disease. On the basis of their work, Becker and others have considered that meridians may be construed as 'transmission lines,' or 'high conductance pathways'.

Hu Xianglong, Wu Baohua and colleagues in Fuzhou have found that lines of low electrical impedance on the skin tend to correspond to the meridian sensations patients feel on receiving acupuncture. They have also shown that points where impedance is low (*low skin impedance points*, or LSIPs) are clearly and reliably distinct from those where it is not. These low impedance points tend to cluster along the traditional meridians, although the relationship between them is still unclear.

# SUMMARY

Basic points to remember on electrophysiology are:

- Cells have electrical polarity.
- Nerves and muscles are electrically excitable.

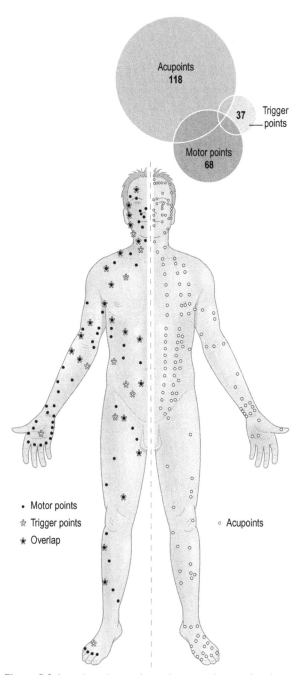

- • Motor points
- ✳ Trigger points
- ✳ Overlap

○ Acupoints

**Figure 5.9** Acupoints, trigger points and motor points: are they the same? Artist's impression of the points on the front of the body, based on standard charts. Although there is some overlap between the three categories of point, they are clearly not identical.

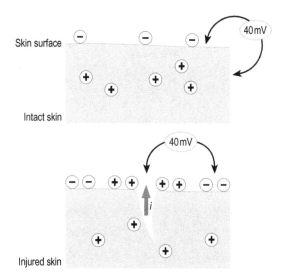

**Figure 5.10** The skin in injury, showing potential difference between injured and uninjured areas, and resulting current.

- • Nerves conduct signals faster if they are thicker or myelinated.
- • Repeated or monotonous stimulation leads to habituation.

Key points on meridians and points are:

- • There is still much controversy over whether acupoints and meridians have measurable electrical characteristics.
- • EA systems depending on electrodermal measurement and its interpretation may be oversimplistic.
- • Points on the body can be described and investigated in a number of ways that are not mutually exclusive.
- • There are (at least) two interwoven levels to acupuncture – the neurophysiological and the meridian/energetic.

## Additional material in the CD-ROM resource

In the electronic version of this chapter, additional material and illustrations can be found on the following topics:

- • Nerve transmission
- • Muscle and the motor unit
- • Types of nerve and peripheral receptors
- • Stimulus and habituation
- • Physical aspects of the CNS
- • Chemical aspects of the CNS
- • Pain and its pathways
- • Electricity, the brain and a synthesis
- • Segments and points
- • The skin and its electrical measurements
- • The electrical properties of acupuncture meridians and points.

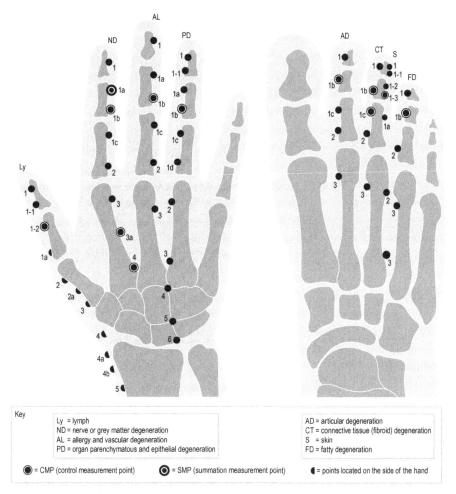

**Figure 5.11** Voll's new vessels: the lymph vessel has 24 points, the others between 4 and 11, on the hands and feet only. (After Voll 1983.)

## Studies on the electrodermal correlates of acupoints and meridians

The CD-ROM resource outlines in 21 brief sections themes that recur in studies of electrodermal correlates of acupoints and meridians. These include:

### 1. Acupoints

- LSIPs (low skin impedance points) occur in many species.
- They do not always coincide with acupoints.
- They are not always tender, but may coincide with areas of referred pain.
- AcPs may vary in both size and location, depending on various factors.
- AcP measurements are relative, not absolute, and differ between individuals.
- Certain points may be located more consistently than others.

- Asymmetry of electrical measurements may reflect pathology.
- Skin conductance (SC) at certain AcPs deviates more from normal values in disease than in health.
- Low SC may reflect chronic pathology (or deficiency), and high SC inflammation (or excess).
- Many factors affect AcP SC readings.
- AcPs may exhibit particular 'bioluminescence' and temperature characteristics.

### 2. Meridians

- Low-frequency sound and light may propagate along meridians, which also exhibit bioluminescence.
- The meridian may be a more consistent electrical entity than the LSIP.
- Stimulating a point on one meridian may affect electrical readings at points both on the same and on other meridians. These changes may reflect an overall shift towards homeostasis.

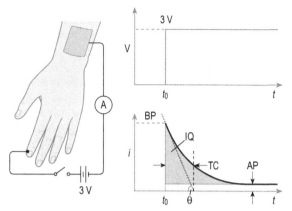

**Figure 5.12** The parameters monitored by the AMI system. (After Motoyama 1980.) When a 3 V impulse is applied for 2 ms at time $t_0$ to a *jing* Well (*sei*) point, the resulting current measured by an ammeter (A) changes rapidly from an initial level (BP, before skin polarisation) to a level some thirty times lower (AP, after polarisation). The shaded area represents the total charge during polarisation (IQ). The time required for ion transfer during polarisation is shown as TC. See text for further explanation.

- High SC zones may correspond to the meridian sensations experienced by acupuncture patients.
- Some meridians may be more electrically active than others.

### 3. Neurophysiology
- Skin conductance measurement depends upon nerve function.

## RECOMMENDED READING

*A stimulating account of the electrical characteristics of cells and tissues:*
Charman RA 1998 Electrical properties of cells and tissues. In: Kitchen S, Bazin S (eds) Clayton's Electrotherapy. WB Saunders, Philadelphia (10th edn), 31–46

*There are many good neuroscience textbooks. An excellent one that I discovered after writing this chapter:*
Haines D 2002 Fundamental Neuroscience. Churchill Livingstone, Edinburgh (2nd edn)

*Introductions to the more rarefied realm of electrical brain function:*
Başar E 1998 Brain Function and Oscillations I: Principles and approaches. Springer, Berlin
Nunez PL, with Cutillo BA, Gevins AS, Ingber L, Lopes da Silva FH, Pilgreen KL, Silberstein RB 1995 Neocortical Dynamics and Human EEG Rhythms. Oxford University Press, Oxford

Steriade M, Jones EG, Llinás RR 1990 Thalamic Oscillations and Signaling. John Wiley, Chichester

*An erudite account of endogenous antinociceptive mechanisms:*
Sandkühler J The organization and function of endogenous antinociceptive systems. Progress in Neurobiology. 1996; 50: 49–81

*A useful account of segmental acupuncture:*
Bekkering R, van Bussel R 1998 Segmental acupuncture. In: Filshie J, White A (eds) Medical Acupuncture: A western scientific approach. Churchill Livingstone, Edinburgh, 105–35

*A standard work on trigger points:*
Baldry PE 2004 Acupuncture, Trigger Points and Musculoskeletal Pain. Churchill Livingstone, Edinburgh (3rd edn)

*An introduction to the electrical properties of the skin:*
Boucsein W 1992 Electrodermal Acitivity. Plenum Series in Behavioral Psychophysiology and Medicine. Plenum Press, New York

*A standard work with useful material on currents of injury:*
Borgens RB, Robinson KR, Vanable JW Jr, McGinnis ME, with McCaig CD 1989 Electric Fields in Vertebrate Repair: Natural and applied voltages in vertebrate regeneration and healing. Alan R Liss, New York

*One of several similar articles on the putative anatomy of acupoints:*
Heine H Anatomical structure of acupoints. Journal of Traditional Chinese Medicine. 1988 Sept; 8(3): 207–12

*Sources for figures:*
Abrahams PH, Hutchings RT, Marks SC Jr 2003 McMinn's Colour Atlas of Human Anatomy. Mosby, St Louis (5th edn)
Berne RM, Levy MN 2000 Principles of Physiology. Mosby, St Louis (3rd edn)
Bibliographisches Institut 1979 The Way Things Work Book of the Body. Simon and Schuster, New York
Burt AM 1993 Textbook of Neuroanatomy. Saunders, Philadelphia (1st edn)
Chusid J 1982 Correlative Neuroanatomy and Functional Neurology. Lange Medical, California
Motoyama H Electrophysiological and preliminary biochemical studies of skin properties in relation to the acupuncture meridian. Research for Religion and Parapsychology. 1980 June; 6 (2[9]): 1–36
Voll R 1983 850 EAV Measurement Points of the Meridians and Vessels Including the Secondary Vessels. Medizinisch Literarische Verlagsgesellschaft, Uelzen
Williams PL et al 1999 (eds) Gray's Anatomy: The anatomical basis of medicine and surgery. Churchill Livingstone, Edinburgh

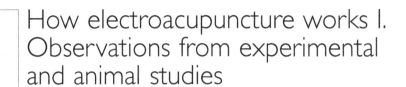
# How electroacupuncture works I. Observations from experimental and animal studies

This general overview of the experimental acupuncture research literature is broadly divided into sections on the body and the brain, including neurochemical and neuroelectric responses to electroacupuncture (EA), then on the wider effects of EA. Particular attention is given to the different parameters of treatment. Other methods of stimulating acupoints and meridians are described, as well as possible adverse effects, and studies on electrical and other acupoint measurements are summarised. Most experimental acupuncture research is on EA, and can teach us much that is useful for clinical practice.

## THE BODY – A CENTRIPETAL APPROACH

### Acupuncture points

Those points that have been researched for their specific EA effects are listed in Table 6.1. However, many of the experimental findings may not have been verified clinically, and so should be considered only as pointers to clinical practice.

### THE EFFECTS OF EA AT AURICULAR POINTS

The concha of the ear is innervated by the vagus nerve (Fig. 6.1), and it is very possible that stimulation anywhere in this area will have similar effects on any of the internal organs. However, some studies do indicate that EA at 'appropriate' points may have more effect than stimulation at 'inappropriate' points. A few possibly specific effects are listed in Table 6.2.

### COMBINING POINTS

Few general conclusions can be drawn from experimental results on combining acupoints with EA. All that can be said

is that combining body and auricular points, or intra- and extrasegmental points, does not always enhance treatment. Some points, such as ST-36, may even enhance particular effects without having any such action when used alone. Some combinations, such as BL-23, ST-36 and Du-14 for immune function, may be worth exploring.

### Left and right

Treating one side of the body may have effects on the other side, or both sides. Bilateral treatment is often the most effective approach, although for some conditions treating the opposite side (contralateral treatment) is used, even supraspinally.

### Segmental patterns

A 'rule of thumb' conclusion on the use of EA at particular points seems to be that local points are more effective than unrelated points, particularly for experimental pain ('local' and 'unrelated' being construed in terms of segments or laterality). The greater effectiveness of local treatment is probably due to its activation of both local and supraspinal mechanisms.

Effects can generally be understood in terms of patterns of innervation rather than meridian connection. Indeed, for EA analgesia (EAA), point specificity may be less relevant than when EA is used for conditions involving autonomic dysfunction or particular patterns of innervation.

### Meridians

The existence of the acupuncture meridians remains controversial. There have been studies of pain threshold changes or magnetic fields along meridian pathways, while radioisotope tracer diffusion has been interpreted in meridian terms. However, none of this research convincingly confirms the existence of meridians, and there are few attempts to explain meridian phenomena neurologically.

**Table 6.1** Effects of EA at body acupoints

| Point | Effect |
|---|---|
| **Ren and Du points** | |
| Du-26 | Enhances sympathetic autonomic activity, may improve adrenocortical function, accelerate awakening of anaesthetised animals (but not necessarily humans) and raise BP when low; also enhances brain oxygen perfusion and electrical activity, so has been used for cerebral ischaemia; has been combined with Ren-24 in treatment of shock, and with GB-30 for experimental pain; some effects in the brain parallel those of KI-1; may inhibit gastric motility |
| Du-20 | Another useful point for acute cerebral ischaemia; has also been used in EAA |
| Du-16 | Has been used for cerebral ischaemia |
| Du-14 | May enhance blood production following chemotherapy |
| Du-8 | Has been used for cerebral ischaemia |
| Du-4 | Has useful immunoregulatory properties |
| Du-1, Du-2, Du-3 | Have been used for local experimental pain |
| **P and SJ points** | |
| P-6 | Has many beneficial effects in experimental acute myocardial ischaemia (may prevent arrhythmia and improve blood pH and viscosity); may raise lowered BP; reduces stress signs in the brain (combined with HE-3); reduces incidence of emesis |
| P-5 | Improves ECG and sinoatrial conduction in acute myocardial ischaemia when combined with P-6 |
| P-4 | Accelerates restoration of heart function in acute myocardial ischaemia; reduces heart rate (alone or with HE-7) |
| P-3 | Promotes recovery from acute myocardial ischaemia |
| P-1 | Improves adrenal function in acute myocardial ischaemia |
| SJ-20 | EHF at this point may increase or reduce hypothalamic activity, depending on the frequency at which it is pulsed |
| SJ-17 | Affects BP and cerebral blood flow |
| SJ-5 | May have more effect on auditory than on visual cortex |
| **HE and SI points** | |
| HE-3 | May reduce signs of stress in the brain (with P-6) |
| HE-4 | Regulatory effect following acute myocardial ischaemia, restoring BP for instance (with HE-7) |
| HE-7 | Reduces heart rate in healthy subjects (with or without P-6); has some effects in the brain opposite to those of KI-1 |
| SI-6 | Improves walking in experimental sprain of contralateral ankle |
| SI-17 | Reduces neurogenic inflammation of brain *dura mater* |
| SI-19 | Depresses BP (with LI-11) |
| **SP and ST points** | |
| SP-4 | Inhibits gastric acid secretion and decreases gastric peristalsis (in obesity) |
| SP-5 | With KI-3, locally useful for arthritis (BL-60 plus GB-40 were less effective) |
| ST-2 | Useful for orofacial pain |
| ST-7 | Useful for orofacial pain (possibly more so than LI-4), although not always |
| ST-25 | Has some effects in the brain opposite to those of KI-1 |
| ST-34 | May inhibit gastric acid secretion (in obesity) |

*Continued*

**Table 6.1** Effects of EA at body acupoints—cont'd

| Point | Effect |
| --- | --- |
| ST-36 | Enhances parasympathetic autonomic activity, and may inhibit some sympathetic activity; thus may decrease cardiac output and stroke volume, and reduce BP; has less effect than P-6 on acute myocardial ischaemia, with some opposite effects in the brain; some effects in the brain are also opposite those of KI-1; tends to normalise gastric motility and electrical activity, as well as intestinal peristalsis; affects pancreatic exocrine secretions; enhances several measures of immune function; may benefit visceral and hind limb pain; frequently used for EAA – usually with SP-6, although also with BL-60 or GB-34 (ST-36 and GB-34 have different effects in the brain); EAA is enhanced if used in combination with LI-4 |
| ST-42 | Intense 20 Hz EA may increase sympathoadrenal medullary function (this does not occur at ST-36) |
| ST-44 | May be less effective for dental/head pain than local points |
| **LU and LI points** | |
| LU-6 | Reduces haemoptysis (expectoration of blood) in tuberculosis |
| LI-4 | May enhance some sympathetic autonomic activity (with inhibitory effects on bladder contraction in urination); may be useful in cerebral ischaemia; attenuates amphetamine-enhanced activity in the brain; one of the most effective acupoints for generalised EAA: usefully combines with ST-36; although raises dental pain threshold, may not be as effective as local points for dental/head pain, and may be ineffective for gum/lip pain |
| LI-5 | May inhibit some parasympathetic activity (such as cardiac sinus arrhythmia) |
| LI-10 | May have some effect on dental pain; combined with LI-4, may increase cardiac output |
| LI-20 | May be useful for dental pain |
| **KI and BL points** | |
| BL-21 | Accelerates restoration of heart function after acute myocardial ischaemia |
| BL-23 | Affects kidney and liver function more than Du-14, reducing renal blood flow; may reduce or enhance bladder contraction |
| BL-28 | May increase bladder contraction |
| BL-32 | Has been used for EAA in gynaecological surgery |
| BL-60 | May result in generalised EAA, combined with ST-36 |
| KI-1 | May depress activity in some thalamic and midbrain areas |
| KI-3 | With SP-5, locally useful for arthritis (BL-60 plus GB-40 were less effective); enhances renal blood flow |
| **LIV and GB points** | |
| LIV-2 | May have some effect on arthritis of the knee (more than ST-36), but little effect on neuropathic pain |
| LIV-8 | May have some useful immunosuppressive effects |
| LIV-14 | Increases bile flow (combined with GB-24, both on right side) |
| GB-3 | Useful for dental pain |
| GB-24 | Increases bile flow (combined with LIV-14, both on right side) |
| GB-30 | May restore cortical activity in cerebral ischaemia; a strong analgesic point when used on the painful side |
| GB-34 | May inhibit some forms of sympathetic autonomic activity, but less so than ST-36; useful for lower body pain (sometimes combined with ST-36); decreases activity in sphincter of Oddi |
| GB-37 | May have more effect on visual than auditory cortex |

Abbreviations: BP = blood pressure; HR = heart rate; EAA = EA analgesia; ECG = electrocardiogram; EHF = extremely high frequency.

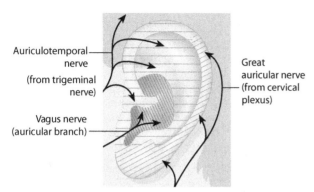

**Figure 6.1** Innervation of the ear. The ear is supplied by three afferent nerves: the trigeminal, vagus and great auricular (from the cervical plexus). (After Oleson 1998.)

Hints on this come from research on representations within the brain of different parts of the body, indicating that meridians may well exist centrally, rather than as a peripheral network around the body.

## Peripheral details

Acupuncture is invasive. The tissue trauma involved initiates a process of local inflammation, with release of histamine and other substances from *mast cells*.

Needling has various electrical effects:

- A current of injury is generated, lasting for up to 48 hours.
- Needle retention in non-uniform tissue results in minute electrolytic effects.
- Needle manipulation may lead to piezoelectric effects and weak low-frequency currents.
- Needling muscle will result in short bursts of activity at up to 2 mV.
- Needling into warm tissue also creates a small current, which can be affected by 'lifting and thrusting'.

| **Table 6.2** Effects of EA at auricular acupoints | |
| --- | --- |
| **Point** | **Effect** |
| Gall bladder (*erdan*) | May induce gall bladder contraction or biliary tract peristalsis |
| Heart (*xin*) | EHF at this point may increase or reduce hypothalamic activity, depending on the frequency at which it is pulsed |
| Lung (*fei*) | More effectively raises pain threshold (PT) in various locations than sympathetic or *shenmen* |
| Sympathetic (*jiaogan*) | May have a slight inhibitory effect on some sympathetic activity |

Heating a needle may itself have electrical effects, while the electrical properties of needles made of different materials may vary.

A causal connection between electrical changes at stimulated acupoints and the state of internal organs, although sometimes posited, is as yet unproven.

## *Deqi* and the nerve fibres

*Deqi*, the sensation experienced by the patient when needled, is strongly emphasised in Chinese acupuncture, even as a prerequisite to EA. It can be elicited by manual acupuncture (MA), EA, transcutaneous electrical acupoint stimulation (TEAS) and pTENS (transcutaneous electrical nerve stimulation, TENS, using a small diameter probe) and will differ at acupoints (AcPs) and non-AcPs. *Deqi*-elicited action potentials (APs) are mainly conducted by type II and III deep muscle afferents, so *deqi* is strongest at the dozen or so major acupoints that are densely innervated with such fibres. It is also stronger in muscles with abundant muscle spindles. Thus an intact afferent nerve pathway is essential for the *deqi* experience, and also for EA to be effective.

However, there is considerable disagreement on the role of type IV (or C fibre) afferents. Clinically, very strong stimulation that recruits C fibres may not be acceptable, while in some surgical situations, when EAA is combined with drugs, it may be quite appropriate. Furthermore, whereas low-frequency (LF) TENS/TEAS also involves activation of type III fibres, conventional high-frequency (HF) TENS/TEAS is mediated predominantly by Aβ fibres.

In the ear the role of the vagus nerve is central, functioning synergistically with the great auricular and cervical sympathetic nerves. The vagus has also been implicated in some actions of P-6 and ST-36, with those of P-4 and ST-21 mediated by sympathetic nerves.

From the acupoints in the periphery, afferent fibres enter the spinal cord. Within the spinal cord, EA activates both local loops and supraspinal pathways up to the brain.

CD ROM

**The brain**

Many parts of the brain have been implicated in the mechanism of EA. These are elaborated in detail in the CD-ROM resource under the headings:
- Jigsaw pieces 1. The forebrain and associated structures
- Jigsaw pieces 2. The brainstem and cerebellum
- Jigsaw pieces 3. Limbic structures and the basal ganglia

## THE NEUROCHEMICAL MAP

There is a huge amount of experimental research on the neuropharmacology of EA, outlined in detail in the CD-ROM ⊙ resource. This chapter offers a short overview of three neurochemical groups frequently associated with EA.

# Neuropeptides I: the opioid peptides

The analgesia that results from morphine and EA appears similar in many respects. Many studies have shown that naloxone, an opioid antagonist, counters the analgesic effect of EA (and sometimes MA, TENS and CES) without necessarily abolishing it. The timing of naloxone application relative to EA is important: in general, naloxone given prior to EA decreases or blocks EAA; if given before maximal EAA it partially antagonises it; if given after EAA is established, has only a partial or little effect.

Furthermore, some forms of unpleasant (noxious) stimulation, for instance at Du-26, may be only partially opioid mediated. None the less, opioid peptides do appear to be involved in EAA in many parts of the brain, although segmental stimulation may not activate these supraspinal pathways. Opioid peptides are probably also activated peripherally by EA treatment for arthritis, and even hypertension. Centrally, they mediate the effects of EA on blood viscosity and pressure: blood pressure may be raised or lowered by EA, depending on circumstances, and naloxone reverses both these changes. Naloxone also counters EA's effects on epilepsy, gastric acid secretion, and growth hormone level.

## β-ENDORPHIN

The opioid peptide considered responsible for many of the effects of EA is β-endorphin (βEP). However, βEP within the spinal cord does not appear to play a major role, while levels of the peptide within the cerebrospinal fluid (CSF) and in the blood may or may not change in response to EA. Thus βEP appears to play more of a neurotransmitter role in the brain than in the spinal cord, and rather less of a neurohormonal role in the blood and periphery.

## THE ENKEPHALINS

There appears to be a two-way relationship between the enkephalins (Enk) and EA in the brain: EA raises Enk levels in various parts of the brain, while prevention of Enk degradation by the enzyme enkephalinase enhances EAA. In animal studies, levels of both leu-enkephalin (LE) and met-enkephalin (ME) vary with EA in different parts of the brain, increasing or decreasing depending on the overall state of the subject. However, when CSF levels of ME are low, as in patients with recurrent pain, they may not change even when EA is effective, and it is possible that raised levels of ME may actually inhibit EAA.

In the spinal cord the enkephalins, particularly ME, are central to the mechanisms of EA. They show different patterns of release in response to different treatment parameters (on one or both sides of the body, locally or distally, at high or low intensity).

## THE DYNORPHINS

The dynorphins (Dyn) play a larger role in the spinal cord than in the brain with EA.

### More neuropeptides

The CD-ROM resource contains detailed information on studies involving neuropeptides:

- Neuropeptides 2. The pituitary peptides
- Neuropeptides 3. The circulatory peptides
- Neuropeptides 4. The gastrointestinal (gut) peptides
- Neuropeptides 5. The hypothalamic hormone releasing peptides
- Neuropeptides 6. The miscellaneous peptides

# The monoamines

The catecholamines noradrenaline (NA, norepinephrine) and adrenaline (Adr, epinephrine) are important in stress, nociception and antinociception, and thus inevitably implicated in many effects of EA. Changes of NA (and Adr) levels in different parts of the brain, and in response to manipulation of α and β receptor function in brain, spinal cord and periphery, are described in the CD-ROM ⊙ resource version of this chapter. βEP plays a role in noradrenergic processes, and NA is yet another neurotransmitter that appears to be involved in tolerance to EA.

The third catecholamine, dopamine (DA), is found particularly in the basal ganglia of the brain. If levels are low, EA may increase them, but if they are increased (by stress, in the prefrontal cortex for example), EA can lower them. Results vary, depending particularly on the intensity of EA used, but also possibly on the frequency. Activation of different DA receptor types also complicates the picture and, as with NA, there appear to be bidirectional influences between endorphinergic and dopaminergic processes. DA changes have been found locally at acupoints after EA.

Although histamine is more often considered for its role in allergy than as a neurotransmitter, both $H_1$ and $H_2$ receptor antagonists such as promethazine and cimetidine may attenuate EAA, depending on dosage or stimulation intensity.

Serotonin (5HT) plays a crucial role in many of the effects of both EA and TENS. Peripherally, in the stomach, 5HT may increase or decrease in response to EA, and in the blood 5HT tends to increase with EA. 5HT in the spinal cord is also implicated in EA: a descending serotonergic pathway mediates several forms of analgesia in the trigeminal nucleus and spinal cord. As with NA, initial changes in 5HT may not continue with repeated EA treatments. Similarly, the 5HT precursor 5HTP, available in some nutritional supplements, may enhance EAA or reverse EA tolerance initially, but attenuate EAA if given repeatedly.

Importantly, as with the endorphins and naloxone, reversal of many of EA's 5HT effects after some minutes of stimulation is not possible, indicating that they are maintained by non-serotonergic mechanisms. At least one of these involves the endorphins themselves. There appears to be, in Han Jisheng's words, a 'compensatory functional interrelation' between opioid peptides and 5HT: if levels of both are high following EA, then generally there is excellent analgesia, but this is moderate if only one or the other is high, and poor if neither is.

## Acetylcholine

Acetylcholine (ACh) is another important mediator of EA, and it has been claimed that there is more cholinergic innervation at AcPs than at non-AcPs. Both ACh and acetylcholinesterase (AChE, the enzyme that breaks down ACh) have been applied to the skin at acupoints, with clinically interesting results. In the blood, levels of both ACh and AChE may increase or decrease with MA or EA.

ACh may be responsible for EA transmission in primary afferents. In different regions of the brain, both muscarinic and nicotinic ACh receptors may be involved in EA. ACh and DA mutually interact in EAA, with further interactions between ACh and the opioid peptides, NA and 5HT, along with other neurotransmitters.

**More neurochemicals**

The CD-ROM resource contains further details of studies involving other groups of neurochemicals under the headings:
- The amino acids
- Purines: adenosine and adenosine triphosphate (ATP)
- Second messengers: calcium and the cyclic nucleotides
- Loose ends: nitric oxide (NO) and prostaglandins (PG)

## The neurochemistry of EA tolerance

If EA or TENS is repeated too frequently, tolerance can develop and treatment becomes less effective. Tolerance develops at different rates in different species, and tolerance to stimulation at one frequency (e.g. 2 Hz) does not entail cross-tolerance to stimulation at another (e.g. 100 Hz). In general, tolerance builds more rapidly to HF, low-intensity stimulation (EA, TENS) than to LF, high-intensity EA or TENS, and possibly more rapidly with HF EA than with HF TENS. Not all EA effects are subject to tolerance.

Tolerance may develop because of peripheral or central mechanisms. Centrally, enkephalins may become depleted. Other neurochemicals released by prolonged opioid activation may also play a part, including NA and cholecystokinin (CCK). 5HTP, the 5HT precursor, may partially reverse EA tolerance.

## THE ELECTRICAL MAP: NEUROELECTRIC RESPONSES TO EA

Considerable research has been done on EA using the methodology of *evoked potentials* (EPs). These are electrical voltage changes, usually measured from the scalp, in response to peripheral stimulation. EPs have been used to investigate the effects of EA on pain, and to differentiate between EA and MA effects, those of deeper and more superficial needling, or of EA/TENS and various drugs (including placebo).

Locally, different regions within the brain respond to EA with their own 'favoured patterns' of discharge, potentially useful but not yet fully explored information when considering stimulation parameters to use with EA/TENS. In general, firing rates increase, decrease or remain unchanged in response to noxious stimulation or pathological state, with EA tending to reverse these changes.

More is known about how the EEG changes in response to acupuncture (both EA and MA), and medication. EA, for example, appears to act like an analgesic, markedly reducing EEG pain responses. Enhanced $\alpha$ power may be a prognostic indicator for good treatment response. Some hypnosis-like changes in the EEG may occur only with relatively strong LF EA (1–2 Hz) and intramuscular needle insertion, and not with higher frequencies or *very* strong stimulation.

## FURTHER EXPERIMENTAL OBSERVATIONS

### EA and pain

EA developed originally in China as a means of treating pain, first postoperative and intraoperative, and then other forms of acute and chronic pain. Thus much experimental research is devoted to the subject of EA and pain. EA results in reduced pain ('hypoalgesia') rather than absence of pain (analgesia), and certainly not in anaesthesia (absence of sensation).

Without consciousness, there is no pain. EA/TEAS may in fact have more influence on the affective than on the sensory dimension of pain. However, EA also clearly affects the sensory level. The levels of experience involved may depend on where EA is applied. The generalised analgesia that can result from EA may begin peripherally, extending to the trunk later. However, better EAA (EA analgesia) may be attainable when EA is itself applied on the trunk rather than peripherally.

Many different ways of attempting to measure pain objectively have been employed in EA research. These include flexion, blink and H reflexes, heart rate variability and the jaw-opening response to tooth pulp pain. This latter method shows that results are likely to be better for canine and premolar pain than molar pain, with different results depending in part on whether local or distal points are stimulated, and possibly less effect on soft tissue (gum) pain than on dental pain itself. Other ways of assessing pain include tail-flick latency and hot plate tests. They do not all involve the same mechanisms, and many factors may affect results, including variation in individual responsiveness. Measuring analgesia is not straightforward.

Pain threshold (PT) studies indicate that sometimes PT change is global rather than restricted to a particular target area, and that EA/TENS may affect pain but not other sensory thresholds. Interestingly, TENS may have a regulatory effect on PT, not just raising it if low, but also reducing it if high.

Response to clinical and experimental pain may well differ (even in the same person at the same time). Thus studies on experimental pain may not be relevant when it comes to clinical pain. Experimentally, however, EA may increase PT more when applied at AcPs than at non-AcPs.

The vast majority of EA/TENS experimental pain studies model nociceptive pain. Neurogenic pain is explored in only a handful of reports. Their results could well be important for the clinical application of EA and TENS.

Pruritis (itching), which is closely related to pain, may respond to LF TENS applied distally, and HF stimulation locally. Brief intense stimulation may be helpful as an alternative intervention. LF and dense-disperse (DD) mode stimulation have also been used.

## EA and the cardiovascular system

EA has autonomic effects quite distinct from those due to analgesia. EA can improve heart function, regulating blood pressure, heart rate, arrhythmia and ventricular fibrillation. Applied at P-6, as well as at other points along the Pericardium meridian and some other acupoints, the benefits of EA in an animal model of acute myocardial ischaemia (AMI) have been explored in some detail. EA appears to regulate coronary microcirculation and possibly relieve microvascular spasm. Stimulation at a variety of frequencies appears to be effective, and strong stimulation may not always be required.

EA regulates blood pressure (BP). If BP is low, EA will tend to increase it. On the other hand, if BP is already raised, EA may well lower it. EA/TEAS may not greatly change normal BP. This has been shown for acute myocardial ischaemia and haemorrhagic shock and stress, for example. If EA is itself painful or stressful, it may increase BP, but EA that reduces pain may also lower BP.

Du-26 (and P-6) have been used to raise BP. ST-36 is the point most researched for its hypotensive properties, but some ear points may also be useful. As with P-6 EA for acute myocardial ischaemia, a wide range of stimulation parameters may be effective with ST-36 EA. TENS on the arm may increase BP, and on the leg lower it, although these changes are small.

P-6 EA may increase or decrease heart rate to maintain cardiovascular homeostasis, often in line with changes in BP. In general, EA and TENS have frequently been shown to reduce heart rate. However, they do not always affect it. EA (at ST-36 or ST-36 with GB-34) may be unlikely to in the presence of severe tachycardia. Auricular, P-6 and ST-36 EA may all reduce or prevent arrhythmia, although ST-36 EA may not be effective if arrhythmia is severe. Auricular and P-6 EA may both reduce the likelihood of ventricular fibrillation.

## EA and the brain

EA can protect the brain following acute cerebral ischaemia. This has been demonstrated using electrical measurements (EP and EEG), and by detecting changes in levels of neurochemicals such as nitric oxide, endothelin, angiotensin and nerve growth factor, as well as by monitoring improvements in cerebral blood flow. In some conditions, EA has been found to regulate blood vessel diameter to maintain balance. *Dumai* points have been used frequently, as well as points such as GB-30, LI-4, LI-11 and ST-36. EA may have greater effects than MA on cerebral blood flow and heart rate.

## EA and circulation

Several forms of stimulation, including EA, TEAS/TENS and spinal cord stimulation (SCS), may increase peripheral vasodilation. Indeed, such vasodilation may contribute to pain relief. It appears to be mediated by 5HT, as well as peptides such as VIP and calcitonin gut-related peptide (CGRP).

The enhanced peripheral blood flow that occurs with EA may lead to a reduction in inflammatory oedema and enhance repair of skin lesions. Circulation (and tissue repair) may also improve within some internal organs. Even within teeth, EAA can contribute to maintaining microcirculation (whereas, with standard local anaesthetics, dental pulp blood and lymph vessels may become constricted and congested).

Strong stimulation is likely to lead to vasoconstriction. Changes with MA differ from those with EA. Both may induce a short-term vasoconstriction, followed by a longer-lasting vasodilation, but on different timescales.

EA has been found to alter levels of several blood constituents, as well as red blood cell membrane characteristics.

## EA and thermal effects

Peripheral temperature changes accompany changes in microcirculation, and occur with MA, EA and TENS. With MA, temperature changes may depend on where the needle is inserted and how it is manipulated, and can be different, even opposite, in different patients. Temperature changes may occur on both sides of the body, or mainly one, in response to unilateral MA.

Results are not dissimilar with EA. Bilateral changes and even generalised warming can occur if treatment is not uncomfortable, but are often preceded by an initial cooling. Global temperature increase may be a useful prognostic indicator that a patient will respond well to treatment. EA tends to have a regulatory effect: if temperature is initially high it may be reduced, if low it may be increased, with little effect on intermediate temperatures.

There are contradictory reports on the generalised thermal effects of TENS/TEAS. Birger Kaada found that comfortable motor level TEAS (at LI-4/~SI-3, with 2 Hz continuous stimulation, CW, or 2–5 Hz trains of 100 Hz) increased skin temperature in patients with peripheral vascular insufficiency. Such changes may not occur in asymptomatic subjects. Initial cooling may be found, as with EA. Locally, temperature tends to increase, although long-term cooling has also been reported. These effects depend on where stimulation is applied, and what parameters are used.

## EA and autonomic function

EA can both activate and calm the sympathetic side of the autonomic nervous system. Stressful or uncomfortable electrostimulation of any type will activate peripheral adrenergic mechanisms. This may account for the initial cooling or raised plasma NA found with some EA, for example. On the other hand, EA and TENS may also counter some effects of both short- and long-term stress.

In general, non-stressful LF EA/TENS appears to have sympatholytic (sympathetic-calming) effects, and distal points such as ST-36 may be less sympathotonic (sympathetic-activating) than some points on the torso. In some circumstances, there may be a correlation between subjective pain reduction and decreased sympathetic activity. A more difficult problem is whether some of the effects of EA result from parasympathetic excitation rather than sympathetic depression, or vice versa. The balance of their involvement appears to vary, depending on the measure, condition or system being targeted (blood pressure, heart rate, gastric acidity or tissue repair, for instance).

## EA and the immune system

Immune reactions are especially evident when injury is involved, as with needling or some forms of moxibustion. Both humoral and cellular immune function may be affected by EA and TENS. EA appears to have useful biphasic regulatory effects on both, although sometimes repeated treatments are needed before these become evident.

EA may affect blood levels of several types of globulin, interleukin, and other immune-related substances. Following immunisation, it can accelerate antibody production. Thus TENS and auricular EA may prevent and reverse stress-induced humoral immunosuppression.

Since the 1950s it has been known that EA can restore a reduced leukocyte (white blood cell) count. Its effects on different types of leukocyte, such as lymphocytes and neutrophils, vary in different studies. Phagocytosis is enhanced by EA, and leukocyte adherence to vascular endothelial cells reduced. EA can enhance natural killer (NK) cell cytotoxicity. EA may also have useful immunosuppressive effects – against mitogenic induction of lymphocyte proliferation, for instance.

ST-36 is the most used point in EA immune studies, sometimes in combination with SP-6, *lanweixue* (M-LE-13) or other points. A variety of stimulation parameters have been investigated, although without any clear conclusion on their relative usefulness.

Some EA immune effects are opioid mediated, although there are immune effects of EA that appear to be mediated peripherally not only through opioid pathways, but also both sympathetically and parasympathetically. Centrally, opioid peptides such as LE and βEP are also involved, as well as catecholamines such as NA. However, EA immune responses may not be based on the same opioid mechanisms as EAA, particularly where central and peripheral βEP

is concerned. ACTH/cortisol release, as well as segmental reflex mechanisms, is also implicated.

## EA and tissue repair

EA accelerates healing of experimental skin ulcers, and prolongs survival of musculocutaneous skin flaps more effectively than MA. TENS may be more effective still, although the reason for this is unclear. Segmental HF high-intensity TENS may be the most appropriate form of TENS to use.

EA may increase neuron survival after lesion, and also promote regeneration of peripheral nerve. Early treatment is essential. Even spinal cord repair may be enhanced if EA is given very shortly after injury. Different types of nerve fibres may recover at different rates. In general, some residual afferent EA pathway is still necessary to achieve any benefit.

## EA modulation of organ function

### DIGESTIVE SYSTEM

In general, EA reduces raised gastric acidity, although in healthy subjects it may increase it after a brief initial decrease. EA may concurrently increase gastric secretion of bicarbonate and sodium. EA may also affect gastric blood flow, and is protective against a variety of stress-induced gastric changes, including ulceration. Both MA and EA influence gastroelectric activity and peristalsis, although not all the different techniques of MA have the same effect. Stimulating limb and abdominal points also leads to different results.

Both EA and MA also affect intestinal motility. In horses, EA has been used for faecal impaction, spasmodic or flatulent colic and paralytic ileus/rectal paralysis, and in piglets for diarrhoea. As in the stomach, EA may reduce manifestations of gastrointestinal stress. It may also enhance peristalsis inhibited by morphine.

In animals in shock, or with severe digestive illness, both EA and transcranial TENS may enhance levels of some liver metabolic markers, while MA may improve liver enzyme function.

EA may reduce gall stone formation, although not necessarily serum cholesterol levels. EA at both auricular and body points can induce gall bladder contractions and bile secretion. Interestingly, EA effects on activity in Oddi's sphincter (which controls flow from the common bile duct into the duodenum) appear opposite in omnivores/carnivores and herbivores; the overall effect in all cases is to increase bile flow into the duodenum. However, effects on bile flow at different acupoints in the same species may also be opposite: in healthy humans, the gall bladder contracts in response to MA at *dannangxue* (M-LE-23), 1–2 *cun* below GB-34, while with GB-40 MA it relaxes.

### RESPIRATORY SYSTEM

EA appears to have regulatory effects on various neurochemical markers in asthma, asphyxiation and experimental pleurisy, although with minimal effects in healthy volunteers.

At LU-6 and P-6, it may also reduce haemoptysis (coughing up blood) due to tuberculosis.

## URINARY SYSTEM

EA has a regulatory effect on some aspects of kidney function. However, segmental (BL-23) stimulation may reverse the effects of distal point stimulation on kidney function in some situations.

Bladder function involves micturition centres in the posterior hypothalamus and medulla, as well as local feedback loops. Thus auricular stimulation and even such seemingly unrelated points as LI-4 may regulate bladder contraction and urine excretion. More locally, EA at BL-23 and BL-28 may have different effects, and these may also depend on the pathology involved.

## REPRODUCTIVE SYSTEM

EA may speed up the waves of electrical activity that sweep through the uterus at most times, even after uterine denervation. Thus EA may enhance uterine blood flow. While the pain of dysmenorrhoea may be reduced by both EA and TENS, this may not, surprisingly, affect intrauterine activity – or can even increase it.

Very strong EA (at LI-4 and SP-6, linked across the body rather than ipsilaterally) induced abortion in some rats, although offspring born to the mothers who did not abort appeared quite healthy.

## EA AND THE ENDOCRINE SYSTEM

### Insulin and blood sugar

In diabetic animals, comfortable 50 Hz EA at BL-23 and ST-36 significantly lowers plasma glucose levels, with improvement in various other diabetes-related measures. TEAS may be less effective. Strong EA (15 Hz) at Ren-12 may also reduce plasma glucose, even when normal, although not in insulin-dependent diabetes. This effect appears to be mediated by βEP and adrenal activation.

### The reproductive system and the sex hormones

EA may affect sex hormones via both the hypothalamo-pituitary-gonadal axis and local reflex pathways. One result of this is that it may induce ovulation, as can MA and other forms of electrical stimulation.

The effects of EA on luteinising hormone (LH), gonadotrophin-releasing hormone (LHRH or GnRH), corticotrophin-releasing hormone (CRH), progesterone, oestrogen, oestradiol, testosterone, dehydroepiandrosterone (DHEA), prolactin and follicle-stimulating hormone (FSH) have been researched, with many appearing to be mediated by βEP. As so often, EA and related methods regulate levels of several of these hormones, increasing or decreasing them depending on circumstance. Thus EA is potentially useful for both female and male infertility problems, as well as for promotion of labour.

## THE THYROID AND PARATHYROID

EA and other electrostimulation methods may influence both thyroid and parathyroid function.

## EA and drug withdrawal

Acupuncture, and particularly EA, has been investigated quite extensively for its effects on drug withdrawal. Many neurotransmitters are involved in addiction and withdrawal, particularly the endogenous opioids and dopamine.

Both HF and LF auricular EA and their variants have been shown to reduce withdrawal behaviour and affect both CSF and plasma neurochemical levels in a number of animal studies. While LF EA may activate the endorphinergic system in relieving pain, HF auricular EA for treating abstinence syndrome may involve enkephalinergic mechanisms. Indeed, it has been suggested that the enkephalinase inhibitor D-*phenylalanine* (DPA) may alleviate withdrawal symptoms associated with endorphin depletion. If withdrawal is stressful and rapid (as when precipitated by naloxone in opiate addiction), EA may not be powerful enough to suppress all the ensuing symptoms and stress-related biochemical changes.

Most of the experimental research has been carried out on opiate addiction, although there are also studies (some using MA rather than EA) on cocaine, amphetamine and alcohol, for example.

## PARAMETERS OF EA AND THEIR EFFECTS

### The effects of intensity

Stimulation may be strong or gentle, depending on how many and what type of nerve fibres are recruited. There are advocates of both approaches. Very strong (noxious) stimulation applied to AcPs or non-AcPs can produce a generalised analgesia. One possible mechanism for this has been called '*diffuse noxious inhibitory control*' (DNIC) (see Ch. 7 for more details). In this model, even non-painful EA may sometimes have generalised effects if pain is already present. Usually though, less strong EA has only a localised (segmental) effect. The neuroscience of both strong and weak stimulation has been explored. Clearly, not all EA has to be uncomfortable!

Stronger stimulation at most frequencies will activate the sympathetic nervous system, raising BP and heart rate, and potentiating some forms of cardiac arrhythmia. Less strong LF stimulation may reduce BP and moderate arrhythmia. Only less strong EA is likely to enhance parasympathetic activity, encourage relaxation and so increase temperature generally. Strong stimulation may exacerbate inflammation.

The electrical responses in the brain to strong and weak EA have been explored. Although strong stimulation appears necessary for some pain-related effects, weaker EA may actually enhance some vision-related activity, for example. Stronger stimulation may also induce a longer-lasting analgesia, whereas weaker stimulation may more effectively inhibit some neurogenic pain.

Box 6.1 summarises some of the effects of strong (painful) and less strong (non-painful) stimulation.

**Summarising the effects of intensity**

| Painful | Non-painful |
|---|---|
| *deqi* acupuncture | superficial or other forms of acupuncture |
| connective tissue massage | light massage |
| heat (moxa cone) | warmth (note: different nerve fibres for warmth/heat) |
| cold | cool |
| less acupoint-specific | more acupoint-specific |
| A$\delta$ & C nociceptive fibres | A$\beta$ & C mechanoreceptor fibres |
| $\beta$EP$\uparrow$ | GABA$\uparrow$ galanin$\uparrow$ oxytocin$\uparrow$ |
| sympathetic tone$\uparrow$ | sympathetic tone$\downarrow$ |
| intensity more important than frequency | more frequency-dependent effects |
| **Pain alleviation:** | |
| relatively generalised | relatively localised |
| *intensity* component more affected | *discomfort* component more affected |
| pain reduction | anxiolysis and well-being |

[Based on a presentation by Thomas Lundeberg]

## The effects of frequency

### THE BEIJING STUDIES

Han Jisheng's Beijing group has demonstrated that frequency is also a key parameter. At least some of the different brain nuclei involved in 2 Hz, 15 Hz and 100 Hz EA have been delineated. In addition, it is clear that 2 Hz EA is mediated by spinal cord $\mu$ and $\delta$ opioid receptors, 100 Hz by $\kappa$ receptors, and 2/15 Hz DD mode by all three.

In the spinal cord, met-enkephalin is released in 'good responder' rats with 2 Hz EA. The more recently discovered endorphin, endomorphin-1, also appears to be involved in 2 Hz EA at spinal level. In the brain, enkephalin synthesis within the hypothalamic *arcuate nucleus* is particularly important for LF EA.

15 Hz EA is mediated spinally by dynorphin, although there may be some differences between mice and humans in the precise mechanisms involved. Other spinal cord neurotransmitters implicated in 15 Hz (and 100 Hz) EA include substance P and *angiotensin II*.

In the spinal cord, Dyn is released in good responders with 100 Hz as with 15 Hz EA. Dyn also plays a role in 100 Hz EA in the brain. It mediates 100 Hz EA suppression of opioid withdrawal symptoms and 100 Hz TEAS amelioration of spinal spasticity. CCK, *orphanin* and other neurochemicals within the brain and spinal cord are also implicated in 100 Hz (but not 2 Hz) stimulation. However, 5HT does not appear to have frequency-specific effects. The brain regions involved with 2 Hz and 100 Hz EAA are, in general, very different.

An important difference between LF and HF EA is that the former has a generalised analgesic action, whereas that of the latter is mainly local. Clearly, with such differences, EA is not just an indiscriminate noxious or stressful stimulation.

2/15 Hz DD mode, mediated by all three types of opioid receptor in the spinal cord, may be more effective in some circumstances than either 2 Hz or 100 Hz EA (both during and after treatment). Thus, unless the optimal frequency is known, 2/15 or 2/100 Hz DD can be used for a synergistic effect between spinal cord ME and Dyn; 2.5–3 seconds of each frequency is optimal.

### OTHER RESEARCH

#### Low frequency
Thin peripheral nerve fibres can respond to stimulation only at low frequencies. Thus nociceptive C fibres may fatigue even at 5 Hz, and pain signals may be blocked at 15 or 20 Hz. Higher frequencies may not improve this effect. Correspondingly, LF may modulate activity more than HF EA in some regions of the brain.

The effects of LF EA on pain tend to last longer than the stimulation itself (although this may not be the case for 8 Hz EA). Very low frequencies, such as 0.2 Hz, may be less effective than those in the 2–8 Hz range. LF EA appears to be mediated by $\mu$ and $\delta$ opioid peptide receptors, although other neurotransmitters are also involved. It also tends to lower BP. Correspondingly, LF EA/TEAS may lower heart rate, and even *entrain* it. Yoshiaki Omura considers that optimal frequency for motor level stimulation should be about the same as the patient's heart rate. There is also some Russian research on using the patient's own respiratory rhythm as the basis for treatment.

#### Medium frequency
The effects of two intermediate EA/TENS frequencies, ~10 Hz and ~15 Hz, differ from those of 2 or 100 Hz in some respects, and possibly involve non-opioid mechanisms.

#### High frequency
HF EA (around 80–200 Hz) is, in general, only partially blocked by the opioid antagonist naloxone. Dynorphin, the catecholamines (NA and DA) and 5HT are probably involved. However, the catecholamines and 5HT are also responsible for some LF EA effects.

It is usually considered that HF EA has a short-term and predominantly segmental effect on pain threshold, in contrast to the longer-lasting and more generalised effects of LF EA. However, this conclusion has not gone unchallenged.

50–60 Hz is considered an optimal frequency for *conventional TENS* (CTENS, defined in Box 6.2) by some authorities. Effects tend to be rapid in onset, and may not – at least in a single session, and in healthy subjects – involve the opioid peptides. However, results are different in acute or chronic pain patients, or with prolonged or repeated TENS. The role of dynorphin in CTENS has not been greatly investigated outside China, but 5HT and substance P have been considered as implicated in HF TENS.

Somewhat surprisingly, CTENS above a certain minimum intensity was found in some studies to have greater effects on circulation and tissue healing than LF TENS. HF stimulation, particularly if strong, tends to increase blood pressure. As a crude generalisation, though, LF EA or TEAS/TENS has more of a warming effect than HF stimulation. However, spasticity responds better to HF than LF TENS.

## THE EFFECTS OF FREQUENCY – CONCLUSION

In general, the consensus is that that LF EA, TEAS or TENS (<10 Hz) produces effects that are mediated by opioids such as βEP and Enk, whereas HF stimulation effects involve other opioids, such as Dyn, and possibly non-opioid mechanisms as well.

# Other treatment parameters

## COMBINATIONS

Box 6.2 lists some definitions.

The effects of CTENS/TLEA are primarily segmental, whereas those of ALTENS/CEA are both segmental and non-segmental. Contralateral effects may be found with both. However, only ALTENS is usually reported as being endorphin dependent. ALTENS/CEA is sometimes considered more effective than CTENS/TLEA. Different frequencies can be combined simultaneously – CTENS local to ALTENS stimulation may permit stronger stimulation than would normally be acceptable. Intermittent LF 'trains' of HF

pulses may be more effective than CTENS, particularly when applied segmentally. This sort of stimulation (sometimes, confusingly, called ALTENS) is opioid mediated, unlike CTENS.

As explained in Chapter 3 of the CD-ROM ⊚ resource, any waveform can be analysed as a combination of sine waves at different frequencies and amplitudes. Thus, if there are unknown frequency-specific effects, a 'shotgun' multifrequency approach – with rectangular pulses, for instance – may be more effective than using a simple sine wave. However, when using TENS/TEAS, signals are anyway distorted by the skin, so arguments in favour of one waveform rather than another may be misleading, and pulse duration may well be a more important variable. If this is long, treatment effects may continue for some time after stimulation has ceased. If short, effects may be minimal, or last only during treatment. The optimum pulse duration to use will depend on other stimulation parameters, how far apart electrodes/needles are positioned, and so forth.

Experimental research on DC stimulation is fragmentary, although hints can be gleaned from some of the older literature on galvanic treatment of psychological conditions. DC needling has been used experimentally to treat tumours.

## TIME AND TIMING

In general, lasting after-effects are found with more intense EA/TENS stimulation, particularly at low frequencies and with longer pulse durations. Analgesic effect may decrease, however, at very low frequencies.

The duration of analgesia may be increased by extra-segmental ALTEAS, even when this has little direct impact on pain by itself. Some circulatory effects of LF EA may last longer than the analgesia it induces. On the other hand, the effects of CTENS or TLEA are usually coincident with the stimulation itself, with a rapid onset and only a brief after-effect. It is possible that pain levels fluctuate after some treatments, rather than changing consistently in the same direction. A key finding is that the effects of CEA and ALTENS generally have a delayed onset. Both onset latency and after-effect depend on supraspinal pathways.

Treatment duration is itself an important variable. For CTENS, 30 or even 60 minutes may be optimal, whereas 30 minutes suffices for ALTENS/CEA analgesia to build, and 30–45 minutes ensures adequate poststimulation analgesia. Longer treatments may be counterproductive. For burst and DD modes, 20 minutes is likely to give better results than 10 minutes of stimulation. Results with handheld pTENS are not altogether consistent. In some studies, best results were obtained with stimulation for around 10 minutes, which is clearly not very useful clinically.

As with treatment duration, repeating treatments too often can be counterproductive. Nevertheless, effects are cumulative. When treating pain, at least initially, two or even three treatments a week should be given. Even in cases of severe pain, it is probably best not to repeat 30-minute treatments more than three to four times daily.

---

**BOX 6.2**

**Definitions**

- *Conventional TENS (CTENS)* is HF (50–200 Hz), low-amplitude (10–30 mA) stimulation, with short pulse durations. It is perceived as relatively gentle (sensory level).
- *Acupuncture-like TENS (ALTENS)* uses lower frequencies (2–5 Hz) at higher amplitudes (15–50 mA), with longer pulse durations, is perceived as relatively strong and may activate muscles (motor level).
- TEAS, or TENS applied at acupoints, can similarly be divided into *CTEAS* and *ALTEAS*.
- *TENS-like EA (TLEA)* is HF low-intensity EA, with short pulse durations, and *Conventional EA (CEA)* is LF high-intensity EA, using longer pulse durations.
- TLS (TENS-like stimulation) refers to CTENS/CTEAS or TLEA, ALS (acupuncture-like stimulation) to CEA or ALTENS/ALTEAS.

---

**BOX 6.3**

Cranial electrostimulation

---

Cranial electrostimulation (CES) has long been explored as a means of inducing analgesia, anaesthesia, or therapeutic effect. Electrodes may be positioned over the forehead and occiput, just in front of or behind the ears, or on the ears themselves. However, apart from the obvious division into two 'families' of CES, with electrodes positioned either 'fore and aft' or transversely, the actual locations used for stimulation might well be less significant than the electrical parameters of the stimulation.

Stronger forms of stimulation tend to be applied over the forehead (even directly over the eyelids) and occiput, and the milder ones between the temples, ears or mastoids. Different parts of the brain are influenced directly, as well as via the cranial nerves, with resulting changes in both the EEG and evoked potentials (EP).

Initially, frequencies of around 100 Hz were used, although it has been suggested that a slower, rhythmically repetitive stimulation may be more relaxing. Strong stimulation at much higher frequencies (up to 166 kHz, for example) has been employed, usually for surgical electroanaesthesia. Much gentler CES has also become popular, with effects even when the currents applied are below the threshold for sensory stimulation. With these more subtle methods, even seemingly minor changes in output waveform or frequency can have considerable effects.

One form of CES, termed SPES (subperception electrical stimulation) by its developer, the Welshman Ifor Capel, has been researched in great depth. To overcome skin impedance differences, its charge-balanced 10 Hz signal is applied via earlobe needle electrodes. Like LF EA, although at much weaker intensities, SPES analgesia is slow in onset, and with an after-effect that may last for several hours. Along with other forms of CES, its impact is clearly cumulative. Like auricular EA, it affects appetite and also drug withdrawal symptoms in animals.

Many forms of CES have been shown to induce relaxation. Gastrointestinal motility, muscle spasticity and tremor may all be altered, as may heart rate and blood pressure. However, with some of the more aggressive forms of CES, stress markers may increase, particularly during surgery. CES has also been investigated for its effects on motion sickness.

The effects of CES on the different major neurotransmitters have been explored. Even though SPES, for example, provides non-stressful subthreshold stimulation, it increases noradrenaline (NA) turnover, and even raises levels of circulating cortisol. Neurochemical changes with the different forms of CES are by no means uniform, however, nor their interaction with different drugs.

---

Finally, treatment needs in some sense to match the condition being treated. The appropriate stimulation parameters may alter as a disorder passes through its different phases. The example is given of experimental arthritis, in which initially both 10 Hz and 100 Hz were effective against severe pain reactions, while after a few days only 10 Hz was helpful.

Box 6.3 details the use of cranial electrostimulation (CES).

# THE MEANS WHEREBY

## Manual acupuncture or electroacupuncture?

EA and MA differ both in mechanism and effect. However, given the variety of EA approaches, the results of reviewing experimental research should be taken only as pointers to appropriate clinical practice, and not necessarily as hard and fast evidence.

As might be expected, the peripheral and central effects of EA differ from those of simple retained needling. This is evident at both neurochemical and neuroelectrical levels, as well as in studies on experimental pain, cerebral circulation and biliary function. There are many reports that the effects of EA are greater than those of MA involving manipulation. Importantly, this appears to be the case for changes in both central and peripheral (plasma) endorphins, as well as other neurotransmitters. EEG changes also differ with EA and MA, while cortical evoked potentials are more marked with EA.

EA may raise pain threshold more than MA, and the analgesia that results from EA is more pronounced, prolonged and widespread than that due to MA. Changes in blood flow and oedema are likely to be greater with EA than MA. Thus EA tends to enhance tissue repair – including that of nerves – more than MA. Its effects on the immune system, gastric acidity, muscle spasticity and even experimentally induced itch are also greater. EA may also reduce the duration of experimental cardiac arrhythmia more than MA.

However, there are studies, on brain oxygenation, pituitary enzyme release, muscle function in patients with cerebral ischaemia, pain threshold and analgesia, where the effects of EA and MA have been shown to be comparable. There are also studies where the effects of MA are superior to those of EA. The *deqi* sensations conveyed by thinner nerve fibres (types III and IV) may be elicited more readily with MA than EA, for example. Equally, Du-26 MA may more effectively enhance cardiac activity than EA at the same point. In some animal studies, changes in progesterone or body weight were greater with MA. In others, MA had greater effects on pain threshold, temperature changes (even fever), infection and salivary flow. Several of these differences appear to be due to sympathetic activation by stronger MA, although tissue damage resulting from vigorous MA may be responsible for some of them. Although there are practical difficulties with such strong manipulation during EA, adding some manipulation during EA may potentiate the effects of both.

## The needles

In EA, needles inserted in acupoints are usually connected in pairs to an EA device (the circuit completed through the body). However, groups of needles can be connected, positioned either along a meridian, or in a particular area. Focused needling is also possible, with the needle tips close together (Fig. 6.2).

## To TENS or not to TENS?

EA and TENS are very similar, but not the same. For one thing, although surface stimulation can activate nerves even 4 cm beneath the body surface, much less current is needed to achieve this when using needles that already penetrate the skin barrier, with its high electrical impedance. For this reason, EA may be less uncomfortable than TENS, although anxieties about invasive stimulation may make EA a more stressful experience.

Strong deep stimulation is endorphinergic, but strong TENS is less likely to be. EA had greater effects on pain threshold than TENS in some studies, although, curiously, latency to EAA was less than that to TENS analgesia in one study on low-intensity LF stimulation.

EA may be more effective than TENS for wound repair, muscle spasticity and for both the symptoms and biochemical markers of diabetic neuropathy. However, Han Jisheng's Beijing group found that EA and TENS have similar time courses and response to naloxone, and that tolerance to one form of stimulation at a given frequency reduced analgesia induced by the other form at the same frequency. Thus there appears to be little difference between them in terms of antinociception or the neural mechanisms involved. Their effects on some aspects of immune function, gastric acid secretion, even psychosis and drug withdrawal may be similar.

On the other hand, tolerance to HF EA may be greater than to HF TENS, and TENS may have more effect on experimental pain than EA (perhaps because larger electrodes enable higher currents to be used, resulting in recruitment of additional afferent fibres without excessive stimulation of nociceptive ones). TENS has also been found to be more effective than EA for improving circulation and skin-flap survival.

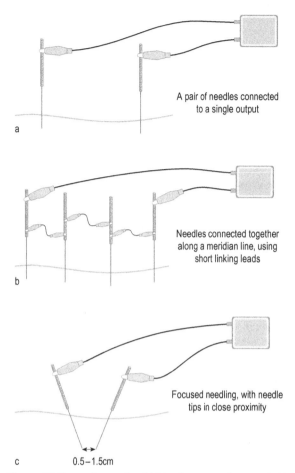

a — A pair of needles connected to a single output

b — Needles connected together along a meridian line, using short linking leads

c — Focused needling, with needle tips in close proximity — 0.5–1.5cm

**Figure 6.2** Connecting needles. (a) Needles are usually connected in pairs to an EA device (the circuit completed through the body). (b) However, groups of needles can be connected, positioned either along a meridian or in a particular area. (c) Focused needling is also possible, with the needle tips close together (0.5–1.5 cm, with the needles angled towards each other).

MA had superior effects to TENS when only the former was familiar to the subjects in one study. MA (at Du-26 in anaesthetised dogs) was also superior to TENS in increasing cardiovascular activity. In humans, MA had a greater effect on temperature than HF TENS. On the other hand, both LI-4 ALTEAS and CTEAS had a greater effect on muscle H reflex than 15 minutes of MA at the same point.

## OTHER METHODS OF STIMULATING ACUPOINTS AND MERIDIANS

### Heat and cold

Moxibustion traditionally constitutes a major part of acupuncture practice. There have been many experimental studies on this method of heating acupoints, as well as others looking at various electrical methods of producing heat, from electro-cautery to 'electric wind'. There is probably little difference between such methods as moxibustion, incandescent heat and 'microwave acupuncture' so far as their heating effects go, although some modern methods are more convenient than the traditional ones.

Cold as well as heat has been applied at acupoints to stim-ulate immune function. Cold, in the form of ice massage or a cooling spray, applied at acupoints/trigger points, affects pain levels.

## Microwaves

Microwave acupuncture has been investigated for its effects on pain, although it is not always clear at first glance whether this is thermal or athermal stimulation. As with EA, it may induce a temperature *drop* along a meridian from the treated point.

## Millimetre waves (extremely high frequency, EHF)

This form of non-thermal stimulation, applied at acupoints, appears to reduce hypersecretion of gastric acid and so pro-tect against peptic ulcer, as well as accelerate ulcer repair. Acupoint EHF also enhances immune function, and has been used in treating experimental tumours. However, prolonged treatment will have a reduced or even opposite effect, as it does for ulceration.

Acupoint EHF regulates some stress-related neurochemical changes, and also autonomic function. Its effects on the EEG, experimental pain and some cardiovascular parameters have been investigated. Individual *'sensor reactions'*, including sensations of heat or cold, changes in pulse rate or intestinal peristalsis, have been used as a guide to what output frequency to use (as these changes are supposed to indicate some form of 'resonance', such individualised EHF treatment is sometimes called 'microwave resonance therapy', MRT).

## Light

Weak, athermal visible light or infrared radiation applied at acupoints may affect the ECG and EEG, as well as serum levels of chemicals such as acteylcholinesterase (AChE). Continuous and intermittent light may affect blood glucose levels quite differently.

## Low-intensity laser and polarised light

'Laser acupuncture' (LA) is applied non-invasively, or some-times via an optic fibre threaded through a hollow needle. It has been shown to alter regional cerebral blood flow significantly in various parts of the brain associated with nociception. However, the effects of low-intensity laser (or light) therapy (LILT) on pain and on the role of the endorphins in LA are both unclear. None the less, response to ST-36 LA has been found useful as a pretest for the epidural dosage required for gastrectomy performed under combined epidural/acupuncture analgesia. There are also interesting studies on pain in animals, in one of which LA analgesia was potentiated by a cocktail of amino acids (L-tryptophan, D-phenylalanine, D-leucine) and other chem-icals (acetylcholine and insulin). LA also has cardiovascular effects – on heart rate and other ECG parameters – and may influence haemoglobin levels.

The benefits of LA for tissue (nerve) repair have been demonstrated in experimental studies. LA may both inhibit and reverse degenerative changes in denervated or inac-tive muscle. Partial recovery of sensation following trauma has occurred (in a dog) following use of polarised light at acupoints. LA also has a beneficial effect on a number of immune parameters.

Some comparative studies indicate that LA, MA, EA and TENS have similar effects, others that LA is more or less effective than MA. In general, results in experimental and animal studies do appear better with traditional needling. Research has also been carried out with varying stimula-tion parameters. Pulsing LA at different frequencies, for example, may have different effects on pain or urinary glucocorticoids. Intriguingly, pulsed at LF (<10 Hz), absorption of 780 nm laser light may be greater at LI-4 than at a non-point.

## Low-intensity pulsed electromagnetic fields (PEMF)

There is little experimental research on applying PEMF in the field of acupuncture. Changes in 5HT have been noted in observational studies, and also alterations in awareness (when PEMF is combined with CES) and in immune function, but these need to be confirmed by more formal research.

## Permanent magnets

Given the popularity of small permanent magnets as a means of stimulating acupoints, it is really quite surprising how little experimental research has been carried out on this modality. There is some evidence of immune effects, that very weak magnets may affect the propagated sensation of flow along meridians (PSM), and that magnets may affect muscle function via changes in local microcirculation.

## Vibration

HF (100 Hz) vibration has useful clinical applications. Like EA and TENS, HF vibration may relieve clinical pain, but without affecting sensitivity to non-painful stimuli (such as heat). Again like EA and TENS, LF (2 Hz) vibration may have an extrasegmental effect on experimental pruritis, but HF vibration only a relatively localised one. However, contra-lateral effects can occur at various frequencies.

Again as with electrical stimulation, HF vibration takes effect more rapidly than LF vibration. Importantly, duration of effect may be greater with clinical than experimental pain. Effects on pain threshold are probably associated with changes in blood flow.

## Sound

There is little experimental research on the effects of sound applied to acupoints. Some has been carried out on the Qi Gong machine described in Chapter 10, and also within the Five Element framework. Combining sound with electrical stimulation can affect body temperature.

## Ultrasound

Very-low-intensity ultrasound may affect electrical activity at auricular acupoints. Applied at ST-36, ultrasound has been found to affect threshold to both body and stomach pain (in rabbits), and circulation in the human leg. At BL-67, ultrasound resulted in occipital lobe functional magnetic resonance imaging (fMRI) changes indistinguishable from those obtained with BL-67 MA. The depth of stimulation appeared to be a key factor.

## POSSIBLE ADVERSE EFFECTS OF STIMULATION

- EA, together with some forms of CES and other methods of electrical treatment for pain, does not necessarily dull sensitivity to other potentially harmful stimuli. However, if a nerve is slightly injured during EA treatment, its threshold to subsequent stimulation may be reduced. In general, though, even repeated treatments do not appear to affect nerve conduction characteristics adversely.
- Exacerbation of pain may indicate that descending inhibitory pathways are impaired in some way (this is less likely to occur with CES).
- Levels of stimulation that are excessive for a given individual may trigger potentially harmful stress responses and should be avoided. Strong muscle stimulation can also temporarily damage muscle fibres, while any treatment that leads to muscle movement may affect tissue uptake or distribution of locally or systemically administered substances. This may not always be desirable.
- The combination of deep needling with strong treatment is not advised at some points (such as Du-3). Spinal or paraspinal points should be used cautiously, as they may reduce heart rate.
- Bronchoconstriction may be an unwanted effect of auricular treatment in rats, and this may be a possibility in some human patients too.
- Points on the throat are generally considered contraindicated for electrotherapy. One reason for this is potential airway restriction. However, although this can indeed occur with HF TENS, LF stimulation may actually serve to open the airway (although effects on BP and heart rate need to be considered as well).
- HF EA/TENS may theoretically inhibit or delay ovulation. LF-induced vasodilation, in contrast, can sometimes result in headache.
- As a generalisation, symmetrical biphasic waveforms produce more effective stimulation and fewer side-effects than others. Needles should not be reused following non-charge-balanced EA.
- Adverse skin reactions with TENS electrodes are more likely with smaller electrodes and longer treatments.
- Although DC and other EA methods have been used to treat tumours, and there is no direct evidence that EA has any carcinogenic effects, it should be used only with caution in patients known to have cancer.
- From animal studies, and on the basis of 'resonance' theories about how EA/TENS work, LF stimulation should be used with caution in young children, whose brains have not yet matured.

Box 6.4 considers the vexed question of epilepsy.

---

**BOX 6.4**

**The vexed question of epilepsy**

Strong rhythmical stimulation in any sensory modality is liable to induce an epilepsy-like response in susceptible individuals. This is less likely to occur at frequencies less than around 15 Hz. However, any sign of rhythmic myoclonic jerks occurring in time with applied stimuli (or at a harmonic of their frequency) should be viewed as a signal to stop treatment immediately.

EA has in fact been found to reduce experimental epilepsy and convulsions in many animal studies, as has MA. However, both may, if strong and applied inappropriately to points on the head, exacerbate a pre-existing tendency to seizure. Strong EA used for prolonged periods in surgery may thus trigger seizures. This adverse effect has actually been harnessed, EA being used to induce convulsion as a less damaging alternative to electroconvulsive therapy (ECT).

Even low-intensity CES, such as SPES, which also has useful antiepileptic effects, may trigger epilepsy in very susceptible individuals. Very weak permanent magnets (10–20 G), which again may attenuate epilepsy, can also sometimes induce an attack if applied to the head.

Epilepsy is perhaps more likely to be triggered if electrical stimulation is combined with certain drugs that themselves can induce seizures. Patients will be more vulnerable either in the early stages of taking such drugs, or when withdrawing from them.

# FACTORS HAVING POSSIBLE ADVERSE EFFECTS ON STIMULATION

## The state of the patient

- *Yang xu* patients may not respond well to strong stimulation that has a cooling effect.
- Stress and anxiety may reduce treatment effectiveness. Anxious or stressed patients may also be less able to tolerate electrical stimulation.
- In cases of peripheral neurogenic pain, stimulating the damaged nerve can sometimes reproduce the pain rather than reducing it.
- Diabetes and Parkinson's disease may reduce some treatment effects in some patients.
- Patients with recent cerebral haemorrhage should be treated cautiously.
- The practitioner should always determine if a patient has been fasting, or has recently eaten a large meal. The importance of adequate nutrition to optimise the function of several neurotransmitters implicated in EA should not be underestimated.

## Drug interactions

- Those on anticoagulant medication (and this may include drugs such as aspirin, or alternatives like gingko biloba or garlic) should not receive strong stimulation to the head.
- Caffeine (and theophylline) may reduce the effectiveness of HF EA/TENS.
- Monosodium glutamate (MSG) may also reduce treatment effectiveness.
- Any drug that enhances spontaneous EEG rhythms within a particular frequency range may potentiate the effect of strong EA or TENS at similar frequencies.
- L-dopa may interfere with EA, but some selective serotonin reuptake inhibitors may improve response to EA.
- Antihistamines may possibly counteract EA. Together with cortisol-like agents, calcium channel blockers, angiotensin-converting enzyme (ACE) inhibitors and MSG, they may also interact with the CES treatment SPES.

## Other treatments and environmental factors

- It has been suggested, but not verified, that prolonged prior exposure to electricity may reduce the effectiveness of microcurrent or CES. Concurrent exposure to strong emissions from other devices (even computer screens, mobile telephones or hearing aids) may not be advisable when using these relatively subtle methods.

- Another unverified observation is that prior or concurrent electrotherapy may interfere with the more finely tuned methods of traditional acupuncture.
- TENS and EA will interfere with other sensitive electronic apparatus, such as cardiac pacemakers or ECG monitors. Until recently, therefore, their use has been totally contraindicated in pacemaker patients or those being monitored. Research now shows that, provided needles/electrodes and the stimulator unit itself are carefully positioned well away from the pacemaker or ECG leads/unit, problems are not inevitable. However, such treatment should be undertaken only with proper safeguards.

# EXPERIMENTAL MEASUREMENTS

## Electrodermal measurements at acupoints and trigger points in response to treatment: in search of the objective

A number of EA systems enable the practitioner to locate points that give unusual electrical readings (generally of skin conductance, SC), treat the points, and then take further measurements to demonstrate that readings have changed. It is generally assumed that electrical properties of acupoints tend to normalise with treatment. Measurements may also be used prognostically. There are claims that the effectiveness of EA may depend on the prior bioelectric characteristics of associated acupoints, for example.

Pressure and heat have also often been used to gauge treatment response, as have other well-known approaches such as muscle testing and pulse taking. All of these methods involve interaction between subject/patient and practitioner, and nearly all involve muscle activity by the latter. This inevitably limits their objectivity. None the less, in the hands of a well-trained and experienced practitioner, and within the total context of the healing encounter, they can be useful.

If an acupoint is stimulated in some way, its electrical characteristics may well change. Changes that occur at other, non-treated AcPs are likely to be more significant. However, in studies where such changes were found it is often not stated whether measurements were carried out solely at AcPs where they would be expected, or at other unrelated points (or non-points) as well. In some cases, changed electrical readings at acupoints do seem to reflect changes in associated internal organ function.

One of the most influential EA-based diagnostic systems has been electroacupuncture according to Voll (EAV), named by its inventor, Reinhold Voll. There are surprisingly few experimental studies on its validity or repeatability, and to my knowledge Voll himself never conducted any.

In basic research on EAV, different groups have found:

- Both SC and its change over time (indicator drop, ID) are strongly affected by the electrode material used.
- SC and ID are reproducible only if repeated within about 20 minutes.

- SC varies considerably between different points.
- SC varies with how long pressure is exerted on a point, as well as the time interval between repeated measurements at the same point.
- Readings vary greatly between different subjects.
- Readings do not clearly distinguish between normal subjects and patients.
- Measurements of SC at a series of points within a short period by different testers will not agree (results are specific to the subject/tester interaction).
- Readings vary more between testers than between subjects.
- Blinded and unblinded tests give different results.
- When 'remedy testing' (Ch. 10), homeopathic and placebo remedies have different effects on both SC and ID.
- Results of the remedy test depend on how pressure is applied to the point, and are likely to be artifacts.
- More consistency between operators was found with 'quadrant' conductance measurements, but readings did not correlate with BP differences.

Thus the tester is very much part of the process, and results will depend on both conscious and unconscious factors influencing pressure at the probe/skin interface.

From my own involvement in a small but very time-consuming study, it seems that:

- ID readings appear to be a pressure artifact.
- SC varies more with age and skin condition than at different points of the same type (e.g. *jing* points) in the same subject.
- Point location can vary within quite a short time.
- SC measurements are reasonably repeatable when heavy pressure is applied to the probe.

This is clearly not a method that gives useful results in the hands of an untrained tester.

## Measuring temperature

Temperature and SC increases may occur together when *qi* arrives in an area of experienced pain (*bi*) in response to acupuncture. Infrared thermography may thus be useful for assessing regional and acupoint temperature changes in response to treatment.

### ELECTRICAL IMAGING METHODS

Kirlian photography (see Ch. 10) produces images that purport to represent the body's bioelectric field and reveal both acupoints and meridians. Unfortunately, the beautiful images of Kirlian photography are more likely to be the product of physical artifact than psychophysiological changes. As a result, experimental Kirlian research gives very little useful information about acupuncture, although there may be correlations between hand-to-hand electrical skin resistance and the images obtained, and MA may (sometimes) affect these images.

Julian Kenyon has found one variant of the Kirlian method to be far less consistent than the Vega Segmentalelectrogram (itself a variant of Voll's original quadrant conductance measurement method), with by far the most repeatable results from the Motoyama AMI device (see Chs 5, 10).

With 'electronography,' a system developed by Ioan Dumitrescu and colleagues in Romania, a single impulse of known characteristics is used rather than the complex random discharge of Kirlian photography. It is claimed to give more reproducible results, and to detect nearly 90% of points tender on palpation.

## Measurements of magnetic fields

Magnetic fields within the EEG $\theta$ and $\alpha$ frequency ranges are emitted from the hands of some healers. Magnetic changes have also been detected in other parts of the body when acupoints are stimulated in various ways.

## SUMMARY

Some key points in this chapter are:

- There is considerable experimental research indicating that EA at different acupoints has different effects
- The existence of the acupuncture meridians remains controversial
- Many opioid peptides and other neurotransmitters are directly affected by EA and heavily implicated in its systemic effects
- Extended use of EA can cause tolerance, with reduced effectiveness
- EA has autonomic, regulatory effects, quite distinct from those due to analgesia
- There is a correlation between treatment intensity and sympathetic activation
- LF and HF stimulation activate different neuro-transmitters
- EA and MA differ, both in mechanism and effect.

 Additional material in the CD-ROM resource

In the electronic version of this chapter, additional material can be found on all the topics mentioned here. Further subjects include the interpretation of reducing and reinforcing in EA, and the effect of magnetic fields on tester sensitivity in such systems as muscle testing, the VEGA test and some dowsing methods.

## RECOMMENDED READING

*Useful introductions to the neurophysiological research on EA, and acupuncture in general, can be found in landmark textbooks such as:*

Pomeranz B, Stux G 1989 (eds) Scientific Bases of Acupuncture. Springer, Berlin

Schoen AM 1994 (ed) Veterinary Acupuncture: Ancient art to modern medicine. American Veterinary Publications, St Louis

Stux G, Hammerschlag R 2001 (eds) Clinical Acupuncture: Scientific basis. Springer, Berlin

*A wonderful collection of papers from major Chinese symposia:*

Zhang XT (Chang HT) 1986 (ed) Research on Acupuncture, Moxibustion and Acupuncture Anesthesia. Science Press, Beijing

*The collected works of Han Jisheng, a colossus in the history of EA research:*

Han JS 1987 The Neurochemical Basis of Pain Relief by Acupuncture. A collection of papers 1973–1987. Beijing Medical University, Beijing

Han JS 1998 The Neurochemical Basis of Pain Relief by Acupuncture 2. Hubei Science and Technology Press, Wuhan

*A full and detailed report on one particular version of cranial electrotherapy stimulation (CES):*

Capel I 1997–98 SPES: the science and history of sub-perception electrical stimulation. An interview with David Mayor. The Electrotherapist. 1997 Winter; 4(3) 6–20; 1998 Spring; 5(1): 7–22; 1998 Summer; 5(2): 11–22

*A thought-provoking account of acupoint measurement methods:*

Tiller WA 1989 On the evolution and future development of electrodermal diagnostic instruments. In: Energy Fields and Medicine: a study of device technology based on acupuncture meridians and chi energy. John E Fetzer Foundation, Kalamazoo, MI, 257–328

*Sources for figures:*

Oleson T 1998 Auriculotherapy Manual: Chinese and Western systems of ear acupuncture. Health Care Alternatives, Los Angeles (2nd edn)

# Seven

How electroacupuncture works II.
Gathering the threads – from
observations to mechanisms
and models

This chapter outlines some of the theories that have been proposed to explain electroacupuncture (EA). They are presented under three main headings: neuroscience, biophysics and traditional Chinese Medicine (TCM).

## HOW EA WORKS IN TERMS OF NEUROSCIENCE

*Blockade* of peripheral nerves, the *gate control theory* of segmental inhibition (Fig. 7.1), and more complex supraspinal pathways and further 'gates' have all been invoked as explanations of how EA and transcutaneous electrical nerve stimulation (TENS) work.

### Pathways and peptides: constellations of the inner sky

The ascending and descending pain inhibitory pathways are activated by peripheral stimulation methods such as EA and TENS. One way of understanding these is through a complex and elegant theory of acupoint and non-acupoint analgesia systems and their checks and balances, developed by Takeshige Chifuyu. His idiosyncratic view of the role of the pituitary peptides is highlighted in the CD-ROM ⊙ resource.

### Neuropharmacology: the endorphin emphasis

Endogenous opioid peptides and other neurotransmitters play a critical role in EA. The chapter in the CD-ROM ⊙ resource places particular stress on the difference between the effects of intensity (Bruce Pomeranz) and frequency (Han Jisheng), and clarifies the importance of serotonin (5HT) at all stimulation frequencies. Han's account of circuitry in the brain, the *'mesolimbic loop'*, is also outlined.

## Understanding the treatment of addiction

The CD-ROM ⊙ resource outlines the possible roles of the various major neurotransmitters in addiction, with obvious implications for methods such as EA and cranial electrotherapy stimulation (CES) that can significantly alter their levels in different parts of the brain.

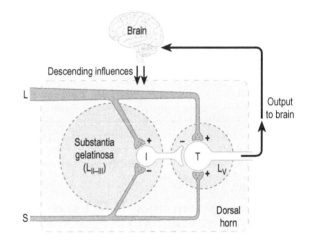

| Afferent input | I cell effect | T cell effect | T cell output |
|---|---|---|---|
| L | + | + | 0 |
| S | + | + | ++ |
| L + S | 0 | + | + |

I cell, activated by L, inhibits T cell; inactivated by S, does not inhibit T cell.

**Figure 7.1** The gate control theory of pain. (Adapted with permission from Walsh 1997 and Fields 1987.) The dorsal horn of the spinal cord, showing in schematic form large (L) and small (S) diameter afferents, an inhibitory interneuron (I) within the substantia gelatinosa (laminae II–III), and lamina V, where L, S and I all synapse with the transmission cell T, whose output signals pain to the brain.

## EA as exercise: the muscular connection

The parallels and divergences between the effects of EA and exercise on neurotransmitters and clinical conditions – from hot flushes to hypertension, and depression to pain – are another basis for understanding the effects of EA.

## Diffuse noxious inhibitory control (DNIC)

The widespread pain suppression that results from strong (noxious) stimulation virtually anywhere in the body is termed DNIC, diffuse noxious inhibitory control. This endorphin-mediated phenomenon has to be clearly differentiated from the effects of non-noxious stimulation. Other endorphin-mediated forms of acupuncture may also be relatively independent of where stimulation is applied.

## The new in neuroscience: broadening the view

Reality is not simple, and cannot be straitjacketed into a single theory. Neuroscience is developing rapidly, with the potential for a broader view that integrates some of the models that we have already.

## Neurotransmitter frequency coding

An attractive hypothesis is that different frequencies of electrical stimulation might be used to 'tune' levels of the various neurotransmitters. Examples are given in the CD-ROM ⊙ resource of how different neurochemicals can indeed be released, even within the same neuron, using this approach. However, frequency is not the only parameter involved, and the picture is probably considerably more complex in clinical situations.

## Long-term potentiation (LTP) and long-term depression (LTD): chronic pain and EA

Memory-like or resonant processes within the central nervous system ('*long-term potentiation*', LTP) may be responsible for some aspects of chronic pain, while opposite processes ('*long-term depression*', LTD) may be responsible for some of the effects of EA and TENS, particularly when these are applied at lower frequencies and amplitudes.

## Calcium, kindling and chaos

In health, adaptability and a homeodynamic balance between excitation and inhibition are maintained. Increased intra-cellular calcium is associated with LTP, '*kindling*', and a number of resultant pathological processes that appear to entail reduced variability in endogenous electrical activity. EA and kindling involve quite different, if not contrary, neurotransmitter mechanisms. Varying EA parameters in different ways may be an important avenue to explore in the future.

## Body brain resonances

Rhythmic stimulation can lead to central, non-humoral resonance effects, particularly within the cerebral cortex, and particularly when the applied stimulation is at one of the 'invariant resonance modes' of the brain. Whether it is possible to test who is a '*strong reactor*' to acupuncture, which frequencies may be most effective when treating chronic pain, and whether different frequencies of EA will elicit different reactions from the different brain hemispheres are explored in the CD-ROM ⊙ resource version of this chapter. Other questions include whether or not it is appropriate in a single treatment session to combine acupuncture with other therapies such as music, or intense EA stimulation for symptomatic relief with more subtle traditional approaches. Indeed, is the 'information content' of acupuncture more or less important than its intensity? Some frequency correspondences for different meridians or types of acupoint are listed, as proposed by various French and Japanese authors.

# HOW EA WORKS IN TERMS OF BIOPHYSICS

The effects of EA and other electrotherapeutic interventions may be explained not just at the macro level of neurophysiology and neurochemistry, but also at the micro level of biophysics. The two may not be mutually exclusive, but even complementary.

## Biophysical possibilities

The CD-ROM ⊙ resource offers a brief explanation of the effects of needling in terms of the 'current of injury', followed by outlines of Robert Becker's theory of *glial DC transmission* and Björn Nordenström's theory of *biologically closed electric circuits*, the latter being possibly more in tune with the classical Chinese view of meridians. Other biophysical explanations of acupuncture are mentioned, although it seems unlikely that any of these can really encompass the subtleties of *qi* and the meridians. Harold Saxton Burr's patterning fields, the meridians as a framework for embryological development, and various rather more tenuous theories of acupuncture in terms of energy flow, wave motion or 'bioplasma' are also discussed.

The effects of pulsed electromagnetic fields (PEMF) on various neurotransmitters and pineal gland function are touched on, as well as the possible non-specific stress response to long-term low-intensity PEMF exposure.

There is also a brief account of how Becker's work and other research have been used in an attempt to give some kind of rationale for microcurrent treatment methods. Finally, the more satisfying theories of James Oschman and Ho Mae-Wan on body circuitry, *tensegrity* and quantum coherence are explored.

## Biophysical microresonance

Frequency 'resonances' may well play a part in our relationships to the world about us as well as to other people (including healers and patients). Some biophysical resonance theories are surveyed, including Liboff's and Lednev's ion resonance theories, work on nuclear magnetic and even DNA resonance, and stochastic resonance. Protein and enzyme resonance changes in the cellular membrane may well explain some of the differences and similarities between the biological effects of low-frequency electrical and magnetic fields. On the basis of these various approaches, ~16 Hz appears to be a potentially useful frequency to use, while 10 seconds would seem to be around the optimum time to continue stimulation if resonance is to occur.

## Resonant recognition and subtle energy

Irena Cosić's 'resonant recognition model of macromolecular bioactivity' (RRM), with its exciting implications for low-intensity laser (or light) therapy, if not EA, is juxtaposed with Jacques Benveniste's 'metamolecular' biology. Both explore the electromagnetic 'signatures' of substance, building bridges between different realms at the forefront of science, yet with immediate applications in terms of therapy.

## THE TCM ACCOUNT OF HOW EA WORKS

The language of TCM has not been well used to explain or describe EA and its effects, yet the roots of EA in traditional acupuncture should not be forgotten if it is to avoid becoming merely another standardised technique applied in mechanical fashion. Different authors' views on the *yin–yang* nature of stimulation (polarity, frequency, duration, modality and waveform) are compared, with the inevitable conclusion that there appears to be little agreement among them, particularly on the question of what parameters can be used to tonify (reinforce) and which to sedate or reduce. In the end, it may well be that traditional labels like 'tonification' and 'reduction' are not applicable when it comes to using EA based on neurophysiology. However, it may be helpful to consider at least some neurological findings in holistic *yin–yang* terms, even if these analogies cannot be taken too far.

## SUMMARY

Some key points in this chapter are:

- There are at least two levels of description: the gross, measurable, *taught* body of biomedicine and the subtle, less palpable, *experienced* body of the more traditional forms of acupuncture
- These descriptions are complementary, one powered by electrical and chemical energy, the other transfused by information patterns of flow and change and oscillation
- The acupoints themselves may be used in treatments directed at both levels.

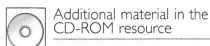

### Additional material in the CD-ROM resource

In the electronic version of this chapter, additional material can be found on psychological explanations of EA, together with a discussion of the placebo effect.

## RECOMMENDED READING

### Neuroscience
*Useful overviews can be found in:*
Bensoussan A 1991 The Vital Meridian: A modern exploration of acupuncture. Churchill Livingstone, Edinburgh
White AR 1999 Neurophysiology of acupuncture analgesia. In: Ernst E, White AR (eds) Acupuncture: A scientific appraisal. Butterworth-Heinemann, Oxford, 60–92

*Takeshige Chifuyu's collected papers, like those of Han Jisheng, offer a heady insight into the scientific investigation of EA:*
Takeshige C 1992 Synaptic Transmission in Acupuncture Analgesia. Showa University School of Medicine, Tokyo

*Grey Walter's work on rhythmic stimulation and its effects in the brain is fundamental to an understanding of body brain resonance:*
Walter VJ, Grey Walter W The central effects of rhythmic sensory stimulation. Electroencephalography and Clinical Neurophysiology. 1949 Feb; 1(1): 57–86

*An in-depth view of acupuncture, resonance and the brain, including some testable hypotheses:*
Mayor DF CNS resonances to peripheral stimulation: is frequency important? Journal of the Acupuncture Association of Chartered Physiotherapists. 2001 Nov; 29–63

### Biophysics
Becker RO 1990 Cross Currents: The promise of electro-medicine, the perils of electropollution. Jeremy P Tarcher, Los Angeles
Nordenström BEW 1983 Biologically Closed Electric Circuits: Clinical, experimental and theoretical evidence for an

additional circulatory system. Nordic Medical Publications, Stockholm

*An interesting book that includes applications of Becker's research in the field of acupuncture:*
Cantoni G, Pontigny JA 1989 Recherche Scientifique Française et Acupuncture. Maisonneuve, Sainte-Ruffine, France

*An alternative view of much of the material covered here:*
Oschman JL 2000 Energy Medicine: The scientific basis. Churchill Livingstone, Edinburgh

*A good explanation of biophysical resonance:*
Liboff AR Bioelectromagnetic fields and acupuncture. Journal of Alternative and Complementary Medicine. 1997; 3(Suppl 1): S77–S87

*A wonderful excursion beyond the boundaries of both neurophysiology and biophysics:*
Cosić I 1997 The Resonant Recognition Model of Macromolecular Bioactivity; theory and application. BioMethods 8. Birkhäuser Verlag, Basel

**TCM**
*Virtually the only non-specialist book that I know that looks in a balanced way at acupuncture and TCM theory:*
Birch SJ, Felt RL 1999 Understanding Acupuncture. Churchill Livingstone, Edinburgh

*Sources for figures:*
Fields HL 1987 Pain. McGraw-Hill, New York

# Eight

## Does electroacupuncture work? Evaluating the controlled trials

Adrian White

Electroacupuncture (EA) has become a standard tool of research into the mechanisms of pain and pain control. There is plentiful evidence that stimulating nerve endings with appropriate electrical signals can produce important changes in the nervous system, particularly the release of neurotransmitters, and laboratory studies indicate that it is better than placebo at reducing experimental pain. However, patients want to know whether EA will help their pain or other symptoms, for which evidence from clinical trials is needed.

## OUR SYSTEMATIC SEARCH AND ITS PARAMETERS

We undertook a systematic search to identify any trial that would help answer the question whether electroacupuncture is effective in clinical practice, in the electronic database Medline and in relevant sections of standard textbooks. We also searched our own files by hand, which included individual papers and collections of conference abstracts.

We included all studies that used electrical stimulation of needles inserted into the skin in the treatment of clinical conditions or for surgical procedures, as long as a clinical outcome was measured. Thus we ignored papers that reported only changes in serum parameters or other physiological measurements. We included studies in which EA was combined with manual acupuncture (i.e. when only some of the needles were stimulated electrically) even though a positive result cannot be definitely attributed to the EA. We included only investigations that had a control group for comparison, so that we could exclude at least the effects of time. The control group could receive either some different intervention or no intervention at all.

Usually the control group was treated in parallel (i.e. recruited simultaneously), though we did include studies where it was possible that the groups may have been treated in sequence, for example in EA for surgery.

We found a number of studies that seemed at first sight to be comparisons of EA, but in fact both groups received EA and differed in some other treatment, such as a drug; we excluded these studies since they test the effect of the drug, not the EA. We included studies in which control groups were given EA using different parameters. We intended to include studies in English, French, German and Chinese, since colleagues were willing to translate them, but in practice all the papers that appeared to meet our criteria were published in English. We did not have the resources at the time to retrieve all the original papers to consider them in this review, so had to decide from the title which studies were the most promising. Resources subsequently became available and the additional studies were read, after translation if necessary. The extracted data are summarised separately in the CD-ROM ⊙ resource.

Quality was measured only by assessing the internal validity of the trials, that is, how likely it was that the result was reliable. We did this by noting whether the authors reported having randomised participants and compared their baseline variables, whether they reported details of dropouts and withdrawals, whether the person who measured the changes in the patients was blinded, and finally the sample size. We approached this conservatively, so that when the precise information was missing, we assumed that that quality criterion was not met.

We summarised the authors' own description of the study outcomes. We should comment here on different possible interpretations when an outcome in the EA group was statistically 'no different' from the comparison group. The meaning depends on what intervention the comparison group received. If the comparison group had no treatment, then the words 'no different' mean 'no effect', but if the comparison group had an active treatment, then EA is also effective. However, we were careful not to claim that the effects of EA and another active treatment are truly 'equivalent' as that requires a true equivalence study, which has to be designed in a special way, for example when calculating sample size and analysing the data.

As always with acupuncture research, there are difficulties with the idea of 'placebo'. Most authors who describe using 'placebo EA' usually connected the needles by wires to an inactivated EA apparatus, which might flash or buzz to give the impression it is active. The credibility of this treatment was assessed in one trial and was not perceived as different from true treatment. In order to make the control more realistic, some workers increase the current to a perceptible degree, sometimes then reducing it and providing some explanation with the aim of convincing the patient that the treatment is continuing. What patients are told about the intervention is critical as it is likely to influence their beliefs and their response to the placebo. Typically, they are told that the treatment 'uses a frequency that cannot be felt'. In all cases, what the patients are told should be reported in the publication. Another point we should note about this type of placebo control is that, because it involves inserting needles, it is unlikely to be completely inert. Therefore we prefer to call it 'sham' EA rather than placebo. A control intervention may be sham on two counts: first because the stimulation is sham, and second because the sites where the needles are inserted are sham (i.e. not acupuncture points).

# FINDINGS OF CLINICAL STUDIES

Our searches located over 400 references to trials of EA, and the titles of about a quarter of these suggested they might meet our inclusion criteria and be of acceptable quality. Finally, 71 studies were included in this review and are summarised in Table 8.1. Most of the remainder have also been summarised, together with other reports held in the Needham Research Institute, and the summaries can be accessed in the CD-ROM ⓞ resource.

The findings are arranged in Table 8.1 according to the clinical condition treated. The studies are spread over a wide range of conditions, and for most conditions there are not enough studies to be able draw any conclusions, the exception being EA for surgical and procedural analgesia. They also used a range of control interventions, which address different questions about the effectiveness of EA.

## EA versus sham or weak EA, at true site

The basic question as to whether the electrical stimulation has any effect over and above the effect of needling (also called the 'specific' efficacy of electrical stimulation, or its efficacy beyond placebo) is addressed by comparing EA with either sham EA or weak EA given at the same sites. Assuming that the patients in both groups are successfully blinded, any difference in the outcome must be due to the electrical stimulation alone.

The table shows that there are only two studies with this design. Genuine EA was superior to weak EA in the treatment of chronic pain according to Mao, although the study was non-randomised and the sample size was small. EA was superior to sham EA in the treatment of diabetic neuropathy, but blinding could have been compromised since this was a crossover study.

## EA compared with manual acupuncture, at true site

In a study that compares EA with manual acupuncture without any pretence at EA apparatus, blinding is impossible. Therefore, this design tests the combination of specific effects of EA as well as its non-specific effects, which include factors such as patient expectation.

EA was superior for back pain in three studies, although in the first two studies the form of EA that was used was atypical. For neck pain, Lundeberg found no immediate analgesic effect of EA compared with MA, and another study, which was seriously limited by very small groups, found no difference between the effects of EA and MA. There was no difference between these forms of treatment for Sjögren's syndrome, for preventing dysmenorrhoea, or for postoperative nausea and vomiting. In the last study both treatments were superior to no treatment. EA was not superior to superficial needling of the correct points in the treatment of acute stroke, but neither intervention was more effective than standard treatment alone. Comparing EA with minimal acupuncture at true points, Emery used local skin prick as the control intervention in a study of ankylosing spondylitis, but this study is not convincing since the treatment course consisted of only three sessions, which seems very inadequate for a condition like ankylosing spondylitis.

## EA at true points compared with sham/weak EA at sham points

This design tests two variables at the same time: site and stimulation. If EA at the correct site is more effective than sham EA at the sham site, one can conclude in a general way that electrical stimulation has some effects, but it is not clear whether these effects occur only at acupuncture points. True-site EA was effective for nausea and for fibromyalgia in high-quality studies. True-site EA showed a small effect in asthma, but did not prove superior in studies for the treatment of chronic pancreatitis, for psoriasis, for stroke or in two studies on drug dependence. Though this evidence is promising and obviously justifies further research in nausea, fibromyalgia and asthma, the overall balance of results is negative. It is impossible to argue convincingly that those trials that were negative chose inappropriate conditions, or tested an inappropriate form of EA.

## EA compared with active TENS, at the same site

This design comparing EA with active transcutaneous electrical acupoint stimulation (TENS) tests the effect of the needle insertion, and participants cannot be blinded. Any difference between the outcomes in the two groups could be a combination of the specific effects and the expectations that patients and therapists have of needles compared with rubber pads. Only one study, in the treatment of back pain, found EA to be superior. One study found a strong trend that was not statistically significant in treating nausea, and the remaining three found no difference for chronic pain, back pain and osteoarthritis. Both EA and TENS were superior to the drug meperidine for postoperative pain, but this report is difficult to interpret.

## EA compared with superficial needling

Superficial needling is often used as a sham treatment in trials of manual acupuncture, but it is not very appropriate for testing EA as there are many differences between the interventions. Any difference in the outcomes could be due to the electrical stimulation, the needle site, the depth of insertion, possibly needle stimulation by hand, and the expectations of the participants. No difference was in fact shown in any of the studies for a variety of indications including stroke, neck pain, tinnitus, smoking cessation and postmenopausal symptoms.

## EA at true points versus EA at sham points or wrong points

This design was the most frequently found. At first sight it looks like a test of the effect of EA, because naturally EA has to be given at the appropriate points. However, strictly speaking it is also a test of needling correct sites: the needles themselves might have an effect quite separate from the effects of electrical stimulation. Therefore positive results cannot be cited as rigorous evidence in support of EA. We have combined the studies that use sham points with those that use wrong points in this review, although it is possible that they have different effects. In three studies of addiction, EA at the correct points was superior but in one it was no different. The correct point treatment was also superior for nausea, for osteoarthritis of the knee, for neck pain, and for preparation for colonoscopy. It did not prove superior for back pain or, using auricular points, for postmeniscectomy pain. The balance of this evidence, some of it of high quality, is therefore in favour of the effectiveness of needling correct points.

## EA versus standard medication

Several studies have compared EA with standard medication: it was better than methadone withdrawal from heroin in one study, but inferior to standard medical detoxification in a second. It was not as effective as cinnarizine for tinnitus, although this is difficult to interpret since cinnarizine is not a generally accepted medication for tinnitus. Two studies found EA no different from medication for postoperative nausea, in one case cyclizine and in the other prochlorperazine. Similarly, EA appeared to be no different from amitriptyline in the effect on depression in all three studies for this condition, though lack of clear diagnostic criteria and other quality problems prevent firm conclusions. Evidence from a single trial of moderate quality suggests that EA can enable patients with schizophrenia to reduce their antipsychotic medication without adversely affecting the clinical outcome. EA with standard medication was better than standard medication alone for angina.

Several studies on pain during and after surgery have compared EA with standard analgesics: it was either no different or superior to standard treatment with fentanyl, or with opioids for preoperative pain. For postoperative pain, it was superior to pentazocine and to opioids in one study, and no different in another. On its own, EA was inferior to lidocaine (lignocaine) for dental surgery but the combination of EA and lidocaine was best of all.

## EA versus standard care

Other studies have compared EA plus standard care with standard care alone for a variety of indications. This is a pragmatic design that tests the effect of integrating EA in normal therapy, but any benefit may be simply due to the placebo effect. For drug dependence, two studies comparing EA with medical withdrawal reached opposite conclusions. For alcohol withdrawal, EA was superior to standard counselling in the short term, but this difference was not maintained and may have been a chance finding. EA was superior to exercises for back pain, superior to splint for temporomandibular joint pain, and probably better than physiotherapy for neck pain, although the study concerned is not easy to interpret. EA was equivalent to hypnotherapy for male impotence, and inferior to biofeedback for tinnitus. For postoperative pain, EA was superior to standard care in two studies, but this result was not confirmed in a third. EA was no different from standard medication for depression, schizophrenia or angina.

## Other comparisons

Scarsella and colleagues found that, for surgery, giving EA at local points in addition to LI-4 was superior to using LI-4 alone. A few studies have compared low-frequency with high-frequency EA. Thomas and colleagues found EA at 2 Hz superior to 100 Hz in the long-term treatment of back pain, but the same was not true for dysmenorrhoea or for short-term relief of neck pain. EA appeared, in one study, to have a similar effect to moxibustion on breech presentation and both were superior to no treatment. EA was better than no intervention in five other studies, relating to alcohol dependence, nausea, temporomandibular pain, and urinary incontinence.

Other studies tested EA as an adjunctive therapy, in which standard care was given to both groups. EA was superior to standard rehabilitation for stroke patients in three studies but not in another more recent one. EA was a useful adjunct in treatment of neurogenic bladder.

# CONCLUSION

On balance, the present evidence from clinical trials does not provide support for the therapeutic value of EA as used in clinical practice. This appears to be 'lack of evidence' rather than 'lack of effect': the only two trials that used the ideal design, comparing EA with placebo EA at correct sites, appear to suggest that EA does have an effect, though this evidence is not high quality. A number of the studies have been performed in medical conditions that are highly resistant to other forms of treatment, such as tinnitus, chemical dependency or chronic pain; such trials may be performed more out of consideration for desperate patients than as a realistic trial of EA. Large trials that compare EA and sham EA for potentially responsive conditions such as nausea or osteoarthritis of the knee should provide more firm evidence for the role of EA in clinical care.

## SUMMARY

Some key points in this chapter are:

- There are insufficient studies in most conditions to allow a conclusion on the effectiveness of EA
- For surgical and postoperative pain the balance of evidence suggests that EA is no less effective than standard analgesics, and better than no treatment
- EA may be superior to sham EA given at sham sites, at least for some conditions, but there is no evidence that it is superior to superficial needling

- EA at the correct sites does seem superior to EA given at incorrect sites, although this effect may be due to the needle alone
- EA appears no different from amitriptyline for depression
- Overall, the evidence is promising but not sufficient to be able to conclude that EA has significant clinical effects.

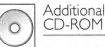 Additional material in the CD-ROM resource

The CD-ROM version of this chapter expands slightly on the studies of EA for surgical and procedural analgesia, but is otherwise almost identical to this.

# RECOMMENDED READING

*A masterly review that remains largely up to date:*
Thompson JW 1998 Transcutaneous electrical nerve stimulation (TENS). In: Filshie J, White A (eds) Medical Acupuncture: A Western scientific approach. Churchill Livingstone, Edinburgh, 177–92

*A refreshing look at the modern approach to acupuncture:*
Ulett GA 1992 Beyond Yin and Yang: How acupuncture really works. Warren H Green, St Louis, MO

*A systematic survey of the topic of EA, though does not include the latest findings:*
White A 1998 Electroacupuncture and acupuncture analgesia. In: Filshie J, White A (eds) Medical Acupuncture: A Western scientific approach. Churchill Livingstone, Edinburgh, 153–75

**Table 8.1** Clinical studies

| Topic and Reference | R | BAS | DRO | BLI | N = | Points used | Parameters | Duration (total no) | Control (s) | Main measure(s) | Results* sig only | FU | Comments |
|---|---|---|---|---|---|---|---|---|---|---|---|---|---|
| *Addiction* | | | | | | | | | | | | | |
| *Smoking cessation* | | | | | | | | | | | | | |
| Parker 1977 | + | − | + | (+) | 41 | Auric (Lung, shenmen) | 2/100 Hz | 20' (6) | 1) Wrong pt + EA 2) True pt press needle 3) Wrong pt press needle | Reported abstinence | No difference | 6 wks | |
| Martin 1981 | (+) | − | + | − | 128 | Auric (Lung, shenmen) + LI-4 | 4 Hz, 0.05 ms (LI-4) | 20' (1) | Auric | Reported abstinence | No difference | 6 mths | Indwelling needle |
| Waite & Clough 1998 | + | + | + | + | 78 | Auric (Lung) | 4 Hz | 20' (1) | Sham + EA | Urinary cotinine | True pts > sham pts | 6 mths | Indwelling needle |
| He 1997 | + | + | + | − | 46 | Auric (3), body (3) | 3 Hz,0.1 ms (body) | 20' (6) | Wrong pt + EA | Serum cotinine | True pts > wrong pts | 3 wks | Indwelling needle |
| White 1998 | + | + | + | + | 76 | Auric (Lung) | 100 Hz | 20' (3) | Sham pt + sham EA | Withdrawal symptoms | No difference | 14 days | |
| *Heroin alcohol withdrawal* | | | | | | | | | | | | | |
| Leung 1977 | + | − | + | + | 18 | Auric (Lung), SP-6 | 125 Hz | 20–40' (8) | Sham pt + sham EA | Response | No difference | None | Trend in favour of EA; pilot study, difficult to interpret |
| *Heroin withdrawal* | | | | | | | | | | | | | |
| Wen & Teo 1975 | − | (+) | + | − | 70 | Auric (Lung), SP-6 | 125 Hz | 30' (twice daily) | Methadone withdrawal | Urinary drug | EA > methadone | 12 mths | |
| Tennant 1976 | − | + | + | − | 54 | Auric concha | 7 Hz | 15–20' (daily) | Medical detoxification | Morphine withdrawal score | EA < medical detox | None | Staple used; high dropout rate |
| *Alcohol withdrawal* | | | | | | | | | | | | | |
| Rampes 1997 | + | + | + | + | 59 | Auric (3) | 100 Hz | 30' (6) | 1) Wrong pts + EA 2) Nil** | Craving score | True pts = wrong pts > nil (8 wks) | 6 mths | No difference at 24 wks |
| *ENT* | | | | | | | | | | | | | |
| *Tinnitus* | | | | | | | | | | | | | |
| Marks 1984 | + | (+) | + | + | 14 | Body, auric | 6–10/100 Hz | 20' (2) | Skin prick (sham pt) | VAS, tinnitus matching | No difference | None | Crossover, 3 wk washout; results not supported by other measures |
| Podoshin 1991 | + | + | + | − | 60 | Body, auric | 6–10/100 Hz | 30' (10) | 1) Biofeedback 2) Cinnarizine 3) Placebo biofeedback 4) Placebo tablets | Severity rating | Biofeedback > EA > other groups | None | Small group size |
| *Neurosensory deafness* | | | | | | | | | | | | | |
| Yarnell 1976 | − | 0 | + | − | 38 | SI-19, SJ-21, GB-2, LI-4 | 8–10 Hz, 0.5 ms | ?? (10–20) | Untreated ear | Audiogram | No difference | None | |
| *Sjögren's syndrome* | | | | | | | | | | | | | |
| List 1998 | + | (−) | + | − | 21 | Local, body (14) | 2 Hz | 30' (20) | MA | Salivary secretion | No difference | None | |

*Continued*

**Table 8.1** Clinical studies—cont'd

| Topic and Reference | R | BAS | DRO | BLI | N = | Points used | Parameters | Duration (total no) | Control(s) | Main measure(s) | Results* sig only | FU | Comments |
|---|---|---|---|---|---|---|---|---|---|---|---|---|---|
| **Gastrointestinal** | | | | | | | | | | | | | |
| *Constipation* | | | | | | | | | | | | | |
| Klauser 1993 | – | 0 | + | – | 8 | BL-25, LIV-3, LI-4, ST-25 | 10 Hz | 25' (6) | Nil** | Stool frequency, transit time | No difference | None | Crossover study, control first |
| *Nausea (chemotherapy)* | | | | | | | | | | | | | |
| Dundee 1987 | + | 0 | – | – | 10 | P-6 | 10 Hz, 0.25 ms | ?? (3–5) | Sham pt + EA | Sickness | True pt > sham pt | None | Multiple crossover |
| Shen 2000 | + | + | + | + | 104 | P-6, ST-36 | 2–10 Hz 0.5–0.7 ms | 20' (5) | 1) Sham pts + sham EA 2) Nil** | Vomiting | EA > sham > nil | 9 days | |
| *Nausea (postoperative)* | | | | | | | | | | | | | |
| Ghaly 1987 | + | – | + | + | 31 | P-6 | 10 Hz, 0.25 ms | 5' (1) | 1) Nil 2) MA 3) cyclizine | Nausea and/or vomiting | EA = MA = cyclizine, all > nil | 6 hrs | EA 10 Hz for 15 min, and EA 1000 Hz increased nausea |
| Ho 1990 | + | + | 0 | – | 100 | P-6 | 3 Hz, 0.75 ms | 15' (1) | 1) Nil 2) TENS at P-6 3) Prochlorperazine | Vomiting | EA = drug = TENS; EA > nil | 3 hrs | |
| *Chronic pancreatitis pain* | | | | | | | | | | | | | |
| Ballegaard 1985 | – | 0 | + | + | 13 | Auric + body (100 Hz to segmental pts) | 2 Hz | 30' (5) | Sham pts + sham EA | Pain rating diary | No difference | None | |
| **Musculoskeletal** | | | | | | | | | | | | | |
| *Back pain (chronic)* | | | | | | | | | | | | | |
| Lehmann 1986 | + | – | + | – | 53 | Body | 2–4 Hz | 30' (6) | 1) TENS 2) Sham TENS | Summary score | No difference | 6 mths | |
| Edelist 1976 | + | – | – | + | 30 | BL-25, BL-57 | 3–10 Hz | 30' (3) | Sham pt + EA | Pain score; examination | No difference | None | |
| Lisenyuk 1992 | – | – | – | – | 75 | Periosteal | 3–100 Hz 0.1 ms | 25–30' (2–6) | MA | Time to discharge | EA > MA | None | Idiosyncratic therapy |
| Ghoname 1999 | + | 0 | – | – | 60 | Segmental (10) | 4 Hz, 0.5 ms | 30' (9 × 4) | 1) Needles (true pt) 2) TENS 3) Exercises | Pain score, activity | EA > needles, TENS and exercise | None | Idiosyncratic therapy; multiple crossover |
| Thomas 1994 | + | + | + | – | 30 | Selected from 6 local, 3–4 distal | 2 Hz | 30' (1 or 10) | 1) MA 2) EA 100 Hz | Activity, pain | EA 2 Hz > EA 100 Hz or MA | 6 mths | Patient preference after trial of all 3 |

| Study | | | | | n | Points | Stimulation | Time (sessions) | Control | Measure | Result | Follow-up | Comments |
|---|---|---|---|---|---|---|---|---|---|---|---|---|---|
| **Craniomandibular disorders** | | | | | | | | | | | | | |
| List 1992 | + | + | + | – | 110 | Local MA + EA to LI-4, ST-36 | 2–3 Hz, 0.2 ms | 30' (6–8) | 1) Splint 2) Nil | Symptom rating | EA > both controls | None | |
| **Fibromyalgia** | | | | | | | | | | | | | |
| Deluze 1992 | + | + | + | + | 70 | LI-4, ST-36 and 6 other body | 1–99 Hz scan | 30' (6) | Sham pt + weak EA | Pain threshold | EA > sham | None | |
| **Knee osteoarthritis** | | | | | | | | | | | | | |
| Yurtkuran 1999 | + | + | + | + | 100 | GB-34, ST-34, ST-35, SP-9 | 4 Hz, 0.1 ms | 20' (10) | 1) TENS 2) ice 3) sham TENS | Pain, stiffness | All interventions > sham TENS | None | Some patients from pain analysis |
| **Rheumatoid arthritis (knee)** | | | | | | | | | | | | | |
| Man 1974 | – | – | – | + | 20 | GB-34, ST-43, SP-9 | ?? | 15' (1) | Sham pt + EA | Pain rating | True pts > sham pts for over 1 mth | 4 mths | Steroid injection to other knee |
| **Neck pain/arthritis** | | | | | | | | | | | | | |
| Emery 1986 | + | 0 | – | + | 10 | 'Standard' (6) | 'Low frequency' | 20' (3) | Skin prick (true pt) | Range of movement, pain | No difference | None | Ankylosing spondylitis; crossover study; 3 wk washout |
| Loy 1983 | – | (+) | + | – | 60 | Body (2–6) | 'Intermittent, biphasic' | 30' (19) | Physiotherapy | Range of movement, global | EA 87% physio 54% improved | None | No statistics |
| Lundeberg 1991 | + | – | 0 | – | 58 | GB-20, LI-3, Du-14, Du-16, Du-20 | 2 Hz, 0.2 ms | 40' (1) | 1) MA 2) Superficial 3) EA 100 Hz | Pain rating, affective, sensory | No difference | None | Immediate effect only |
| Matsumoto 1974 | – | – | + | (+) | 24 | Most tender | ?? | 5' (3–10) | 1) MA true pt 2) EA sham pts (3–5) other combinations | Index of pain, activity etc | EA = MA; true pt > sham pt | None | Group size = 4 |
| **Pain (chronic musculoskeletal)** | | | | | | | | | | | | | |
| Cheng 1987 | (+) | – | – | – | 131 | 'Standard' (6) | 4/100 Hz, 0.1 ms | 20' (up to 12) | TENS (Codetron) | Pain relief | No difference | 4–8 mths | Wide range of conditions; TENS superior at FU |

*Continued*

**Table 8.1** Clinical studies—cont'd

| Topic and Reference | R | BAS | DRO | BLI | N = | Points used | Parameters | Duration (total no) | Control (s) | Main measure(s) | Results* sig only | FU | Comments |
|---|---|---|---|---|---|---|---|---|---|---|---|---|---|
| Mao 1980 | – | + | + | – | 26 | Appropriate | 8–15 Hz, 40 ms | 45' (7) | Weak EA (true pts) | Pain, activity | EA > weak EA | 2 wks | First arm of crossover study |
| Shinohara 1986 | – | | | – | 117 | Local pts (6–8) | 3 Hz, 0.5 ms | ??' (1) | 1) MA 2) direct current EA (7s) | Numerical pain scale, 3 days | No statistical comparison | None | Trend appears in favour of EA |
| *Neurological* | | | | | | | | | | | | | |
| *Acute stroke* | | | | | | | | | | | | | |
| Hu 1993 | + | + | + | – | 30 | Scalp, body | 9.4 Hz (scalp), DD (body) | 10' scalp, 20' body (14) | Nil** | Neuro deficit, Barthel | EA > nil for neuro deficit only | None | Non-significant trend in favour of EA |
| Naeser 1992 | + | + | + | + | 16 | Body, scalp, auric | 1–2 Hz (limb + scalp) | 20' (20) | Sham pt + sham EA | Motor evaluation | No difference | None | |
| Gosman-Hedström 1998 | + | (+) | + | + | 104 | Body (10) | 2 Hz (limb) | 30' (20) | 1) Superficial 2) Nil** | Neuro score, Barthel | No difference | 12 mths | |
| Johansson 1993 | + | + | + | – | 78 | Body (10) | 2–4 Hz (limb) | ??' (20) | Nil** | Nottingham Health Profile | EA > nil | 12 mths | |
| Si 1998 | + | + | + | + | 42 | P-6, LIV-3, LI-4, SP-6, Du-20, Du-24 | 5/45 Hz | 30' (until discharge) | Nil** | Chinese Stroke Scale | EA > nil | None | |
| *Diabetic peripheral neuropathy* | | | | | | | | | | | | | |
| Hamza 2000 | + | + | + | – | 50 | Nerve + segment pts (10) | 15/30 Hz, 0.5 ms | 30' (9) | True point, EA turned off | Pain VAS, SF36 | EA > control | None | Crossover, 1 wk washout |
| *Neurogenic bladder* | | | | | | | | | | | | | |
| Cheng 1998 | + | + | + | – | 60 | BL-32, Ren-3, Ren-4 | 20–30 Hz, 0.2 ms | 15' (as required) | Nil** | Time to bladder control | EA > nil | None | Early spinal injury |
| *Peripheral nerve injury* | | | | | | | | | | | | | |
| Hao 1995 | – | – | – | – | 108 | Local pts | 3 regimes each session | 30' (30) | Oral vitamins | Electromyography, sensation | EA > control | None | No outcome data |
| *Obstetrics and gynaecology* | | | | | | | | | | | | | |
| *Breech correction* | | | | | | | | | | | | | |
| Li 1996 | + | – | + | – | 111 | BL-67 | ?? | 30' (daily up to 6) | 1) Moxa 2) Nil | Version to vertex | EA = moxa, both > nil | None | |

| Study | | | | | n | Points | Frequency | Duration (n) | Control | Measure | Result | Follow-up | Comments |
|---|---|---|---|---|---|---|---|---|---|---|---|---|---|
| *Postmenopausal symptoms* Wyon 1995 | + | – | + | – | 24 | Body (12) | 2 Hz (some) | 30' (10) | Superficial acup | Diary of flushes | No difference | 3 mths | Crossover + free choice final mth |
| *Dysmenorrhoea* Thomas 1995 | + | 0 | + | – | 19 | BL-32, SP-6, SP-9, Ren-4 | 2 Hz | 20' (2 each) | 1) MA 2) EA 100 Hz 3) Periosteal acup | Pain score, choice of mode | No difference | 3 mths | |
| *Incontinence* Kubista 1976 | – | – | (–) | – | 60 | BL-57, KI-11, ST-36, Ren-6 | 8 Hz 0.5 ms | 30' (1) | 1) Nil 2) Placebo suppository | Urethral-closing pressure | EA > both controls | None | EA superior on some items |
| **Psychiatric** | | | | | | | | | | | | | |
| *Depression* Yang 1994 | + | – | – | – | 41 | Body (11–13) | 80–100 Hz (some) | ?' (36) | Amitriptyline | Hamilton | No difference | 6 wks | Multicentre study |
| Luo 1985 | + | + | – | – | 47 | Du-20, yintang (M-HN-3) | 1.3–1.5 Hz | 60' (30) | Amitriptyline | Hamilton | No difference | None | |
| Lou 1990 | + | + | – | – | 241 | Du-20, yintang (M-HN-3) | 2 Hz | 45' (36) | Amitriptyline | Hamilton | No difference | 2–4 yrs | |
| *Schizophrenia* Zhou 1997 | + | – | – | + | 40 | Body EA + reduced drugs | 180 Hz, 0.5 ms | 15' (36) | Standard medication | Clinical rating scales | No difference | None | Fewer adverse effects in EA group |
| **Respiratory** | | | | | | | | | | | | | |
| *Asthma* Christensen 1984 | + | + | – | + | 17 | BL-13, LI-4, Ren-17, Ex-17 (dingchuan, M-BW-1) | 4/100 Hz | 20' (10) | Sham pts + sham EA | Peak flow, medication | EA > sham at 2 wks only | None | Modest, temporary effect |
| **Surgery** | | | | | | | | | | | | | |
| Brandwein 1976 | + | – | 0 | – | 184 | Appropriate local + distal | ?? | During | 1) Lidocaine injection 2) EA + lidocaine | Pain rating | Combination > lidocaine > EA | None | Dental root surgery |
| Cahn 1978 | + | – | + | + | 90 | 10 body | 12 Hz, 10 ms | 10' before + during | Sham pt + EA | Ease; symptoms | True pts > sham pts | None | Gastroscopy |
| Taub 1979 | + | – | 0 | + | 51 | LI-4 | 60 Hz | 20' + during | Non-penetrating + EA | Dentist and pnt rating of analgesia | No difference | None | Dental surgery; control needle non-penetrating |

*Continued*

**Table 8.1** Clinical studies—cont'd

| Topic and Reference | R | BAS | DRO | BLI | N = | Points used | Parameters | Duration (total no) | Control (s) | Main measure(s) | Results* sig only | FU | Comments |
|---|---|---|---|---|---|---|---|---|---|---|---|---|---|
| Masuda 1986 | − | + | 0 | − | 24 | SJ-6, GB-14, LI-4, ST-2 | 2–3 Hz | 30' + during | Standard anaesthesia | Fentanyl requirement | EA better than standard | 1 wk | Retinal detachment |
| Kho 1991 | + | + | + | − | 29 | Body and auric | 10 Hz, 0.7 ms | 30' + during | Standard fentanyl | Fentanyl requirement | EA better than standard | 6 days | Retroperitoneal lymph node dissection |
| Scarsella 1994 | − | − | 0 | − | 200 | LI-4, local | 60–350 Hz | 25' after | EA at LI-4 only | Pain rating | EA local pts > EA LI-4 only | None | Dental surgery |
| Poulain 1997 | + | + | 0 | − | 250 | P-6, GB-39, SP-6, auric (shenmen) | 40 Hz | 20–25 min | Standard analgesia | Need for fentanyl | EA superior | 5 days | Cancer surgery; EA also superior for recovery |
| Wang 1997 | + | + | + | − | 59 | ST-36, ST-37 | 2 Hz | 20–25 min | Meperidine 50 mg | Pain rating | No difference | None | Colonoscopy; EA fewer side-effects |
| Stener-Victorin 1999 | + | + | 0 | − | 150 | LI-4, SJ-5, ST-29, ST-36, Du-20 | 2/80 Hz, 0.2 ms (ST-29 100 Hz) | 30' before + during | Alfentanil IV | Pain rating | No difference | 2 hrs | Oocyte aspiration |
| *Postoperative analgesia* | | | | | | | | | | | | | |
| Strom 1977 | + | − | − | + | 21 | Auric (Knee) | 2 Hz | 2' (1) | EA auric (shoulder) | Flexion, extension | No difference | 1 wk | Meniscectomy; group with poor extension improved more with EA |
| Facco 1981 | + | + | 0 | − | 34 | GB-26, ST-36, SP-6, auric (shenmen) | 5–10–15–50 Hz | 40' preop | Pentazocine 30 mg | Pain relief; lung function | Pain no difference; function EA superior | 5 hrs | Hysterectomy |
| Martelete 1985 | + | − | − | − | 72 | Appropriate for operation | 1 Hz | Postop, 30'(1) | 1) Drug (meperidine) 2) TENS | Pain rating | EA and TENS > drug | 2 hrs | Results difficult to interpret |
| Lapeer 1987 | + | − | − | − | 18 | LI-4, SP-6 | 0.6 Hz | During + 15' after | Pethidine inj + N₂O | Pain rating + drug diary | No difference | 10 days | Dental surgery |
| Wang 1988 | + | − | − | − | 36 | Auric (Lung and sanjiao) | 2–20 Hz | 10' (twice daily × 14) | Nil** | Coughing pain, lung function | EA > nil | 7 days | Thoracotomy; all pts injected with vitamin B after EA |
| Christensen 1989 | + | + | + | + | 20 | BL-32, Du-2, Du-4 | 10/100 Hz, 0.32 ms | ?? (1) | Nil** | Pethidine requirement | EA > nil | 3 hrs | Major gynae surgery; EA from wound closure |
| Christensen 1993 | + | + | + | − | 50 | BL-32, ST-36, SP-6, Du-2, Du-4 | 10/100 Hz, 0.32 ms | Per-op (1) | Nil** | Pethidine requirement | No difference | 4 hrs | Major gynae surgery; EA started preop |

| | | | | | n | | | | | | | | |
|---|---|---|---|---|---|---|---|---|---|---|---|---|---|
| *Miscellaneous* | | | | | | | | | | | | | |
| *Angina* | | | | | | | | | | | | | |
| Zamotrinsky 1997 | + | + | + | – | 20 | Auric (Heart) | 3 Hz, 1.5 ms | 15' (10) | Nil** | Angina attacks, exercise ECG | EA > nil | Up to 21 days | Also biochemical marker |
| *Male impotence* | | | | | | | | | | | | | |
| Aydin 1997 | + | – | + | – | 60 | KI-6, ST-30, ST-36, Ren-4, Ren-6 | 3 Hz | 20' (12) | 1) Hypnotic suggestion 2) Oral vitamin placebo | Verbal report | No difference | 3–12 mths | |
| *Psoriasis* | | | | | | | | | | | | | |
| Jerner 1997 | + | + | + | + | 56 | Body + auric | 10–20 Hz | 20' (20) | Sham pt + sham EA | PASI score | No difference | 3 mths | |

Note: full details of the references listed can be found on the CD-ROM companion to this book.

Abbreviations: BAS = baseline variables compared; BLI = assessor blind; DRO = dropouts and withdrawals reported; FU = follow-up after intervention; NS = no significant difference (re-analysis); pnt = patient; pt = point; R = randomised.
+ Criterion met, – criterion not met, () criterion not applicable or partly met.
?? Insufficient information.
**Patients in all groups also received standard therapy.
†Some information from duplicate publication (Luo 1998).

# CHAPTER
# Nine

## Acupuncture in clinical practice: an overview

## 9.1 PSYCHOLOGICAL AND NERVOUS CONDITIONS

Acupuncture, working at the interface of body and mind, can affect both of these. In this subchapter, psychological conditions are considered first, and then central nervous system disorders.

## PSYCHOLOGICAL CONDITIONS

### Anxiety

Morbid or chronic anxiety is common, sometimes taking the form of panic attacks. It can aggravate somatic problems, and is often associated with increased muscle tension.

Although acupuncture has often been used as a treatment for anxiety, it is surprising how few electroacupuncture (EA) or transcutaneous electrical/acupoint stimulation (TENS/TEAS) studies there are on anxiety. These methods have been used for exam nerves, and for anxiety as a concomitant of chronic fatigue syndrome; they may also reduce anxiety associated with conditions such as chronic pain or depression, or during drug or alcohol withdrawal. EA and TEAS appear to have comparable effects on anxiety, with TEAS more acceptable and effective for some patients.

**Points used** In traditional Chinese Medicine terms, there are different sorts of anxiety and various point combinations may be used. *Dumai* vessel points may be particularly useful, while cranial electrotherapy stimulation (CES) generally uses points either side of the head, rather than along the midline.

**Parameters used** From the EA studies on anxiety, no conclusions can be drawn on optimum parameters. However, from what is known about the rapid onset of high-frequency (HF, ~100 Hz) stimulation effects, and the anxiolytic benefits of non-painful stimulation, gentle 100 Hz currents

may be appropriate. Low-intensity stimulation at ~10 Hz, or even 0.5 Hz, has been used with CES.

### Phobias

Phobias are a particular form of anxiety. A simple protocol, for either manual acupuncture (MA) or microcurrent pTENS (handheld probe), has been developed by Corinne Groom. TEAS too has been used in the treatment of phobias.

**Points used** It may be sufficient to use very simple major points, such as KI-3, LIV-3, ST-36 and the auricular 'Fear' point on the dominant side (Groom), or LI-4 and Du-20 (Yamashita) to treat phobia.

**Parameters used** Weak- or moderate-intensity low-frequency (LF) stimulation may be appropriate.

### Depression

Depression affects many people at some stage in their lives. It may occur alone, or in association with other conditions or events, including virtually any chronic illness, cancer, menstrual disorders, childbirth, menopause, or drug abuse or withdrawal.

Acupuncture has often been used as a treatment for depression, with EA, CES, TENS and laser acupuncture (LA) all being used to treat depression associated with other conditions, particularly drug and alcohol abuse and withdrawal. EA and CES have also been used for various forms of depression on its own, as has millimetre wave acupoint irradiation (microwave resonance therapy, MRT, or extremely-high-frequency stimulation, EHF).

**Points used** Nine studies from the same group of researchers predominantly used points on the cranial portion of the Governor Vessel. Auricular points were used in one study. CES often uses non-specific auricular application.

**Parameters used** LF EA has been used predominantly when treating depression; ~100 Hz is more common in CES studies.

## Manic-depressive psychosis

EA and MA have both been used in the treatment of the depressive phase of drug-resistant manic depression, with MA possibly being more effective. Although mania is commonly mentioned in standard TCM textbooks, EA should probably be used only cautiously during manic phases of bipolar depression.

## Schizophrenia

Schizophrenia generally involves psychotic delusions and auditory or somatic hallucinations. It can occur at any age from adolescence onwards, but only 25% of cases progress to chronic schizophrenia. Symptoms of schizophrenia may be associated with mania or depression (as in schizoaffective disorder), but schizoid and paranoid personality types should not be confused with schizophrenia as such.

Acupuncture has been used for the treatment of schizophrenia or its accompanying hallucinations, with the suggestion that the more frequent the attacks and the more chronic the condition, the less effective the treatment becomes. EA and LA in particular have both been used, with EA and TEAS giving similar results in one study.

Despite the usual methodological criticisms of Chinese studies, reviewers have concluded that both needle acupuncture (MA or EA) and LA may be effective in the treatment of schizophrenia. EA has even been used in instances of what traditionally would have been considered as transitory 'possession' by some unwelcome entity.

CES has also been used as an adjunctive therapy in chronic schizophrenia.

**Points used** Treatment is predominantly to the head, on the Governor Vessel (Du-15, Du-20, *qinxu*, *yintang*), or the Small Intestine (SI-19), *sanjiao* (SJ-15, SJ-17, SJ-19, SJ-21), or Gall Bladder (GB-15, GB-18) meridians, at extra points (*taiyang*) or scalp points. Additional points for specific syndromes are rarely mentioned, although SJ-21 and SJ-17 have been used for auditory hallucinations.

**Parameters used** At least two studies used extremely strong EA stimulation (up to 60 mA in one, and sufficient to cause head and neck spasm in the other). LF or HF frequency appears to have been used (at strong intensities in the same two studies), but insufficient detail is available from most reports to draw any general conclusions on usage. As for LA, very-low-power HeNe has been most used, with the laser sometimes held a considerable distance from the treated point.

## Neurosis

Neurosis differs from psychosis in that the ability to distinguish reality from fantasy is unimpaired, even if symptoms are out of proportion to external circumstances. These symptoms may be somatic or psychological and can blight behaviour and social relationships. Hysterical neurosis may involve various physical 'conversion symptoms' that do not match those of known somatic illnesses.

Acupuncture has been used for various neurotic conditions. In particular, there have been attempts to treat neurosis or its manifestations using EA and CES. There is also a long history of using electrotherapy in the treatment of hysterical paralysis. EA or TEAS is quite often used for this condition, whereas CES has been employed for 'chronic hysteria'.

**Points used** For hysterical paralysis, KI-1 has been used, together with points on the paralysed limb. For obsessive–compulsive disorder, points on the head have been used.

**Parameters used** Strong if not painful stimulation was used in studies on hysterical fainting and paralysis, but more gentle stimulation for obsessional neuroses. However, stronger stimulation may aggravate neurotic conditions. This may occur with EA, as well as CES, particularly with higher frequencies (40–60 Hz as against 5–15 Hz, for example).

## Sleep disorders

As well as insomnia, which affects huge numbers of people, there are other extreme forms of sleep disturbances: somnambulism (sleep walking), night terrors (in children, particularly) and narcolepsy (irresistible drowsiness occurring several times daily). Sleep pattern and quality are important indicators of internal equilibrium and health. Both may worsen with age.

Acupuncture and related interventions seem to be particularly helpful to the disturbed sleep–wake cycle, with improved sleep a 'beneficial side-effect' in many studies of acupuncture. In particular, EA has been found to improve the disturbed sleep that occurs with or following drug withdrawal. EA to reduce pain during surgery may likewise improve postoperative sleep. Most types of acupuncture have been used to treat insomnia, including EA, TEAS, LA and magnets or copper/zinc metal contacts applied to acupoints.

An interesting application of EA has been in preventive or remedial treatment for shift workers, pilots or those on long sea voyages. 'Magnetic acupuncture' has also been used for computer operators doing shift work. EA has been used as a treatment for somnambulism.

CES has also been used to treat sleep disturbance problems. As with EA, somnolence during CES treatment has been reported, as well as changes in sleep pattern when CES is used for other conditions, particularly drug withdrawal.

Other electrotherapy methods for sleep problems include microwave auriculotherapy, EHF acupoint stimulation and so forth. Eeman's circuits can also be used.

**Comparisons** Acupoint probe stimulation (pTENS) and MA gave comparable results in one study, although the former took effect more rapidly, while the brief stimulation required was more acceptable to patients. In several reports on the use of both EA (percutaneous electrical nerve stimulation, PENS) and MA for low back pain, sleep quality improved more with EA than MA. EA was also more effective than TEAS for disturbed sleep in one schizophrenia study.

**Points used** The few EA and LA studies clearly favour the use of cranial or auricular points, as in CES, with the occasional addition of HE-7, traditionally for insomnia, or other major points such as LI-4. The magnet and copper/zinc contact studies use body points, such as back *shu* points together with major points such as GB-34 and SP-6, or the master and coupled points of the eight extra meridians.

**Parameters used** Given the association of delta EEG frequencies (0.5–3 Hz) and deep sleep, one would expect LF stimulation to be used predominantly. However, dense-disperse (DD) mode and frequency scanning (pulsed, however, at LF) have also been used. In the CES studies, 100 Hz is, as so often, the most common frequency, although two studies used 30–40 Hz, another 350 Hz. Two that did make use of lower frequencies (Achté 5–10 Hz, and Frankel 15 Hz) reported negative results. Robiner, testing 6, 10, 12 and 18 Hz, noted that, whatever frequency was applied, the brain responded in much the same way (with frequencies of 5–6 Hz in subcortical structures and 8–10 Hz in the cortex).

## Stress and relaxation

Stress and anxiety are closely related. Generally, we can adapt to a certain amount, depending on our make-up and lifestyle, but if we become overwhelmed by stress, any number of different conditions can ensue, from chronic pain to gastrointestinal upset, asthma, high blood pressure, insomnia, and depression. Muscular tension and acupoint/ trigger point (TrP) tenderness may be an early warning sign of stress.

Many experimental studies show beneficial effects of EA on stress-induced symptoms, including acute emotional stress, cardiac arrhythmia and ventricular fibrillation, raised blood pressure and viscosity, gastrointestinal dysfunction and immune deficit. Similar benefits have been reported for CES and acupoint MRT.

Relaxation is often a key to preventing the effects of stress. The monotonous rhythm of LF stimulation, as in EA, may be particularly relaxing. EA has been used to relax patients with pain problems and to counter work-related stress, and even that induced by fasting. As with anxiety, though, it is surprising how few studies have specifically addressed the effects of EA on stress. More attention has been given to stress and relaxation in studies on electroacupuncture analgesia (EAA), where EA, possibly more than MA, may have a role in reducing the effects of stress, as well as intra- and postoperative pain.

EA and TENS/TEAS have been found to have a relaxing effect in dental work and childbirth. Many authors have reported that EAA reduces the stress response of patients undergoing surgery (and even of the fetus, during labour). Some studies have also indicated beneficial changes in biochemical stress measures, suggesting that *combining* acupuncture analgesia (AA) (or TENS) with standard neuroleptanalgesia may be particularly useful.

CES is an anxiolytic and relaxing treatment. Like EA and TENS, it has been used in the treatment of stress, including stress secondary to other medical conditions. It has been used for its relaxing effects in the treatment of drug withdrawal, as well as of non-abstinent alcoholism. As with EA, it has found a place as a preventive treatment for work-related stress.

**Points used** Major points for relaxation such as LI-4 and LIV-3, the 'Four Gates' (*siguan*), are obvious candidates here. MRT has been applied at points on head and neck (GB-20, BL-10, SI-16, for example). Bilateral auricular or mastoid stimulation is the rule in CES. An interesting variant on standard EA practice is Allen Chen's method of treating points sequentially, starting at the head (with Du-20 and *yintang*) and working downwards in repeated sweeps, using major points such as GB-20, P-6 or P-7, ST-36 and KI-3 (bilaterally).

**Parameters used** Some authors have sought to correlate LF stimulation, LF electroencephalogram (EEG) and relaxation (a 'parasympathetic' response), and HF stimulation, HF EEG and activation (a 'sympathetic' response). Thus LF EA, as well as 0.5 Hz CES, has been used for relaxation and stress treatments. However, HF CES has also been used, and others have found that in dental work, for instance, HF (99 Hz) TENS may be experienced as more relaxing than LF. High-intensity LF (or HF) may well be experienced as stressful.

# DISORDERS OF THE CENTRAL NERVOUS SYSTEM

## Cognitive and behavioural dysfunction of presumed organic origin

### DOWN'S SYNDROME
Mental disability can sometimes be quite severe in this genetic disorder. There are clearly limits to what Chinese medicine can achieve, although in one controlled MA/EA study improvements in attention and memory were noted.

### MEMORY AND ATTENTION: ATTENTION DEFICIT DISORDER (ADD)
There is at least one anecdotal account of acupuncture improving concentration and memory in 'normal' schoolchildren, but very few reports of EA being used for ADD as such. However, TENS has been utilised for an attention deficit hyperactivity disorder case labelled as 'encephalitis', and CES for ADD, both primary and secondary.

**Points used** Kiran Phalke has used *yintang* and the auricular Hippocampus point in normal children. CES is applied bilaterally to or behind the ears. Scherder's group has applied TENS electrodes according to their standard protocol: paraspinally at T1–T5 level.

**Parameters used** ADD and attention deficit hyperactivity disorder (ADHD) may involve EEG 'low-frequency pathology', with deficits in the 12–14 Hz range. One CES study on

ADD, however, found no clear differences between results when using three completely different sorts of stimulation.

## NEURASTHENIA

Neurasthenia covers a group of symptoms resulting from some functional nervous system disorder, usually due to prolonged and excessive expenditure of energy. It is marked by a tendency to fatigue, lack of energy, back pain, memory loss, insomnia, constipation and loss of appetite. In TCM, neurasthenia involves disturbance of memory, cognition and sleep, with further symptoms according to syndrome differentiation.

Neurasthenia has been treated with EA, and also with magnets applied to acupoints. Electrosleep, the Russian precursor to CES, has been used for 'cardiovascular neurasthenia'.

**Parameters used** Meg Patterson has suggested that, in treating neurasthenia with CES, lower frequencies (5–10 Hz) should be used for 'hypersthenia' and higher frequencies (20–25 Hz) for 'hyposthenia'.

## HEAD INJURY

Following initial concussion and amnesia, chronic symptoms such as headache and dizziness, irritability, insomnia and poor concentration, anxiety or depression may develop. Chronic subdural haematoma may result in fluctuating changes in consciousness and impaired intellectual function.

Acupuncture (EA, LA, moxibustion) has been used in both acute and chronic stages of brain injury, with benefits even in quite severe cases (coma). CES has been applied after brain operations to improve mental function.

**Points and parameters used** There is little evidence as yet on optimum stimulation parameters. LF EA at head points has been used for coma.

## DEMENTIA

Some of the symptoms of dementia are very similar to those of depression, or those that result from head injury. Acupuncture has been studied for its effects on dementia, particularly the more remediable 'cerebrovascular dementia' due to arteriopathy rather than that due to degenerative disorders such as Alzheimer's disease or Huntington's chorea. Vascular dementia, whether due to atherosclerosis, multiple 'silent' infarcts deep within the brain or cervical problems, is a contributory cause in well over half of all cases of senile dementia, particularly in men. It is considered as a form of Wind-stroke in TCM.

The treatment of senile dementia has been explored by Scherder's Dutch group in a series of publications on TENS. Treatment may enhance some aspects of visual and verbal short-term and long-term memory and fluency, general behaviour and independence and rest–activity rhythm, but not necessarily affective functioning. Results are also short lived.

**Points used** Scalp points, and head points such as GB-20, Du-20 and *sishencong* (M-HN-1) have been used in studies of EA for dementia. Scherder's group applied a pair of TENS electrodes 2 cm either side of the spine, at the T1–T5 level,

this being one source of sympathetic afferents to the brainstem. Adjunctive points tend to be selected according to TCM principles, although ST-36 has been shown to be potentially useful in experimental research.

**Parameters used** Most researchers have used LF EA. Scherder's group has explored HF trains or alternating 2 Hz and 100 Hz every 90 minutes (TENS).

# Motor disorders originating in the central nervous system

## SPASTICITY

Spasticity may be characterised as an abnormal muscle state in which stretch reflexes are usually hyperactive, flexion reflexes are hyperactive, and dexterity and strength are decreased. It is the most common symptom of cerebral palsy, and is the result of damage to motor centres in the brain during late pregnancy, birth, or early infancy. It may be associated with other conditions as well.

Treatment of spasticity has become an important and well-documented specialty in electrotherapy. Electrical muscular stimulation (EMS) is often used to reduce spasticity, particularly when combined with physical therapy re-education. Acupuncture has been similarly combined, with both EMS and intensive rehabilitation. Umlauf has emphasised exercising the affected part *during* EA/LA. TENS and vibration may also be helpful. Whatever method is used, improvement is likely to be slow. Treatment may need to be continued for months, and for several hours at a time (overnight, for instance). If it is interrupted for long periods, benefits may be lost.

CES and auricular acupuncture, as well as scalp acupuncture, have been used in the treatment of spasticity. One group found that CES has greater effects on cerebral palsy spasticity when it is more severe.

Although there are few controlled studies of acupuncture for cerebral palsy, a number report good results with MA (scalp MA increases cerebral blood flow in these patients). Yoshiaki Omura, however, has suggested that EA may be more effective as a treatment for spasticity than either MA or TENS. Auricular EA may improve circulation in affected extremities, at least temporarily.

LA has often been used for cerebral palsy, sometimes in combination with magnetotherapy and other forms of acupuncture, usually with continuing rehabilitation. Better results are reported if treatment is started when children are younger. Low-power laser diodes can be used regularly at home, under practitioner supervision, by parents of young children.

EA, TEAS and LA have been used in the treatment of spinal spasticity. When spasticity is due to spinal cord injury (at or above T8), it can be associated with 'autonomic dysreflexia', with an abnormal tendency to raised blood pressure in response to stimulation, for example. Thus such patients should be monitored during treatment, particularly if already hypertensive.

**Points used** Cerebral palsy is the result of damage to motor regions in the brain. Thus the scalp motor area or other scalp points are often used. Different practitioners use different combinations of head and limb points. Thus Wojciech Filipowicz has applied LA, with a basic formula of LI-4, ST-36 and Governor Vessel points (Du-4, Du-14, Du-20), adding scalp and further body points for specific indications. Umlauf's basic LA formula involved Ren-24, Du-20 and the four points around it, *sishencong* (M-HN-1). Auricular stimulation is another possibility.

As a non-invasive alternative to spinal cord stimulation, EA has been used at Governing Vessel points (together with distal points on leg *yang* meridians and other major points, such as HE-5, and LI-4/LIV-3). Both LA and TENS have been applied at paraspinal segmental points (Margaret Naeser recommends points along the Bladder meridian, for example).

EA and TENS have also been applied at limb points alone, in part for their local effect. In general, intramuscular needling may have more of an effect on spasticity than shallow needling; submotor threshold stimulation of muscle *tendons* may be particularly helpful. With EMS, heterosegmental may be more effective than segmental stimulation.

**Parameters used** In the 1950s, strong tetanic stimulation was used to relax spastic muscles, particularly after spinal injury. More recently, less forceful methods have been used. For instance, tetanising frequencies of around 100 Hz may be used to fatigue and relax the spastic muscle directly, and lower frequencies (individual pulses) to stimulate weakened antagonist muscles. Interrupted trains are popular, for instance frequency 50 Hz, pulse duration 0.5 ms at low intensity (on and off for 2 seconds), or 33 Hz, 0.2 ms (on 7 seconds, off 10 seconds), or 30 Hz, 0.3 ms (5 seconds on, including 2 seconds ramp, and 5 seconds off).

For spinal spasticity, Lojze Vodovnik's group in Ljubljana have used 30 Hz but, having tested a range of parameters (10–1000 Hz, 10–1000 μs), concluded that 100 Hz, 100 μs was optimal.

Three CES studies all used the Liss stimulator (15 kHz modulated at 15 Hz, 500 Hz and 1500 Hz), as did a further study on severe postanoxic spasticity.

With EA and ST-36/LI-4 TEAS too, it seems that dynorphin-mediated higher frequencies (~100 Hz) have a stronger and more rapid effect on spinal spasticity than lower ones (2 Hz, or even 2/100 Hz DD). The effect is cumulative with repeated treatment, which should be daily, or at least three times each week, for the first 3 months.

If spastic muscle is passively stretched, it may go into clonus (repeated spasms) at around 5–7 Hz. It may be that stimulation at around this frequency range should therefore be avoided in general, and frequencies at around 100 Hz used instead. However, some practitioners do find brief (5–10 min) LF EA (or sometimes DD or intermittent stimulation) helpful for spasticity.

## PARKINSON'S DISEASE

Parkinson's disease generally occurs in middle-aged and older people. It is associated with loss of dopaminergic neurons from the substantia nigra in the brainstem.

Malfunction rather than destruction of neurons can lead to a reversible 'parkinsonism', with dyskinesia and tremor. Although resting tremor is the commonest symptom at first, also characteristic are rigidity, slowness and lack of movement.

Acupuncture is traditionally used for Parkinson's disease, which is seen as related to Liver Wind. According to Maciocia, patients with *qi* and Blood deficiency respond better than those with Phlegm-Fire, with *yin xu* patients responding least well. Both MA and EA may provide some clinical benefits in Parkinson's disease and parkinsonism, although researchers disagree on whether EA improves both rigidity and tremor, or only the former. The effects of CES and LA are less certain.

**Comparisons** Scalp EA was found to be marginally more effective than MA in its effects on the muscle activity of patients, and significantly more so than TCM herbal remedies. EA was more effective than Western medication in another small study.

**Points used** Charles Buck has written a useful account of treating Parkinson's disease, giving MA point formulae for the various TCM syndromes involved. However, acupuncture and CES studies, together with Sandyk's work on magnetic fields, indicate that scalp or Governor Vessel points, or both, should be stimulated.

**Parameters used** There is insufficient information to judge what parameters are most helpful. However, experimental research indicates that HF rather than LF EA may be appropriate. As for LA, 632 nm, the wavelength of the HeNe laser, may be particularly appropriate.

## TREMOR

Tremor occurs in a variety of conditions. It can be a difficult symptom to treat, but a number of EA studies indicate benefit for some varieties of tremor. Auricular stimulation with pTENS, CES and low-intensity scalp magnetic fields, as well as simple dry needling of trigger points in the neck and shoulder area, have been investigated.

**Points used** Conditions in the tremor studies are not similar enough to be able to draw conclusions. In leg tremor, both local points and CES have been used, in stroke, both proximal and distal points, and in paroxysmal tremor following lightning strike, P-6.

**Parameters used** Tremor normally occurs at around 10 Hz, pathological tremor being slower, at 3–6 Hz in Parkinson's disease. Both LF (1–2 Hz) and HF ('dense') have been used in the EA treatment of tremor.

## PARALYSIS I. MUSCLE WEAKNESS IN UPPER MOTOR NEURON DISEASE AND POLIOMYELITIS

**Upper motor neuron disease** Motor neuron disease includes conditions such as amyotrophic lateral sclerosis (ALS), with muscle weakness, hypertonia and abnormal tendon reflexes, but usually without sensory loss. In one German survey, acupuncture was the most used form of complementary and alternative medicine for ALS. Despite this, the conventional wisdom is that attempting to stimulate weakened muscles in the presence of CNS damage is not likely to be useful.

There are reports of EA stimulation via locally implanted electrodes and pulsed magnetic fields being used in the treatment of ALS. In one EA study, Roya Monajem used points for deficient *qi* and Blood, and to strengthen muscle, and a frequency of 10 Hz, appropriate for building slow muscle. There may be a link between strong electric shock and the site of origin of motor neuron disease, so strong stimulation should be avoided.

**Poliomyelitis** Poliomyelitis can result from viral damage to the cerebrum or cerebellum, but classically follows inflammation of the anterior horns of the spinal column, leading to muscle weakness and flaccid paralysis of one or more limbs. Many who have had the disease in the past still suffer the consequences. According to Giovanni Maciocia, acupuncture may be helpful for postpolio paralysis only if treatment is started early, but some EA studies indicate that benefits for the muscular sequelae of polio are still possible some time after the initial stages.

*Postpolio syndrome*, with similarities to *fibromyalgia* or *chronic fatigue syndrome*, may ensue even years after the initial viral infection and seeming recovery. EA and static magnetic field stimulation of trigger points have both been used to treat this condition.

**Points used** Although motor points by definition cannot be found in denervated muscle, acupoints may still be present if sensory nerves are undamaged. Thus there is no contraindication to EA for paralysis, although if there is sensory as well as motor denervation then progress will be difficult. Muscle atrophy (*wei bi*) may improve using contralateral treatment. Local meridian points in the affected muscles to regulate the flow of *qi* are also recommended for *wei bi* when using EA, with particular emphasis on *yangming* (Stomach and Large Intestine) points. However, Gu's studies using two rows of linked needles aligned along the most affected meridians indicate that specific acupoint stimulation may not be necessary, at least for sequelae of poliomyelitis. Paraspinal (*huatuojiaji*) segmental points are also used.

**Parameters used** In general, strong regular electrical stimulation, particularly in the *early* stages of paralysis, may result in spasm and so should be avoided. It would seem appropriate to use gentler, irregular or changing stimulation parameters instead. However, for the *sequelae* of polio, stronger EA may be required than for those of stroke, reducing the amplitude as the condition improves. From the studies, it seems that LF is more used than HF.

To encourage more natural muscle activity, attempts have been made to mimic normal motor unit activity with the applied stimulation. Thus LF low-intensity stimulation, with long interruptions between elicited contractions, has been recommended, short treatments being repeated several times daily. Although 100 Hz has also been used for denervated muscle, one recommendation is that frequencies > 50 Hz should not be used if denervation is present. For direct treatment of denervated muscle, triangular or sawtooth waveforms with long rise times have been employed.

## PARALYSIS II. PARALYSIS DUE TO SPINAL CORD INJURY

Spinal cord injury (SCI) can affect both motor and sensory function. Treatment may be directed towards repairing injured nerves or preventing muscular atrophy, or both.

Experimentally, both EA and low-intensity laser/light therapy (LILT) may enhance spinal cord regrowth after injury. However, emphasis after the acute phase should always be on rehabilitation rather than the hope that the original injury will recover. Unassisted, spinal cord axons do not tend to regrow significantly once completely transected.

Both MA and EA have been used for traumatic paraplegia, with good results claimed, given perseverance. Changes are observed in limb temperature, as well as spasticity, muscle strength and atrophy. Exercise and early intervention are important. Electrical stimulation of muscle during immobilisation can help maintain muscle mass and function.

CES and LILT may be of benefit for SCI. However, LILT may require many hours of daily treatment to be effective.

**Points used** In MA, EA, TENS and LILT studies, local stimulation of the spinal cord appears to be one aim, either directly using Governor Vessel meridian points (interspinal spaces above and below the level of the lesion) or via paraspinal (*huatuojiajia* or Bladder meridian) points. Distal points on the Bladder meridian are also used.

Points are sometimes used for their TCM functions, as with GB-39 and GB-34, the *hui* points for marrow and tendons respectively, or points on Spleen and Stomach meridians to nourish the muscle tissue. Other points also have their rationale, such as GB-30, an important point for leg problems. Conception Vessel points are occasionally used, presumably in part for their effect on the bladder. EA at Du-2, Du-4 and Du-14, with moxibustion at Ren-4, are suggested for traumatic paraplegia in one textbook. Another author suggests that EA should be used firstly at ST-31, ST-32, ST- 36 and ST-41, with secondary use of BL-36, BL-37, BL-40, BL-54, BL-57 and BL-60. Willem Khoe's point selection very much echoes that evident in the CD-ROM resource ⊛ database: BL-37, BL-40, BL-57, BL-60, GB-30, GB-31, GB-39, LIV-3, ST-36, ST-41, SP-6, SP-7, with additional points such as BL-24, BL-25, BL-26, Ren-4 and Ren-6. However, he also states that treating the scalp motor area will result in more rapid improvement.

A very different protocol for paralysis has been proposed by Chen Tiwei, inventor of a Chinese version of the Japanese SSP system (the WT-100 Quick-Cure apparatus). For upper limb paralysis, one electrode is held on P-6, and the other on all the hand *jing* points in turn. ST-36 is used in the same way for lower limb paralysis.

**Parameters used** LF (or burst LF) EA appears to be commonly used, though with little indication on intensity.

---

**BOX 9.1.1**

**Paralysis and muscular disorders**

Paralysis refers to complete or incomplete loss of the voluntary movement of a certain part of the body. Like spasticity, it can occur as a result of traumatic or degenerative changes in motor pathways at different levels in the nervous system. Within the CNS, damage may occur in the brain or spinal cord, as in upper motor neuron disease, stroke or paraplegia. When it occurs in the anterior horn of the spinal cord, it results in the flaccid paralysis of polio. Interruption of peripheral efferent pathways through compression entrapment can lead to conditions such as facial paralysis. Myasthenia gravis is due to degeneration at the neuromuscular junction, whereas muscular dystrophy is associated with abnormal changes in the structure of the muscle itself, with the nerves remaining intact. All these conditions, except the last, result in denervation of muscle. Flaccid paralysis is one form of *wei bi*, or atrophy syndrome, for which acupuncture is traditionally used.

There is controversy on the usefulness of stimulating denervated muscle electrically. Even partially denervated muscle will be less responsive than normal muscle, and standard electrotherapy is demanding on both patient and practitioner. Treatment is important early on to prevent muscle atrophy, but cannot reverse atrophy that has already occurred.

However, both electrotherapy and acupuncture have long histories of being used with some degree of success for various forms of paralysis, presumably depending on some retention of nerve excitability after the initial acute phase of the condition (~3 weeks). LA too may have a role in promoting regeneration and reinnervation of denervated skeletal muscle. Although peripheral efferents may enter a state of 'hibernation' if their supply from the spine is cut off, this may not result in true denervation: with considerable perseverance, it may be possible to reawaken the nerve supply. If the nerve no longer responds, treatment must focus on the muscle itself.

---

Box 9.1.1 details the treatment of paralysis and muscular disorders.

## MULTIPLE SCLEROSIS

Symptoms of multiple sclerosis include weakness, numbness, spasticity or paralysis in one or both arms or legs, blurred vision, vision loss or other eye problems such as nystagmus, dizziness, imbalance, difficulties with bladder and eventually bowel control, intention tremor and lack of coordination while walking. This condition runs an erratic course, with unpredictable remissions lasting sometimes for many years.

Multiple sclerosis is the result of demyelination in the CNS, and the conventional view is that electrostimulation for the resulting spasticity will not produce lasting benefits.

EA, pTENS, TENS, acupoint microcurrent stimulation, EMS, spinal cord and magnetic field stimulation all have their advocates, but once muscle atrophy has occurred electrostimulation will not reverse it.

In TCM terms, MS is considered the result of an invasion of external Dampness, in later stages accompanied by Blood stasis. Early treatment is considered most helpful.

TENS, used to treat pain in multiple sclerosis, has been found to have unexpected benefits for sensation, muscle tone and balance as well. Bladder dysfunction may also be helped by TENS. EMS (20 Hz, for 1 hour) over peripheral nerves can temporarily reduce clonus and rigidity. pTENS has been considered helpful for foot and leg pain and foot or wrist drop.

**Points used**  Both scalp and limb acupoints are used for EA, the former for their systemic effect, the latter for more localised effect on, for instance, limb spasticity. Similarly, TENS or EMS applied directly over peripheral nerves has been used to reduce spasticity.

**Parameters used**  Slow muscle fibres are initially affected more than fast fibres in multiple sclerosis. Thus, in one early EMS study, 60 Hz sine wave stimulation was found to be more beneficial than 5 Hz or 10 Hz in slowing atrophy. In his EA case reports, Hoang used 200 Hz. However, there are few indications on what parameters to use on the scalp.

## EPILEPSY

Brain injury or dysfunction from many different causes can result in epilepsy. Epileptic seizures may be generalised or only partial, with some forms of epilepsy being non-convulsive. *Status epilepticus*, in which seizures continue for more than 5 minutes, constitutes a medical emergency.

Acupuncture has traditionally been used in the treatment of infantile febrile convulsions, epilepsy, and even status epilepticus. There are several studies of EA for epilepsy, with some claims that it is more effective than MA.

LA has been used to halt epileptic seizures since 1972. More specifically, seizure frequency in children with cerebral palsy has been reported as reduced when treated at home by their mothers with a 5 mW red beam diode laser.

There are parallels between epilepsy and some sorts of migraine. Many epileptics, like migraine sufferers, appear to be particularly sensitive to external stimuli. Both static and varying magnetic fields may elicit epileptiform activity in the brain, as well as prevent experimentally induced seizures.

**Points used**  In experimental studies, Du-3, Du-4, Du-8, Du-16, Du-24 with Ren-24 and other Governor Vessel points have been used to treat experimentally induced convulsions, with better results using midline points than points such as BL-60 or LIV-3. KI-1 and Du-26 are points for which indications also traditionally include convulsions, as is GB-12. MA to Du-26, for example, has been used successfully for iatrogenic drug-resistant seizures. However, strong stimulation to head points may aggravate epileptiform activity in the brain, and midline points such as Du-20 and Du-26 have also been used in 'EA convulsive therapy' for schizophrenia. Thus these points appear to have a bidirectional effect, depending on the condition being treated and the excitability of the underlying brain structures (HF stimulation of the motor cortex, which straddles the midline just anterior to Du-20, is particularly likely to induce seizure).

**Parameters used** LF rather than HF EA has been used in the treatment of epilepsy.

Regularly repetitive strong stimulation, particularly at points near or on the head and at high frequencies, should be avoided. However, although strong stimulation to the head may exacerbate epileptiform activity in the brain, strong stimulation at lumbar Governing Vessel points may inhibit it. A number of studies have utilised strong-intensity stimulation, but in my view this should be instigated cautiously, and only after an initial trial at lower intensity.

**Note**

Before treating any patient for epilepsy or convulsions, the relevant sections in Chapters 6 and 12 should be reviewed.

**9.1** Summary of relevant studies in the electronic clinical studies database (number of studies)

| Condition | EA | Other | Condition | EA | Other |
|---|---|---|---|---|---|
| **Psychological conditions** | | | Dementia (general or non-vascular) | 5 | 11 |
| Anxiety | 6 | 51 | Dementia (vascular) | 10 | 3 |
| Phobia | 0 | 6 | Drug abuse (cognitive function) | 0 | 3 |
| *Depression* | | | Learning and mental performance in the healthy | 0 | 5 |
| Manic depression | 6 | 2 | | | |
| *Schizophrenia* | 18 | 26 | Coma | 9 | 1 |
| *Neurosis and personality disorder* | | | *Ataxia – Parkinson's – Chorea* | | |
| Neurosis | 2 | 9 | Ataxia and related conditions | 1 | 1 |
| Hysteria | 6 | 7 | Parkinson's disease | 15 | 2 |
| Obsessive–compulsive disorders | 3 | 2 | Parkinsonism | 1 | 4 |
| Personality disorder | 0 | 2 | Dystonia and spasmodic torticollis | 3 | 8 |
| *Psychosexual disorders* | | | Other forms of tremor | 3 | 4 |
| Male sexual dysfunction | 5 | 7 | Chorea | 1 | 1 |
| Female sexual dysfunction | 2 | 1 | Tourette's syndrome | 1 | 1 |
| *Sleep disorders* | 10 | 57 | *Paraplegia – spinal injury* | 34 | 18 |
| *Stress and relaxation* | 2 | 13 | *MS – polio – ALS* | | |
| **Central nervous system conditions** | | | Multiple sclerosis | 4 | 8 |
| *Cerebral palsy and spasticity* | | | Poliomyelitis | 13 | 3 |
| Cerebral palsy | 11 | 24 | Postpolio syndrome | 1 | 1 |
| Spasticity (other) | 1 | 10 | Motor neuron disease | 1 | 0 |
| *Cognitive and behavioural deficit* | | | Amyotrophic lateral sclerosis | 2 | 1 |
| Down's syndrome | 3 | 5 | Syringomyelia | 1 | 0 |
| ADHD, encephalitis and developmental disorders | 15 | 5 | *Epilepsy – convulsions* | | |
| Chronic fatigue syndrome and neurasthenia | 7 | 11 | Epilepsy | 12 | 16 |
| | | | Convulsions due to other causes | 3 | 2 |
| Head/brain injury | 3 | 15 | Proconvulsive treatment | 3 | 1 |

# SUMMARY

Some key points in this chapter are:

- Various forms of EA have been used successfully for depression, stress and insomnia, but studies on EA for anxiety are relatively few
- Paralysis is frequently treated with EA, with treatment more effective if commenced as early as possible
- In paralysis associated with denervation, treatment is best focused on soft tissue and muscle
- Epilepsy can be treated with EA and MA, but with considerable caution as regards the intensity of treatment.

## Additional material in the CD-ROM resource

In the electronic version of this chapter, additional material is presented according to the headings here, on psychosexual disorders and also on less commonly treated conditions such as phobias, post-traumatic stress disorder and amnesia, cognitive dysfunction resulting from drug abuse, cerebral palsy, dystonia, ataxia, chorea and Tourette's syndrome. Parallels between 'neurasthenia' and chronic fatigue syndrome are also examined.

# RECOMMENDED READING

*An introductory discussion on anxiety, depression, pain and acupuncture:*
Mayor DF The hurts, the angst, the blues. Making sense of pain, emotion and psychopathology. European Journal of Oriental Medicine. 1998 Summer; 2(5): 8–17

*EA for depression – one of several studies by this group:*
Luo H, Meng F, Jia Y, Zhao X Clinical research on the therapeutic effect of electroacupuncture treatment in patients with depression. Psychiatry and Clinical Neurosciences. 1998 Dec; 52(Suppl): S338–S340

*A useful review of acupuncture for schizophrenia:*
Beecroft N, Rampes H Review of acupuncture for schizophrenia. Acupuncture in Medicine. 1997 Nov; 15(2): 91–4

*Many Italian doctors in the 1970s were open-minded, often combining acupuncture with a psychoanalytic approach:*
Frigoli D, Ciniselli G [Group acupuncture and mobilization of long-term psychotic patients]. Minerva Medica Riflessoterapeutica. 1978 Dec 22; 69(62): 4317–27

*One of Chen Kezhen's pithy review articles on all types of acupuncture:*
Chen KZ Insomnia. International Journal of Clinical Acupuncture. 1995; 6(3): 289–94

*A thoughtful account of Parkinson's disease by Charles Buck:*
Buck C Acupuncture and Parkinson's Disease. Journal of the Acupuncture Association of Chartered Physiotherapists. 2000 Oct; 25–9

*Three views of acupuncture and epilepsy:*
Rosted P Repetitive epileptic fits – a possible adverse effect after transcutaneous electrical nerve stimulation (TENS) in a post-stroke patient. Acupuncture in Medicine. 2001 June; 19(1): 46–9

Wu D [Mechanism of acupuncture in suppressing epileptic seizures]. Journal of Traditional Chinese Medicine (Zhongyi Zazhi). 1992 Sept; 12(3): 187–92

Xue CC, Xie HS, Ruan QC, Cheng YD, Luo DL Electric acupuncture convulsive therapy. Convulsive Therapy. 1985; 1(4): 242–51

# 9.2 STROKE AND CEREBROVASCULAR DISEASE

*John L Stump, with David F Mayor and a contribution by Pekka J Pöntinen*

> This subchapter outlines the types of stroke and the uses of acupuncture in both prevention and rehabilitation

## CAUSES AND TYPES OF STROKE

Stroke, or cerebrovascular accident (CVA), is the most common cause of severe handicap in the world's adult population. About half of stroke survivors are left with neurological impairment and physical disability. Strokes are caused by disruption in blood supply, either outside or within the brain, damaging cells by depriving them of oxygen.

Since strokes can be prevented by early treatment, symptoms of impending stroke must be taken seriously. They may include brief episodes of hearing loss, nausea, one-sided numbness or *paraesthesiae*, falling without reason, difficulty in swallowing or speaking, throbbing headache, amnesia, visual disturbances, loss of comprehension, muscle control or coordination, and dizziness.

There are two broad categories of stroke: ischaemic strokes, and strokes due to haemorrhage. The majority of strokes are ischaemic; the less common haemorrhagic strokes are more deadly.

### Ischaemic stroke

Ischaemia is the term for reduced blood supply to any part of the brain. Oxygen-starved cells stop functioning properly, either temporarily or permanently depending on the degree of ischaemia and its duration. If the blood supply is cut off completely, cells die within minutes, forming an infarct.

Ischaemia may be due to thrombosis, embolism, small vessel arteriopathy, or spasm of a cerebral vessel. Transient ischaemic attacks (TIA) cause brain cells to pause in their normal functioning, usually for minutes, but sometimes for almost 24 hours. Once the blood supply is restored, cells revive and bodily functions recover. Symptoms vary, depending on where blood flow is reduced (in the *carotid* or *vertebrobasilar* arterial systems), and there is no loss of consciousness.

### Haemorrhagic stroke

This stroke is triggered by haemorrhage that occurs when an artery ruptures, spilling its contents into surrounding tissue. The major pathogenic causes are hypertension and cerebral arteriosclerosis. Aneurysm is a common cause, particularly in subarachnoid haemorrhage, when the rupture is usually due to high blood pressure or trauma, or both.

## Stroke: the varieties of neurological impairment

Several factors influence the outcome of a stroke: its type, the extent of brain damage and, most importantly, where the damage occurs. Hemiplegia is often the most obvious symptom. Paralysis of the right side of the body occurs when the stroke has damaged the left side of the brain, and vice versa, as fibres cross over (decussate) between the brain and the rest of the body. Typically, people with left brain damage will have difficulty with speech and language, whereas people with left hemiplegia have spatial– perceptual deficits, or impaired ability to judge distance, size, position, movement speed, form and the relationship of parts to the whole.

## STROKE REHABILITATION

Despite permanent tissue damage, most surviving stroke patients improve to some extent over time. The purpose of a formal treatment programme is to assist in and accelerate this recovery process. Recovery can be divided broadly into two phases. In the early phase, from within a few hours to as long as months after a stroke, many patients experience a partial or even a complete reversal of their neurological impairments. The body is most receptive to rehabilitative therapies during the first 6 months after a stroke, and patient and family members need to work closely with a stroke rehabilitation team. In the later phase, after the 6-month point, restoration of function may well continue for up to 2 years or more after a stroke.

## ACUPUNCTURE AND STROKE

Traditionally, acupuncture is important at all stages of stroke – as a preventive measure, immediately following stroke, in the convalescent stage, and for the later sequelae.

Box 9.2.1 details the effects of acupuncture on the cerebrovascular system.

### Acupuncture as a preventive measure

Traditionally acupuncture has always had an important preventive role. Hypertension, dizziness, headache, memory loss and difficulties in understanding can all presage stroke, as well as being associated with other forms of cerebral insufficiency such as vascular dementia and TIA. According to Russian studies, initial signs of cerebral insufficiency may be associated predominantly with essential hypertension or with atherosclerosis. Those in whom hypertension predominates may suffer from an overactive sympathetic nervous system, and be responsive

**BOX 9.2.1**

**Acupuncture's effects on the cerebrovascular system**

Most experimental research on stroke has focused on the effects of electroacupuncture (EA) in animals with acute cerebral ischaemia (ACI), a model for both TIA and ischaemic stroke. There is less research on experimental models of haemorrhagic stroke. The following general conclusions can be drawn:

**Blood pressure**

Acupuncture may markedly reduce both systolic and diastolic blood pressure (BP). However, in some models of ACI, BP is low. In this case, Du-26 EA may increase it once more.

**Cerebral blood flow**

From a growing number of studies it is clear that acupuncture can affect cerebral haemodynamics, improving microcirculation and ameliorating tissue anoxia in the brain. Stimulation of the circulation superficially may also have an effect on blood flow within the brain.

The effects of EA on cerebral circulation alter to maintain a degree of physiological balance. Thus, following ischaemia, EA at many different points (including LI-11, ST-36 and Du-26) may *increase* cerebral vasodilation. On the other hand, EA *reduces* pial arteriolar diameter in rats with acute haemorrhagic hypotension.

Blood viscosity improves. Strong EA within 10 days of stroke tends to regulate (though not normalise) plasma levels of substances involved with platelet clumping and atheroma formation. Interestingly, levels may change more with 0.3 Hz EA given between 7 and 9 a.m. than the same treatment at 7–9 p.m.

**Brain damage and oedema**

Experimentally, EA can protect against brain damage in the ACI model, reducing infarct size, whether applied at GB-30, LI-4, Du-8/Du-16 (7 Hz continuous stimulation, or 15 Hz paused for 10 minutes out of every 30), or at Du-20/Du-26 (3.85/18 Hz DD). Clinically, in patients with cerebral infarction, EA at LI-4, LI-11, ST-36 and SP-6 on the affected limbs increases activity in the contralateral parietal cortex (motor and sensory area) and other regions of the brain, including the infarcted area. The area of the infarct decreases as a result.

As well as reducing infarct size, EA at ST-36 may actually foster proliferation of new cells in some parts of the brain. Thus Du-20/Du-26 EA (3.85/18 Hz DD) may up-regulate fibroblast growth factor. Changes in the basal ganglia, limbic system and cerebellum have been noted with EA following ACI, with similar changes in stroke patients.

One cause of cell damage following ischaemia is the oedema that occurs in the ischaemic region of the brain following restoration of circulation. Clinically, oedema has been observed to decrease in patients with cerebral infarction following EA (at points on the affected limbs), and in animals after EA at Du-20/Du-26.

to acupuncture (EA). Atherosclerosis may be more amenable to a combination of acupuncture, physiotherapy and dietary management. Indeed, some authors recommend against electrostimulation in severe atherosclerosis.

Chronic neck problems may also lead to cerebrovascular pathology, as in vertebrobasilar insufficiency (impaired circulation in the vertebral artery and its continuation in the basilar artery at the base of the brain). Neck rotation in such patients may reduce blood flow in the vertebral arteries. This in turn can be responsible for vertigo.

According to Yoshiaki Omura, abnormalities in the common carotid artery may be associated with blood pressure abnormalities within the brain. Resulting circulatory changes within the brain may be responsible for cerebrovascular dementia and vascular headache, including migraine. In TCM, vascular dementia is sometimes considered a form of stroke.

Recurrent TIA has been treated with EA, resulting in more rapid control of symptoms, fewer cases of embolism and greater improvement of haemorheology index and platelet aggregation.

Omura has used MA, TENS and massage to relax spastic musculature in the neck and shoulders and so improve circulation within the brain. Functional abnormalities resulting from impaired circulation should respond rapidly whereas organic problems will not.

Case study 9.2.1 is an example of the treatment of brainstem sensory-motor lacunar infarction.

**Comparisons and combinations** EA gave better results than MA in one study of auricular acupuncture for the initial manifestations of cerebral circulatory failure in hypertensive patients.

LA and EA have been used together for the early stages of cerebral circulation insufficiency, prolonging blood-clotting time in addition to other effects.

**Points used**

*Points on the head:* GB-8, Du-20 and *taiyang* (M-HN-9) have been used with MA for cerebral arteriosclerosis. Du-20 MA is used for prodromal symptoms of stroke.

*Points on the occiput and neck:* GB-20 MA has been used for cerebral arteriosclerosis and TIA and for prodromal symptoms of stroke. GB-20 EA is also used for vertebrobasilar insufficiency due to cervical spondylosis. BL-10 and GB-12, used in MA studies, may be appropriate too.

*Points on the body:* P-6 and LI-4 have been used for early cerebral arteriosclerosis. Points for prodromal stroke symptoms or TIA could include GB-34, LIV-3, LI-4, LI-11 and SP-6. EA at the *huatuojiaji* points has been used for vertebrobasilar insufficiency associated with cervical spondylosis. Moxibustion at ST-36 is a traditional prophylactic treatment for stroke.

## Acupuncture in stroke rehabilitation: an overview

Restimulating and re-educating brain function after stroke is a key to successful recovery. Music, movement, visual

# CASE Study 9.2.1

## Author's experience of brainstem sensory-motor lacunar infarction – fast recovery from complete right-sided hemiplegia
**Pekka J Pöntinen**

The first transient ischaemic attack started with slight vertigo preceded by a hectic period of editorial work and presentations at home and abroad. It was over in a couple of minutes, but 5 minutes later at the tea table the author, a 71-year-old male, experienced a tingling sensation in the right arm radiating to the fingers and a few minutes later also some paraesthesiae and weakness in the right lower extremity, leading to right-sided hemiparesis after a further 10 minutes.

At this time laser therapy (780 nm, < 50 mW, 1 J/point) was applied to the neck and shoulder region (C7/*Dazhui*, Extra 21 (*Huatuojiaji*) at T1 bilaterally, GB-21/*Jianjing*) and paravertebrally at C2–3 bilaterally (2 J/point), over the left carotid artery (9 J) (Fig. 9.2.1), and to scalp midline acupuncture points, from Du-20/*Baihui* to Du-24/*Shenting*, and at Du-26/*Renzhong* (1 J/point). In about 15 minutes sensory and motor function returned to near-normal level and the author took a few steps around his bed. However, the symptoms returned and progressed to nearly complete right-sided hemiplegia, including speech difficulties during a phone call, but with no impairment in consciousness or cognitive tasks.

Laser therapy was now given over the radial artery (9 J). Recovery started in 10 minutes and both sensory and motor functions were back to normal in less than an

hour. The whole episode lasted less than 2 hours and the author returned to his normal email correspondence, sending an urgently needed report to South Africa an hour later. Physical and mental activities continued from the second day forward, as before, without problems. As a preventive treatment acetylsalicylic acid (0.25 g × 1) and warfarin (2.5 mg × 1) were added to the previous programme consisting of peripheral electric stimulation with muscle belt (ABGymnic), occasional laser therapy for muscle care and dietary supplements (glucosamine 1.5 g × 1 and chondroitin 1.2 g × 1) necessary to control hip osteoarthritis.

The author experienced a second attack 4 weeks later in bed early in the morning, awakening with dysaesthesiae and paraesthesiae again spreading towards the fingers and toes in the right side. Immediate laser therapy to the same regions and points as above did not alleviate the symptoms, which gradually progressed to hemiparesis and later during the day in the hospital to complete right-sided hemiplegia with central involvement (double vision, tongue deviation, swallowing and speech difficulties).

There were no abnormalities found in a CT taken 6 hours from the beginning of this attack. No signs of plaques or other abnormalities were found by ultrasound in the carotid arteries, in which blood flow was excellent and vessel wall consistency normal on both sides 4 days later. A possible narrowing in the upper (intracranial) part of the right vertebral artery was suspected. In about 18 hours gradual recovery started in both legs and arms and in 24 hours the grasping force in the right hand was reasonably good, with minimal signs of neurological deficit. Eight hours later the author was able to start handwriting in English, creating the preface to the Farsi edition of his laser book and signing it. Laser therapy continued daily and walking exercises started on the second poststroke day. Electrical stimulation of thigh muscles was started on the third poststroke day and then continued daily. Muscle force in the legs and arms was now normal but some uncertainty still remained when walking. On the fourth poststroke day walking distance during the day reached about 1 km. Back home on the sixth day and thereafter, routines gradually returned to normal, including physical and mental exercises (e.g. walking, cycling, rowing and gardening, as well as piano playing for delicate sensorymotor-auditory training).

Two months later, some minor sensory deficit is still present in the right lower calf and outer side of the foot, probably from peripheral (peroneus) nerve compression while lying on the atonic hemiplegic side during the first evening in hospital. Eight months later (January 2004), the author is still taking acetylsalicylic acid (100 mg daily). In June and July, manuals on Light Therapy were completed in English and German. Skating and ice hockey were started in August with the Oldtimers team to maintain proper muscle coordination

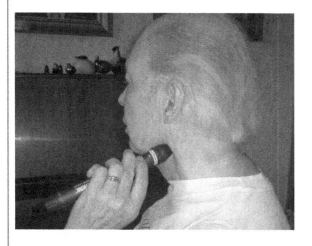

**Figure 9.2.1** Carotid artery irradiation (LILT) following transient ischaemic attack. (Courtesy of Pekka J Pöntinen.)

---

**CASE Study 9.2.1 Continued**

and balance. Sensory deficit was now limited to the outer side of the foot.

Some points of interest and importance are:
- the early start of active and passive peripheral stimulation in order to maintain peripheral sensory and motor input
- photon therapy locally and via the bloodstream to provide extra energy to the hypoxic CNS cells and thus increase recovery from the ischaemic injury

- any extra day in a bed will lead to progressive reduction in the size and accuracy of the corresponding cortical reflexion zone, which in turn will delay motor and sensory recovery and may lead to central pain syndromes
- muscle force can be maintained with passive electrical stimulation applied directly to the affected muscles
- for delicate sensory and motor exercises, playing musical instruments or painting, or both, are of great importance to train both brain hemispheres.

---

retraining and above all peripheral somatic stimulation (touch, acupuncture, TENS) can all be important. In the East, there is a long history of treating stroke with acupuncture. In the last decades of the twentieth century, large numbers of clinical studies were published, apparently supporting the use of acupuncture for stroke. Although the validity of most of these has been questioned, there are in fact more randomised controlled trials (RCTs) on acupuncture for stroke than for any other condition.

The syndromes involved in the TCM treatment of stroke ('Wind-stroke') include *yin* deficiency with Liver *yang* flare-up, Phlegm and *qi* deficiency and Blood stasis. Severe stroke is due to attack of internal organs (*zangfu*) by Wind, with loss of consciousness, coma and aphasia. The main organs affected are the Heart, Liver, Spleen and Kidney. In mild stroke, the meridians alone (*jingluo*) are affected, resulting in hemiplegia, numbness and slurred speech, but without loss of consciousness. An alternative interpretation is that the acute phase is characterised by Wind attacking the *zangfu* and sequelae by attack on the *jingluo*. Initial hemiplegia with muscle spasticity or tension is due to collapse of *yin*, and flaccid paralysis to collapse of *yang*.

Giovanni Maciocia reports that best results are obtained if acupuncture is given within 1 month, and good results if within 3 months, but that stroke is difficult to treat after 6 months, and more so after 1 year. Even without treatment, most stroke survivors improve significantly during the first month after stroke onset, and spontaneous recovery can occur even 6 months later. However, even if the borders of an infarct become fixed after about 3 months, patients may still benefit from treatment. Clearly earlier treatment gives better results.

The benefits that acupuncture may bring to the treatment of stroke have yet to be shown conclusively, given the methodological problems that bedevil acupuncture research. For instance, in one review of 50 RCTs from China on the effectiveness of acupuncture in stroke rehabilitation (a total of 6221 patients), results were highly significant statistically, suggesting that the acupuncture methods used were better than no treatment, conventional treatment and standard acupuncture methods. However, further analysis showed that some of the observed effectiveness in these trials

could be attributed to lack of blinding, publication bias and placebo effect.

Acupuncture, however, encompasses many styles and variations, not clearly differentiated in most reviews. While these reviewers concluded that MA appears to give better results than non-MA, there still seems to be no single optimum treatment approach, and little clear evidence that one approach is better than another. Not only does the variety of treatment need to be considered carefully when reviewing acupuncture studies on stroke, but also the variability inherent in stroke itself and its recovery. Results may depend on degree of disability, on infarct size, or on its depth within the brain.

The treatment of stroke can be divided into *acute*, in its immediate aftermath, *subacute*, during convalescence once the patient's condition has become stable, and *chronic*, when treatment is delayed more than 3–6 months following stroke onset and is directed at the sequelae of stroke, such as hemiplegia.

## ACUTE STROKE

It is still difficult to determine aetiology in around 25% of strokes, and it is against this background that possible roles for acupuncture must be considered. It is clear that stroke responds better when treated early. To protect against free radical damage of neurons, for example, animal research indicates that EA must be initiated rapidly, even within an hour following infarct, and certainly within 6 hours afterwards. After haemorrhagic stroke, however, the situation may be different: to treat too early may be counterproductive. Thus some authorities consider EA contraindicated in the acute stage of cerebral haemorrhage, even though most bleeding ceases within 4 hours and needling thereafter, even at points like Du-15 and Du-16, is unlikely to cause problems.

Margaret Naeser states that the best results with all forms of acupuncture are obtained if initiated within 24–36 hours in ischaemic infarct cases, and after bleeding is controlled in haemorrhagic cases, usually 4–6 hours post onset. Some clinicians start treatment only after the patient's condition has stabilised (~36 hours). Others have taken this approach for EA (at scalp points), but have felt that earlier use of body MA is permissible.

In acute stroke, some authors consider the vascular effects of acupuncture to be the most important, although by the subacute stage (even at 10 days) the damage is done and vascular factors are less likely to be relevant. Thus some TCM authorities consider that it is important immediately following stroke not only to give treatment for resuscitation but also to pay attention to 'removing obstruction from the *fu* organs'.

A more cautious view would be that acupuncture is secondary in the acute stage of stroke, important only to help relieve certain symptoms and signs such as spasm, twitching and coma, and to lower blood pressure. Treatment for the *sequelae* of stroke can then be undertaken, from 2–3 days after an ischaemic stroke, or 7–10 days after haemorrhagic. Some authors suggest that local treatment after any acute injury is best avoided for 48 hours.

Although there is no conclusive agreement on this important issue, EA should be applied only once the cause of the stroke has been clearly diagnosed, and not sooner than 6 hours after haemorrhage.

With MA, results may vary depending on the location and size of the infarct. Not surprisingly, results with EA are poorer in patients with larger infarcts. Although in general larger infarcts have a poorer prognosis, in one RCT on EA for acute stroke it was those with *poorer* neurological and functional status at baseline who improved most.

Brain scans can provide useful corroboration of improvements with EA. In one single case report of haemorrhagic stroke, the disease focus was no longer found with CT examination following LF EA at body points and the right scalp motor area. In a SPECT scan study on ischaemic stroke, EA (6 Hz at ST-36 and ST-37) re-established photon emission from brain areas where it had been reduced in 50% of cases.

**Points used** With tension (collapse of *yin*), points such as KI-1, Du-20, Du-26 and the *jing* Well points are used traditionally to relieve coma, eliminate spasm and lower blood pressure, often with bleeding of the *shixuan* (M-UE-1) points. P-6 and SP-6 may be added for spasm and contraction of the limbs, together with points for hypertension. One EA device manual recommends LIV-3 and ST-40, with Du-20 and Du-26. For accompanying spastic hemiplegia, *yin* meridian points are sometimes emphasised.

With flaccidity (collapse of *yang*), points such as P-6, ST-36, Ren-4 and Ren-6 may be used, often with moxibustion at Ren-8. *Yang* meridian points may be particularly appropriate.

If the disease is severe or it is difficult to distinguish between tense or flaccid pattern, ST-36 and Du-26 can be selected, with other points according to symptoms and signs. These points, together with P-6, have been used for acute stroke. The *huatuojiaji* points level with C2 and C3 may also promote resuscitation.

Joseph Wong recommends points such as LI-4, ST-36, Du-16, Du-20, Du-26 and *sishencong* (M-HN-1), with BL-2, GB-20, ST-9 and Ren-22 to stimulate circulation to the brain.

From the experimental research, it would seem that ST-36 and Governor Vessel points (Du-14, Du-16, Du-20, Du-26) are key points to use for acute stroke. In one

clinical study, for instance, the addition of Du-15 and Du-16 to standard body points improved outcome and shortened treatment duration.

**Parameters used** It is unclear from experimental studies what the optimum stimulation parameters for acute stroke might be. Several reports seem to use midrange frequencies (7–30 Hz) rather than low frequencies. DD has also been used to disperse oedema within the brain.

## Acupuncture treatment for the sequelae of stroke

### APHASIA
Aphasia, impaired spoken or written language, may precede or follow stroke, and can be very difficult to treat. However, good results were reported with LF scalp EA in one controlled study. As with physical exercise during treatment for hemiplegia, the patient should exercise both voice and memory (singing, saying their address, and so on) during scalp MA for aphasia.

**Points used** In traditional MA, points such as HE-5, KI-6 and Ren-23 are used, together with bleeding of the sublingual points *jinjin* and *yuye* (M-HN-20). Other sublingual points, such as *yumen*, have also been used.

Joseph Wong recommends different Gall Bladder points on the scalp for expressive (motor) and receptive (sensory) aphasia, together with scalp points.

### PSEUDOBULBAR PARALYSIS AND DYSPHAGIA
*Pseudobulbar paralysis* (PBP) may be due to damage to nerves linking the cortex and medulla, to multiple lacunae within the brain, or to lesions of the lowermost cranial nerves (IX, X, XII). If it occurs following CVA, the resultant *dysphagia* can interfere with normal eating and drinking, and so impede recovery. Nasogastric feeding may be required, and speech may also be impaired.

A number of different EA point prescriptions have been tried for pseudobulbar paralysis, with Ren-23 (and GB-20) occurring frequently.

MA at GB-20, Ren-23 and points 0.5 cun bilateral and *rostral* to Ren-23 have been used for dysphagia following CVA. GB-20 and Ren-23 are possibly the most used points for the condition.

### HEMIPLEGIA
Hemiplegia is usually the most obvious symptom of stroke. If muscle is not to waste, it must be treated as soon as possible after paralysis sets in. Once atrophy is allowed to occur, it cannot be reversed. Exercise, acupuncture and electrotherapy are all important methods of maintaining the muscle's nerve supply and proprioception (awareness of the body), as well as preventing atrophy of the muscle itself. Peripheral stimulation, even at subliminal intensity, may be a key to speedy recovery after brain injury.

Improvements in paralysis may not be simply in terms of motor function. MA at scalp points was found to improve the weight-lifting capacity of paralysed legs in one experimental study. In another report, 2-year follow-up after 20 sessions of mixed MA and EA treatment (LF EA on the affected limb) indicated patients' improved ability to maintain balance.

EMG (electromyography) measurement of electrical muscle activity amplitude in ischaemic stroke showed that body MA and scalp EA increased its amplitude, but scalp MA did not. Many of the EA studies of scalp acupuncture emphasise the need to make muscles contract, with passive joint movement, for optimum effect.

As with other locomotor disorders, the *combination* of acupuncture with exercise may be important. Many authors emphasise the need for moving the affected limb, actively or passively, during treatment. Scalp needles may be left inserted during physical therapy sessions, for example. Exercise may also be important to maintain proprioception and prevent the development of neurogenic pain, as well as the formation of adhesions. It should not be too strenuous initially, but at the same time should not be avoided for fear of exacerbating spasticity.

Results with scalp needling may be better if sensation is obtained in the affected limb. PSM ('propagated sensation along the meridian') has also been explored in the treatment of stroke using body points. This has particular relevance in the treatment of stroke, where peripheral sensory and motor pathways may need to be maintained pending repair of central lesions. PSM, and recovery, can be encouraged by visualisation and energy awareness exercises that can lend an extra and rewarding dimension to the hard work of rehabilitation.

Margaret Naeser has concluded that if hemiplegia is still severe ('dead limb') and there is no isolated finger movement at 3 months or more after a stroke, then the paralysis is unlikely to improve very much if CT scanning shows a lesion occupying more than half the motor pathway areas in the periventricular white matter, PVWM. However, reductions in spasticity and improved limb circulation are still possible. On the other hand, a significant increase in movement is possible if some isolated finger movement remains and the lesion occupies less than half the PVWM. If there is no paralysis, or only mild hand paresis (partial paralysis), significant increases in finger and hand strength and dexterity can be expected. Thus, in one 1994 study Naeser's group found improvements in hand paresis with EA even 6–8 years after stroke. Other authors have found that EA is ineffective if the lesion is large and deep, bilateral, multifocal or involves the brainstem.

**Points used** Traditionally, if treatment is given within 3 months, points on the *yang* meridians of the affected limb may be used. In one textbook on treatment of paralysis the following are given:

*Upper limb:*
- Main points: SJ-5, LI-4, LI-11, LI-15 (bilaterally)
- Secondary points: P-2, SJ-3, LI-10, *jingbi* (M-HN-41).

*Lower limb:*
- Main points: GB-30, GB-34, GB-39, ST-36 (bilaterally)
- Secondary points: BL-39, BL-60, GB-31, LIV-3, SP-9, ST-31, ST-32, ST-41.

So, for example, one EA device manual suggests LI-4, LI-10, LI-11 and LI-15 for upper limb paralysis, with GB-30, GB-31, GB-34, GB-39, LIV-3 and ST-36 for the lower limb. Another recommends SJ-5, LI-4, LI-11, LI-15 and BL-23, GB-30, GB-34 and GB-39, respectively. Another variant for EA might be two to three points from LI-4, LI-6, LI-10, LI-11 (upper limb) or GB-30, GB-34, SP-6 (lower limb), together with scalp points. Other *yang* meridian points are possible, such as LI-14 or BL-40. *Huatuojiaji* points can also be important. Concentration on pairs such as LI-11 and LI-15, or SJ-5 and LI-15, for the upper limb, with ST-32 and ST-36 for the lower limb, is another possibility if your EA device has only one or two outputs. Others suggest taking three pairs of points from SJ-5, LI-4, LI-11, LI-15 and GB-30. In one systematic review of controlled studies of stroke, SJ-5, GB-34, LIV-3, LI-4 and LI-11 were the most commonly used points.

After 3 months, if there is no muscle wasting, one standard approach is first to reduce points on the healthy side and then to reinforce points on the diseased side, using the same points each side, or possibly just the *yang* meridian points on the affected side. If atrophy is present, treatment should be as for *wei* syndrome, reinforcing points such as BL-20, BL-21, ST-36, SP-6, Ren-11 and Ren-12.

Some very detailed accounts of points useful for EA treatment of paralysis, based on physiological rather than TCM principles, have been given by Wong. Points are selected for paralysis of individual muscle groups – for example, BL-11(−) and GB-21(+) for difficulty in raising the shoulder, or BL-16(−), BL-43(+) and SP-20(+) to lower the shoulder. A number of non-traditional points based on Western medical principles are included. Sometimes points at either end of a paralysed muscle will be selected.

For the paretic or spastic hand, *jing* Well, *baxie* (M-UE-22) and other commonly used shallow points on the hand and wrist may be stimulated, with a combination of microcurrent and LA (Naeser). For foot drop, corresponding points would be *jing* Well and *bafeng* (M-LE-8), with points such as BL-60, KI-3, KI-6, GB-40, LIV-4, ST-41 and SP-5.

Scalp regions are frequently used for hemiplegia–the middle 2/5ths of the motor zone and hand motor zone, for example.

**Parameters used** When using EA for muscle stimulation in stroke rehabilitation, muscle contraction is usually emphasised. Thus DD and intermittent modes have been recommended; 2 Hz or 2–4 Hz CW is also appropriate.

## SPASTICITY

Spasticity may be characterised as an abnormal muscle state in which both phasic (rapid) and tonic (slower) stretch reflex thresholds are decreased so that reflexes appear hyperactive and strength is reduced. Spasticity can occur in opposed muscle groups at the same time, resulting in rigor.

If untreated, spasticity can result in permanent muscle and joint contracture. Spasticity goes hand in hand with hemiplegia following CVA, and is the most prominent problem for many stroke victims.

Initially following stroke, the paralysed limb may be flaccid and unresponsive to touch. Spasticity and reflex spasm may increase as the ratio of slow to fast muscle fibres rises, hopefully then to diminish as normal movement is re-established. Recent hemiplegia, in which there may be increased excitability in response to electrical stimulation, may be differentiated from late stage hemiplegia, when response is reduced due to inactivity.

Significant increases in finger and hand strength and dexterity can be expected even if acupuncture is not started till after 3 months if paresis is mild, but little change in range of movement is likely with severe spasticity. In such severe cases, acupuncture may still maintain circulation to the limb, prevent contractures and keep the extremities warm. It is unlikely to be effective once muscle has become fibrosed and permanent contracture has set in. However, HF EA at Governor Vessel points may be more effective for poststroke spasticity than that following spinal trauma, perinatal cerebral damage or Parkinson's disease.

As with paralysis, electrotherapy (CTENS in particular) has important contributions to make in the treatment of spasticity. In cases of extreme spasticity, some authors have cautioned against HF stimulation, or even against EA altogether except at particular points well away from the area concerned. Others have suggested EA should not be used when the limb is rigid (rigor).

Case study 9.9.2 gives a personal perspective on poststroke electroacupuncture.

**Comparisons** Yoshiaki Omura has suggested that EA may be more effective for localised spasticity than either MA or TENS. It is not clear whether this is the case for spasticity following stroke.

**Points used** Joseph Wong recommends BL-6, GB-17 and Du-22 for stimulation of the basal ganglia, Du-16 and Du-26 for stimulation of the medulla, and *huatuojiaji* points or BL-41–BL-52 for stimulation of the spinal nerves, among other points.

Contralateral points have been used during the early, flaccid stage of paralysis, with stimulation to the antagonistic muscles on the paralysed side once spasticity has developed. Treatment of antagonist muscles for spasticity is a time-tested approach in Western electrotherapy. The effects of CTENS may last longer if applied heterosegmentally.

If spasticity is severe, it has been suggested that EA should be limited to points such as Du-6 and *naoqi* (M-BW-29), both points indicated for seizures. Governor Vessel points (Du-2, Du-6 and Du-15) were emphasised in one clinical report of spasticity due to various causes.

**Parameters used** Some authors have found brief (5-minute) LF EA to be helpful for spasticity in the lower leg. However, frequencies as low as 2–3 Hz are not often used.

Because spasticity is sometimes considered to result from an increase in the proportion of slow muscle fibres once muscle is denervated following stroke, HF stimulation to retard this increase might be appropriate. This is in keeping with Han Jisheng's emphasis on HF stimulation for spasticity. In the stroke studies that focus on treating spasticity, it does seem that most clinicians use EA at around 10–15 Hz, 20–25 Hz or 100 Hz, rather than at lower frequencies.

## PAIN
Central pain, due to damage to the pain pathways within the brain, may occur in up to 8% of stroke patients. Impaired circulation in unused muscle can lead to ischaemic pain, the pain of oedema, and to neurogenic pain because of damage to poorly nourished nerves within the muscle. Neurogenic pain may also arise because of lack of afferent input to the central nervous system from the muscle.

In particular, if the arm is paralysed, it becomes a 'dead weight' pulling on the shoulder. Once muscles holding the shoulder joint in place lose their tone, subluxation of the joint becomes increasingly possible, resulting in further injury, not only to the joint and surrounding muscles, but to nerves as well. In turn this can lead to the development of '*shoulder-hand syndrome*,' a form of complex regional pain disorder (CRPD). Shoulder pain retards rehabilitation and can lead to complete disuse of the affected arm. It may occur in as many as 40% of stroke patients, and is especially prevalent in the first few weeks after leaving hospital.

Electrical stimulation is often used to prevent and treat shoulder pain after stroke. The authors of a Cochrane review on this approach found that stimulation reduced the severity of glenohumeral subluxation, and so improved pain-free range of passive humeral lateral rotation, but without significantly affecting upper limb motor recovery or spasticity. Pain incidence and intensity were also not directly affected.

Both EA and TENS have been used for shoulder-hand syndrome. The main point used in one EA study was SI-12 (the meeting point of the Small Intestine, *sanjiao*, Gall Bladder and Large Intestine meridians in the supraspinatus muscle). In another, 10 Hz stimulation with triangular waves was applied, at an intensity sufficient to induce muscle contractions. Although this is an EA study, these are parameters typical of the Western electrotherapy approach to treating denervated muscle.

## TREMOR
Tremor following CVA has been treated with EA, in one case first with HF for 10 minutes, followed by 'sawtooth' wave stimulation for 20 minutes, at maximum tolerated intensity. Treatment was given once daily for 7 days, alternating between local and distal points.

## STROKE: SOME GENERAL COMMENTS
**Comparisons and combinations** In the meta-analysis of Chinese acupuncture RCTs for stroke mentioned above, MA was found to be superior to non-manual acupuncture in its effects. Adrian White, in his review of EA for various

# CASE Study 9.2.2

### Poststroke electroacupuncture: a personal perspective
**John L Stump**

On May 2, 1999, I returned from a lecture on acupuncture in Richmond, Virginia, for the International Academy of Medical Acupuncture. My wife, Dianne, and I decided to go out that evening to enjoy the last few minutes of a gorgeous sunset over Mobile Bay while having dinner at LuLu's Place. We finished dinner about 9 p.m. and went home to begin packing for a lecture trip to New Zealand.

By the time we got home we decided to get ready for bed instead of beginning the packing. About an hour after arriving home something went terribly wrong. I could not tell exactly what, but I could not move my right arm. Then my right leg began to go numb. I tried to tell Dianne what was wrong, but the language would not come out correctly. Now, almost in a panic, Dianne called 911 and our next-door neighbour to get help. By the time the ambulance had gotten there, I was out and did not regain consciousness for nearly 2 weeks. During this time, my wonderful wife Dianne had to take care of everything.

She was the only one who knew what I was thinking and put it into effect. I am forever in her debt for that. For without her I'm not sure what would have happened.

Everyone was saying I had a severe stroke, yet I had no symptoms of any problem before the apparent stroke. When stabilised, I was then taken from the emergency care at Thomas Hospital in Fairhope, Alabama to the rehabilitation hospital care at Mercy Medical in Daphne. Dianne called Dr Bob Cowan, a chiropractor and acupuncturist who had been with me at the lecture in Virginia, and asked him to come over to the hospital to see if we could begin acupuncture. Bob, it turned out, would come over from Pensacola, Florida, three times each week to do the acupuncture.

At first he began with the auricular points, *shenmen* and Brainstem, and the *jing* Well points because I still had some tubes attached and could not be moved. In the ensuing weeks, the tubes were removed. Intensive physical, occupational and speech therapy was started, and days turned into weeks before the doctors finally realised, as I had felt, that there must be an explanation why my blood pressure could not be stabilised. My blood pressure would not just spike at around 230/120 for no reason! My neurologist agreed, and the hunt was on as to the reason. They soon brought in an endocrinologist. She had nearly every inch of my body scanned by MRI or CT. Then they found

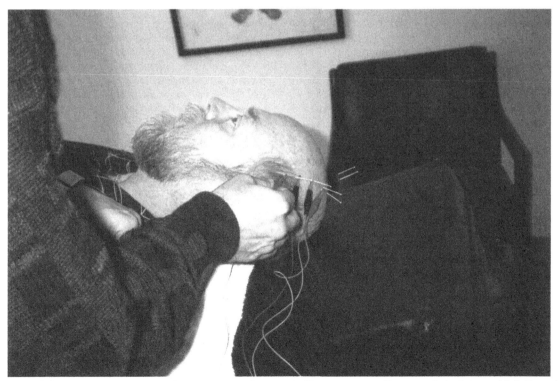

**Figure 9.2.2** John Stump being treated for stroke by Bob Cowan, using EA at scalp points. (Courtesy of John Stump and Bob Cowan.)

*(Continued)*

the culprit, a small tumour that carries a big stick, a pheochromocytoma about 30 mm × 30 mm. This adrenal tumour seemed confined to my right side.

During this time, Dr Bob was continuing to do electroacupuncture on me, but I had to make a decision. The tumour was still not allowing my blood pressure to stabilise, even with all the medication. It was then I decided to go for the surgery. However, another catch: the pheochromocytoma was a very rare tumour, thus a rare surgery, less than 1% nationwide and even more rare in Southern Alabama!

The decision was made to have the tumour removed. Although it was determined to be benign, it was still capable of causing the catecholamines (epinephrine and norepinephrine) to become unbalanced and act erratically. The surgery was scheduled at the Mobile Infirmary and successfully completed on 18 October 1999. As soon as I was able to get out of intensive care and back home, I had Bob come over and resume the acupuncture. Bob had been the best student I had taught, not because he had the best grades, but because he wanted to know the why, when and how of the procedures in acupuncture. Dr Bob Cowan would be a lifesaver for me in more ways than one.

Bob came three times each week to do the acupuncture. He used scalp points (opposite side of stroke), auricular points and *jing* Well points for the first month. Then, as I could move a little, he began to use full body treatment. Balancing the meridians at first was very difficult, for I had very little right pulse to read. He said my tongue looked surprisingly good for what had happened.

During this period, the sessions were about 45 minutes and electroacupuncture was the prime method utilised. The EMI (electromeridian imaging) method was used to check the progress of the meridians each week and he noticed my Kidney meridian begin to come up to an acceptable level after the first 6 weeks of treatment.

My progress had been remarkable. To have survived was first, then there was the adrenal surgery, and now the therapy. Each week there was a little progress. The occupational therapist and the physical therapist asked what we were doing, as I seemed to be responding much better and faster than the other stroke victims, some of whom had much lighter strokes and were much younger.

All of this is not to say that a stroke or apoplexy is not severe and considered so by all practitioners. The loss of motor and sensory function on one or both sides (hemiplegia is a partial paralysis) and the loss of communication (aphasia) can be completely debilitating to some, if not most. This is not to mention the psychological and emotional trauma that must be considered. I know that all of these factors were certainly apparent during my stroke.

This last year has been very difficult and challenging to say the least. Yet it has also been highly inspirational and educational when looking at it from the patient's perspective instead of the doctor's point of view! I am progressing well, all things considered. The major problem I have to overcome now is the hypertensity in my right arm and leg.

Dr Bob reports that the plasticity and the energy flow are much improved. This accounts for the rapid change in my body structure and function during electroacupuncture and chiropractic. Neural feedback systems regulate the muscle tone. The receptors in this system include the Golgi tendon organs at the muscle insertions, but the receptors don't seem be getting the message yet! It is as if I have 75% flexion and only 25% extension on the right side of my body.

Presently, we are continuing the electroacupuncture once or twice per week, chiropractic, exercise and a vast array of naturopathic and homeopathic supplements. Bodywork has been a definite help and will continue to be utilised. The present hurdle to be crossed is the hypertensity and spasticity of the right arm and leg. The fact that I was able to write this account is a testimony for the clarity and cognisance of my mental process. The aphasia is all but gone, and I am sure it will only be a matter of time before I am back to teaching and lecturing.

## Postscript January 2004

It is nearly 4 years since I became involved in this book. At the time, I was not sure I would be able to accomplish the research and writing to make the allocation promised. Recently I resumed lecturing and nearly 2 years ago I began to see patients on a part-time basis. I can no longer do chiropractic manipulation because I lack the use of my right hand. I can do acupuncture with my left hand and I can also use a laser instrument when necessary.

I remembered my *sensei* (teacher) in Japan, Dr Shingo Fukinbara, saying that he knew a blind, one-armed acupuncturist who could palpate and insert the needles as accurately and as smoothly as silk. This he told while teaching us how to manipulate the needle and the pipette. I never forgot those words and they have become an inspiration to me.

I still have the spasticity in my right arm and leg, although to a much lesser degree than 4 years ago. I can now walk without braces but my most difficult problem is still the right arm from the elbow down. I have motor ability and sensory sensation, but both seem to be less than 50% at best. I will continue to try to improve the situation as best I can. Otherwise I seem back to a relatively normal life, although I have not tried some of my favorite pastimes since the stroke, like scuba diving, golf or billiards. I do wish I could return to teaching the Zen Buddhist martial art to which I dedicated much of my time – Shorinji Kempo. However, I do not feel I can adequately teach the movements and techniques and so retired last year after teaching it for nearly 30 years.

I do not think I could have made it back to this stage as quickly or as well without the benefit of Oriental medicine and electroacupuncture.

conditions elsewhere in this book, reports that EA was not superior to superficial MA for acute stroke, and neither was more effective than standard treatment alone. Nor was EA superior to sham EA for stroke, except when lesions as visualised using CT scan occupied less than half the 'brain motor pathway'. However, EA was superior to standard rehabilitation for stroke in three studies, although not in a fourth.

On the other hand, experimental studies indicate that EA may enhance cerebral blood flow more than MA, and the authors of many clinical stroke studies also believe that EA is superior to MA in some respects. In one EMG study of electrical muscle activity, for example, results were better with EA than MA at scalp points. In a further report, EA at scalp points, with or without body points, gave better results than MA for the sequelae of CVA.

**Points used** Governor Vessel and Gall Bladder points on the head are prioritised by various authors. Both experimental and clinical research certainly indicate their usefulness. In particular, many traditional prescriptions use Du-20 and GB-20. Stimulating GB-20, for instance, can dilate arteries and increase blood flow to the brain to reduce ischaemic brain damage. Other occipital points, such as BL-10, or points on the neck (LI-18) may also be important as well.

The use of *huatuojiaji* points is sometimes emphasised; for example, needling those between C1 and C2 can stimulate the superior cervical sympathetic ganglia and improve cerebral circulation. Those level with C4 to C7 can be used for upper limb paralysis, and the L2 to S1 *huatuojiaji* points for lower limb paralysis. Some authors suggest they should not be used before the patient's blood pressure and general condition have stabilised.

Points such as GB-30, LI-4, LI-11 and ST-36 are frequently used in experimental studies. Other points can be added for additional problems, such as ST-4 for facial paralysis. Joseph Wong usefully lists points for various stroke sequelae, including hemisensory deficit and bladder dysfunction, as well as hemiplegia.

Many extra points have been used for stroke treatment too, such as the series of *zhitan* points (M-UE-30, N-UE-27; M-LE-13, N-LE-13, N-LE-18, N-LE-38).

Contralateral needling is particularly common in the treatment of hemiplegia. For example, contralateral MA within 6 months of stroke gave better results than needling the paralysed side in one report. Other MA studies support this conclusion. Alternating points on the healthy and affected side may give even better results.

According to traditional theory, treatment should be staged. Some authorities consider the early stage of stroke to last up to 6 months and the middle stage from 6–18 months, followed by the late stage (up to 3 years). Others allow only 1 month for the acute stage, from the second to sixth month for the middle stage, and from then onwards for the late stage. As already mentioned, much research indicates that 3 months is the watershed between early and subsequent phases.

In the early stage of the disorder, the healthy side may be energetically excess (*shi*) and the paralysed side deficient

(*xu*), and treatment should be directed to reducing the excess until the paralysed extremity can be moved slightly, or registers sensation. A contrary view is that stagnation on the affected side in the early phase warrants reduction.

In the middle stage, stagnation of *qi* is present too, and both sides should be treated, reducing on the healthy side, supplemented with reinforcing on the paralysed side.

In the late stage, emphasis should be on reinforcing the affected side to counter stagnation of Cold and impaired circulation of *qi* and Blood, supplemented with reducing treatment on the healthy side if necessary. Some studies indicate that contralateral needling is most appropriate in the acute stage (or in the early, flaccid stage of paralysis). Others consider that tonification of the affected side is the most important aspect of treatment. With scalp points, there is surprisingly no apparent difference between needling the affected or contralateral side.

Although contralateral treatment is often recommended in traditional theories and MA studies, in most EA studies treatment is concentrated on the affected side. In one report, however, EA contralateral (*juci*) to the affected limb changed both the colour *and* flow rate of nailbed blood flow, whereas ipsilateral EA (*tanci*) treatment changed only the flow rate. In one study, blood flow changes in the brain confirmed the usefulness of treating the healthy side. Bilateral treatment may be better still.

*Yin and yang:* A standard treatment for hemiplegia is to use *yang* meridian points on the affected limb. However, some MA and EA studies have emphasised treating *yin* meridian points. In the very vigorous *xingnao kaiqiao* ('consciousness awakening') MA method, also adapted for EA in some experimental studies, *yin* and *yang* points are alternated in sequence: P-6, Du-26, SP-6, BL-40, ~HE-1 (located somewhat distal to its usual position), LU-5 and LI-4 – each to the point of tears (Du-26) or muscle jerking. Better results are claimed than with standard *yang* meridian and scalp point stimulation, with improvements in several objective measures.

An alternative suggestion is that *yang* meridian points be used within the first 3 months after a stroke, with both *yin* and *yang* meridian points stimulated from 3 to 6 months, and points mainly from *yin* meridians after 6 months.

*Scalp and head points:* As an alternative to treating traditionally located points on the Governor Vessel and Gall Bladder meridian, scalp acupuncture was developed by several different researchers, with roots in the work of Huang Xuelong, who in the 1930s suggested a relationship between the scalp and the underlying cerebral cortex. Since the early studies, various authors have used CT or other scanning methods to locate lesions and therefore the most appropriate scalp points for EA.

Traditional head points such as GB-7 and Du-20, rather than scalp points *per se*, have also been used in MA studies for hemiplegia. In fact there may be considerable overlap between the two systems, particularly in the use of points at or around Du-20. Temporal needling and 'enclosing needling' guided by CT scan rather than fixed-point location are other approaches.

According to one comprehensive review, BL-7, GB-7, GB-18, GB-20, Du-15 and Du-16 are the most commonly used head points, the most frequently used scalp areas being the motor, sensory, foot-kinaesthetic sensory and speech II areas, the most frequently used scalp lines being the anterior oblique line of the vertex-temporal, the posterior-anterior oblique line of the vertex-temporal, and lines I and II lateral to the vertex. No significant difference was found between using the stimulation areas and the standardised scalp lines. In another such review, the most commonly used head points for stroke are BL-6, BL-7, GB-6, GB-7, GB-17, GB-18, Du-20, Du-21 and Du-24, and the most commonly used scalp acupuncture areas are the motor region, sensory region and foot motor sensory region. Better results are obtained by needling points and scalp lines on forehead, vertex and temple than on the occiput. As already mentioned, there is little apparent difference in results when needling the two sides.

However, the meta-analysis of Chinese stroke RCTs suggests that stimulating body points may give better results than needling points on the head. Again, this result may need qualification, depending on other factors. For instance, scalp MA may have less effect on muscle function following ischaemic stroke than body MA or scalp EA. In contrast, scalp MA was superior to body EA when both were combined with acupoint injection in a different report. In a further study, the combination of scalp and body point EA or MA gave better results than scalp points alone, when used for the sequelae of CVA such as paralysis and aphasia. One group, using 'synchronised stimulation' at corresponding body and scalp points, claimed superior results with this combination approach. In yet another study, scalp EA together with acupuncture at body points gave better results than the latter alone.

**Parameters used** When using body points, as with any condition, the basic decision on whether or not to use MA or EA is often based on syndrome differentiation.

Different frequencies of stimulation may have different effects on the cerebrovascular circulation. For instance, in one experimental study sciatic nerve electrostimulation at 50 Hz increased arteriolar diameter in the corresponding somatosensory cortical area by more than 50% (5 Hz by some 30%). This may well be important when treating hemiplegia.

Midrange frequencies (10–15 Hz) at high intensity have been used in some studies. However, in part because the primary symptom addressed is usually hemiplegia, strong LF EA (CEA) is usually employed, from less than 1 Hz to around 6 Hz. In one report, 5–15 Hz was used, and one group has used both 30 Hz and 100 Hz TLEA for acute stroke, although this is less usual. Low-frequency moderate-intensity and DD EA have also been used.

*Parameters for scalp point stimulation:* In most scalp MA studies, it seems that needles are rotated at about 200/minute (3.3 Hz). Variations with mechanised needle twirling include reduction at 300–400/min (5–6.7 Hz) for hemiplegia with aphasia, and reinforcing at 100–150/min (1.7–2.5 Hz) following cerebral haemorrhage, particularly in debilitated patients. Scalp EA with reduction at 300–500/min and reinforcing with 150–200/min have been used as well.

In one comprehensive review of scalp acupuncture for stroke, many papers supported the view that effects increase in proportion to intensity of stimulation. Perhaps because of this, HF (100–200 Hz) EA has sometimes been recommended for scalp stimulation. Val Hopwood and George Lewith used 100 Hz in their study, for example. Others have suggested 20 Hz (0.5 ms pulse duration) or DD. Many studies, though, use LF EA to maximum tolerance on scalp points, as on body points, though 'low frequency' can vary in this context from less than 1 Hz to around 10 Hz. A minority of studies use 'comfortable,' 'mild' or 'low-voltage' stimulation.

*Treatment frequency:* Giovanni Maciocia suggests that acupuncture should be given daily within 3 months of stroke onset, or every other day if treatment is started more than 3 months after stroke, with a break of 1–2 weeks after two months. Margaret Naeser suggests treatment three times weekly for acute stroke, and twice weekly after a month (a total of 20–40 sessions over 2–3 months). Better results are obtained the more treatment is given. In some Chinese hospitals, for instance, stroke patients may be treated twice daily while they are inpatients, returning for further acupuncture once they have been discharged. Even more intensive treatment has been used: in one study on the effects of scalp MA on haemodynamics following stroke, outcome was improved when treatment was given three times daily, rather than twice.

According to the meta-analysis of Chinese RCTs, the median number of treatments given was 30 over a 38-day period. Few Western studies have included such intensive treatment, possibly one reason why results are more equivocal than those from China. TEAS may be a more economically viable intervention for many patients.

*Other possible approaches:* In line with the suggestion that higher frequencies may be more reducing, reduction with 300–500/min (5–8.3 Hz) EA has been used on the

**Cautions on points and parameters used**

Although it is clear that points on the head and neck may be the key to successful treatment of stroke and transient ischaemia, patients should be carefully monitored. Even if acupuncture, and EA in particular, generally has a regulatory effect, untoward vasodilation may not be appropriate following recent menangioma or aneurysm, and vasoconstriction may be unhelpful if the patient is liable to TIA. Thus some authors consider EA contraindicated in the acute stage of haemorrhagic brain trauma or stroke, although scalp MA may be acceptable.

Strong electrostimulation ('faradisation') was inadvertently found to induce further strokes in those who had already suffered an attack by Guillaume Duchenne de Boulogne, one of the founding fathers of Western electrotherapy.

healthy side, and 150–200/min (2.5–3.3 Hz) on the affected side for hemiplegia.

What has not been adequately explored as yet is treatment using frequency parameters derived from EEG readings. If, as the result of stroke or cerebral atherosclerosis, the amplitude of certain frequency ranges in the EEG spectrum is altered, then stimulation, particularly at scalp points, at these same frequencies may be beneficial. Monitoring the effects on the EEG of different stimulation frequencies could open up new therapeutic possibilities.

## CONCLUSION

For all the advances of medical science, stroke remains a leading cause of death and disability throughout the world. Stroke prevention, treatment and rehabilitation are a priority. Although acupuncture has been used for thousands of years for stroke, and many clinical studies on stroke have been carried out, the place of acupuncture, and EA in particular, in integrated medical care for this condition still remains to be substantiated scientifically.

| **9.2** Summary of relevant studies in the electronic clinical studies database (number of studies) | | |
|---|---|---|
| **Condition** | **EA** | **Other** |
| **Stroke** | | |
| Stroke | 126 | 88 |
| Aphasia | 22 | 13 |
| Pseudobulbar palsy | 17 | 11 |
| Spasticity | 5 | 14 |
| Hemineglect | 0 | 4 |
| Hemiplegic shoulder pain and subluxation | 7 | 9 |
| Urinary symptoms | 3 | 1 |
| Bowel symptoms | 0 | 1 |
| Stroke-like symptoms due to trauma | 6 | 4 |

## SUMMARY

Some key points in this chapter are:

- Treatment should be started as early as possible to give the best chance of recovery
- EA has often been used as a preventative measure in patients at risk of stroke
- Contralateral treatment is frequently used in the treatment of hemiplegia with MA, EA being used more frequently on the affected side
- Treatment over a year after the stroke is unlikely to produce significant benefit.

 Additional material in the CD-ROM resource

In the electronic version of this chapter, considerable additional material is presented on stroke and its different types, its treatment with other acupuncture modalities and information on other acupuncture reviews and many specific studies. Other topics include a rapid review of the neurochemical changes involved in protecting the brain against insult, and short sections on hemineglect and the electrical activity of the brain following stroke and its treatment with acupuncture and moxibustion.

## RECOMMENDED READING

*Some reviews of acupuncture for stroke:*
Park J, Hopwood V, White AR, Ernst E Effectiveness of acupuncture for stroke: a systematic review. Journal of Neurology. 2001 July; 248(7): 558–63
Sze FK, Wong E, Or KK, Lau J, Woo J Does acupuncture improve motor recovery after stroke? A meta-analysis of randomized controlled trials. Stroke. 2002 Nov; 33(11): 2604–19
Tang JL, Zhan SY 1999 Is acupuncture effective in stroke rehabilitation? A meta-analysis of randomized controlled trials in China. [Offprint, sent 2001 April 23]

*The last of these, available from the authors at the University of Hong Kong (jltang@cuhk.edu.hk) is rather more positive than the other two, based as it is solely on RCTs from China.*

*Useful pointers for the treatment of stroke are given in:*
Chen A Effective acupuncture therapy for stroke and cerebrovascular diseases. 1. American Journal of Acupuncture. 1993 July–Sept; 21(3): 205–18

*Textbooks containing a wealth of information include:*
Kong Y, Ren X, Lu S 1996 The Acupuncture Treatment for Paralysis. Science Press, Beijing
Lü SJ 2002 Handbook of Acupuncture in the Treatment of Nervous System Disorders. Donica Publishing, London
Wong JY 2001 A Manual of Neuro-Anatomical Acupuncture. Volume II: Neurological disorders. Toronto Pain and Stress Clinic, Toronto

# 9.3 PERIPHERAL MOTOR DISORDERS, THE IMMUNE SYSTEM AND THE ENDOCRINE SYSTEM

*With contributions by Steven KH Aung, J Gordon Gadsby and Lynnae Schwartz*

In the last chapter, motor disorders originating within the central nervous system were considered. Here, peripheral motor disorders are discussed, particularly Bell's palsy, followed by accounts of how EA and related methods can be used in conditions affecting the immune and endocrine systems.

## PERIPHERAL MOTOR DISORDERS

### Facial paralysis – Bell's palsy

Most cases of facial paralysis result from inflammation of the peripheral facial nerve (cranial nerve VII), or its compression due to vasospasm or oedema, generally in the mastoid region. It is often associated with herpes simplex or zoster infection, and precipitated by exposure to draughts on the face. The muscles above the eyes are affected, and pain behind or in front of the ear may precede paralysis.

Bell's palsy is not uncommon, and 80% of patients recover within weeks to months, but the outcome is less favourable in patients aged over 60 years. Ramsay Hunt's syndrome (herpes zoster oticus), in which paralysis is associated with a herpetic rash in or around the ear or on the roof the mouth, offers less than a 20% chance of spontaneous recovery.

The presence of incomplete paralysis in the first week is a favourable prognostic sign. If recovery is delayed, more than a simple neurapraxia (conduction block) may be involved, with axonotmesis, or degeneration of the nerve peripheral to the lesion. In these cases, recovery is likely to be incomplete. As degeneration can set in within a few days, many physical therapists consider early treatment to be important, which is directed at first to relieving pressure on the nerve, in the case of neurapraxia.

In acupuncture too, the emphasis is on early treatment. However, even treatment several years after the initial insult can produce useful results in cases of axonotmesis, if patients are willing to persist with it. At this stage, the aim of treatment is to assist nerve repair and facilitate muscle re-education. In general, interventions such as acupuncture that improve local circulation are likely not only to release local nerve compression but also to assist nerve regeneration. However, stimulation of totally denervated muscle (without sensation as well as movement) is unlikely to give good results.

In TCM, facial paralysis following a stroke is considered as due to internal Wind, and Bell's palsy to external Wind. Acupuncture has traditionally been considered to be very effective for the latter. Manual acupuncture (MA) has also been employed for facial paralysis due to diabetic (motor) neuropathy, particularly of the oculomotor nerve.

Simple manual needling may induce current of injury levels and densities in precisely the range required for nerve regrowth, and some authors state categorically that electrical stimulation should not be used for facial paralysis. Although strong stimulation of denervated muscle can, especially early on, lead to contractures and synkinesis (involuntary muscle movements), gentler electrotherapy is by no means contraindicated after the initial acute phase. Even during the acute phase, electroacupuncture (EA) with carefully controlled parameters, or other forms of acupoint electrostimulation, have been found helpful, although strong ipsilateral stimulation may well be counterproductive.

**Comparisons and combinations** Both EA and transcutaneous electrical acupoint stimulation (TEAS) are more effective than MA, according to some studies, with fewer treatments required, although one researcher found gentle manual vibration of shallowly inserted needles to be as effective as conventional EA.

Combination with moxibustion or far infrared appears to improve results with both MA and EA. The addition of extremely-high-frequency (EHF) stimulation, acupoint injection, (herbal) application or massage again improved the results of EA alone.

**Points used** Initially, few points should be treated. According to one useful review of point selection for EA, two to four acupoints from the affected area are generally used, such as *taiyang* (M-HN-9), with BL-2 or ST-2, for incomplete eye closure. LI-4 and SJ-5 may be used bilaterally as distal points. Other reviewers have suggested ST-4, ST-7, with LI-20 and *taiyang* ipsilateral to the paralysis and LI-4 contralateral. Simple combinations of GB–14-LI-4, ST-2–ST-7 or ST-4-LI-4 have been recommended for use with single-output stimulators.

Looking through the numerous studies, it is clear that local points are used, selected to activate particular paralysed muscles, together with some distal points. The most commonly used points appear to be GB-14, ST-40, ST-6 and ST-7, with LI-4 (indicated > 70 times), followed by SJ-17, LI-20, ST-2 and *taiyang* (> 50 times), BL-2 and GB-20 (> 40 times), SJ-23, SI-18, Ren-24, Du-26 and *yuyao*, with ST-36 (> 20 times). Contralateral treatment appears to be far rarer than treating the affected side. In some studies, different acupoints are used at different stages of the condition.

A rational selection of points might include BL-2, SJ-23, GB-14 and *taiyang* for involvement of the first branch of the facial nerve, SI-18 and ST-1 for second branch involvement, and ST-4 and ST-6 for the third branch. In terms of particular muscle function, BL-2 and GB-14 have been recommended for difficulty in frowning, SJ-23 and GB-14 for difficulty in raising the eyebrow, ST-3 and ST-4 for an inability to smile, with SJ-17, ST-4 and ST-6 as general points. SJ-17 has been emphasised by several authors.

**Parameters used** Strong electrostimulation for long periods should be avoided, especially in the early stages of facial paralysis, or if spasm is already present. Low-intensity EA should be used, just strong enough to elicit muscle contraction, possibly with stronger stimulation at distal points. An alternative might be gentle TEAS, daily initially for 4–5 days, then twice weekly, and so on. However, gentle motor level stimulation is less frequently mentioned than the standard Chinese 'intensity to tolerance' (or even 'maximum tolerance'), with gentle stimulation reserved for elderly or debilitated patients. One study explicitly states that only MA was used in the acute stage, and EA in 'restoration' and 'residual' stages.

On the basis of MA studies, LF stimulation for scalp points may be applied. There is a tendency to use LF, intermittent or DD stimulation, although 20, 50 and even 125 Hz are also mentioned. However, devices specifically for facial paralysis may use quite different parameters. In a wonderfully simple protocol suited to an unsophisticated rural practice, for example, ST-4 and ST-6 were stimulated using one to four ordinary 1.5 V batteries, although such non-charge-balanced stimulation should be used only with caution.

## Facial spasm

Facial spasm, near the eye or elsewhere, can follow facial paralysis and may follow or accompany multiple sclerosis (MS).

Both MA and EA have been used for facial spasm, sometimes with the latter locally and MA at distal points. Laser acupuncture (LA) and magnetic acupoint stimulation have been employed on their own, or combined with other acupuncture-based methods.

## Hiccup

Hiccup is caused by abrupt involuntary spasm of the diaphragm, leading to sudden inspiration and closure of the glottis, with the characteristic sound of hiccupping. The causes of hiccups range from neurological, respiratory, cardiovascular and gastrointestinal to pregnancy, uraemia and neurosis. Persistent hiccups can become debilitating and may require treatment.

MA and EA are quite widely used in the treatment of hiccup, including postoperative hiccup. pTENS and magnetic stimulation have also been explored, as well as TENS (for phrenic nerve stimulation).

**Points used** P-6, BL-17, ST-36 and Ren-12 or Ren-15 are usually recommended for the EA treatment of hiccup.

Other points include BL-2 and *erzhong* (M-HN-2), KI-15, GB-17, GB-20, GB-38, LIV-13, LIV-14, LI-17, ST-19, ST-21, Ren-16, Ren-22 and (for MA) the middle finger *sifeng* point (M-UE-9). Some of these are local to the diaphragm; others might have a direct or indirect effect on the phrenic nerve, such as LI-17, or Yan Liansheng's 'hiccup-relieving' point.

Auricular points are frequently used, presumably because of their inhibitory effect on hiccup via the vagus.

**Parameters used** There is little consistency across studies in the stimulation parameters employed, although intense stimulation is often used at some point during treatment.

## Other peripheral motor disorders

There are many forms of peripheral motor disorder. Localised muscle atrophy can result from spinal disc herniation, for example. The area may be surrounded with needles, *jing* points on the affected meridians and GB-34 stimulated (with MA or EA). Local scars can be 'bridged'.

Paralysis may result from peripheral nerve trauma. EA has been used to treat this in adults and infants, points being selected on the basis of TCM concepts or according to the nerve pathway, and LF or intermittent stimulation being employed. Other forms of peripheral paralysis or weakness that have been treated using EA include those due to multiple neurogangliitis, occupational poisoning or Guillain–Barré syndrome. Segmental abdominal zoster paresis has been treated with TENS.

# THE IMMUNE SYSTEM

The immune system is involved in most human ailments. Its fundamental function is to distinguish 'self' from 'not self', and to defend against the latter if potentially harmful. The immune system may be compromised, or hypoactive, leading to infection or conditions such as AIDS, cancer or chronic fatigue syndrome (CFS). It can also become hyperactive, leading to allergic responses to things not normally harmful, or may fail to distinguish self from not self, resulting in autoimmune disorders.

## The effects of acupuncture and its variants on the immune system

Traditionally, acupuncture is considered as supporting the body's upright *qi* and expelling external pathogens. By its very nature, therefore, immune enhancement is one of its major functions.

The immune system is activated by any invasion, and needling of course is no exception. As with its effects on the autonomic nervous system (ANS), those of EA on the immune system appear to be bidirectional and homeodynamic, countering, for example, the immunosuppressive effects of chemotherapy, or calming hypersensitivity to challenge by chemical antigens. EA may also have immune effects in apparently healthy humans – a pointer to its possible prophylactic use, for instance, prior to or during surgery.

EA and TENS affect both humoral and cellular immune functions, the latter via neurotransmitter receptors on lymphocytes, for example. EA, possibly more than MA, may enhance leukocyte counts generally, including those of lymphocytes and neutrophils, or lower them where there is local inflammation or a generalised defence reaction to toxins. Furthermore, EA may increase phagocytosis and reduce fever.

Moxibustion has traditionally been used for many conditions that would today be considered the result of immune dysfunction, and its immunological mechanisms have been explored in many studies. Electrically heated needles, acupoint EHF (MRT), LA and even small magnets applied to acupoints have all, in experimental studies, been found to enhance immune function. EHF treatment and acupoint magnetic stimulation have been used clinically.

Like EA, EHF and LA/LILT (low-intensity laser therapy) have a regulatory effect on immune function. In particular, LAA during surgery appears to enhance immune response. Pekka Pöntinen and others have proposed that preoperative LILT, by effectively controlling postoperative pain and inflammation, may have immune protective effects, which is particularly important in cancer patients.

## Some examples of the immune benefits of acupuncture and its variants in different circumstances

### TISSUE REPAIR
A number of electrotherapy modalities have been used in the treatment of infected wounds, including TENS, low-voltage DC, LILT and pulsed electromagnetic fields (PEMF).

EA, with its effects on microcirculation and immune function, can be used preventively in acute injury, as well as when wounds are slow to heal. In one Russian study, for example, its effects were found to be superior to those of LILT or narcotic management for infected wounds. In a Chinese study, the therapeutic effect of LA on infected facial wounds was the same whether or not antibiotics were used in addition. Other interventions for enhancing tissue repair and immune function include electrically warmed needles and EHF.

## The compromised immune system – infection and its prevention

Public health officials may be concerned about possible infection from inadequate sterile procedures in acupuncture, but acupuncture is in fact frequently used in the treatment of both acute and chronic infection. Historically, it has even been used in China for cholera, and more recently for malaria, and there is evidence from animal studies that this may not be as outrageous as it seems. Indeed, EA may enhance antibody production in response to some immunisations.

Acupuncture, but EA possibly less than MA, has a febrifugal effect. EA has been found to accelerate recovery from influenza, for example, and has also been used preventively.

The symptomatic treatment of mumps with MA and TENS is worth noting, as is the fact that mumps has also been treated with auricular MA alone.

LILT has been used to improve immune function in enuretic children with a tendency to urinary tract infections, as well as for recurrent herpes simplex. Whether LILT could prevent herpes zoster (shingles) has not yet been explored, although it has been used for the itch of chickenpox, for shingles (LA at immune-enhancing points, as well as locally) and for postherpetic neuralgia.

Sonopuncture has been used for different herpes infections, and for lymphadenopathy associated with infectious mononucleosis (glandular fever). However, it should be remembered that ultrasound is often considered to be contraindicated in acute infection (or malignancy).

Although acupuncture is frequently used in the treatment of those with HIV and AIDS, EA is not often considered, perhaps because the condition is primarily a Deficient not a Full one, in TCM terms. In a comprehensive article on HIV/AIDS, Nicholas Haines has suggested using EA (intermittent 5–8 Hz) at SP-2 and SP-3, in conjunction with MA at SP-9 and ST-8, for Spleen *qi xu* with Damp. Some studies also report benefits treating HIV-related peripheral neuropathy with EA, as well as postherpetic neuralgia in HIV patients. Cranial electrotherapy stimulation (CES) has also been tried to help those with HIV cope more effectively with the stresses this condition induces.

Case study 9.3.1 describes the use of ion-pumping cords and TEAS in a paediatric patient.

## The compromised immune system – oncology

### TREATING CANCER
Various forms of acupuncture may have a useful and important role to play in cancer treatment, although always in association with input from other health professionals:

- in immune support
- for pain relief (including peri- and postoperative analgesia)
- to counter the side-effects of chemo- and radiotherapy
- in terminal care
- and – not to be forgotten – in rehabilitation.

The effects of acupuncture on immune-related leu-enkephalin (LE) have been suggested as a rationale for its use in oncology (D-phenylalanine, the enkephalinase inhibitor, may enhance the inhibitory effect of acupuncture on sarcoma cell growth, for instance). Changes in cellular immune function with acupuncture have also been documented in cancer patients. High levels of oestradiol ($E_2$) associated with mammary hyperplasia may be associated with immune inhibition, setting the scene for possible development of cancer later on. EA has been found to reduce levels of $E_2$ and its inhibitory effect on immune function. Low-cost local treatment of tumours using DC stimulation through needles, as developed by Björn Nordenström, is being used more and more in China. It is also being combined effectively

# CASE Study 9.3.1

## Electrical stimulation of acupuncture points and meridians in paediatric patients I
### Lynnae Schwartz

Specific English language descriptions of clinical experience using electrical stimulation of acupuncture points and meridians in paediatric medicine are few. Infants and young children present many challenges for the acupuncturist wishing to use EA, for reasons that include:

1. For infants and children, the *qi* tends to be superficial along the channels and at specific points, easily manipulated by *tuina* or very shallow needle technique. EA may be too strong a stimulus relative to the depth and strength of the infant's or child's *qi*, with the theoretical potential to aggravate disease driving it deeper into the body.

2. The placement of needles through the skin is typically not acceptable to the awake younger child.

3. Needle placement after induction of anaesthesia in children circumvents problems of patient acceptance, but may compromise efficacy.

4. Experienced practitioners may perceive *deqi* (PSM) even if their patient is sedated, anaesthetised or unable to cooperate, but there exist no validated measures to assure that *deqi* has been reached in patients unable to communicate.

5. There are no dose–response curves published for EA in paediatric patients, with little knowledge of effective intensities, frequencies, patterns of stimulation, duration or validated outcome measures for EA administration.

In summary, published English language experience for electrical stimulation of acupuncture points and meridians in infants, children and younger adolescents is limited. Such stimulation can be used, but much is not yet understood, including dose–response, optimal patterns and timing of stimulation, physiological effects, indications and patient selection, optimal point combinations, interactions with standard allopathic medical management, and contraindications specific to a paediatric population. Additional published case material as well as prospective clinical trials and physiological investigations are needed before recommendations can be made concerning routine use of electroacupuncture in paediatric patients.

The following case example is offered to illustrate these issues in paediatric practice.

## Case I

A 6-year 9-month-old, 19.4 kg boy with advanced HIV-1/AIDS, CDC classification B2, came as scheduled for his third outpatient acupuncture based treatment, accompanied by his father. The father's goal was to improve his son's immune status through acupuncture-based treatments, offered in addition to standard medical management of AIDS and secondary infections. The patient's HIV-1 infection had led to progressive loss of health, falling CD4 cell count and rising viral load assays despite aggressive and consistent antiretroviral medications and treatment of intercurrent infections. Additional medications included granulocyte colony stimulating factor (GCSF). Review of symptoms (ROS) was notable for lack of specific complaints. He attended school, had friends and enjoyed a stable home life with his father. Physical examination at his first visit (10/97) revealed thin habitus, an engaging and focused personality, a toe-in gait under orthopaedic treatment with braces, and oral candidiasis. Pulses were thin but palpable, diminished bilaterally in the third position, with perhaps only a slight decrease in *qi* on the left compared to the right side. Tongue examination was positive for a red tip, normal coating and no quiver. Palpation of meridians and selected points/areas was remarkable for lack of reaction.

Treatment 1 was as follows:

- ion-pumping cords without needles – LIV-3 (red clip) to LI-4(black clip) – gently taped to skin at each acupoint
- 002 needle to right LU-7
- *tuina* massage at *yintang*
- meditation and quiet rest for10 minutes
- *tuina* massage to back *Shu* points, especially BL-20 and BL-23

The patient found the treatment to be relaxing, and returned in 1 month for a second treatment. At that visit, he looked well despite a further decline in his CD4 cell count with a rising viral load. The ROS was remarkable for his good appetite and energy, doing well in school and no acute complaints. The physical exam was unchanged except for pulses suggesting diminished Spleen *qi* and superficial Lung *qi*, with an increased heart rate suggesting Heat/susceptibility to external pernicious influence.

Treatment 2 consisted of:

- ion-pumping cords with 002 needles very superficially placed in LU-7 (black clip) but placed only on the skin at KI-6(red clip), retained for 12–15 minutes, during which the patient fell into a light sleep
- *tuina* massage to back *shu* points and *yin* channels of the lower extremities. Tension was noted on the right from BL-13 to BL-20, and a sensation of emptiness in the *yin* channels.

Returning in 1 week for a third treatment, he was less well but not toxic or medically unstable. His ROS was positive for symptomatic oral thrush, loose stools, a 24-hour history of low-grade fever, and mild symptoms of upper

*(Continued)*

## CASE Study 9.3.1 **Continued**

respiratory infection. Vital signs included a temperature of 38.9°C, heart rate of 113–120 and blood pressure of 112/66. He was in no acute distress, and had no evidence of haemodynamic or metabolic instability. Prior to acupuncture he was seen and examined by his primary paediatrician, who requested that the patient go to the emergency room for laboratory tests and intravenous antibiotics immediately following a brief acupuncture treatment. Acetaminophen was given for fever. Pulses were decreased in the left third position, with superficial Lung *qi*, and thin character overall. He was tender to palpation at LU-7, KI-6 and Ren-15, LU-1–LU-2 and all along the *renmai* (Conception Vessel).

Treatment 3 was as follows:

- an ITO-F3 electroacupuncture unit with lead wires connected to rubber electrodes, each containing a 3000 G magnet (Fig. 9.3.1), was applied transdermally to stimulate LU-7 and KI-6 bilaterally, arranged so that one lead connected the ipsilateral points, with the (+) electrodes to KI-6; intensity and frequency were adjusted to patient comfort, maintaining a constant (continuous) stimulation pattern
- 002 needle to Du-23.

He immediately fell deeply asleep, and remained so despite termination of stimulation and needle removal after 20 minutes. Vigorous stimulation after 60 minutes of sleep provoked little change in status. After 90 minutes he was alert enough to be carried to the emergency room, where he received intravenous antibiotics and fluids, with discharge home late that night. Blood and other cultures were ultimately negative; he soon became afebrile and back to his usual level of health until 2 months later, when he developed severe mucositis requiring prolonged hospitalisation.

### Discussion

1. Our initial treatment goal was nurture the *yin* with gentle stimulation of *yinqiao renmai*. Improving pulse examination and the development of reaction upon point palpation suggested some success without apparent adverse effect.
2. Electrical stimulation of these same points resulted in prolonged, deep sedation, suggesting that the treatment was too strong for the patient's *qi*. His disease (external pernicious influence) could have been driven deeper, with potential for serious infection in this already immunocompromised and medically fragile boy.

(A second case is described in Section 9.13.)

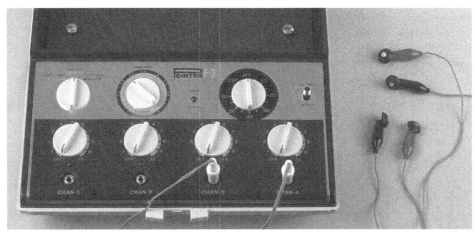

**Figure 9.3.1** ITO electrical stimulation unit and electrodes with 3000 G magnets attached. Magnets are placed on indicated acupuncture points. Stimulation is titrated to patient comfort and clinical effect. Alternatively, the electrodes may be attached to inserted needles, if acceptable both to the child and the parents. A maximum of four channels (eight needles or electrodes) may be stimulated simultaneously.

with chemotherapy. With the aid of ultrasound and other scanning methods, even non-superficial tumours have been treated with this sort of approach. Of course, this is a specialist area, and such methods should not be attempted without proper guidance and training.

From the CD-Rom ⊙ database, it would seem that EA, TEAS, LA/LILT and EHF potentially have a part to play in improving immune function and quality of life in cancer. In general, such treatments applied for relatively *short* periods appear to work with the body, rather than against it. The potentially carcinogenic effects of *prolonged* exposure to various forms of electromagnetic fields have been reviewed many times.

## CANCER PAIN

Physically, cancer pain can be unremitting and excruciating, although it is often controllable with conventional medication. However, medication does not always control pain, and frequently leads to side-effects in cancer patients. Neuropathic pain, often arising as a result of chemotherapy, can be particularly intractable.

Many different physical interventions, including MA, EA, TENS, LILT/LA and even direct brain stimulation have been attempted for cancer pain. Low-intensity microwave stimulation has been claimed to have both an immediate and also a cumulative effect on cancer pain. There are also good indications that EA, TENS and LA may be helpful, though the results of some studies show pain relief diminishing rapidly with time, and others demonstrate no effects on cancer pain.

Case study 9.3.2 is an example of the use of EA in cancer pain.

Whatever the misgivings on the use of electrotherapy in cancer, EAA has been used in many operations for resection (partial excision) of tumours, without apparent adverse effects. This approach has been applied for cancer of the brain, jaw, oesophagus, larynx, thyroid, breast, stomach,

---

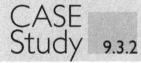

# CASE Study 9.3.2

**Electroacupuncture: an integrative clinical perspective I**
**Steven KH Aung**

In my medical clinic in Edmonton, Alberta, I utilise acupuncture for most of the conditions recognised by the World Health Organization (WHO) as well as several other conditions, including cancer pain, chronic fatigue syndrome, fibromyalgia, immunodeficiency and various psychological illnesses. In my opinion – based on over 30 years of intensive clinical experience – acupuncture is an effective and safe approach to symptom control. I consider my practice a complementary or integrative model, since I have been comprehensively trained in both traditional Chinese medicine and biomedicine, with special training in geriatric medicine. Most of my patients are elderly and most are suffering the pain and discomfort of various difficult medical conditions, such as osteoarthritis and cancer.

In general, according to my own clinical practice, the indications for electroacupuncture are the same as for classical acupuncture. The relevant acupuncture points to be stimulated are selected after a biomedical and traditional Chinese medicine dual diagnosis has been performed. I may also use various 'electrical' techniques in diagnosis, notably, the Accu-O-Matic (see Fig. 10.2 on page 283). The Accu-O-Matic allows the practitioner to measure the electrical resistance of special energetic acupoints (known as *jing* Well points) in relation to the surrounding tissue. It is also a treatment device for stimulating points of relatively high resistance with electrical energy of negative polarity and points of relatively low resistance with a positive input. It is especially useful in paediatric and other cases where needling may be inadvisable.

I use basic electroacupuncture in approximately 90% of my clinical treatments, since most of my patients are suffering from chronic medical conditions. This therapy involves the application of electrical pulses of varying frequency and intensity from an electrical device through wires to the inserted needles. It produces a stronger stimulation than the mere insertion of needles. Moreover, it allows the electrical stimulation to be adjusted according to what is required for specific conditions. In terms of traditional Chinese medicine, this is beneficial not only for controlling pain but also for harmonising the *qi* of patients. It may be applied by various devices, including the four-channel outlet ITO IC-4107 model, which is commonly used in clinical practice (Fig. 9.3.2). Generally, I believe that a low-frequency and low-intensity pulse is indicated for normal pain control (for stimulation of endorphin and other neurotransmitter release), whereas a higher-frequency and higher-intensity pulse is indicated for various chronic disorders involving the central nervous system (in order to stimulate enhanced serotonin release).

The overall treatment goals are the same as for classical acupuncture – namely, to relieve pain and to harmonise the *qi* of patients. Patients generally feel good during their electroacupuncture treatment session, finding their 15–60-minute experience of being 'hooked up' to the device to be relaxing. Initially, the treatment procedure is the same as for classical acupuncture. The relevant acupoints are selected and the needles are inserted with the appropriate tonifying or sedating manipulation. Once the *'deqi'* sensation has been obtained on each needling site, the wires of the electroacupuncture device are clipped to the needles and the appropriate frequency and intensity of current is applied.

I generally treat severe cases on alternate days for the first week or two, until the patient reports a satisfactory response. I then schedule a treatment once every 2 weeks, then once a month, until the patient no longer

*(Continued)*

requires therapy. Unresponsive, difficult cases are referred back into the biomedical system for further assessment. Some patients may decide to purchase a portable electroacupuncture device for self-care purposes (see Fig. 9.11.4 on page 229). It is the responsibility of the physician or therapist to train patients how to use these devices in the proper manner.

In conclusion, electroacupuncture is one of the most valuable ancillary therapies within the discipline of medical acupuncture and in integrative primary care. Like classical acupuncture, it helps control pain and harmonise the total health of the patient. It is also a relaxing, energising experience for most patients. The basic electroacupuncture I practise is an efficient, cost-effective approach.

I have selected two brief cases examples to illustrate my basic approach to electroacupuncture.

## Case 1

The first case involves a 65-year-old woman experiencing colon cancer with metastasis to the bone, liver and lungs. This patient was referred to me on the basis of her severe pain in the lower abdomen and back. She also complained of fatigue and poor appetite. She was, in fact, dying of cancer. The traditional Chinese medical diagnosis indicated that her pain was due to severe Damp-Heat in the Lower Burner (*jiao*), or bowel area. I prescribed a number of relevant points on the Stomach meridian, including ST-40 (removal of Damp), ST-44 (for pain in the Lower Burner) and ST-25 and ST-37 (for general colonic pathology). P-6, a point on the Pericardium meridian, was prescribed to help control her nausea, and LI-11 to remove Heat. In addition a number of points on the Governor Vessel (Du-4 and Du-14) and the Conception Vessel (Ren-4, Ren-6, Ren-12 and Ren-17) were prescribed. In the traditional Chinese systems, the Governor and Conception Vessels are important in enhancing the vital energy of patients and uplifting their spirit.

The wires were connected and a pulse of low frequency (4 Hz) and intensity (intermittent) was applied for 30 minutes. The wires were connected as follows: ST-25 + ST-40, ST-37 + LI-11, P-6 + ST-44, (bilaterally) and Du-4 + Du-14, Ren-4 + Ren-12, Ren-6 + Ren-17

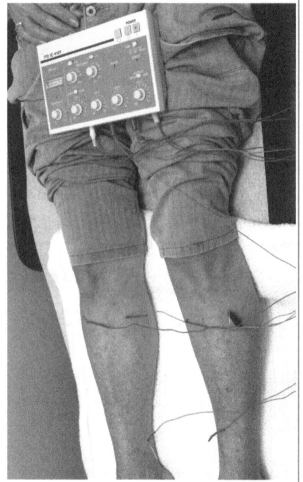

**Figure 9.3.2** Ito IC-4107 EA device in use. Note use of different coloured leads, and how needles from each output are connected ipsilaterally.

(connected along the midline of the body). After the first treatment the patient reported less pain and fatigue. Subsequent treatments over the next few months produced the same result. This served to enhance her quality of life, although the patient eventually died owing to the severity of her cancer.

(See Subchapter 9.12 for Steven Aung's second case.)

---

uterus and other organs. EAA has also been applied during DC tumour treatment for thyroid adenoma, and for laser treatment of skin cancer.

TENS has been used during cancer surgery, though less commonly than EAA, as has transcranial electrotherapy (TCET, a stronger form of CES), in combination with low-dose local analgesia and other medication. Given the immune suppression that results from radiotherapy, and the aggravated immune depression that can then follow operative procedures and the use of anaesthetics, methods such as EA or TCET that can support immune function seem particularly appropriate for cancer patients.

Postoperatively, MA and EA may potentially be helpful not only for pain but also for postoperative sequelae such as hot flushes following castration in men with prostate cancer. TCET has also been employed postoperatively to enhance recovery. However, although there is no indication that very-low-intensity stimulation can adversely affect cancer, and brain stimulation has been used for relief of intractable cancer pain, experimentally the latter was also found to increase metastatic activity dramatically in one study. It would therefore clearly seem sensible to err on the side of caution when treating cancer patients with CES/TCET.

Some researchers have even cautioned against using any form of electrical stimulation in patients with cancer. Because of the uncertainties surrounding long-term effects of many forms of electrotherapy, it should be used only with extreme care, if at all, in the early stages of cancer. In later stages of cancer, however, when life expectancy is anyway diminished, treatments that can improve quality of life with minimal side-effects, such as CES, EA, TENS or LILT, may be very helpful.

## RADIOTHERAPY AND CHEMOTHERAPY: COUNTERING IATROGENESIS

In the 1950s, some French acupuncturists believed that MA became less effective in patients who had been subjected to ionising radiation. However, both EA and MA have been employed for the prevention and treatment of chemo- and radiotherapy side-effects, including *xerostomia*, vasomotor symptoms (hot flushes) and nausea or loss of appetite.

MA has been used for radiation-induced oedema in patients with breast and cervical cancer, while moxibustion can be effective against chemotherapy-induced leukocytopenia. EA has been used similarly in animals, and EA to ST-36 has been used to improve gastrointestinal function in chemotherapy patients.

Non-invasive TENS, CES, acupoint MRT and LILT/LA have all been investigated, as well as polarised light, singlet oxygen and magnetic stimulation. Intraoral LILT, for example, has been used successfully in RCTs for chemotherapy-induced mucositis (inflammation of the mucous membranes) in patients undergoing bone marrow transplants. LA too has been used to counter the side-effects of chemotherapy and radiotherapy, and even for cerebrovascular insufficiency associated with the Chernobyl accident. However, some authors consider LILT contraindicated in patients subjected to chemo- or radiotherapy, and others suggest that these may reduce the effectiveness of magnetic field treatments, or that magnets should not be applied to skin recently exposed to radiation.

In conclusion, the potentially useful effects of various sorts of acupoint stimulation on patients given radio- or chemotherapy fall into three main categories:

1. countering leukocytopenia (lowered white blood. cell count), with positive effects on other blood constituents as well.
2. tissue repair, preventing necrosis and fibrosis – particularly of salivary glands or mucous membranes.
3. improving circulation and reducing oedema.

In addition, the well-known antiemetic effects of P-6 stimulation are important.

There may be advantages in applying treatment prophylactically, as well as after radio- or chemotherapy.

Case study 9.3.3 is a randomised placebo-controlled pilot study on neuroelectric acupuncture (NEAP or TEAS) for pain, nausea and vomiting and fatigue in palliative care.

## ACUPOINT MEASUREMENT, THE 'DIAGNOSIS' AND 'CAUSES' OF CANCER

Changes in electrical skin potential and resistance occur in cancer, both at acupoints and more generally. Acupoint temperature may also change when cancer is present. Many systems have been devised for detecting electrical and temperature changes in breast cancer, although without reference to acupuncture.

Trying to find patterns of meridian imbalance in heterogeneous groups of cancer patients is probably not a worthwhile approach, although ryodoraku might be useful in monitoring changes over time in individual patients. More work needs to be done to determine whether electroacupuncture according to Voll (EAV) and similar methods can really detect 'premalignancy', and differentiate between cancer and other conditions, or just indicate imbalance in a general sense.

## The hyperactive immune system – allergy and transplants

The immune hyperresponsiveness that leads to allergy or sensitivity may be associated with a tendency to electrical kindling in the brain. This itself may reduce response to more subtle forms of treatment, or be part of a wider 'sensitivity', to light, noise, or even particular weather conditions or electrical frequencies.

Thus, if allergy is the result of the immune system being conditioned into hyperactivity, then it may be possible to 'recondition' it using LF EA, or other simple methods. There are studies on EA for hypersensitivity, allergic shock response to chemical anaesthesia, allergic rhinitis and other respiratory allergies.

Both AA and TENS have been used for allergic patients as an alternative to anaesthesia using drugs, not infrequently for dental interventions. LILT, like MA, has been used to enhance acceptance of donor skin grafts, enhancing the effect of immunosuppressive treatment.

In EAV and some related methods (Ch. 10), higher acupoint conductance readings may indicate an allergic response. Voll even created a new 'allergy meridian'. Thus EAV, the Vega Test and allied systems have been used to test for allergy. It is claimed that the Vega Test, like EAV, might even be helpful in determining the correct homeopathic dilutions for desensitisation. However, such methods remain unproven and the British Allergy Foundation, for instance, does not consider that Vega Testing gives repeatable results. A more standard method of testing for allergy is the skin-prick test.

Occasionally, electrical hypersensitivity may be part of the picture in allergic patients, and this should always be borne in mind when using non-traditional acupuncture methods.

# CASE Study 9.3.3

## Neuroelectric acupuncture for pain, nausea and vomiting and fatigue in palliative care: a randomised placebo-controlled pilot study
J Gordon Gadsby

## Introduction

The objective of this study was to determine the potential role of neuroelectric acupuncture (NEAP), also known as acupuncture-like transcutaneous electrical nerve stimulation (ALTENS), in helping to improve the quality of life for terminally ill patients in a palliative care setting. The study design followed a double-blind randomised controlled trial protocol within a hospice setting.

Fifteen patients admitted for symptom control were randomly allocated to receive standard treatment, standard plus NEAP or standard plus placebo. The main outcome measures were assessed using the EORTC QLQ-C30 Quality of Life Questionnaire. The results of this study showed that the symptoms of pain, nausea and vomiting were not significantly improved in this group of patients, who were already receiving large amounts of opiates and antiemetics, but that symptoms of fatigue showed some improvement, the relative risk of this improvement being 8 times that of placebo and 16 times that of standard controls. The overall quality of life was also improved, the relative risk being twice that of placebo and 2.7 times that of standard controls.

It is difficult to draw conclusions on the basis of such a small pilot study, but the initial indications, suggesting the beneficial effects of neuroelectric acupuncture on the quality of life and fatigue experienced by the terminally ill patient, would appear to warrant further investigation in the future. This study would also suggest that the beneficial effects observed in treating this fatigue might also be usefully explored for the treatment of chronic fatigue syndromes.

## Summary of clinical manifestations

The inclusion criteria were that patients should have pain, or nausea and vomiting symptoms, or both, be in the age range 35–75 years and be of Caucasian origin. Exclusion criteria included all patients unwilling to provide informed consent, those too ill to cope with 30 minutes of treatment, patients with an on-demand pacemaker, premenopausal women, patients with vomiting due to intestinal obstruction, raised intracranial pressure or iatrogenic causes, and those who had previously received TENS or ALTENS treatment.

## Diagnosis

Terminally ill cancer patients suffering from the three main symptoms usual at this stage of their illness – pain, nausea and vomiting, and fatigue – were randomly admitted to the study. There were 14 female patients and 1 male patient, with ages ranging from 38 to 74 years and with a diagnosis of terminal cancer, comprising 6 breast, 3 colon, 2 pancreatic, 2 kidney, 1 stomach and 1 cervical.

## Treatment goals

These were to improve the symptoms of pain, nausea and vomiting, and fatigue, together with an overall improvement in the quality of life estimations on a physical, psychological and spiritual level.

## Treatment plan

Patients were entered into the trial following an independent assessment by a clinician and completion of a consent form, the EORTC QLQ-C30. On entry, patients were randomly allocated trial therapies, via the sealed envelope method of colour-coded allocation cards, to receive active NEAP, placebo NEAP or no NEAP ('no NEAP' standard control) in addition to recognised conventional therapies for pain and antiemesis. Daily biophysical measurements of body electrical resistance readings pre- and post-treatment were taken using a standard multimeter and handheld electrodes. Daily real or placebo ALTENS treatments were given, using a colour-coded system of leads corresponding to the colour code allocation card.

## Treatment procedures

### Points used

The use of acupuncture point P-6 for electroantiemesis is well accepted in the literature and the use of LI-4 for electroanalgesia is a standard procedure within both traditional and Western acupuncture systems.

### Method of application

A pair of lightly gelled carbon vinyl electrodes (size 4 cm$^2$) was attached to the patient: one to the acupuncture point P-6 and one to the point LI-4 of the dominant hand (and secured with tape). The leads were then attached to a V-TENS™ stimulator (see Fig. 11.2 on page 313).

### Treatment parameters

The pulse rate was set at 2 pulses per second with a symmetrical biphasic pulse wave in continuous mode, pulse duration at 200 microseconds, amplitude at 2.5 on the unit output scale and the timer at 30 minutes as the duration of each treatment.

---

### CASE Study 9.3.3 Continued

#### Course of treatment

The course of treatment comprised five consecutive daily 30-minute treatments.

#### Summary of outcome

The results of this study showed that the symptoms of pain and nausea and vomiting were not significantly improved in this group of patients, who were already receiving large amounts of opiates and antiemetics, but symptoms of fatigue showed an improvement, the relative risk of this improvement being 8 times that of placebo and 16 times that of standard controls. The overall quality of life was also improved, the relative risk being twice that of placebo and 2.7 times that of standard controls.

#### Discussion

The aim of this study was to start to assess whether there may be a role for neuroelectric acupuncture in helping to improve the quality of life for terminally ill patients, the rationale being that neuroelectric acupuncture treatment at 2 p.p.s. for 30 minutes has been shown to produce a marked increase in gene expression of beta-endorphins and met-enkephalins, with a subsequent reduction in pain and nausea/vomiting and a return of homeostasis. The main objectives of this study were first to assess the effectiveness of this non-invasive therapy, as an antiemetic and analgesic, as an adjunct to conventional care, and secondly to record biophysical measurements of electrical resistance in cancer patients and to compare them with measurements in non-cancer controls.

The results outlined above did not reach statistical significance and, if NEAP did have an effect on pain or nausea in palliative care, it is doubtful that a study with five patients per arm would be large enough to detect it. The trial is therefore underpowered and so there is a high probability that it may have failed to detect differences, particularly in view of the heterogeneous population.

The initial observations and analyses would also appear to support the theory that biophysical measurements of electrical resistance recorded in cancer patients and in comparison with measurements in non-cancer controls indicate significant differences, up to 40 times normal – the implications of which are not fully known at this time. It had been suggested that the readings of high electrical resistance in terminally ill patients may be due to a high intake of opiate medication, but this was not supported by a comparison of the retrospective dose drug estimations for individual patients.

It was also expected that the three randomly assigned treatment groups at baseline would have no significant differences. However, it appears, from the retrospective drug estimations, that patients assigned to the real treatment were taking significantly larger quantities of daily opioids than those receiving the placebo or the standard control.

Finally, although the pilot study showed several interesting observations within palliative care in respect of the global quality of life and the symptoms of fatigue, the main objectives of using neuroelectric acupuncture to alleviate pain and nausea and vomiting were not demonstrated within this small pilot study. However, the observations on the treatment of fatigue are most interesting, which may have wider implications within the field of chronic fatigue states and also help to explain the improvement many patients with such fatigue states experience after a course of NEAP or electroacupuncture using high-intensity low-frequency stimulation.

---

On the basis of one MA case report, because similar pathways may be activated by both acupuncture and opiate drugs, it has also been proposed that acupuncture be used cautiously in those with morphine hypersensitivity.

## Autoimmune conditions

Scleroderma is a systemic connective tissue disorder that may affect the gastrointestinal tract as well as the skin itself, and is frequently preceded by Raynaud's phenomenon. Like Raynaud's itself, it has been treated using EA and TENS. EA was found to improve measures of both cell-mediated and humoral immunity in this condition.

Another connective tissue disease is systemic lupus erythematosus (SLE), in which arthralgia and sun-sensitive skin lesions may sometimes be accompanied by fever.

Acupuncture has been used for both SLE and localised lupus. Methods include EA and LA, although far-infrared stimulation may need to be used with care in this condition, as in MS.

In rheumatoid arthritis (RA), acupuncture may enhance immunoglobulin levels. LILT can decrease the level of circulating immune complexes and reduce synovial lymphocyte levels.

**Points used in immune conditions** ST-36, alone or in combination with SP-6 or *lanweixue* (M-LE-13), is the most used point in EA immune studies. Many other combinations have also been found helpful. From experimental studies, Du-4 may be useful for hypersensitivity to challenge by some chemical antigens, and Du-26 has been used for toxic shock (anaphylaxis). LIV-8 may also have its uses, as may BL-20, ST-25, ST-37 or Du-15.

Phil Rogers and his colleagues suggest the following points for immunostimulation: BL-11, BL-20, BL-23–28, GB-39, LI-4, LI-11, ST-36, SP-6, Ren-12 and Du-14. In general, clinical studies of EA and other acupoint interventions for immune problems tend to use these points, together with others based on TCM diagnostics and local points as appropriate.

The most commonly used points to counter the effects of radio- and chemotherapy appear to be those for tonifying Blood and *yin*, together with some of these general points. From the experimental studies, ST-36, Du-14 and BL-23 may be effective points for chemotherapy.

Rogers considers BL-47 as immunosuppressive, and for use in autoimmune conditions suggests BL-23, LI-4, LI-11, ST-36, Du-14, BL-23, BL-40, with BL-23, ST-36 and SP-6 for SLE, in particular. He also lists Du-14 and ST-36 as antifebrile points. Manik Hiranandani proposes the same points for immune support, adding Du-20 and LU-7 (MA to Du-20 has been used to reduce fever accompanied by convulsions in infants, for example). Josef Bahn has a different list, subdividing the points into those useful for humoral immune stimulation (BL-60, LIV-3, LI-4, LI-11, ST-25, ST-36, SP-6 and Ren-12) and those for cellular immune stimulation (BL-11, BL-23, BL-24, BL-25, BL-26, BL-27, BL-28 and Du-14). Willem Khoe suggested the following points could increase leukocyte activity, and phagocytic response in particular: BL-23, LIV-3, LI-4, LI-11, ST-36, SP-6, Du-4 and Du-14. For SLE, he recommended 60 seconds of 1 W ultrasound at local points (ST-3, Du-25) for malar 'butterfly erythema', and 2 Hz EA to points such as P-4, ST-25, ST-42, SP-6, SP-9, Ren-6 and Ren-12 for articular symptoms.

From the few cancer studies with detailed entries in the ⊕ database, it would seem that points in the region of the tumour are used, as well as distal points on associated meridians and major points such as LI-4 and ST-36. For cancer pain, local and *ashi* points again are used, as well as *huatuojiaji* and back *shu* points, and major points like P-6 and LI-4. In one review, Steven Aung recommends points such as HE-7, P-6, LI-4, SP-6, Du-4 and Du-20 for controlling cancer pain (with EA if it is severe). Of course, treating directly over a tumour site should not be undertaken lightly, and many authorities consider needling over the site of cancer to be absolutely contraindicated. Contralateral treatment may be an option.

Some interesting work has been done on exposure of the thymus gland to EHF stimulation in both tuberculosis and rheumatoid arthritis (the spleen was also stimulated in RA). LILT too has been applied to the skin over the thymus, reducing immune overactivity in adults, but with only an insignificant effect in children.

**Parameters used in immune conditions** LF, DD and HF EA may all enhance immune function. A frequency of 10 Hz, a good candidate for an 'antistress frequency', may enhance immune function if stress is a factor, although Willem Khoe consistently recommended 1 or 2 Hz EA for use in acute infections. When treating patients with cancer, it may also be worth remembering that brain tumours at least are associated with reduced EEG variability; therefore fixed-frequency stimulation may not be the most appropriate method to use.

From the little data available, it would seem there is a tendency to use LF or DD EA, with some HF or intermittent TENS, in treating cancer or cancer pain. Both low- and high-intensity EA and TENS have been used experimentally to enhance immune function. Theoretically, the Arndt–Schulz law could well be important: use lower intensities to stimulate immune function, stronger ones to damp it down.

Immune enhancement with EA may take a few days of regular treatment to gain momentum, and this should be borne in mind when designing a treatment protocol. In treating cancer pain with TENS, it has been suggested that stimulation for 6–7 hours each day may be required to allow pain medication to be reduced.

Phil Rogers recommends treatment once or twice weekly for autoimmune conditions. For acute infection, an appropriate treatment interval might be more like 4–6 hours. For wound healing, Pekka Pöntinen suggests that TENS three times daily for 30–45 minutes, possibly in conjunction with LILT, should control any infection within 2 weeks.

# THE ENDOCRINE SYSTEM

The endocrine glands considered here are the pituitary itself, master gland of the endocrine system, and those glands with which it is intimately connected: the thyroid, parathyroids, pancreas and adrenals. For the sake of simplicity, each gland and its conditions are considered separately.

## The pituitary gland

Apart from conditions involving disruption of the feedback loops between the pituitary and other endocrine glands, the main pituitary disorders that have been treated using acupuncture involve pituitary growth hormone (GH), although here too there can be a feedback loop involving the pancreas and blood sugar levels Thus EA to LI-4 may increase serum GH levels in patients with chronic pain, but not in normal subjects (although 20 Hz auricular EA did increase plasma GH in healthy women). Conclusions are difficult, as serum GH may in any case rise in response to stress. EA has been used to treat arthritic limb pain due to excess GH secretion and resulting pituitary gigantism (acromegaly).

According to some authors, the pituitary gland plays a pivotal role in the analgesic and some other effects of EA. Yet EAA has been employed during operations for pituitary adenoma. Presumably such surgery leaves intact those parts of the gland needed to maintain hypoalgesia during the operation. However, from Kaada's description of an operation for pituitary tumour, it is clear that the patient was by no means pain free as the tumour was removed.

# The thyroid gland

Hyper- and hypothyroidism can be due to autoimmune or thyroid dysfunction, or to nutritional deficits. In Down's syndrome, for instance, abnormal thyroid hormone metabolism may be corrected by dietary zinc. Hypothyroidism may be associated with myofascial pain, and be a factor in many other conditions.

EA and CES can affect thyroid function (e.g. thyroxine levels). EA and LA have been used for hyperthyroidism in particular, as well as for their effects on thyroid hormones in cases of associated local scleroderma. Acupuncture has been used preoperatively in thyrotoxicosis (hyperthyroidism).

There have been more operations on the thyroid under EAA than on any other endocrine gland, and indeed, in China, acupuncture analgesia (AA) appears to be used mostly for neck and head surgery. On the one hand, it offers certain advantages over conventional anaesthesia. For example, since the patient is conscious, damage to the recurrent laryngeal nerves is less likely. EAA may also be used with hyperthyroid patients when conventional anaesthesia is likely to be problematic due to cardiac involvement and a tendency to fibrillation. On the other hand, AA may be less effective in hyperthyroidism (one indication for thyroid surgery) than in other thyroid conditions, in part because hyperthyroid patients are less likely to relax under treatment.

Thus AA combined with low-dose drug anaesthesia has been used in hyperthyroid cases. In China, this has become routine since 1991. Thyroid surgery using AA has been performed in the West too: for example, thyroid lobectomy has been carried out in Italy, where other forms of electroanalgesia have also been used. EAA for thyroid operations does not in itself appear to affect levels of thyroid hormones unduly.

LA has been used in the treatment of exophthalmic hyperthyroidism, while acupoint EHF has been used for post-thyrotoxic ophthalmopathy. LA has also been used to treat thyroid adenoma, as has electrochemical therapy or 'ECT', local EA using DC current.

## The parathyroid glands

Parathyroid hormone, together with vitamin D and calcitonin, controls levels of serum calcium. Hyperparathyroidism can lead to kidney problems (stones or calcification), bone pain and degeneration, and sometimes peptic ulceration, constipation and depression. Hypoparathyroidism can lead to paraesthesiae and tetany.

EA may have some influence on parathyroid function. AA has been used during parathyroidectomy in patients with primary hyperparathyroidism.

## The pancreas: diabetes and functional hypoglycaemia

Different types of cell in the islets of Langerhans in the pancreas secrete somatostatin, pancreatic polypeptide, glucagon (catabolic) and of course insulin (anabolic). There are complex feedback loops between these, pituitary GH and other hormones or their release factors.

Diabetes mellitus, the most common endocrine disorder of the pancreas, is due to insufficient insulin secretion, resulting in hyperglycaemia, or high blood sugar. Hypoglycaemia, in which insulin overcounteracts raised blood sugar levels, may result from adrenal insufficiency (insulin may itself act as an adrenal stressor).

Some effects of EA and TENS on experimental diabetes and insulin/blood glucose levels were outlined in Chapter 6 (page 67). Depending on the points and parameters used, as well as the initial state of the subject, blood sugar and insulin levels may increase or decrease: in type II (non-insulin-dependent) diabetes, blood sugar tends to fall and insulin to rise, whereas in normals blood sugar tends to rise. Regularly repeated moxibustion too (at ST-36) may increase insulin levels. Acupuncture as an adjuvant method of analgesia has been found to suppress the hyperglycaemic response to surgical stress.

Both MA and EA have been used in the treatment of diabetes. In one review, for instance, it is stated that stouter patients do better than thin ones, and that initially blood sugar levels may rise in response to MA before stabilising later. When it comes to individual clinical studies, in many cases it is the consequences of diabetes that have been addressed primarily, rather than the raised blood sugar that causes them. Thus there are only a few EA studies on raised blood sugar levels in diabetes: two on the application of cold or 'freezing acupuncture', and two on 'biofrequency spectrum irradiation'. Others focus on functional or reactive hypoglycaemia, and the remainder describe changes in acupoint electrical characteristics that occur with diabetes, with one (twice reported) on EAV.

CES has been used in the treatment of diabetic patients, reducing blood sugar levels in type II diabetes. Blood glucose levels may also change in response to skin illumination. Thus LILT has been recommended for diabetes, though again more for its effects on the sequelae of the condition than for the hyperglycaemia itself. LA (at Du-25 and Du-26) has been used to raise low blood sugar levels.

It is likely that acupuncture will be helpful for type II diabetes only, when the pancreas is still able to release some insulin. True type I diabetes is unlikely to respond. However, insulin resistance resulting from regular insulin injections may also inhibit EA effects on blood sugar, and it is possible that diabetes itself may render EA less effective than in normals. Diabetic neuropathy may reduce MA or EA effectiveness when treating herpes zoster or senile pruritis, for instance. At the other extreme, functional hypoglycaemia may result in anomalous responses to EA.

## The adrenal glands

The possible importance of ACTH (adrenocorticotrophin) and the pituitary–adrenal axis for EA was described in detail in Chapter 6 ⊙. Whatever their role in helping us cope with stress or in stress-induced analgesia, it seems that neither is essential for EAA in all circumstances.

Circulatory cortisol, the stress glucocorticoid hormone from the adrenal cortex, may increase, remain unchanged, or decrease in response to EA or TENS, to some extent depending on how long or how stressful the treatment is, the situation in which it is given (surgery, for instance), or what is appropriate to maintain optimum balance. In some situations, cortisol needs to increase, not decrease. Cortisol increases with EA might help reduce swelling or inflammation, or both – in asthma, arthritis, or following a stroke, for example. Raised cortisol (with *reduced* levels of adrenomedullary catecholamines) was also implicated in the beneficial effects of TEAS on some forms of eczema, and, in one report of EA for induction of labour, better results were obtained in mothers whose cortisol levels were raised as a result of treatment. However, cortisol levels remained unexpectedly unchanged in some TENS studies, despite clinical improvements.

On the other hand, excessive cortisol can adversely affect the immune system, and may contribute to fatigue and depression, poor wound healing and osteoporosis, failing memory and dementia, poor sleep quality and many other problems. The beneficial effects of acupuncture in these conditions may be partly mediated by decreases in cortisol. As an example, the excessive serum cortisol levels found in stressed withdrawing addicts may be significantly reduced by auricular EA.

A number of studies have explored the changes in adrenal stress hormones that occur during surgery with EAA, TENS or TCET. In some of these, no marked differences were found between combined electroanaesthesia and routine anaesthesia. In others, the stress of the situation was clearly evident in patients not under general anaesthesia. In some, adrenal hormones increased only marginally, or less than with pharmacological methods, and in a few, levels of adrenal hormones were actually lowered. It seems that inhibition of peripheral adrenergic mechanisms is proportional to the effectiveness of analgesia induced.

Cortisol levels are raised in Cushing's disease. Iatrogenic Cushing's syndrome due to steroid intake may lead to adrenocortical atrophy and hypofunction. EA to ST-36, which may raise endogenous cortisol levels, was found to restore this function, at least partially, in dogs and rabbits, with possible clinical implications for humans (EA to ST-36 can also reduce cortisol already raised by stress). In one case report on iatrogenic Cushing's, auricular EA possibly contributed to relief of tremor and perspiration.

Although corticosteroid treatment may reduce the effectiveness of acupuncture, acupuncture can still be useful under these circumstances. Thus EA may still benefit asthma patients who are cortisone dependent.

As for the adrenal medullary hormones, adrenaline (Adr, epinephrine) and noradrenaline (NA, norepinephrine), levels of these in the blood may increase or decrease with EA, again demonstrating its regulatory action. How levels change may also depend on the points stimulated.

## Other hormones

Gut hormones (gastrin, secretin, cholecystokinin, vasoactive intestinal polypeptide and motilin) can all be affected by EA. The sex hormones are considered elsewhere in this book.

**Comparisons in endocrine disorders** Urinary excretion of glucocorticoids (which raise blood sugar levels) was higher with 2 Hz than with 64 Hz EA in one case report, and in another urinary glucocorticoid levels were higher with EA than with TENS, possibly indicating that treatment was experienced as stressful. From experimental work, it would appear that EA is more effective than TENS for treatment of diabetes and resultant neuropathy. Conversely, LA more effectively increased blood sugar levels than EA in one brief report.

**Points used in endocrine disorders** In EAV, the *sanjiao* meridian is interpreted as representing endocrine function as a whole. Given the complexity of the endocrine system, this is probably simplistic, although acupoints near individual glands might have some local effect, and other points on a meridian whose trajectory is close to a gland might also influence it.

However, direct stimulation over a gland may not always be appropriate. Direct LILT over the thyroid gland can lead to some patients becoming nervous, with tachycardia, tremor and sweating, for instance. In one case MA 'on' the thyroid gland in a patient with transient thyroiditis led to a recurrence of her goitre.

Stimulating points around the margin of the gland has been found useful to reduce thyroid hyperplasia in exophthalmic goitre. Local TEAS is another possible approach.

The *jing* Well points (with Ren-4 for the Directing Vessel and Du-2 for the Governing Vessel) have been used in hyperthyroid patients.

LI-18 is the most frequently point for EAA during thyroid operations. For exophthalmos, LA has been applied at LI-18, together with local points, and for thyroid adenoma at local and segmental points ST-10 and GB-21, with ST-36 as a distal point.

Commonly used points for diabetes include HE-7, BL-13, BL-17, BL-20, BL-23, KI-3, KI-7, P-6, GB-39, LI-4, LI-11, ST-36, SP-6, SP-8, Ren-4, Ren-12, Ren-24, *jinjin* (M-HN-20), *yishu* (M-BW-12) and *yuye* (M-HN-20), with Ren-12 having particular effects on plasma glucose levels. Tseung used BL-40, GB-34, SP-6 and the auricular 'Pancreas' point most consistently in his study. For low blood sugar, LA was used at Du-25 and Du-26 (an example of the importance of Du-26 as a revival point, even given the gentleness of LA), whereas Gregory Chen made more use of back *shu* points and 'BL-17B' (*yishu*, midway between BL-17 and BL-18), together with LIV-3.

**Parameters used in endocrine disorders** Gregory Chen's use of 125 Hz for auricular stimulation in iatrogenic Cushing's syndrome and LF in hypoglycaemia is probably a reflection of standard thinking that HF EA should be used at ear points and LF at body points, and not related to the condition being treated. Tseung and Chen do not make it clear why they chose the particular parameters they did in treating diabetes and its complications.

From the experimental studies, I would expect stronger stimulation (verging on the painful) to increase stress hormone (or blood sugar) levels in those with reserves to allow this, and gentler stimulation to bring them down, depending on the acupoints used. In those with adrenal or pancreatic insufficiency, strong stimulation might have contrary effects. However, there is little clear evidence from clinical studies on the effects of different parameters on the levels of hormones covered in this section.

| **9.3** Summary of relevant studies in the electronic clinical studies database (number of studies) | | |
|---|---|---|
| **Condition** | **EA** | **Other** |
| **Peripheral motor disorders** | | |
| Facial paralysis | 108 | 60 |
| Spasm (tic) | 12 | 15 |
| Hiccup and other diaphragm disorders | 13 | 13 |
| Other/mixed conditions | 16 | 2 |
| Muscle spasm | 2 | 2 |
| Muscle contracture | 1 | 1 |
| Myasthenia gravis | 2 | 0 |
| Ptosis | 1 | 1 |
| Muscular dystrophy | 1 | 2 |
| Scoliosis | 0 | 2 |
| Peripheral nerve injury | 18 | 2 |
| **Immunology** | | |
| Specific infections | 4 | 15 |
| HIV/AIDS | 2 | 3 |
| Autoimmune conditions | 5 | 2 |
| Allergy and sensitivity | 2 | 15 |
| Immune function | 9 | 15 |
| **Cancer** | | |
| Cancer | 17 | 44 |
| Cancer pain | 24 | 26 |
| **Radio- and chemotherapy** | 8 | 30 |
| **Endocrinology** | | |
| Thyroid | 5 | 10 |
| Adrenal | 2 | 0 |
| Pancreas | 12 | 15 |

## SUMMARY

Some key points in this chapter are:

- Better results are obtained with early treatment for facial paralysis, with gentle stimulation likely to be more effective
- Acupuncture appears to have a bidirectional and homeodynamic effect on the immune system
- Acupuncture, and especially EA, has been successfully used to treat acute infections
- EA can be particularly beneficial in pain relief for cancer patients and in countering the effects of chemo- and radiotherapy.

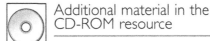 Additional material in the CD-ROM resource

In the CD-ROM resource, in addition to more information on the topics presented here, the following are also covered:

- Peripheral motor disorders: blepharospasm, myasthenia gravis, muscular dystrophy, scoliosis
- The immune system: more technical information, immune function and trauma (surgical or other), chronic fatigue syndrome (also covered in Subchapters 9.1 and 9.12), wound healing (with further information in Subchapter 9.6)
- The endocrine system: aldosterone, the pineal gland.

## RECOMMENDED READING

*Prelude to a rigorous review of acupuncture for facial paralysis:*
He L, Zhou D, Wu B, Li N Acupuncture for Bell's palsy (Protocol for a Cochrane Review). In: The Cochrane Library, Issue 1, 2001. Oxford: Update Software

*An informal but useful review:*
Chen KZ Acupuncture treatment of Bell's palsy (Part 2). International Journal of Clinical Acupuncture. 1994; 5(2): 173–8

*General articles on acupuncture and immune function:*
Bossy J Immune systems, defense mechanisms and acupuncture: fundamental and practical aspects. American Journal of Acupuncture. 1990 July–Sept; 18(3): 219–32

Jonsdottir IH Physical exercise, acupuncture and immune function. Acupuncture in Medicine. 1999 June; 17(1): 50–3

*Detailed survey of the acupuncture literature on immune disorders:*
Rogers PA, Schoen AM, Limehouse J Acupuncture for immune-mediated disorders. Literature review and clinical applications. Problems in Veterinary Medicine. 1992 March; 4(1): 162–93

*TCM views on difficult immune conditions:*
Haines N Treatment by acupuncture: HIV and AIDS. Journal of Chinese Medicine 1994 Sept; (46): 5–19

Lee MH Overview of the diagnosis and treatment of chronic fatigue immune dysfunction syndrome according to traditional Chinese medicine. American Journal of Acupuncture. 1992 Oct–Dec; 20(4): 337–48

*The quiet start to a revolution in the treatment of inoperable cancer:*
Nordenström B Biologically closed electric circuits: activation of vascular interstitial closed electric circuits for treatment of inoperable cancers. Journal of Bioelectricity. 1984; 3(1–2): 137–53

# 9.4 DISORDERS OF THE SKIN AND HAIR, EYE AND EAR, NOSE, THROAT AND MOUTH

*With contributions by Goto Kamiya and Ron Sharp*

This subchapter is in four parts, covering the major specialties of dermatology (the skin and hair), ophthalmology (the eye), otorhinolaryngology (the ear, nose and throat) and stomatology (the mouth). Indications on points and parameters to use are given wherever possible, including those for a selection of less common conditions. This chapter exemplifies the wide range of disorders for which EA and associated techniques may be appropriate.

## DERMATOLOGY: DISORDERS OF THE SKIN AND HAIR

The skin is our boundary with the world, and a key part of the immune system. It may react to outside stressors, irritants, or diet. Many skin conditions have complex pathologies, so that one treatment will not suit everyone, and a single therapy approach is not always appropriate. In particular, underlying immune problems may need to be remedied, as well as core stress patterns. Improving circulation in the skin may also be important.

Acupuncture can be helpful in skin conditions, although reviews indicate that long periods of treatment may be necessary. Skin problems and irritation can sometimes indicate a hypersensitivity to electrical stimulation; treatment responses when using electroacupuncture (EA) and associated methods should be carefully monitored.

### Skin conditions – general

#### PRURITUS (ITCHING)
In TCM, itching is considered predominantly an empty (*xu*) condition, and pain a full one (*shi*). Itching may result from particular skin disorders, from deterioration of the skin with age and from other causes.

Various types of acupuncture have been used, while transcutaneous electrical nerve stimulation (TENS) in particular has been used for generalised pruritus in the elderly, and for pruritus during burn healing.

Manual acupuncture (MA), EA and TENS have been used for uraemic pruritus, EA (4–6 Hz, tolerable intensity, at ST-36 and SP-9 for 2 hours) to reduce pruritus resulting from opioid epidural anaesthesia.

#### ACNE AND ROSACEA
Acne results when the sebaceous glands secrete too much oily sebum.

There are a number of reviews of acupuncture for acne. MA, auricular MA, EA and laser acupuncture (LA) have all been used. Acne is an accepted indication for low intensity light therapy (LILT).

Rosacea is characterised by erythema and telangiectasia with papules and pustules. It has been treated with both MA and EA.

### ECZEMA
Eczema can be endogenous, as in atopic dermatitis (or neurodermatitis) and varicose eczema, or exogenous, as in contact dermatitis.

Acupuncture has frequently been used for eczema, both endogenous and exogenous, in infants as well as adults. EA has been used for dermatitis, using the surround-needling technique, with other points utilised for their immune function. LF intermittent TENS has also been used. Other approaches include cranial electrotherapy stimulation (CES), LILT, extremely-high-frequency (EHF) stimulation and auricular EA combined with local ultrasound ('sonopuncture') directly over the lesion.

The possibility of contact dermatitis when using stainless steel needles or TENS electrodes should not be forgotten.

### LICHEN PLANUS
This itchy dermatosis can be stress related, but may also be associated with infection, or toxic or immunological disturbance. It has been treated with acupuncture, including EA and helium–neon (HeNe) LA, together with LILT.

### NEURODERMATITIS
Strictly, this is a lichenoid eruption limited to the axillary and pubic areas and associated with a nervous disorder. There is considerable overlap between this and 'eczema'. Acupuncture, CES, LA (in children) and acupoint magnetic stimulation have been used. Auricular acupuncture, either MA or EA, is another possibility.

### PSORIASIS
Lesions are usually around elbows, knees, lower back, ears and scalp. However, the entire skin is different from that in non-psoriatics, and not just the specific lesions.

Acupuncture has frequently been attempted for psoriasis, sometimes with good results (generally in uncontrolled studies), and sometimes with little effect (in more rigorous trials). MA, EA and TENS have all been used.

LA has been used for psoriatic arthropathy, its combination with LILT giving better results than either modality alone. For skin lesions, LILT may be used, along with LA at immune points. LILT may be unhelpful if large areas are affected.

## SCLERODERMA

This autoimmune connective tissue disorder affects the skin, and also joints, muscles and internal organs. The skin becomes thicker, harder and more rigid. Localised scleroderma may recover spontaneously, but generally the condition is slowly progressive.

Various forms of electrotherapy, MA, EA and plum blossom needling have been used for scleroderma, and LA in perinatal infantile scleroderma.

## URTICARIA

Acupuncture has long been used to treat urticaria. Cupping has also been used. EA and LA are other approaches.

## BITES AND STINGS AND BURROWING MITES

Direct stimulation of the bite, whether with high-voltage DC, piezoelectric shocks, or even moxibustion, may reduce inflammation and toxic response.

EA has been used to initiate healing in a long-standing spider bite wound, using surround needling. Scabies in humans has been investigated using EAV.

# Viral infections

## HERPES ZOSTER

Herpes zoster (shingles) causes pain and itching in the affected dermatome. Eye involvement may occur if the ophthalmic division of the trigeminal nerve is involved. The severe pain of postherpetic neuralgia may ensue.

Traditionally, herpes zoster is considered amenable to acupuncture and traditional Chinese herbal medicine (TCHM). MA in the acute phase (within 24–72 hours of onset) may hasten recovery and reduce the incidence of postherpetic neuralgia. Relief is less if treatment is delayed.

MA usually involves surround needling, plus treatment according to the pathogenic factors and meridian pathways involved. Plum blossom needling is also common, sometimes with cupping. Simple bleeding of auricular and body points has been used, as well bleeding locally or around the lesions.

EA with surround needling is also used for acute herpes zoster.

Moxibustion, LA and LILT have been employed to treat acute herpes zoster. Because pain can flare up in response to the slightest touch, the laser probe should not contact the skin locally (although, surprisingly, the contact mode has been considered preferable for postherpetic neuralgia).

Whether MA, EA or LA/LILT is used, it seems that the rash, pain and itch subside rapidly provided treatment is started early enough, with a low incidence of postherpetic neuralgia.

## HERPES SIMPLEX

'Cold sores', or 'fever blisters', caused by the HSV-1 strain, are usually self-limiting, though may become recurrent. Genital herpes, caused by the HSV-2 strain, is not only extremely painful, but may also predispose to cervical cancer. Even though antiviral drugs reduce the duration of an attack, remission may be lengthened and recurrence reduced with acupuncture.

MA has been used for both oral and genital herpes, and LILT for both cold sores and herpetic stomatitis. LILT is also claimed to shorten episodes and lessen relapse rate.

## VIRAL WARTS

Warts may last for up to 2 years. Deep MA to the 'mother wart', moxibustion or 'electrothermal acupuncture' and vitamin B12 acupoint injection have all been used, as has intermittent sonopuncture (ultrasound). Such local treatment does not necessarily prevent recurrence.

# Fungal infection

*Tinea pedis* has been treated with EA, *tinea capitis* (of the head) by MA and blood letting at acupoints near the posterior auricular vein. *Mycosis fungoides*, a rare and potentially fatal skin condition, has been treated with MA.

LA and far infrared have been used for fungal skin conditions.

# Cosmetology and scar tissue

## FACIAL TREATMENT

MA and EA, needling either directly into wrinkles or at local acupoints, have been employed for 'face lifts'. Some practitioners also use scalp needling, and others emphasise body points. Microcurrent treatments are frequently offered in beauty salons, although results, as with acupuncture, are only temporary.

## SCAR TISSUE AND ADHESIONS

Scars may cause problems. They may become painful if a neuroma forms at the site of injury. They may physically lessen the effectiveness of electrotherapy. They may also have non-local effects as, for example, in trigger points that refer pain elsewhere. Chronically infected scars may also cause referred pain.

To minimise scar formation, electrical (anodal), LILT or ultrasound stimulation can accelerate healing and reduce scar formation following injury. Ultrasound may improve the quality of scars, and applied at acupoints has been recommended for keloids. Results with LILT may be better still.

Short scars may be treated at each end only, and longer ones at points along their length, at *ashi* or trigger points within it, or on either side of the scar (compare Figs 9.6.1b-i and 9.14.1a on pages 162 and 260).

EA may both accelerate healing and reduce scar formation. However, vigorous EA may not be appropriate near recently healed scars, and extensive adhesions may be a contraindication to EAA, although gentle motor-level stimulation can usefully stretch tissue and improve circulation. EA has been employed for intestinal adhesions, as well as local scar pain. For local analgesia, TENS can also be applied.

Very-low-intensity microcurrent stimulation (of negative polarity) has been used over adhesions, either via handheld probes or via Ag/AgCl surface electrodes. This is less invasive than EA, and is suitable for points within the scar (or at either end of larger scars).

Like microcurrent, LA/LILT (or even just a red LED) is non-invasive and can be used over the scar. LA has been used for acute abdominal pain caused by adhesions. LILT may accelerate remodelling of scar tissue.

## VITILIGO AND HYPERPIGMENTATION

Vitiligo is characterised by patchy loss of skin pigmentation. Steroids and narrow-band ultraviolet-B (UVB) light therapy are usually suggested.

MA has been used but, while this may halt progression, it is less likely to reverse the condition. It has also been treated with EA.

Chloasma has been treated with MA, bleeding and cupping, as well as moxibustion and acupoint injection, and ear point pressure. Hyperpigmentation has often been treated with LILT, and sometimes with herbal-based cosmetics. Surprisingly, EA has been claimed to help pigmented naevi.

# The hair

## ALOPECIA AREATA

Alopecia may be amenable to physical treatments. Previously, ultraviolet light was considered helpful, and other electrical methods have been employed, although the condition is usually self-limiting.

Acupuncture has often been used because of its effects on microcirculation. Plum blossom needling is also common, directly to the scalp as well as paraspinally. Both of these approaches may be combined with electrical stimulation of the needles.

**Comparisons** Experimentally, EA may be more effective than MA in reducing itch, and cutaneous field stimulation, a variant of EA, more effective than TENS. EA was more effective than MA for lichen planus.

For alopecia, electric plum blossom needling may be more effective than ordinary plum blossom needling.

**Points used** Surround needling with EA is appropriate for many skin conditions. A number of points are used repeatedly for a range of skin complaints, including LI-4, LI-11, ST-36, SP-6 and SP-10.

A simple MA protocol with gentle stimulation is useful in the treatment of a variety of skin conditions, utilising LIV-3, LU-7, LI-4, Du-20 and *sishencong* (M-HN-1) supplemented with auricular Lung and Adrenal. This could be adapted for EA in recalcitrant cases.

Contralateral 'counterirritation' may be helpful for pruritis. However, local (intrasegmental) stimulation is probably more effective. Results indicate that high-frequency (HF) TENS or vibration is best applied intrasegmentally at, or proximal to, a pruritic area, whereas low-frequency (LF) TENS, or 60 Hz vibration, may be useful extrasegmentally or contralaterally.

For acne, Khoe suggests auricular EA at the Lung, Internal secretion and Adrenal gland points, adding the External nose point for rosacea. For eczema, he recommends auricular EA at the points for the Lung, Large Intestine, Occiput and Adrenal gland.

For neurodermatitis, one Chinese auricular acupuncture textbook suggests EA at *shenmen*, Liver, Spleen, Endocrine, Subcortex and Lung points, or the Lung, *shenmen*, Adrenal and Occiput points, together with the appropriate auricular area. In addition to surround needling, body points such as LI-11, ST-36, SP-6 and SP-10 can be added.

A similar protocol can be used with LILT for eczema. Hiranandani suggests LILT with LA at acupoints such as LU-5, LU-7, LI-11, SP-10, Du-14, Du-20 and auricular *shenmen*, Lung and Internal secretion points. For transcutaneous electrical acupoint stimulation (TEAS), he suggests LU-5 (+), LU-7 (-), bilateral LI-11 and SP-10 (at 5 Hz), and auricular *shenmen* (+) and Lung (-) (at 100 Hz).

For psoriasis, Hiranandani suggests non-contact scanning of the lesion with LILT, plus LA at points such as LU-7, LI-11, ST-36 and SP-6, for their immune function.

For scleroderma, both EA and LA can be applied at local points. Kaada used his standard combination of LI-4 and ~SI-3 with TENS. Immune points may also be used.

For MA treatment of urticaria, points such as LI-11, ST-36, SP-6 and SP-10 are most commonly used. LI-11 has also been used for LA.

For herpes zoster, surround needling with EA is used most frequently, with *huatuojiaji* or other paraspinal points (either in the affected dermatome, or in those immediately above and below it), or sometimes points such as LIV-3 and LI-4. Points for the immune system, auricular points for the affected area, and points along the affected meridian have all been used.

For herpes simplex, direct LILT is normally used, sometimes with local acupoints or immune points.

For clusters of viral warts, EA using positive stimulation to the 'mother wart', and a negative return needle along the involved meridian, has been suggested.

For alopecia, EA is generally used locally, with points for blood deficiency or immune function. Electric plum blossom needling and LILT have been applied locally but, for MA, GB-8, GB-20, SJ-23 and *yintang* have been recommended, with points such as LIV-3 and P-6, as appropriate.

In one study of alopecia, tenderness at preselected groups of ear points was used to determine which to treat. The groups included *shenmen*, Endocrine, Thyroid, Neurasthenia, Adrenal and 'Grey matter' ear points for alopecia areata, and *shenmen*, Gonads, Endocrine, Thyroid and Adrenal points for male pattern baldness. Khoe, however, used Kidney, Lung and Internal secretion ear points for LF EA treatment of alopecia. Surround needling, local and paraspinal plum blossom needling, and other acupoints to improve scalp circulation (such as GB-20 or local *ashi* points) are commonly used.

**Parameters used** Experimental studies indicate that 100 Hz may be more effective than 2 Hz or 200 Hz for itching when using TENS or vibration locally (vibration may be more effective than TENS). For extrasegmental stimulation, 2 Hz EA or TENS is more effective, although DD EA or 60 Hz vibration may have some extrasegmental/contralateral effects.

Stronger, even noxious, stimulation may be more effective than that of low intensity. Whereas brief noxious TENS may be useful, LF EA for 20 minutes may be needed for extrasegmental effects (although HF EA locally will reduce itching within a few minutes).

For acne, Margaret Naeser suggests LILT at only 1–2 J/cm². 

For neurodermatitis, local surround needling with EA at 8.3–10 Hz is suggested in one Chinese auricular acupuncture textbook. This was used in EA studies by Liu Jixian, and corresponds to Iliev's use of 8–12 Hz for both lichen planus and alopecia.

For scleroderma, LF seems appropriate, whether EA or TENS, given its effects on microcirculation. HeNe was used in two LA scleroderma studies.

For vitiligo, LF and HF and DD EA have all been used. 

For alopecia, Emil Iliev used ~10 Hz (alpha) frequency EA (as also for lichen planus).

# EYE DISORDERS

Vision does not exist in isolation: all sensory inputs converge and interact in the cerebral cortex, and other sensory stimuli influence visual perception. Acupuncture is no exception.

There are a number of reviews and accounts of acupuncture for eye conditions. However, the more rigorous of these show no firm evidence that acupuncture should be the primary therapy for any of them.

## Amblyopia, asthenopia and amaurosis

Reduced visual acuity (amblyopia) has many causes. Results with MA treatment are not always clear cut, and the condition may also become refractory to repeated treatment.

EA has been used for dysbinocular amblyopia, and TENS for low visual acuity following congenital cataract extraction. Microcurrent too has been used for 'poor vision'.

Amaurosis (blindness without obvious lesions), in particular hysterical amaurosis, has been treated with HF electrotherapy, congenital idiopathic blindness with EA.

Asthenopia (easily tired eyes) is a consequence of the heavy visual emphasis in our culture. EA has been used for this, particularly in the former Soviet Union.

## The optic nerve and visual pathways in the brain

Electrical stimulation of the retina can produce visual effects. With TENS, this has been used both diagnostically and therapeutically for optic nerve atrophy.

Brain injury can affect vision. Unilateral cortical lesions may cause an inability to perceive objects on the contralateral side. This 'visuospatial hemineglect' has been treated with TENS: stimulating the neck or hand on the neglected side may bring temporary improvements. 'Cortical blindness' has been treated with EA.

Optic neuritis may occur in various conditions, and lead to optic atrophy and blindness. Until recently, it was thought such atrophy was irreversible. However, many recent experimental studies demonstrate that the partially damaged optic nerve may recover to some extent when subjected to DC electric fields or LILT. Optic neuritis and partial (not total) optic nerve atrophy have been treated with acupuncture, including MA and EA.

TENS has been used for partial optic atrophy, as for amblyopia and visual field disturbance. Indirectly stimulating the optic nerve with TENS was also of benefit in patients with more central nerve damage associated with cerebrovascular aneurysm, or with hypertensive hydrocephalus.

EHF has been used to restore function in the damaged optic nerve.

## The retina

Acupuncture has been used for chronic retinal conditions, including retinitis pigmentosa, retinal arterial occlusion and central serous retinopathy. EA in particular has been used for retinal conditions, including chronic arterial occlusion.

TENS, as well as EA, may be useful for retinitis pigmentosa and macular degeneration, especially when associated with impaired circulation in the head and neck.

Microcurrent at acupoints around the eyes has been used for macular degeneration.

## Colour blindness

There are inherited forms of colour blindness, and acquired forms secondary to excessive use of alcohol and tobacco. Colour vision may be transiently affected by mood and general state of health, or permanently by optic neuritis.

Colour blindness has been treated with MA, as well as EA. Colour vision has been reported to improve using ryodoraku-style treatment. Case study 9.4.1 is an example of this.

## The shape of the eye

Ametropia, a general term for alterations in the shape of the eye, includes myopia, hyperopia and astigmatism. It has been treated with a combination of auricular medicated plasters and plum blossom needling.

### MYOPIA

Conventionally, myopia is correctable only with glasses and laser surgery. The condition tends to worsen until around the age of 30 years. However, juvenile and adolescent myopia have been treated with auricular acupressure. Pressure, either directly or indirectly to 'pellets' or seeds (sometimes medicated) affixed at the points, may be combined with auricular point injection.

EA is claimed to enhance visual accommodation. Both EA and electric plum blossom needling have been used for myopia.

Myopia in children and adolescents has been treated with LA. Hiranandani suggests LA, with ultrasound as

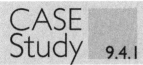

## CASE Study 9.4.1

### Ryodoraku electroacupuncture therapy for colour blindness
**Goto Kimiya**

In recent years, with the rapid progress of visual displays such as personal computers in the home, school and office, eye diseases such as asthenopia have also been on the rise. Increased reports of eye disease have not been matched by an increase in treatment reports. There are especially few reports about the treatment of colour sensation abnormalities, the majority of which are not even discovered until medical checks at school.

Colour blindness is considered a hereditary and incurable condition. Therefore, very few clinical studies exist.

### Colour blindness

Colour blindness and partial colour blindness are said to be products of X-linked recessive inheritance. Sex-linked inheritance can be understood in terms of combinations of male and female genes. Male colour sensation gene types can present as normal or colour blind. Female colour sensation gene types can present as normal, carrier of colour-blind gene, or colour blind. Males have a 5% incident rate of colour blindness, and females a 0.02% rate. A father's genes will pass only to his daughter. However, a mother's genes can pass equally to either son or daughter.

### Materials and methods
#### Examination

The 'Color Sensation Abnormality Test Book for School' and 'Ishihara Color Sensation Abnormality Test Book' were used to evaluate colour blindness.

#### Devices

The following devices were used: a neurometer (device for measuring and adjusting sympathetic nerve excitation), a ryodoraku autonomous regulatory device MR Shin-Kan (a unique autonomous regulatory needle holder used in ryodoraku therapy), a cluster needle, a low-frequency electrical stimulator, and no. 5 acupuncture needles (50 mm and 30 mm).

### Treatment techniques

1. Cluster needle technique: stimulating skin until it becomes red.
2. Retained needles technique: 10–20 minutes.
3. Electroacupuncture technique: using MR Shin-Kan, 200 μA, connected from the cathode for 7 seconds.
4. Electro jyakutaku technique (electro sparrow pecking method): insertion and piston stimulation of Showa Shin-Kan needle.
5. Low-frequency electrical stimulation: for roughly 15 minutes.

The most effective stimulation is the combination of EA and retained needles.

### Treatment points

The core points for all vision abnormalities and eye problems are BL-10, GB-20, BL-18, LI-4, LIV-2, ST-3 and GB-37. Extra points include Nakatani Eye point A, which is 1/2 cm lateral to GB-1, with 45° insertion towards the opposite jaw, and Nakatani Eye point B, halfway between SJ-21 and GB-1, inserted towards Du-15 at the base of the skull. Electroacupuncture technique is used on Nakatani A and B points.

### Oriental perspective

The Kidney Essence, Liver Blood, and *qi* and Blood from the Spleen and Stomach all nurture the eyes and support vision. Eye disease presents upon the diagnosis of Liver and Kidney *yin* deficiency and Spleen and Stomach deficiency. The Chinese Classics state that the Liver controls the muscles and ensures the free flow of *qi* and Blood. The eyes are the 'opening' of the Liver, and the nails its 'flowering'. It is important to regulate the Liver channel for any problem involving the eyes.

Table 9.4.1 shows the eye and channel correspondences.

**Table 9.4.1** Eye and channel correspondences

|  | Yin | Yang | Colour | Eye | Ryodoraku | Disorder |
|---|---|---|---|---|---|---|
| Wood | Liver | Gall Bladder | Blue | Iris | F2/F5 | Glaucoma |
| Fire | Heart | Small Intestine | Red | Corners | H3/H4 | Conjunctivitis |
| Earth | Spleen | Stomach | Yellow | Eyelids | F1/F6 | Jaundice |
| Metal | Lung | Large Intestine | White | Cornea | H1/H6 | Cataract |
| Water | Kidney | Bladder | Black | Pupil | F3/F4 | Inner eye |

*(Continued)*

## CASE Study 9.4.1 Continued

### Treatment
### Case 1
*Name: AH; age: 8; sex: male*

After a school eye exam with the Ishihara Color Sensation Abnormality Test, the patient was found to suffer from severe colour blindness. The same test was administered at my clinic before the first treatment, resulting in only 3 out of 12 plates being identifiable.

The first ryodoraku measurement (Fig. 9.4.1) showed F2, F6 and F4 all excited and H4, H6 and F1 all inhibited. It is observed that the excitation of F2 and F6 and the inhibition of F1, H4 and H6 are related to the eyes. It can be interpreted that the feeble functions of the Stomach and Spleen are inadequate to nourish the eyes.

### 1. Treatments 1 to 5

General regulatory treatment using cluster needle with low-frequency connection was used on Du-4 and Du-12, as Child regulatory points, with Ren-12 to regulate the Spleen and Stomach. Retained needles for 10 minutes were used on Nakatani eye point A, Nakatani eye point B and LI-4.

### 2. Treatments 6 to 10

General regulatory treatment was the same as above, with the addition of BL-18, BL-20 and BL-23. Retained needles for 10 minutes with a low-frequency 3 Hz pulse were used on Nakatani eye point A, Nakatani eye point B, and LI-4 (Fig. 9.4.2).

### 3. Treatments 11 to 15

General regulatory treatment was the same as 2 above, with the addition of Ren-12 and Du-20. Retained needles were the same as above.

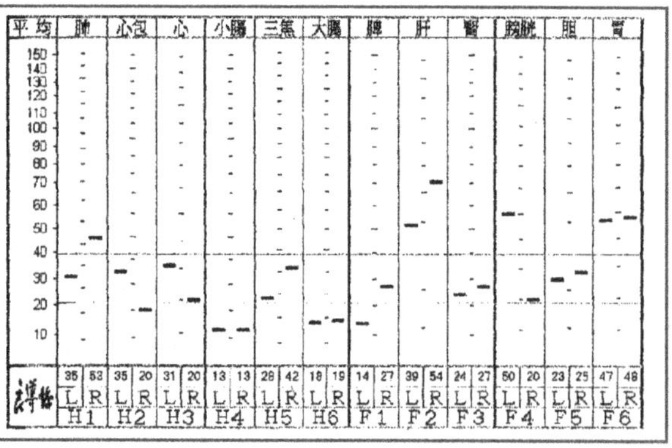

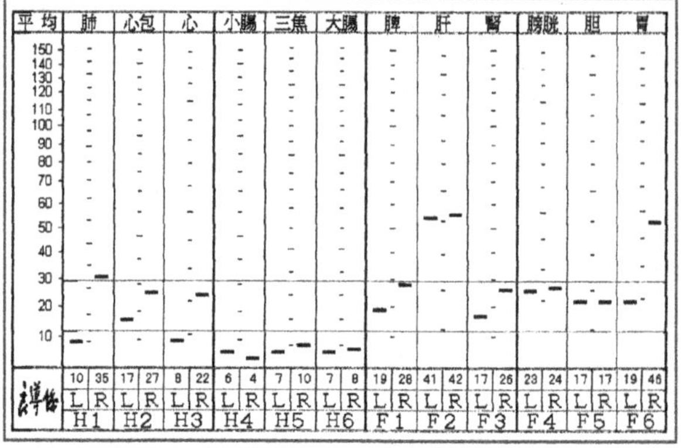

**Figure 9.4.2** Ryodoraku chart: measurement 10.

### 4. Treatments 16 to 19

General regulatory treatment was the same as 3 above, with the addition of BL-10 and GB-20. Retained needles were the same as 2 above, with the addition of GB-37 and LIV-2 (Fig. 9.4.3).

### Results (Table 9.4.2)

The Ishihara Color Sensation Abnormality Test was administered at my clinic before the first treatment, with the result that only 3 out of 12 plates were identified correctly. Treatments three times per week improved the score from 3 to 6. From treatment 7, in order to prevent the results from being detrimentally affected through recollection, the test book was changed to 'Hiragana Test Book.' An improvement to 8 out of 12 was recorded by the 19th treatment. After a 7-month break, a check was made to evaluate long-term effectiveness. Prior to receiving treatment, the patient scored 8 out of 12 to confirm the success of the treatment for colour blindness.

### Discussion

The cells that detect colour, the red, green, and blue cone cells, are located behind the retina. It is generally thought

**Figure 9.4.1** Ryodoraku chart: measurement 1.

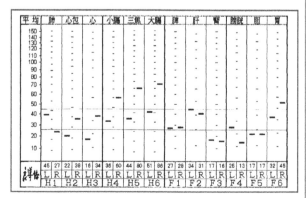

**Figure 9.4.3** Ryodoraku chart: measurement 19.

## CASE Study 9.4.1 Continued

**Table 9.4.2** Colour blindness results chart

| Treatment number | Date | Before (B) or after (A) treatment | 25 | 2 | 5 | 8 | 3 | 9 | 6 | 4 | – | 58 | | | Pt — Number of correct identifications (out of 12) |
|---|---|---|---|---|---|---|---|---|---|---|---|---|---|---|---|
| 1 | 14 | B | 25 | 2 | 52 | 3 | 33 | 8 | — | — | — | 55 | 53 | 56 | 3 |
| | Aug | A | | | | | | | | | | | | | |
| 2 | 15 | B | | | | | | | | | | | | | |
| | Aug | A | 25 | 2 | 5 | 3 | — | 8 | — | 10 | — | 56 | — | 54 | 4 |
| 3 | 18 | B | 25 | 2 | 5 | 3 | — | 8 | — | — | — | 28 | 10 | — | 4 |
| | Aug | A | | | | | | | | | | | | | |
| 4 | 20 | B | | | | | | | | | | | | | |
| | Aug | A | 25 | 2 | 5 | 35 | 3 | 9 | — | — | — | 53 | 96 | — | 6 |
| 5 | 21 | B | | | | | | | | | | | | | |
| | Aug | A | 25 | 2 | 5 | 8 | 3 | 9 | — | — | — | 53 | 96 | — | 7 |
| 6 | 27 | B | | | | | | | | | | | | | |
| | Aug | A | 25 | 2 | 5 | 36 | 3 | 9 | — | — | — | 56 | 96 | 21 | 6 |
| 7 | 28 | B | や | ら | — | — | — | は | — | — | — | — | い | — | 3 |
| | Aug | A | や | ら | — | よ | — | は | — | — | — | — | — | に | 3 |
| 8 | 6 | B | や | ら | — | よ | — | — | — | — | — | — | い | — | 3 |
| | Sept | A | や | ら | — | よ | — | は | — | — | — | — | い | に | 4 |
| 9 | 20 | B | や | ろ | ら | — | — | は | — | — | — | — | い | に | 5 |
| | Sept | A | や | ろ | ら | よ | — | は | — | — | — | — | い | に | 5 |
| 10 | 4 | B | | | | | | | | | | | | | |
| | Oct | A | 25 | 3 | 5 | 3 | 6 | 85 | — | — | — | 56 | — | 26 | 3 |
| 11 | 11 | B | 25 | 2 | 6 | 5 | 3 | 9 | — | — | — | 56 | — | — | 5 |
| | Oct | A | 25 | 2 | 5 | 8 | 5 | 56 | — | 98 | 80 | 50 | 53 | — | 4 |
| 12 | 18 | B | 25 | 2 | 5 | 3 | 8 | 9 | — | — | — | 50 | 53 | 56 | 5 |
| | Oct | A | 25 | 2 | 5 | 3 | 50 | 9 | — | 89 | — | 56 | 66 | 51 | 5 |
| 13 | 8 | B | 25 | 2 | 5 | 3 | 50 | 9 | — | — | — | 59 | 58 | 50 | 5 |
| | Nov | A | 25 | 2 | 6 | 3 | 36 | 9 | — | — | — | 56 | 58 | 51 | 4 |
| 14 | 15 | B | | | | | | | | | | | | | |
| | Nov | A | 25 | 2 | 5 | 3 | 3 | 9 | — | 51 | — | 59 | 56 | 21 | 6 |
| 15 | 16 | B | | | | | | | | | | | | | |
| | Nov | A | 25 | 2 | 5 | 8 | 3 | 9 | 10 | — | — | 55 | — | 11 | 7 |
| 16 | 23 | B | | | | | | | | | | | | | |
| | Nov | A | 25 | 2 | 5 | 8 | 3 | 9 | — | — | 0 | 56 | 16 | 11 | 6 |
| 17 | 29 | B | 25 | 2 | 5 | 8 | 3 | 9 | — | 19 | — | 50 | 13 | 11 | 7 |
| | Nov | A | 25 | 2 | 5 | 8 | 3 | 9 | — | 10 | — | 58 | 50 | 11 | 8 |
| 18 | 6 | B | 25 | 2 | 5 | 8 | 3 | 9 | — | 10 | — | 56 | 15 | 51 | 7 |
| | Dec | A | 25 | 2 | 5 | 8 | 3 | 9 | — | 10 | — | 58 | 51 | 15 | 8 |
| 19 | 13 | B | | | | | | | | | | | | | |
| | Dec | A | 25 | 2 | 5 | 8 | 3 | 9 | — | 16 | — | 58 | — | 91 | 8 |
| 20 | 28 | B | 25 | 2 | 5 | 8 | 3 | 9 | 5 | — | — | 58 | — | — | 8 |
| | Jul | A | | | | | | | | | | | | | |

Key: Shaded area indicates a correct identification; A: test made immediately *after* treatment; B: test made immediately *before* treatment.

---

**CASE Study 9.4.1 Continued**

that colour blindness is the result of underdevelopment or hypofunction of cone cells. The different types of colour blindness relate to the different colours of cells. Until recently, colour blindness has been considered to be an incurable hereditary dysfunction. However, many reports on treatments of colour blindness have demonstrated that electroneedling stimulation is able to increase or restore eye function to normal levels.

In the *Journal of Autonomic Nervous Society*, Dr Sasagawa Kyugo, Professor Emeritus of Kyoto University, reported that it is said that colour blindness is incurable because the excitation of photoreceptor cells is naturally low and the situation continues for life. However, it is possible to activate photoreceptor cells by practising electroneedling stimulation on Nakatani eye points A and B. One course of treatment comprises 20 visits. If an effective result is not achieved in this period, it is advised that the patient cease treatment for a period of several months. A further course of treatment is then likely to be more effective.

Is relapse likely after treatment? There are, of course, individual reactions in the post-treatment phase. In cases of light affliction, the speed of improvement is fast, and the improved condition stable. In more severe cases, there may be a need for repeated check-ups and sustained treatment. Any eye-related problem, but colour blindness in particular, responds best to treatment at a young age (i.e. at primary or middle school age rather than high school or later).

If a patient can recognise a character correctly, this does not necessarily mean there has been recovery. The Color Sensation Abnormality Test Book is not perfect. There are patients who can recognise characters correctly when reading through red glasses. It was therefore considered that the patient's colour sense improved only to a certain extent if they could recognise the character correctly.

**Conclusion**

In this case, F2 was improved on the ryodoraku chart. In Chinese medicine, and also in ryodoraku, it is said that the eyes are the 'flowering' of the Liver. I have arrived at the conclusion that the improvement of F2 (Liver) is effective in improving eyesight and colour blindness.

---

an alternative. However, ultrasound is usually contraindicated for treatments directly over or near the eye, and proper precautions should be observed when using low-powered lasers near to the eyes.

### HYPEROPIA

Hyperopia (hypermetropia) has been treated with acupuncture in 'youngsters' (using implanted needles at ear points), and also with TENS.

## Glaucoma

In most types of glaucoma, intraocular pressure is raised, resulting in damage to the eye and loss of vision.

Acupuncture is sometimes used for glaucoma, and auricular EA has been used for experimentally induced ocular hypertension. Both MA and EA can reduce intraocular pressure in the short term in healthy volunteers, and a number of clinical studies have shown that EA may reduce intraocular pressure in some cases.

## The muscles of the eye

### STRABISMUS (SQUINT)

In children, lack of muscle coordination can result in 'concomitant strabismus'. In adults, 'paralytic strabismus' is usually due to lesions of the nerve supplying the affected extraocular muscles.

Concomitant strabismus has been treated with acupuncture, plum blossom needling and EA. Oculomotor nerve

injury has been treated with MA, as has outright paralytic strabismus.

### NYSTAGMUS AND OTHER OCULOMOTOR DISTURBANCE

Involuntary movements of the eye (nystagmus) may be congenital, or accompany inner ear (vestibular) dysfunction.

In one experimental study on congenital nystagmus, MA at points in the sternocleidomastoid muscles was found to modify the pattern of eye movements in some patients. Clinically, MA has been used for nystagmus, including congenital nystagmus with associated oscillopsia (apparent movement of objects).

## The eyelids and conjunctiva

Conjunctivitis may be acute or chronic, and inflammation may also involve the cornea (keratitis). In the elderly, this may result from dry eyes (keratoconjunctivitis sicca, or xerophthalmia).

Conjunctival irritation is virtually the only ophthalmic condition for which Filshie and White consider acupuncture may be of any real benefit. Both EA and LA have been used for conjunctivitis. Khoe has recommended probe stimulation (pTENS) with a ryodoraku-style neurometer.

Auricular MA with blood letting has been used for acute conjunctivitis.

Acupuncture may be helpful for dry eyes. For conjunctivitis sicca, auricular MA or the combination of auricular with body points may be useful. Using the same protocol for dry eyes that was successful for xerostomia, but with MA rather than electrical stimulation, one study showed promising results in four patients with dry eyes from various causes. LA too has been used for conjunctivitis sicca, and was found to be as effective as MA for this.

LA with LILT has been used for both ulcerative palpebritis and stye. It was also helpful in a case of lagophthalmus (incomplete closure of the eyelid) following meningitis. Red LED irradiation has been used for dark areas and puffiness under the eyes, as has microcurrent.

## Other eye conditions

LF EA to auricular points has been recommended for ophthalmic herpes.

Ophthalmitis, potentially sight-threatening inflammation of the whole eye, has been treated with MA.

Blocked tear ducts in a 9-month-old infant have been treated with LA. In adults, a traditional treatment for epiphora (excessive watering of the eyes) is warm needling at BL-1.

**Comparisons in ophthalmology** Electric plum blossom needling is claimed to give better results than manual plum blossom needling for myopia and concomitant strabismus.

However, in one study on myopia, LA was found to be more effective than electric plum blossom needling, and in another its effects on cerebral blood flow were 'more or less superior' to those of EA. In the treatment of conjunctivitis sicca, LA was as effective as MA.

Auricular electrostimulation and HeNe LA have been combined in treating amblyopia.

**Points used in ophthalmology** The most used local points for eye problems are BL-1, BL-2, SJ-17, SJ-23, GB-14, GB-20, ST-1 and ST-8, with around 15 non-meridian local points also used (especially *taiyang* (M-HN-9) and *yintang* (M-HN-3)). Similar points have been used for such disparate conditions as myopia and conjunctivitis.

BL-1 has been used for chronic central angiospastic retinopathy, for example. Zheng Qiwei, in his overview of points for EA, suggests *taiyang* (M-HN-9) with BL-2 or ST-2 for incomplete eye closure.

Distal points LIV-3 and LI-4, BL-60 and GB-37 are most frequently selected. Auricular points are recommended by some authors.

Van Nghi and colleagues recommend purely distal points for analgesia in eye and other face and neck operations: P-6, GB-37, LIV-3, LI-4 and ST-36. Points are selected according to the operation site. Others have used GB-14, ST-2, ST-5, *yintang*, *taiyang* with SJ-5 or SJ-6, LIV-2, LIV-3, LI-4, ST-36 and auricular points. Walied Abdulla's group, in their series of TENS studies, used points according to their dermatomal innervation.

**Parameters used in ophthalmology** Given that electrical activity in the retina peaks at around 2 Hz, and bearing in

mind that LF rather than HF stimulation can increase peripheral circulation, 2 Hz might be an appropriate frequency to enhance vasodilation in arterial retinopathy. In one collection of case reports, on diabetic optic neuritis and glaucoma, both DD and intermittent EA (i.e. with a LF component) gave better results than either LF or HF alone.

# DISORDERS OF THE EAR, NOSE AND THROAT (ENT)

## The outer ear

Most acupuncturists are familiar with the microsystem of acupoints on the pinna developed by Paul Nogier in the 1950s. Other points within the ear canal itself have also been detected electrically.

Otitis externa has been treated with a combination of 50 Hz with VHF or UHF 20 mT (200 G) PEMF, combination treatment giving better results than either 50 Hz or UHF/VHF alone.

## The middle ear

### OTITIS MEDIA

Acute otitis media is usually the result of Eustachian tube obstruction following nose and throat infections. It can lead to a chronic suppurative form, glue ear, or mastoiditis and chronic conductive hearing loss.

Both ordinary otitis media and aerotitis media (barotitis) in aviation personnel have been treated with MA.

Acupuncture can give symptomatic relief for earache, although the underlying cause must also be addressed. Local LA at SI-19, SJ-17, SJ-21 and GB-2, and distally at SJ-3, SJ-5, GB-41, LI-4 and ST-44, has been suggested. Naeser recommends local points, including SI-19, SJ-21 and GB-2. Khoe has used ultrasound at SJ-17 and directed into the ear canal itself for this.

### MIDDLE EAR DEAFNESS

For middle ear deafness, Khoe recommended a combination of EA with ultrasound and then pTENS at points within the ear canal. He advocated endaural ultrasound particularly for patients scheduled for stapes immobilisation.

## The inner ear

### SENSORINEURAL DEAFNESS

Sensorineural deafness may accompany ageing (presbycusis) or Ménière's disease, or result from trauma or tumour. Unilateral hearing loss may be due to acoustic neuroma or the use of certain drugs.

There are continuing anecdotal reports of MA's usefulness for deafness, for instance with scalp needling, yet controlled research has shown that MA does not produce statistically significant improvements in hearing, and may even result in *poorer* hearing levels following treatment. There have been a number of negative reviews on acupuncture (mostly MA) for sensorineural deafness.

EA has been used for hearing loss and sensorineural deafness. There have been both experimental and clinical studies on the effect of EA on antibiotic-induced ototoxic auditory damage.

In one early review of ryodoraku-style EA, it was claimed to be effective in 68% of cases of hearing loss.

LA has been used in the treatment of deafness, including sensorineural deafness in infants.

## TINNITUS

Tinnitus is usually associated with inner ear problems, but may result from central disorders, and is sometimes associated with temporomandibular joint disorder and ipsilateral chronic muscle tension.

Both acupuncture and TENS have been used. Direct electrical stimulation of the eardrum and mastoid area was recommended as long ago as the nineteenth century.

There are reports of MA helping tinnitus, especially if *deqi* reaches the affected ear. In general, though, studies are not optimistic.

In a review of randomised clinical trials on tinnitus published up to 1998, no benefits were found for the six acupuncture studies. In another recent review of six RCTs (four on MA, two on EA), acupuncture was again not shown to be useful. However, Filshie and White did concede that EA might be more effective than MA, if used within a comprehensive management programme, although treatment may need to be long term for any sustained effect.

LILT directed within the auditory meatus or to the skin around the ear (with stronger irradiation) has been used for tinnitus. As with electrical stimulation, LILT may be helpful for tinnitus caused by acute or chronic acoustic trauma to the inner ear, or stress and consequent muscle spasm, but not that due to damage within the brain.

EHF has been used in the treatment of auditory nerve damage.

Whatever method is attempted, benefits are likely to be slight; if there is only minimal early improvement in response to treatment, it is probably not worth persevering. Despite these conclusions, studies on electrotherapeutic methods for tinnitus continue to be published.

## Ménière's disease and the sense of balance

Ménière's disease originates in the labyrinth of the inner ear, and typically consists of deafness, tinnitus and vertigo. The symptoms of acoustic neuroma are similar, but in Ménière's there is often prolonged remission, and the condition can be self-limiting.

Acupuncture has traditionally been used for Ménière's disease, with MA at both body points and ear points. EA, ultrasound and acupoint injection have also been explored.

## VERTIGO AND MOTION SICKNESS

Vertigo (dizziness) may occur as a result of most ear conditions, as well as many others of central or peripheral origin. Dizziness may be a sign of general electrical hypersensitivity.

MA may be helpful for motion sickness, and for dizziness associated with neck muscle tension, or balance disorders following whiplash injury. Deep needling on the neck has been used for 'spinogenic' dizziness ('cervical vertigo'). MA has also been employed for migraine-related vertigo, as part of a comprehensive treatment programme, and for vertigo resulting from abnormal blood pressure. Auricular acupuncture has been used for vertigo, in particular that due to head injury. Scalp MA has been utilised for various forms of vertigo.

Although in one uncontrolled study EA did not benefit postural vertigo associated with cervical spondylosis, and in some studies was less effective than warm needling or other acupuncture methods, it has been found helpful for this particular symptom particularly in combination with other modalities such as massage or moxibustion. It has been used to reduce dizziness following stroke, and for treating vertigo due to hypertension.

pTENS has been considered for central (neurovascular) equilibrium disturbances. Motion sickness has been treated with TENS to P-6, as have other types of nausea.

Microcurrent TENS (MENS) has been used for idiopathic vertigo, using a probe in each ear canal in conjunction with stretching and positional exercises. Intra-aural LA has been found to be useful for cochleovestibular dysfunction.

MA, bleeding and cupping have been combined for cervical dizziness due to narrowing of the cervical foramina restricting vertebral arterial flow. The total symptomatic effective rate was claimed to be 96.4%. Points bled included Du-14, Du-15, Du-16 and Du-20.

## Other ear problems

Ear pain (otalgia), like postural vertigo, may be referred from the neck. This has been considered an indication for pTENS.

## The nose

### ANOSMIA

Hyposmia and anosmia (reduced or absent sense of smell) have been treated with acupuncture, and with EA in particular. When due simply to nasal congestion, they may respond to local pTENS. Auricular MA may also modify olfactory acuity, and occasionally acupuncture may induce an aversion to certain smells. There are acupuncture-based exercises designed to improve breathing and the sense of smell.

### RHINITIS

Chronic nasal inflammation (rhinitis) may result from sinusitis, nasal blockage or continuous exposure to inhaled allergens, dust or other air pollutants. Allergic rhinitis may be seasonal or perennial. It may progress to sinusitis or chronic rhinitis, and can significantly affect a person's life and character.

Both MA and acupoint injection have been used for hay fever and other forms of allergic rhinitis, as have moxibustion and bleeding. Auricular MA, acupressure and plaster therapy have also been employed, as well as ECIWO ('embryo containing the information of the whole organism') MA, along the second metacarpal. Even moxibustion directed locally to the nostrils has reduced symptoms of house dust mite allergy. Although there is a strong clinical impression that acupuncture is of benefit for hay fever, this is not supported by the existing evidence.

LF EA has been recommended for allergic rhinitis. EA has also been combined with stellate ganglion blockade in the treatment of nasal obstruction, with effects on the skin temperature of the nose.

MENS probes applied at acupoints, as well as intranasally, have been used for rhinitis.

LA has been used both experimentally and clinically for allergic rhinitis, and specifically for hay fever (pollinosis), although results may only be temporary. For chronic rhinitis, Naeser uses ST-40 as well as LI-4 and LI-20. She has found that exposing the nostrils to LILT can be helpful, either daily or on alternate days if acute, or 2–3 times weekly if chronic. Clearly, proper precautions need to be observed in using even low-powered laser so near to the eyes, especially in children. However, non-laser narrow-band red light therapy within each nostril has also been shown to be useful for both seasonal and perennial allergic rhinitis.

### SINUSITIS

Sinuses drain poorly, and easily become infected. Poor drainage can lead to chronic sinusitis.

MA has been used for acute and chronic sinusitis, the balance of evidence suggesting that acupuncture may be helpful for chronic sinusitis.

EA or TEAS based on hand-to-hand or foot-to-foot electrical resistance measurements has been used for some sinus problems. In particular, LF EA has been used for sinusitis pain, at a combination of local and distal acupoints.

Frontal sinusitis has been suggested as an indication for pTENS.

LA has been used for both acute and chronic sinusitis. One method would be to apply laser at local points such as SI-18, GB-14, ST-2 and ST-3, with distal points LI-4 and the combination of LI-11 with SP-10. Intranasal LILT is also possible; LILT and magnetic stimulation have also been combined.

Vibratory stimulation may relieve sinus pain. Hiranandani has found the combination of LA with local ultrasound to be more effective than LA alone, and the Qi Gong machine has been used to clear sinus headache.

Case study 9.4.2 details the treatment of a male patient with chronic sinusitis and facial pain.

### OTHER CONDITIONS

The common cold is a standard indication for acupuncture in Chinese textbooks.

For a head cold, Khoe has suggested that ultrasound on local points can give rapid effects, and also recommended

EA at BL-13, LI-4, LI-20 and Du-23 for sneezing and rhinorrhoea. Both MA and pTENS may be effective too. A simple treatment for coryza would be daily LF EA at LI-20 (bilaterally) and LI-4 (–) with *yintang* (+), or pTENS at the same points.

The common cold may also respond to LA, which has been used as well at LI-20 and *bitong* (M-HN-14) for nasal obstruction or discharge when treating bronchitis.

Snoring associated with mucosal congestion has been treated with MA at LI-20.

## The throat

The throat is generally taken as including the pharynx, larynx and tonsils.

### THE PHARYNX

Sore throat has been treated with MA, and chronic pharyngitis with MA combined with acupoint compresses, or local *ashi* point injection.

Intraoral LILT has been used for acute pharyngitis. LA too has been used for rhinopharyngeal infection. LA may be more effective for inflammatory ENT conditions if treatment is started early.

### THE VOICE AND LARYNX

MA has been used for dysphonia (vocal impairment) with possible effects on vocal cord 'polyps'. MA has also been used as an alternative to botulinum toxin injection for spasmodic laryngeal adductor dysphonia, and has formed part of a comprehensive treatment approach for unilateral paralysis of the recurrent laryngeal nerve. MA at LI-4 and P-8 may reverse laryngospasm.

Electrical stimulation of the throat is generally considered to be contraindicated, both because of the risk of laryngospasm and the possibility of affecting blood pressure via the carotid baroreceptors. However, low-intensity pTENS over the tracheo-oesophageal groove may actually *increase* glottic aperture as frequency is increased from 10 to 30 Hz, although further increases eventually lead to glottic closure.

### THE TONSILS AND OTHER LYMPH NODES

Tonsillitis is considered to be an indication for ryodoraku and, with faucitis, is listed as amenable to EA in the manual of one auricular EA device.

Following tonsillectomy, MA, EA, pTENS and TENS have been used for postoperative pain. While MA (begun *after* conventional anaesthetic induction) was unsuccessful for postoperative nausea in children in one report, EA (in the recovery room) was helpful.

**Comparisons in ENT** Huang Yiqing regarded EA as more effective than medication for hay fever. Kaslow and Lowenschuss considered that pTENS could achieve results more rapidly than MA.

One study on allergic rhinitis suggested that the combination of intranasal LILT and acupuncture was superior to either

# CASE Study 9.4.2

## A male patient with chronic sinusitis and facial pain
### Ron Sharp

This patient first presented with facial pain from an infected frontal sinus, and also had an inner ear infection and hay fever. For a period of over 2½ years, he had had great difficulty in clearing his nose, which always felt blocked, and so had difficulty with breathing. Aggravating factors included excess dry/damp atmospheres, pollens and any strong smelling substances.

His previous history included nasal problems since childhood with many minor surgical procedures and injections. In addition he had asthma, mild eczema, headaches and occasional migraine. His eyes were often irritable and there was occasional dizziness. He tended to get recurrent infections and always had profuse sweating.

Previous treatments included nasal sprays, injections, sinus washes and local cocaine probes to the anterior ethmoidal nerves. Only with strong analgesics, resting in an upright posture and keeping his head still, was relief gained from pain. The ENT consultant had planned surgery (fenestration) to promote irrigation of the nasal cavity.

Tongue examination showed a large dry red cracked tongue, with a thin sticky white irregular coat and a red tip. The general pulse was slippery, fine and fast with Earth in excess (*shi*), and Fire in deficiency (*xu*). On palpation, there was tenderness over GB-14, ST-2, *yintang* and *taiyang* (Extra points).

The treatment plan was to relieve the pain and restore fluid metabolism, primarily of the nasal cavity. The first treatment was symptomatic, to judge the patient's energetic response and tolerance to acupuncture. *Yintang* (Extra point), bilateral ST-2 and left LI-4 were needled, with the needles retained for 10 minutes after *deqi* was achieved.

Two days later, after a slight post-treatment healing crisis lasting 4–5 hours, the first treatment was repeated with the needles retained for 20 minutes, using even method by agitating the needles every 5 minutes. One week later, the patient's mucus was moving and there was less pain. Treatment that day was *yintang* and bilateral LI-4,

with left ST-44 added, as the eyes were a little inflamed. Needles were retained for 20 minutes, with even method.

This treatment gave good pain control but increased mucus production, so the treatment was changed to combat this. Bilateral *bitong* (Extra point) was exchanged for *yintang*, with the others remaining, all for 20 minutes. That treatment cleared the mucus, but did not help the pain, which returned to its previous level.

This resulted in a dilemma. The treatment either produced good pain relief with increased mucus production or cleared the mucus with an increase of pain. In consultation with the ENT consultant, we decided to concentrate on the pain relief. I decided to use electroacupuncture for more pain control. The first treatment was LI-4, LI-20, bilaterally for 20 minutes at 200 Hz, with an intensity that was just comfortable, checked every 5 minutes to maintain the intensity and to control any accommodation to the treatment.

The patient had a very strong reaction to this change, which also exacerbated his migraine. After two more attempts had the same effect it was decided to refrain from electroacupuncture, as it appeared that the treatment was too powerful and was not controlling his pain.

The next few sessions managed to control the pain using LI-4, LI-20, bilaterally with even technique. In general the pain was well controlled, but only for about 7–10 days, not really good enough to plan a discharge date.

We decided to try laser as he really found acupuncture uncomfortable, and used it on LI-4, LI-20 bilaterally, and left auricular *shenmen*, for 1 minute at each point. The laser worked well to control pain, but the effect lasted for only 4 days. Since the patient could not attend for treatment indefinitely, we needed to adopt another strategy: that of home treatment on a daily basis, allowing me to concentrate on the systemic approach to clear his channels and to attempt to address the cause.

I used a piezoelectric wand stimulator for home pain control. This worked very well with one treatment of three charges every 2 days on *yintang* and LU-7, bilaterally. After 4 weeks treatment by him for pain control and me toning up his immune system with acupuncture, he was discharged for review by the ENT team, who actually discharged him as well. On follow-up 6 months later he still had good pain control with only one application of the wand per week and he had not had a chest or sinus infection in the previous 6 months.

method alone. Pothmann and Yeh found MA was more effective for sinus problems in children than LA.

**Points used in ENT** For otitis media, whether using EA, LA or ultrasound, SJ-17 is used most frequently, plus other local points (for EA or LA) such as SI-19, SJ-21 and GB-2.

Deep needling at ST-7 may dilate the Eustachian tube. Distal points such as KI-3, SJ-3 and LI-4, or others according to TCM differentiation, are sometimes used in addition. For middle ear deafness, Khoe also recommended auricular points such as Kidney, Occiput, External ear and Cochlea.

For sensorineural deafness, the same local points are favoured, along with Du-15. Distal points such as BL-23, SJ-5 and LI-4 are most used, as well as distal points on the Gall Bladder meridian.

For tinnitus, the most common local points are SI-19, SJ-17, SJ-21 and GB-2. Distal points include SI-3, SJ-5 and LI-4. Auricular EA daily or every other day has been suggested for tinnitus and reduced hearing, using such points as Subcortex, Endocrine, Liver and Kidney, with the intensity depending on whether the condition is more *xu* or *shi*.

For vertigo and Ménière's disease, SI-19 and SJ-17 have been used, with cervical paraspinal points and even endaural points. Khoe also used LF EA bilaterally over the minor occipital nerve (*anmian*, N-HN-54?) and at auricular points, his modality of choice being ultrasound over ST-9 and in the ear canal. For motion sickness, P-6 is the most researched point.

Endaural acupoints within the external ear canal may be more effective than auricular points for inner ear problems. There are few studies for inner ear deafness using standard auricular points, though more tinnitus studies use ear points. Scalp vertigo and auditory areas have been stimulated bilaterally for tinnitus and deafness as part of a comprehensive treatment approach.

Local points such as BL-2, LI-20 and *bitong* (M-HN-14) or *yintang* (M-HN-3) can be useful for nasal problems, including congestion, with distal points LI-4 and LI-11. Auricular points, particularly the Internal nose point, can be effective. As Alexander Macdonald states, almost any acupoint or trigger point in the area can relieve a blocked nose rapidly. However, in a study, of eight acupoints traditionally considered to improve nasal breathing, only LI-20 was effective when air-flow resistance was measured in patients with nasal congestion.

Most rhinitis (or anosmia) studies are based on stimulation of LI-20, whether with MA, EA, pTENS, LA or ultrasound, sometimes with other local points as above, or local *sanjiao* points, GB-2, GB-20, LI-19 or Du-26. Distal points generally include LI-4, often BL-13, and sometimes LI-11, ST-36 or Du-14. For allergic rhinitis, local acupoints such as LI-4, LI-20, Du-23, Du-24, Du-25 and *yintang* have been used, with LILT to the nose externally and points of general action such as SP-10.

For sinusitis, the most common local points are SI-18, BL-2, LI-20 and *yintang*, sometimes with GB-20, Du-19 or Du-20, and others according to the affected sinus. LI-4 is the most frequent distal point. The combination of LI-11 with SP-10 has also been suggested.

For throat problems, SI-16, LI-18, ST-9, Ren-22, Ren-23 or other local extrameridian points are used (sometimes with BL-10 or GB-20), with distal points for their TCM indications, such as KI-3, KI-6, LU-7, LI-4 or SP-6.

A similar combination of local LILT and distal LA (LU-6 and LI-4) is used for tonsillitis.

**Parameters used in ENT** Tian Zhenming suggests using daily 2 Hz EA with strong stimulation in acute otitis media, moderate stimulation every other day if chronic. For middle ear deafness, Khoe recommended 2 Hz for body points, but 50–100 Hz at ear points.

For inner ear deafness, LF EA is employed most often. For tinnitus, DD and intermittent (LF trains) seem to be more used than CW LF. The changing AlphaStim signal was used, as well as a frequency sweep through the whole audio range, in one TENS study. For vertigo and Ménière's disease, both LF and HF have been used.

There is little indication from the studies on which parameters of EA (or LA) are most likely to be helpful for rhinitis, although HeNe lasers were used almost exclusively for LA. Intranasal LILT (5 mW 670 nm) is suggested by Naeser.

For throat problems, LF EA seems the most commonly used modality.

# Oral disorders

## APHTHOUS STOMATITIS
Recurrent aphthous ulcers, or 'canker sores', are painful, but self-limiting. They are often stress related, but may also be caused by sodium lauryl sulphate (detergent) in toothpastes.

Recurrent aphthous stomatitis has been treated with EA, ryodoraku (probe) stimulation directly to the ulcers, and LA. LA may not be so effective for a chronic condition. Hiranandani suggests using infrared LA at distal points, with LILT locally and oral B complex vitamins. Pöntinen recommends a HeNe or diode laser locally.

## DENTAL STOMATOLOGY – THE GUMS
MA has been used for chronic gum discomfort in periodontal disease.

EA has been found first to decrease, but then to increase immunoglobulin G (IgG) in the gingival trough (around the tooth).

LILT has been used to reduce pain and bleeding in gingivitis and for herpetic stomatitis.

## ORAL PAIN AND OTHER CONDITIONS
LF EA at both local (ST-5 and ST-7) and distal (ST-36) points was used in one case of cenaesthopathy (abnormal sensations in various parts of the body, with malaise) following pulpectomy.

TEAS has been used for mouth pain (stomatodynia).

## THE SALIVARY GLANDS
A dry mouth (xerostomia) may result from anxiety, adverse drug reactions or acute infection, as well as various autoimmune conditions. It may also follow radiotherapy of the head or neck, and can lead to difficulties in speech articulation and swallowing. Most studies on all types of xerostomia treatment have been criticised for their poor quality.

MA has been shown to increase salivary flow, although non-painful LF EA does not (and EA may actually decrease salivary flow already stimulated by chewing, whereas MA has no such effect).

Overall, evidence suggests that acupuncture may be helpful for various forms of xerostomia, although it may not alleviate dry mouth as a side-effect of medication.

There is little difference between MA and EA in their effect on xerostomia due to Sjögren's syndrome. TEAS (the Codetron device) and TENS have been used for xerostomia.

## THE TONGUE

Glossodynia has been treated using TENS to the tongue, the Liss microcurrent stimulator, and Russian 'electrosleep' (CES). EA has been used for 'glossopharyngalgia'.

## THE LIPS

LILT has been used for cheilitis. Acupuncture analgesia (AA) has been used for pain relief while draining abscesses of upper and lower lips (using P-6, ST-2 and ST-44), and for corrective lip surgery.

**Comparisons in oral disorders** Clinically MA and EA appear comparable in their effect on dry mouth due to Sjögren's syndrome (although in experimental studies on xerostomia, MA may be more effective).

**Points used in oral disorders** For stomatitis, local intraoral stimulation predominates, with LA at local points such as ST-6 and at distal points such as LI-4, ST-36 (and LU-7 or Du-14), or at auricular points. In dental stomatology, local points can be used according to the underlying odontons affected, with LI-4 as the preferred distal point.

For xerostomia, EA at ST-7 or local extrameridian points has been combined with MA at local and distal points. For parotitis, LA at SJ-17, ST-6 and (other) *ashi* points has been used, with other points according to TCM indications.

For tongue (taste) and lip conditions, local TENS and LA have been used, as well as stimulation at ear points or a special point 1.5 *cun* posterior to Du-20.

**Parameters used in oral disorders** LA (mostly HeNe) is used in preference to EA for stomatitis but there is little information on other helpful parameters in stomatology. For periodontitis and other gum conditions, perseverance is necessary if treatment is to be effective.

In one xerostomia study, 2 Hz EA was employed, but most studies have used MA. Long-term but less frequent treatment may be required to maintain improvement.

## SUMMARY

Some key points in this chapter are:

- EA is frequently used for skin disorders, for instance with 'surround needling' or non-contact LILT
- Acupuncture treatment in the acute phase of shingles may hasten recovery and reduce the incidence of postherpetic neuralgia
- There is no evidence to suggest that EA should be used as a primary therapy in eye disorders
- Colour blindness appears to be treatable with EA and ryodoraku
- Although results with RCTs of the treatment of tinnitus with EA are inconclusive, this continues to be a highly researched topic
- EA and MA are often used with success in the treatment of vertigo and Ménière's disease.

### Additional material in the CD-ROM resource

In the CD-ROM resource, in addition to more information on the topics presented here, the following are also discussed:

- Dermatology:
  —Piezogenic papular pain, nappy (diaper) rash, pemphigus, ichthyosis, tissue reduction (electrolipolysis), disorders of perspiration
  —Hair removal (epilation), hair colour
- Ophthalmology:
  —Nyctalopia and night blindness (in brief), cataract, blepharitis, ophthalmic surgery
- Otorhinolaryngology:
  —Auditory pathways in the brain, iatrogenic dizziness
  —Vasomotor (non–allergic) rhinitis, atrophic rhinitis, nasal surgery
  —Sialadenitis, chronic parotitis, iatrogenic laryngospasm, tonsillectomy
- Stomatology:
  —Procedural pain, Melkersson–Rosenthal syndrome, chronic oral infection, salivary gland surgery, speech disorders.

**9.4** Summary of relevant studies in the electronic clinical studies database (number of studies)

| Condition | EA | Other | Condition | EA | Other |
|---|---|---|---|---|---|
| **Dermatology** | | | Glaucoma and cataract | 4 | 7 |
| General | 0 | 1 | Strabismus | 2 | 4 |
| Pruritis | 5 | 9 | The eyelids and conjunctiva | 1 | 17 |
| Acne | 3 | 4 | Other/mixed eye conditions | 5 | 11 |
| Eczema and dermatitis | 11 | 20 | **Otology** | | |
| Lichen planus | 1 | 1 | The outer ear | 0 | 3 |
| Psoriasis | 2 | 6 | The middle ear | 2 | 5 |
| Urticaria | 1 | 3 | The inner ear – deafness and hyperacusis | 19 | 21 |
| Vitiligo | 4 | 1 | Tinnitus | 8 | 43 |
| Herpes zoster | 10 | 25 | Ménière's disease, vertigo and related disorders | 8 | 12 |
| Herpes simplex | 0 | 6 | Vestibular stimulation (motion sickness) | 0 | 2 |
| Other viral conditions | 1 | 4 | **Nose and throat** | | |
| Fungal conditions | 1 | 1 | THE NOSE | | |
| Other/mixed conditions | 4 | 17 | Anosmia | 1 | 1 |
| Hair (alopecia) | 7 | 13 | Rhinitis | 10 | 41 |
| **Cosmetology – scar tissue** | | | Sinusitis | 2 | 14 |
| Adhesions and scar tissue | 7 | 8 | Other nasal conditions | 1 | 2 |
| Cosmetology | 3 | 1 | THE THROAT | | |
| Perspiration | 0 | 1 | The pharynx, larynx and trachea | 8 | 21 |
| **Ophthalmology** | | | The tonsils | 1 | 9 |
| Vision (general) | 1 | 0 | **The mouth** | | |
| Amblyopia, asthenopia and amaurosis | 2 | 10 | The oral cavity: stomatitis and other | | |
| The optic nerve | 10 | 9 | conditions | 1 | 13 |
| Muscles of the eye | 4 | 2 | Dental stomatology | 2 | 9 |
| Retinal disorders | 7 | 17 | The salivary glands | | |
| Colour blindness | 3 | 3 | *Xerostomia* | 3 | 19 |
| The shape of the eye | | | *Other* | 1 | 6 |
| *Myopia* | 13 | 18 | Taste and the tongue | 2 | 1 |
| *Hyperopia* | 0 | 2 | The lips | 0 | 1 |

# RECOMMENDED READING

*A simple method outlined:*

Rosted P The use of acupuncture in the management of skin disease. Alternative Therapy in Clinical Practice. 1996 July–Aug; 3(4): 19–24

*A useful descriptive review:*

White SS 1994 Acupuncture for dermatologic disorders. In: Schoen AM (ed) Veterinary Acupuncture: ancient art to modern medicine. American Veterinary Publications, St Louis, 269–76

*A cautionary tale:*

Fisher AA Allergic dermatitis from acupuncture needles. Cutis. 1986; 38(4): 226

*One of Willem Khoe's informal accounts of his creative approach to acupuncture:*

Khoe WH Dermatologic conditions successfully treated with acupuncture. American Journal of Acupuncture. 1976 Oct–Dec; 4(4): 362–4

*A realistic assessment:*

Liu Q (Liu C), Deng YC, Li L, Lin GZ Evaluation of acupuncture treatment for sensorineural deafness and deafmutism based on 20 years' experience. Chinese Medical Journal. 1982 Jan; 95(1): 21–4

*A readable, if technical, paper:*

Johnson M, Ashton H, Marsh R, Thompson JW Songs, rockets and whistling kettles: electroencephalographic changes in drug related auditory disturbances and treatment with acupuncture and transcutaneous electrical nerve stimulation. Acupuncture in Medicine. 1993 Nov; 11(2): 98–102

*A downbeat systematic review:*

Park J, White AR, Ernst E Efficacy of acupuncture as a treatment for tinnitus: a systematic review. Archives of Otolaryngology. 2000 April; 126(4): 489–92

*One of a series of MA studies on xerostomia:*

Dawidson I, Angmar-Mansson B, Blom M, Theodorsson E, Lundeberg T Sensory stimulation (acupuncture) increases the release of calcitonin gene-related peptide in the saliva of xerostomia sufferers. Neuropeptides. 1999 June; 33(3): 244–50

This subchapter outlines the use of EA in pregnancy and childbirth, in gynaecological problems involving infertility and menstruation, and in breast disorders.

There are probably more books on acupuncture for women's conditions and childbirth than for any other applications. There are also many review articles on acupuncture in obstetrics and gynaecology. Controlled studies of acupuncture for obstetrics are of variable quality, whereas those on gynaecological conditions are somewhat better. Both tend to have consistently positive results.

# OBSTETRICS

## Pregnancy

### RISKS IN PREGNANCY

Treatment for morning sickness with manual acupuncture (MA) in early pregnancy appears to be without serious adverse effects. However, all forms of electrotherapy are generally contraindicated, not because of known adverse effects, but because their safety has not been established beyond doubt. Thus electroacupuncture (EA), transcutaneous electrical nerve stimulation (TENS) and probably cranial electrotherapy stimulation (CES) should not be used during the first trimester, except with great care for hyperemesis. It is important to remember that EA can induce labour, and could theoretically cause cervical dilatation and uterine contractions.

From the fourth month of pregnancy onwards, there is less risk of harm to the fetus, and some electrostimulation methods may be used, although again with care. In particular, strong stimulation on the legs and abdomen should be avoided.

In general, low-intensity laser therapy/laser acupuncture (LILT/LA) should be applied only away from the pregnant uterus, and any form of magnetic field treatment is probably best avoided during pregnancy and lactation until more is known about its effects.

### PAIN RELIEF AND SURGERY DURING PREGNANCY

More than a third of women experience back pain during pregnancy. Pelvic and back pain have been treated with MA, the results being superior to those of group physiotherapy sessions. TENS has been used for 'meralgia paraesthetica' of pregnancy (pain and paraesthesiae in the outer surface of the thigh), although this may also respond to simple MA.

### MORNING SICKNESS

Nausea occurs in 50–80% of pregnancies, continuing beyond 20 weeks in 10%. Vomiting occurs in 50%, sometimes with little warning.

There are many reports on EA, TENS and acupressure for nausea in pregnancy. While in one study P-6 TENS appeared to benefit both nausea and vomiting of pregnancy, acupressure and MA have sometimes been found more effective for nausea than vomiting. Transcranial electrotherapy (TCET, a stronger form of CES) has been used in the treatment of more severe vomiting (hyperemesis gravidarum).

**Points used** The major point to use is P-6. Adding different acupoints results in little added benefit as far as nausea and vomiting go, although they may have other useful effects. Traditionally, such points include BL-20, BL-21, ST-21, ST-25, ST-36, Ren-12, Ren-13, the combination of LIV-3 and LI-4, and SP-4 for dyspepsia and gastritis. Auricular points such as *shenmen*, Sympathetic, Liver and Stomach, may also be used.

P-6 LA has been recommended for symptomatic relief of nausea and vomiting (904 nm, 10 Hz, 3 mW for 30–40 seconds, every 5 minutes until an adequate response is obtained), with the suggestion that LA should be used in pregnancy only if symptoms are severe.

**Parameters used** While John Dundee's group found that 10–15 Hz TENS for 5 minutes every 2 hours was optimal, others have suggested using LF bursts of 100 Hz (200 µs pulse duration) for 5–60 minutes every 2 hours. In view of the supposed balancing effects of 10 Hz stimulation, Dundee's protocol is probably preferable, increasing treatment time if it is ineffective.

### CIRCULATORY DISORDERS OF PREGNANCY

Pregnancy-induced hypertension (toxaemia) is potentially life threatening for both mother and fetus if allowed to progress to eclampsia (convulsions). It has been treated both with TCET and LA, in one study at HE-7, P-6 and ST-36 (10–15 seconds/pt, power unspecified). MA has been used for eclampsia and pyelonephritis associated with toxaemia.

### FETAL PRESENTATION

Breech presentation makes for a more difficult birth, and in the West is generally considered an indication for Caesarean section.

Traditionally, moxibustion at BL-67 has been used for 'version' (turning the baby). Better results are obtained if fetal movement is felt during treatment and if treatment is initiated before 34 weeks' gestation (though version may still occur even after 37 weeks).

Although caution suggests that LILT should not be used during pregnancy, towards term LA at BL-67 has often been used as an alternative to traditional moxibustion. The two have even been combined. In one interesting study, HeNe LA at BL-60 (unilateral) was as effective as at BL-67 (bilateral). EA has also been used for version.

**Comparisons**  In one study, EA was found to be marginally more effective than moxibustion (though not significantly so), whereas in another it was less helpful than moxibustion. LA, on the other hand, seems more consistently superior to moxibustion (with the combination of the two being more effective than either alone).

**Points used**  BL-67 is the most commonly used point.

**Parameters used**  There is little guidance on effective parameters to use with EA. One possibility might be to modulate EA intensity to mimic the effect of intermittent heating of the point, although some Chinese authors predictably recommend using the strongest tolerable current.

> **Caution**
> Given the effectiveness of traditional moxibustion, this should be attempted initially unless suitable LA equipment is available. EA should be attempted only if this fails. Given the possibility, albeit unlikely, of disrupting the placental circulation when the baby turns, treatment should be carried out in consultation with the supervising midwife.

# Labour

## MISCARRIAGE AND PREMATURE LABOUR

Preterm labour may occur as a result of poor uterine or fetal circulation (placental insufficiency), or both. TENS (paravertebrally, for instance) has been found to improve circulation, increase activity and prolong gestation, with a positive impact on the health of the fetus. TCET with interferential currents has also been used to improve fetoplacental circulation, as well as levels of oxygen and other gases in the mother's blood. MA, EA, TENS, TCET and LA have been used to prevent miscarriage, and EAA during cerclage of the cervix.

Towards the end of pregnancy, when labour is imminent, both EA and TEAS have been considered helpful in preparing the mother for birth, reducing anxiety, normalising both CNS and autonomic activity, lessening early onset pains, and contributing to a better delivery.

**Points used**  EA studies are too heterogeneous to draw any useful conclusions, although there are TCM arguments for using SP-4. Paraspinal TENS would appear to be justifiable for placental insufficiency. Starting at the 36th to 37th week of pregnancy, Nikolay Zharkin uses points that mildly tonify the uterus and also calm the spirit, such as HE-3, HE-5, HE-7, HE-9, BL-13, BL-31–BL-34, P-6, P-7, LIV-3, LI-4, ST-25, SP-1, SP-6, Ren-6, Du-20 and *yintang*.

**Parameters used**  Gentle LF EA would seem to be appropriate, rather than any form of strong stimulation. Thus Zharkin uses EA (at 3–6 Hz), but recommends that sessions should not last longer than 10 minutes. LF EAA (at just below discomfort level) of 'local' (torso) points was used in a study on cerclage, although in many EAA gynaecological studies these are given HF stimulation.

## INDUCTION OF LABOUR

Induction of labour occurs frequently in the Western world. As an alternative to drugs, EA has been used in women who have had prior Caesarean section or ovarian surgery. Given during the final weeks of pregnancy, it may shorten the first stage of the ensuing labour.

It is sometimes hard to tell from induction studies what type of acupuncture (MA or EA) was used. However, there appears to be a preference for EA, which is considered to be more effective by some authorities. In one induction protocol, for example, MA was used at LIV-3, LI-4, SP-6 and SP-10 until contractions began, at which point EA was used to maintain them until delivery. Reinhold Voll recommended LF probe TENS (pTENS) at EAV points BL-50, BL-50-1 and BL-50-2. In an American acupuncture sourcebook from the early 1970s, SP-6, SP-15, Ren-2, Ren-3 and Ren-4 (but not Ren-5) were suggested, with 12 V pTENS for 15 seconds every 3–4 minutes, or 100–300 Hz 9–12 V EA. The recommendation was given that EA at points close to the uterus should not be combined with oxytocin, to avoid tetanic contractions, although oxytocin could be used if EA failed, or could be combined with pTENS. A similar caution has been voiced against combining electrostimulation of auricular Uterus and Bladder points with oxytocin.

TENS has been used to stimulate uterine contractions. Indeed, experimental electrical stimulation of the uterus was carried out as long ago as 1911.

Case study 9.5.1 details the use of electroacupuncture in obstetric care.

## UTERINE INERTIA

Fatigue during childbirth can prolong labour, and is the cause of many Caesarian sections. Electrostimulation for 'tedious labour' and haemorrhage (for instance, in cases of placenta praevia) has been known since the nineteenth century. There are several studies of EA for 'labour fatigue' (uterine inertia) from Eastern European countries. TENS, TCET and LA have also been used.

**Points used**  LI-4 and SP-6 are by far the most commonly used acupoints for induction, whether with MA or EA, although in a number of studies Ren-2, Ren-3 and/or Ren-4 were added, and occasionally local (BL-32) or distal (BL-60, BL-67) Bladder meridian points, and other points according to TCM differentiation.

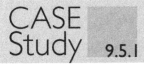

# CASE Study 9.5.1

## Electroacupuncture in obstetric care
**Sarah Budd**

Acupuncture has been practised by the midwives in the maternity unit in Plymouth since 1988. Initially, the service was set up to cater for women wishing to reduce the amount of drugs they used for pain relief in labour, or to find a treatment that would be an alternative to, or complement, conventional induction of labour. This then evolved into a busy outpatient service for pregnancy-related conditions.

Electrostimulation was found to be preferable to manual stimulation of the needles for induction of labour and pain relief in labour. Not only does it enhance the effect of the needles more comfortably over what could be a long period of time, but it also allows the woman to have some control over the amount of stimulation she is receiving through the needles (Fig. 9.5.1), something that is very useful during painful contractions.

### Electroacupuncture to induce labour

The most common indication for induction of labour is when pregnancy has gone beyond 40 weeks' gestation.

Management by obstetricians varies, with some intervening at 41 weeks and others waiting until 42 weeks. The usual method is to use hormonal pessaries, which many women prefer to avoid where possible. Acupuncture is a very useful alternative.

The main points used to initiate contractions are *hegu* (LI-4) and *sanyinjiao* (SP-6) with electrostimulation for 20 to 30 minutes, followed by turning the patient on to her left side, and using BL-31 and BL-32, again with electrostimulation for 20 minutes. Other points for imbalances indicated by a TCM diagnosis may also be added when appropriate.

*As a caution*, it is important to note that pregnant women can have a tendency to faint if lying flat on their backs, because of pressure from the baby on the inferior vena cava causing postural hypotension. It is therefore advisable to sit them up as much as is comfortable for the first points, and stay with them where possible.

### Electroacupuncture for pain relief in labour

In the Chinese texts the points SP-6 and LI-4 are recommended. When women are in active labour, however, they usually like to move around and adopt several positions, which makes these points difficult, so at the maternity unit in Plymouth it was decided to use the ear points Uterus, *shenmen* and Endocrine, as they are less restrictive (see Fig. 9.5.1).

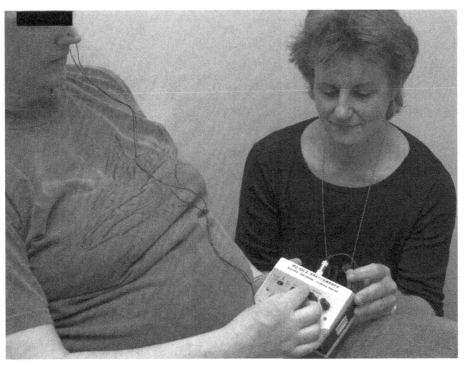

**Figure 9.5.1** Electroacupuncture in childbirth. Sarah Budd giving instruction in the use of the WQ10C2 device for auricular stimulation. (Courtesy of Sarah Budd. Photograph by Helen Blake.)

One side is used first, whichever the birthing mother prefers, rather than both. It is then possible to use the other side if the labour is long and the ear becomes sore, particularly if needles fall out and have to be replaced.

The points are needled with 12.5 mm (0.5 inch) needles, which are taped down. They should be inserted about 2–4 mm, depending on angle of insertion (a 'flatter' angle is better when securing with tape). One electrode is attached to either of the top points, Uterus or *shenmen*, and the other to Endocrine at the bottom. It may be a good idea to place a cotton wool ball between the two electrodes so that they cannot touch and 'short out,' which is not only very uncomfortable but also quite likely if the woman is moving around a lot.

It does not take very long for the acupuncture to take effect, usually within 10 to 20 minutes, and when all is going well, it is a wonderful sight as the women are so much more relaxed. Sometimes, the midwives have almost been caught out, when they have not expected a woman who is so calm to suddenly start pushing!

If the contractions become less frequent in labour, it is a good idea to try to enhance them with some of the points above used for induction of labour, adding others as appropriate, such as ST-36 for tiredness or LIV-3 if the cervix does not dilate.

*As with TENS, the signal from the EA stimulator can interfere with the fetal monitor (CTG, or cardiotocograph). Keeping the two as far apart as possible usually resolves this problem.*

## Case 1. Diana – induction of labour

This was a second baby; the mother presented at term plus 10 days requesting acupuncture for induction of labour, as she was booked in for medical induction in 5 days' time. A full case history was taken. TCM diagnosis was of slight Stomach and Spleen *qi xu*.

Treatment:

LI-4 R (+) and ST-36 R (–)
LI-4 L (+) and SP-6 L (–)        Medium frequency 30 Hz
SP-6 R (+) and LIV-3 R(–)        Intensity 1 to 4.5
LIV-3 L (–) and ST-44 L (–)
Then:
GB-21 R (+) and BL-21 R(–)
GB-21 L (+) and BL-20 L (–)    Medium frequency 30 Hz
BL-32 and BL-31                      Intensity 1 to 4.5
    (both bilateral stimulation)
    Went home with seeds on left ear points: Uterus, Endocrine, Stomach, Subcortex and Kidney.
Diana cancelled her next appointment and went into spontaneous labour on the day she was due to go into

hospital for medical induction of labour. She had a normal delivery of a baby girl with a birth weight of 4160 g.

## Case 2. Sally – induction of labour following spontaneous rupture of membranes

This was a first baby; the mother presented at term having had ruptured membranes for 48 hours. This means there is some risk of infection as the membranes normally protect against infection up to a point, so she had been started on antibiotics orally. There were only occasional period-type pains.

Treatment:

LI-4 and ST-36                         Medium frequency 30 Hz
    (both bilateral stimulation) Intensity 3 to 4
Sp-6 and LIV-3
    (both bilateral stimulation)
Then:
GB-21 and BL-32
    (both bilateral stimulation)
BL-31 R (+) and BL-60 R (–)  Medium frequency 30 Hz
BL-31 L (+) and BL-67 L (–)   Intensity 3 to 6
    Went home with seeds on right ear points: *shenmen*, Uterus, Endocrine and Stomach.
    Sally went into spontaneous labour at 6 a.m. the next day and at 9.15 a.m. the cervix was 4–5 cm dilated. She delivered a baby girl at 1.30 p.m., with a birth weight of 3840 g. There was no maternal pyrexia following delivery.

## Case 3. Fran – analgesia in labour

This was a first baby; the mother was admitted to the delivery suite of the maternity unit at 5 p.m. with a history of spontaneous rupture of membranes since midnight, and contractions since 7 a.m. Examined at 6 p.m., when the cervix was 3 cm dilated. Acupuncture commenced for pain relief at 7.18 p.m. The point Du-20 used to relax mind and body, and manually stimulated. Bilateral LI-4 and LIV-3 were added, and all points manually stimulated at 5-minute intervals.

Treatment:

7.45 p.m.: Needles inserted to right ear points:
    *shenmen* and Endocrine    Medium frequency 30 Hz
                                              Intensity 3.5
    Uterus point added             Manual stimulation
All body needles were removed.
8.06–9.25 p.m.: Intensity gradually increased from 3.5 to
    5.5, with cervix dilating to 6 cm at 9.05. Coping well.
10.10 p.m.: Strong urge to push. O/E: cervix fully dilated. Started pushing.
10.32 p.m.: Normal delivery of baby girl, birth weight 3105 g.

*(Continued)*

---

### CASE Study 9.5.1 **Continued**

#### Case 4. Gill – analgesia in labour

This was a first baby; the mother was admitted to the maternity unit delivery suite at 7.20 a.m., membranes having ruptured at 2.45 a.m. On examination at 7.45 a.m., the cervix was 2–3 cm dilated. Gill had a hot bath and some tea and toast. At 8.45 a.m., point Du-20 used for relaxation (manually stimulated), and ear points for pain relief:

Treatment:

8.55 a.m.: Needles inserted to right ear points:

| | |
|---|---|
| *shenmen* and Endocrine | Medium frequency 30 Hz |
| | Intensity 3.5 |
| Uterus point | Manual stimulation |

9.15 a.m.: Intensity increased to 4. Fetal heart fine and contractions good.

9.30 a.m.: Needle to point Du-20 removed. Gill was comfortable, relaxed between contractions.

9.45–11 a.m.: Intensity increased gradually in stages to 4.75. Gill in 'all fours' position, then gets up to go to toilet, and eventually gets into water-birth pool (all acupuncture needles removed).

11.30 a.m.: Normal delivery in water of baby girl, birth weight 3550 g.

---

**Parameters used** Although many of the EA studies use relatively low-frequency stimulation (LF, around 2–8 Hz), some use much higher frequencies (120–500 Hz), and at least one DD (dense-disperse). The emphasis in general seems to be on strong (but non-painful) stimulation. As for TENS, there are too few studies to draw any conclusions. However, it is intriguing that in one Russian report on combined EA and TENS, LF (3–7 Hz) EA with high-frequency, low-intensity TENS (conventional TENS, CTENS) was considered more helpful in slowing down the process of early labour, whereas higher-frequency (3–30 Hz) EA led to induction. Another report from the same Moscow group found that 100–120 Hz TENS could be used to stimulate the uterus, and 30 Hz TENS for relaxation.

#### Recommendation

For induction, use LI-4 and SP-6, with strong but not painful EA (20 Hz has been suggested). Auricular points such as Endocrine, Uterus and *shenmen* may be used too. BL-67 and auricular Bladder point may be added to enhance stimulation (10 Hz surface stimulation of BL-67 alone has been used quite successfully for induction). Daily treatment is essential, and may even be repeated several times each day if necessary.

## PAIN RELIEF DURING LABOUR

Most women in the West request some form of analgesia during childbirth, with the vast majority wishing to remain fully alert and to play an active role as well. Simple, non-sedating low-risk analgesic methods such as TENS, TCET and (perhaps to a lesser extent) EA clearly have a role to play if they can be shown to be effective. Even if EAA and related methods only reduce the need for medication without

major impact on experienced pain, this could nevertheless contribute significantly to a more positive outcome for both mother and child.

EA has frequently been used during labour, although MA *prior* to labour appears to be of little benefit for the pain of labour. Like acupressure and MA, it can have a calming as well as a pain-relieving effect.

Unfortunately, analgesia with EA is rarely complete and not always predictable, and this, together with possible interference with fetal monitoring and the presence of wires that can become an encumbrance, may make EA less convenient than TENS. However, even with these shortcomings EAA has a role to play in labour if used appropriately. Observational studies have found that EA may shorten labour (particularly the first stage), reduce the duration of pain during each contraction, and contribute to the mother's sense of well-being and being in control of the situation.

TENS has frequently been used for pain relief during labour, with few apparent adverse effects on the neonate. Despite some shortcomings, it may be simpler both to set up and operate than EA. Furthermore, many obstetric TENS devices are supplied with a handheld switch for the birthing mother to hold, which can make the procedure feel more controllable. TENS may also encourage the mother to stay mobile longer, and it is telling that in many studies women expressed considerable satisfaction with TENS, even if 'objectively' it gave incomplete pain relief.

TCET has also been used during labour, with minimal adverse effects on the fetus. Whichever method is used, it is important to start treatment for pain relief as soon as possible once contractions have begun.

**Points used** There are many protocols for EA in childbirth. Nguyen Van Nghi and colleagues suggested GB-26, LI-4 and ST-36, but also mentioned other combinations, such as BL-57, GB-28, LIV-2, LI-4 and SP-9, or GB-26, LI-4 and

ST-36, or P-6, LI-4 and ST-36. Recommendations in one early US textbook included ST-44 or ST-36 + SP-6 for the first stage of labour, with points such as LIV-2 or LIV-3 + BL-60, BL-66 or BL-67 for relieving backache and sensations of pressure, and a scattering of other optional points. BL-21, BL-22 and BL-23 were suggested for back pain, and BL-31, BL-32, BL-33 and BL-34 for uterine and perineal analgesia, with Ren-1, Ren-2 and Ren-3 for further perineal or vaginal analgesia. ST-29 or ST-30, directed towards Ren-2, together with Du-1 or Du-2, could be used for rectal pain.

The most used body acupoints appear to be BL-32 and BL-31 on the sacrum, LI-4 and SP-6, with additional points such as P-6, ST-36 and SP-9. Distal points on the BL- meridian are also used sometimes, as is ST-44 if Stomach or Spleen meridian points are stimulated on the abdomen (ST-25, ST-28, SP-14) or in the groin (ST-30). Also listed are *neima* (*neimadian*) and SP-8 on the lower leg. GB-34, LIV-3 and Du-20 occasionally appear. Conception Vessel points are rarely used.

In some EA studies, auricular points were used, either alone or together with body points. The most commonly used points are the Uterus, *shenmen* and Sympathetic points, although points for the Lumbar spine and External genitals also appear. Zita West, for instance, recommends 2.5 Hz EA at Uterus and *shenmen* (and possibly Endocrine) ear points as less inconvenient than body points. However, she also endorses the use of BL-31 and BL-32 to stimulate contractions during the first stage of labour.

Manik Hiranandani has suggested LA (904 nm, 3–4 mW, 10 Hz; 30 seconds/point) at LI-4, ST-36, ST-44, SP-6 and Du-20, repeated if necessary after 5 minutes, every 3–4 hours early in labour, and half-hourly later on, or TENS (8–10 Hz continuous) at ST-36(+), ST-44(−) and SP-6, together with ultrasound.

With TENS, electrodes are generally affixed on the back, a procedure easily carried out without special training, the standard locations being in the T10–L2 dermatomes for the first stage of labour (when pain is mostly due to dilatation of the cervix) using larger electrodes (3 × 9 cm), and at S2-S4 level at the end of the first stage and throughout the second stage (when pain is more from the uterine contractions themselves), with smaller ones (5 cm diameter). However, TENS applied in this way may not be very effective for suprapubic pain, and sometimes pads are affixed suprapubically. Less commonly, TENS (TEAS) has been applied at acupoints rather than just segmentally.

**Parameters used** LF (0.25–10 Hz) EA appears to be used more frequently than HF (50–100 Hz), and strong stimulation ('to tolerance', even as high as 50 mA!) more than low intensity. In one interesting study, low-intensity stimulation was adjusted to the frequency of the mother's heartbeat. In another, a higher frequency (66.7 Hz) was applied dorsally at BL-32, and a lower one (25–30 Hz) ventrally, at ST-30 and SP-14. Occasionally the choice of frequency has been left to the birthing mother after an initial period of LF EA. It is worth noting that poor results were obtained in one early study when very low frequency EA (0.25–075 Hz) was used.

Varying the frequency as labour progresses is more common with TENS than EA. Initial intensity (described as 'low,' 'submotor threshold,' 'comfortable' or 'pleasant') is also sometimes increased as labour progresses, or during contractions. Thus some authors recommend starting with LF (or intermittent) stimulation (for longer-term pain relief), and increasing the frequency as labour progresses or to accompany contractions (HF for a rapid analgesic boost). This is supported by Russian research on premature labour indicating that HF may stimulate contractions as well, lower frequencies being useful for relaxation in between contractions. A number of TENS devices provide a hand-held control so that the mother can easily adjust the output. There is, however, one study in which a medium frequency (10–25 Hz) was used at first, with lower-frequency ALTENS later on. Interestingly, labour duration *increased* with this method, although it has frequently been reported as decreasing when HF TENS is used during contractions. It is unclear whether this has anything to do with the recommendation to avoid 20 Hz stimulation in the 1988 study by Iris Skelton and Michael Flowerdew.

Duration of stimulation can be an issue. In one study, maximal analgesia was attained with LF EA only after 35–45 minutes. In another, however, although it was 40 (10–80) minutes before EA took effect, only 20 minutes of actual treatment were needed to achieve this, the ensuing analgesia lasting for 6 hours. If this is the case, then clearly leads can be disconnected from inserted needles for

**Recommendation**

- First, ensure the birthing mother understands that EA will not 'take the pain away', but may provide considerable *relief*.
- Initially, EA can be useful for relaxation, using 2.5 Hz for 30 minutes, either 'hand-to-hand' (using cylindrical electrodes) or ST-36 bilaterally (via needles or pads). This preparatory treatment can be carried out daily in the period before the due date, or on the day prior to planned induction.
- During labour itself, EA-like TENS is best started early on, preferably at least 30–40 minutes *before* reaching 4 cm dilation (particularly for a first birth). It should also be started 30-40 minutes before any induction procedure.
- If the mother is very anxious, needle ST-36 and SP-6 on one side only, making sure clips and needles are unlikely to be dislodged (some sort of tape can be used to secure them). Again use 2.5 Hz, as strong as is comfortably possible, in the first stage of labour.
- When about 4 cm dilated, discontinue ST-36, and use SP-6 with *neima* (6.5 *cun* proximal to the prominence of the medial malleolus), on one leg only.

**NB:** If your machine has a handheld obstetric switch, it is important the mother uses this during contractions when they become moderate to strong.

(This protocol is based on that suggested by the Society of Biophysical Medicine.)

considerable periods during labour, weakening the argument that EA is not an appropriate intervention because of the inconvenience of trailing wires and possible interference with fetal monitoring.

### AFTER LABOUR (THE PUERPERIUM)

Acupuncture has a role in the treatment of postpartum weakness, particularly in the case of retained placenta. In the nineteenth century, electrostimulation was used to expel the placenta ('afterbirth') following delivery. Simple 10 Hz EA at SP-6 can be helpful for women, with auricular Bladder and Uterus points added if the uterus is lacking in tone (hypotonic), as recommended by the Society of Biophysical Medicine. Other possible points include GB-21, an empirical point when using MA for retained placenta, LIV-3, LI-4, Ren-3 and Ren-4.

EA (HF, at SP-1 and SP-6) has been used for postpartum bleeding, as has TEAS.

## Caesarian section

Caesarian section is routinely carried out under general or epidural/spinal anaesthesia. However, because of the possible adverse effects of chemical anaesthesia on the neonate, AA may have much to contribute here and is, indeed, relatively successful for Caesarian section. EAA (and TCET) are often combined with more conventional methods.

Effects of EAA on the neonate appear to be minimal, compared with those of general anaesthesia. EAA appears to enhance immune function in the newborn and, for similar reasons, EA has been used following labour in premature infants subjected to potentially stressful interventions. In the mother, blood pressure, pulse rate and respiration have been reported as comparatively stable during the operation, with less blood loss than in epidural or local anaesthesia. In one case of uterine haemorrhage during Caesarean section, for instance, EA (at P-6, LI-4, SP-10, Du-20 and Du-26) increased blood pressure and stemmed blood loss within 20 minutes.

For acute postoperative pain, EA, TENS and even implanted wire electrodes have been used. However, although using TENS may help control paraincisional pain, it may not decrease narcotic intake.

Daily 10 Hz EA at SP-6, or the auricular Uterus point if required, has been suggested for faulty involution (return to normal size) of the uterus following Caesarean section.

**Points used** For AA during Caesarean section, the most frequently used points include SP-6, *waima* (*waimadian*, the 'External anaesthesia point' on the lateral aspect of the leg), subcutaneous paraincisional needling, and the 'lip point' combination Ren-24 and Du-26 (in one Japanese study this was replaced by BL-2 and LI-20). Further points such as P-6, LIV-3, ST-36 or ST-39 have quite often been added, sometimes combinations based on Du-4 or Du-6, and occasionally SP-4 or SP-8. Auricular points (*shenmen*, Uterus and Sympathetic) have also been tried. Curiously, given their hypertensive action, in several reports Ren-24 and Du-26 were employed in cases of toxaemia of pregnancy, with no adverse effects.

For postoperative pain following Caesarean section, EA at GB-34, ST-36, SP-4, SP-6, auricular points and also paraincisional needling have been tried.

With TENS, most studies use paraincisional electrodes.

**Parameters used** For Caesarian section, quite a high frequency (e.g. 800 Hz) was used in some studies for subcutaneously inserted paraincisional needles, with LF at distal points. For postoperative pain, CTENS is often applied on each side of the incision.

# GYNAECOLOGY

## Ovulation and fertility

EA has the ability to regulate ovarian function and has been used to induce ovulation. Successful outcomes (pregnancy) with EA have been reported in several studies, the most rigorous being those carried out in Sweden by Elisabet Stener-Victorin's group.

For in vitro fertilisation (IVF) and embryo transfer (ET), optimal endometrial receptivity at the time of implantation is important. Impaired blood flow in the uterine arteries will reduce pregnancy rate. EA at segmentally related points, distally at BL-57 and SP-6 (LF), and locally at BL-23, BL-27 and BL-28 (100 Hz) appears to restore blood flow. The pregnancy rate following ET with acupuncture was higher than without it. Auricular EAA has been used for women undergoing IVF procedures.

Another electrical stimulation method that has been investigated for anovulation is a form of low-intensity scalp TENS (over the frontal lobes).

Electrical skin resistance changes occur with ovulation, in particular at acupoints such as SP-6. If hand temperature rises within 30 minutes of P-6/LI-4 EA, indicating inhibition of sympathetic activity, then the subject is likely to be a good subject for treatment aimed at the induction of ovulation.

**Points used** The local points most frequently used include BL-23, BL-28, BL-32 and Du-4 (but also BL-18 and BL-20) dorsally, and Ren-3, Ren-4 and *zigong* (but also ST-29, Ren-2, Ren-5 and Ren-6) ventrally. Distally, SP-6 is a particular favourite, as well as points on the Bladder meridian (BL-57, BL-60 and BL-62), or SP-9. Other points include P-6, SJ-5, LIV-8, LI-4, ST-36 and Du-20, depending on the practitioner's TCM orientations or which local points were favoured.

**Parameters used** Other than the use of HF EA locally and LF EA distally by Swedish researchers, there seems to be little coherent information available on what electrical settings to use. Clearly, if sympathetic activation is to be avoided, intensity should be comfortable, not too high. However, Chen Boying, a much-quoted authority in this area, has suggested that strong LF EA (4–5 Hz at 7–8 mA) for 30 minutes on 3 consecutive days (days 10–12 of the menstrual cycle) may need to be used. Treatment should be repeated consistently over several menstrual cycles.

## Endocrine effects of EA

EA appears to act to normalise oestrogen levels and, along with TENS and LA, to regulate prolactin secretion. In one study, for instance, LA stimulated both prolactin secretion and lactation.

## The cervix, vagina and vulva

Cervical erosion has been treated with LILT and broad-spectrum irradiation. In one very small study, 400 G (40 mT) magnets in the vaginal area were used for endocervicitis and cervical erosion, with a possible regulatory effect on hormonal imbalance.

For the treatment of vaginitis, local 'sonopuncture' (ultrasound with a vaginal soundhead) has been suggested, together with EA at points such as BL-64, BL-65, KI-11, LIV-8, SP-6, Ren-2 and Ren-3. Vaginal electrodes are available with EAV and some other electrotherapy devices, predominantly for urinary incontinence.

Chronic vaginal discharge (leukorrhoea) may have various causes, with several possible TCM differentiations. If infection and cancer have been excluded, then auricular EA may be tried, or LA to points such as ST-36, SP-6, Ren-1, Ren-2, Ren-4 and Ren-5 (904 nm infrared, 3 Hz or 10 Hz, 15–20 seconds/point, for 5–7 days), or ultrasound (0.5 W, 1.5–3 min) with a vaginal soundhead if the condition is refractory to LA.

For vaginal (as opposed to uterine) prolapse, Nguyen Van Nghi and colleagues recommended EA at KI-14, GB-27, LI-4, ST-36, SP-6, SP-11 and Ren-1.

In leukoplakia vulvae, white patches appear on the delicate skin of the vulva, causing it to become atrophied, drier and shrivelled (kraurosis). The condition has been treated using 'electrothermal' needling. EA with moxibustion (20–30 minutes, at SP-6 and Ren-4) gave 'satisfactory' results in one report.

**Points used** Emphasis in most of the studies is on local points (Ren-1, Ren-2 and Ren-3) or nearby points such as KI-11 or LIV-12, with other points used for associated problems.

## Dysmenorrhoea and other pelvic pain

Various forms of acupuncture have been used for dysmenorrhoea: MA (sometimes on local points such as Du-2), plum blossom needling (at points such as LIV-2, LIV-3, SP-1, SP-4, SP-6 and Ren-4), EA and so on.

According to some authors, EA may be particularly helpful for both acute and chronic pelvic pain (pelvic inflammatory disease). However, electrostimulation may not be appropriate for acute pelvic pain accompanied by purulent discharge. It has been suggested that pTENS at SP-6 may be helpful for both dysmenorrhoea and ovulation pain.

TENS has been used increasingly for primary dysmenorrhoea, although it may not actually affect uterine activity. It not only reduces pain and the need for analgesic drugs, but also other symptoms associated with dysmenorrhoea. Whereas Mannheimer and Whalen found that ALTEAS was not effective for dysmenorrhoea, other studies suggest that HF TENS (at low or high intensity) may be useful.

**Comparisons** In one study on dysmenorrhoea, MA, LF and HF EA, and LF TENS were all found to be effective for the condition, whereas HF TENS was less so. LF EA was reported by the same group as more effective than HF EA in the long-term treatment of low-back pain (not menstrually related). In contrast, HF TENS has been found useful by others, with a trend to giving more pain relief overall.

**Points used** SP-6 and Ren-4 are the most used points in EA treatment of dysmenorrhoea, with dorsal points BL-21, BL-29 and BL-32 also used, and ventral points such as ST-29, Ren-4 and Ren-6. Other points with particular TCM functions, such as GB-34, LIV-3, LI-4, ST-36 and SP-9, are often added.

For more chronic pelvic pain, BL-23 is the most used back point, and Ren-3, Ren-4, Ren-6 and *zigong* the most used abdominal points (with KI-12 and some Stomach meridian points occasionally added), SP-6 and SP-10 being the most common distal points (with LIV-3 and ST-36 also mentioned, depending on the practitioner's TCM perspective).

Points such as BL-31–34, SP-6 and Ren-3 are possibly best avoided in women treated during menstruation for non-gynaecological conditions (although they may well be appropriate for *shi* types of dysmenorrhoea).

TENS for dysmenorrhoea is generally applied on the abdomen, at around ST-25 (in T10–T11 dermatomes) or Ren-2/Ren-3 (T12 dermatome). Pads have also been applied in the lumbosacral region.

**Parameters used** On balance, it would seem logical to use moderately strong LF EA (or ALTENS) when severe pain is not experienced, and HF EA (or CTENS) when it is, bearing in mind that CEA/ALTENS may be more appropriate at distal points, and TLEA/CEA locally. HF EA has been used for chronic pelvic pain as well as dysmenorrhoea, with 150–200 Hz initially, reduced to 60–100 Hz after 10 minutes.

## Menorrhagia

Dysfunctional uterine bleeding has traditionally been treated with acupuncture, and is considered by some as an indication for EA. Uterine bleeding in adults and adolescents has also been treated with LA, and excessive bleeding with 500 G magnets applied at ST-36 and SP-10.

## Irregular and infrequent menstruation

To regulate menstruation, EA at points such as KI-5, KI-6, KI-13, SP-6 and Ren-2 has been suggested, with auricular Fulcrum (Point zero), Internal secretion, Uterus and Ovary points.

In one study, BL-32 LA was used for irregular menstruation. LA (904 nm pulsed at 4.9 or 10 Hz, or 780 nm at 100 Hz) has been recommended at a different selection of points: BL-23, BL-32, KI-3, GB-19, GB-21, ST-36, SP-6, Ren-4 and Du-20, with auricular Internal secretion and Uterus points; treatment is continued over five to six menstrual cycles.

## Other disorders of the uterus and ovaries: uterine prolapse

EA has been recommended for uterine prolapse, with MA (reinforcing) at ST-36 and EA bilaterally at *zigong* (2 *cun* needles directed towards the uterus, stimulated until the patient feels the uterus contract, with *deqi* travelling as far as the vulva, and stimulation then maintained for 15–20 minutes).

## Menopause

There are many parallels between the effects of exercise and those of EA when muscular contraction is involved. As exercise reduces the prevalence of hot flushes in women around menopause, the same could be expected of EA. Indeed, in experimental studies, EA (especially at ST-36) appears to act to normalise oestrogen levels, and thus may have a role to play in the treatment of menopausal symptoms such as hot flushes. EA may also be useful following total ovariectomy in women.

Silver spike point (SSP) therapy (at points such as LI-4, LI-11, SP-6 and ST-36) has been used for menopausal symptoms, as have TCET and LA.

**Comparisons** EA may be more effective than superficial MA for menopausal symptoms.

**Points used** Acupoints such as BL-23, LI-11, SP-6 and Ren-4 have been used in the EA studies. Although these are too heterogeneous to be able to draw meaningful conclusions, experimental research suggests that BL-23 is particularly relevant.

## Gynaecological operations

AA has frequently been used for hysterectomy. In a review of operations in Shanghai hospitals to 1973 it was claimed to be 74% effective for hysterectomy, with 34% having an excellent outcome. AA seems to have retained a role, albeit a minor one, for rather longer in gynaecological surgery than in childbirth through Caesarian section.

Whichever methods of electroanalgesia are used (EAA, TENS, TCET), these are often combined with conventional medication. However, as with EA, TENS in addition to standard anaesthesia may not greatly reduce the stress of procedures involved in hysterectomy, for example. Another combination that merits further exploration is the use of LA to enhance the effectiveness of EAA during hysterectomy.

Other gynaecological operations have been carried out under EAA, such as curettage (also performed under MAA),

hysteroscopy and surgery for ovarian cyst, severe endometritis, ectopic pregnancy, fibromyoma (fibroid tumour), smooth muscle myoma (leiomyoma), Bartholin's cyst, vaginal prolapse and cervical dysplasia.

In some studies, gynaecological operations under EAA were found to be more stressful than those in which the patient was completely anaesthetised, even though cardiovascular function appeared stable. For those with pre-existing cardiac arrhythmias, HF EA at P-6 was found useful in stabilising circulatory function during epidural anaesthesia. However, some authors have recommended that 'electrostimulation anaesthesia' should not be used for gynaecological surgery in cardiac-risk patients.

Interestingly, both MA and EA have been used instead of traditional anxiolytic *pre*medication for some gynaecological operations. TENS has been employed for postoperative pain afterwards; TCET has been used both during such surgery and after it, for postoperative pain. HeNe LA has been used in conjunction with MA and moxibustion for the long-term sequelae of tubal ligation.

**Points used** Points such as BL-32 have frequently been used for EAA during gynaecological operations. For dilatation and curettage, Van Nghi and colleagues recommended points such as GB-34, LI-4, ST-36 and SP-6, and for curettage with tubal ligation P-6, GB-26, LIV-3, ST-36, SP-11. Others have used LIV-3 with LI-4, SP-6, Ren-2 and Ren-4 for curettage. Earlier Chinese studies on tubal ligation focused on BL-32, SP-6 and the lip points Ren-24 and Du-26, as well as auricular points (*shenmen*, Uterus and Endocrine points in particular) and paraincisional needling. Extra points such as *zhaguan* and *neima* were also used.

For EAA during hysterectomy, BL-32, GB-27 and GB-28 (and less commonly GB-26), SP-6, Du-4, Du-6 and *neima* have been frequently used, with adjunctive points such as P-6, GB-34 (to accompany the proximal Gall Bladder points), LI-4, ST-36, SP-8, and even some head points. Occasionally the Ren-24/Du-26 combination was used too. Van Nghi and colleagues proposed acupoint injection for hysterectomy at BL-23, BL-25, BL-34 and Du-1, together with AA at P-6, GB-26, ST-36, SP-6, SP-11 and Ren-6.

For EAA during other gynaecological operations and investigations, BL-27, BL-28, BL-32 or corresponding *huatuojiaji* points are frequently used. SP-6, with or without ST-36, is also popular, as is paraincisional needling. Ren-3 and Ren-4 also appear, as do other local points such as GB-28 or ST-29. P-6, GB-34, LIV-3 and/or LI-4 may be added. Auricular points may be combined with body points, or used alone.

For postoperative pain after hysterectomy, EA has been used in a number of studies, particularly at BL-32, ST-36, SP-6, Du-2 and Du-4, but also at other points familiar from the EAA hysterectomy studies, such as GB-26. TENS and LA at ST-36 have also been used. Following other gynaecological operations, TENS has been applied paraincisionally or at acupoints such as LI-4.

**Parameters used** For tubal ligation, many different parameters were explored, with one report finding DD to be more effective than continuous wave (CW) stimulation, for example. In general, HF was used locally (e.g. at BL-32, GB-27 or ST-26 and ST-29) and at ear points, with LF at lip points or distal points such as SP-6.

For hysterectomy, torso points are generally stimulated with HF, and distal points with LF, although in one 1984 report 10 Hz was used for both local points (BL-32, GB-24 and GB-28) and head points (*zhongjiao, xiajiao*).

Postoperatively, the local HF/distal LF pattern is evident again, although 2/100 Hz or 10/100 Hz DD is also used, combining the two frequencies in a different way. In one study, as was common in Italian EAA research for a while, a gradually increasing frequency pattern was employed, starting at 5 Hz then working up to 50 Hz.

In EAA for other gynaecological operations, the same pattern of HF segmental and LF distal stimulation can be seen. Postoperatively, 2/100 Hz DD appears to be more common, and possibly more effective than either frequency on its own.

## THE BREAST

Various forms of acupuncture (MA, EA, LA and different methods of heating) affect prolactin levels and have been used both to encourage and inhibit lactation. Galactorrhoea has even been reported as an unexpected side-effect of MA for pain following mastectomy (at paravertebral segmental points, contralateral LI-4 and trigger points such as SI-11).

Mastitis has been treated with MA, EA and related methods. Premenstrual breast pain has been treated with MA, brief EA and LILT. Local magnet application, combined with herbal remedies, has also been suggested.

Mammary hyperplasia (fibrocystic breast disease, mastosis) has been treated with MA, EA and 'refrigeration acupuncture'.

Cyst treatment, lumpectomy and mastectomy have been carried out under AA.

**Points used** *Huatuojiaji* points have been used in MA treatment of fibrocystic breast disease.

Local points such as ST-15, ST-16, ST-18 and Ren-17 have been used in EA, LA and other studies on breast conditions using non-traditional interventions. Other points used include GB-34, LIV-3 and LI-4, ST-36, ST-40 and SP-10, depending on the underlying TCM pattern(s) detected.

## SUMMARY

Some key points in this chapter are:

- Trials of acupuncture for obstetrics and gynaecological conditions tend to have consistently positive results
- Electroacupuncture is generally contraindicated in the first trimester of pregnancy
- The frequent use of P-6 for morning sickness and BL-67 for breech presentation is borne out by experimental and clinical trials
- Treatment for breech presentation is best undertaken in consultation with the midwife
- EA and TENS, with established protocols, are now an established part of the labour process
- EA has been successfully used to regulate and induce ovulation.

### Additional material in the CD-ROM resource

In the CD-ROM resource, in addition to more information on the topics presented here, the following are also discussed:

- Elective abortion, episiotomy, partial asphyxia of the baby during childbirth
- Tubal ligation, vaginoplasty and other surgery under EAA
- Interactions with contraception and hormone replacement therapy (endocrine effects are covered in Chapter 6)
- Premenstrual syndrome
- Kraurosis vulvae
- Postmastectomy oedema.

| **9.5** Summary of relevant studies in the electronic clinical studies database (number of studies) | | |
|---|---|---|
| **Condition** | **EA** | **Other** |
| **Late pregnancy** | | |
| Foetal malposition | 5 | 29 |
| Other complications of late pregnancy | 5 | 18 |
| **Induction and labour** | | |
| Preparation for labour | 0 | 1 |
| Induction of labour | 23 | 15 |
| Elective abortion | 5 | 1 |
| Pain relief in labour | 38 | 91 |
| Other aspects of labour | 2 | 7 |
| **Infertility and ovarian function** | | |
| Infertility | 15 | 14 |
| Infertility (animal studies) | 2 | 0 |
| Menopause (natural and induced) | 7 | 6 |
| Endocrine effects and ovarian function | 5 | 1 |
| Tubal function | 1 | 1 |
| **Menstrual disorders** | | |
| Dysmenorrhoea and premenstrual syndrome (PMS) | 6 | 33 |
| Pelvic inflammatory disorder (chronic pelvic pain) | 2 | 23 |
| Mixed or other menstrually related pain | 1 | 2 |
| Other menstrual/uterine disorders | 7 | 14 |
| **Breast and genital disorders** | | |
| Mammary disorders | 20 | 15 |
| Genital disorders | 2 | 19 |

## RECOMMENDED READING

*Useful textbooks:*
Tureanu V, Tureanu L 1999 Acupuncture in Obstetrics and Gynecology. Warren H Green, St Louis, MO
West Z 2001 Acupuncture in Pregnancy and Childbirth. Churchill Livingstone, Edinburgh

*Another useful account:*
Zharkin NA Acupuncture in obstetrics: part two. Journal of Chinese Medicine (Hove, England). 1990 Sept; (34): 14–19

*A non-acupuncture approach to induction:*
Theobald GW 1973 The Electrical Induction of Labour. Butterworth, London

*An excellent review of acupuncture and fertility:*
Stener-Victorin E 2002 Acupuncture in reproductive medicine: overview and summary of recent studies. In: Sato A, Li P, Campbell JL (eds) Acupuncture: Is there a physiological basis? Satellite Symposium of the 34th World Congress of the IUPS, held at Auckland College of Education, Auckland, New Zealand on 24 August 2001. Elsevier Science, Amsterdam, 149–56

This chapter is divided into four main sections: on systemic and peripheral circulation (e.g. blood pressure, peripheral vascular disorders), the heart (coronary heart disease, arrhythmias), circulation and healing (ulcers), and surgery and the cardiovascular system.

## SYSTEMIC AND PERIPHERAL CIRCULATORY EFFECTS

### Blood pressure

Our blood pressure (BP) varies all the time, depending on our overall patterns of behaviour, how active we are or our emotional state. It generally increases with stress and pain.

Taken together, experimental studies indicate that electroacupuncture (EA) has a regulatory effect that depends upon the initial circulatory status of the patient, both in the acute situation (acute myocardial infarction, haemorrhagic shock, defensive hypertensive reactions) and in chronic cases.

### HYPERTENSION

The root cause of sustained high BP, or hypertension (≥ 140/90 mmHg), is usually increased peripheral vascular resistance due to arteriolar contraction and loss of elasticity. Hypertension may also result from disorders of the adrenal glands and kidney.

It is very difficult to achieve adequate BP control with single-drug treatment in most patients. Provided, however, that good BP control can be maintained by non-pharmacological means, large-scale studies have shown that antihypertensive medication can safely be withdrawn in older persons without evidence of cardiovascular disease and with a BP less than 150/90 mmHg.

There is some clinical evidence that acupuncture can help reduce high BP. Some studies indicate that benefits may last for a year, or even longer. Results with acupuncture are better when hypertension is treated early, and where antihypertensive medication has not been used over a long period. Acupuncture clearly has the potential to play an important role in the treatment of hypertensives, particularly if combined with lifestyle and dietary advice.

In one uncontrolled study, manual acupuncture (MA) at BL-2 markedly increased the excretion rate of urine and sodium, with a hypotensive effect. In another, one session of MA at GB-34 and ST-36 was found to reduce both systolic and diastolic BP significantly in patients with essential hypertension, as well as plasma renin levels. MA appears to lessen the impact of stress on BP.

EA can be used at 'homeostatic' points such as LI-11, ST-36 and SP-6, together with auricular EA at the *shenmen* (+) and Heart (−). Should BP drop too far, simple nail pressure at Du-26 may remedy the situation. An even simpler treatment with low-frequency (LF) stimulation at handheld or footplate electrodes, or both, reduced high BP in 50% of patients for some 8–14 days following treatment.

Experimentally, BP is reduced by cranial electrotherapy stimulation (CES) and its variants. The usefulness of CES (electrosleep) as a treatment for hypertension has been explored in children, adolescents and adults with early stage hypertension.

Low-intensity laser therapy (LILT) has been used to control BP, with laser acupuncture (LA) instead of EA at points such as LI-11, ST-36 and SP-6, together with auricular *shenmen* and Heart points, and other adjunctive points as required.

**Points used** EA in general appears to have a regulatory effect on BP. However, certain acupoints may have more specific effects. Many experimental studies using EA on ST-36, for example, indicate that it has a depressor (BP-reducing) effect, whereas painful EA (whether at P-6, LI-4 or Du-26) has a pressor effect. Low-intensity EA at SI-19, or at P-6 (alone, or together with P-5) has been found to have a depressor effect.

SJ-17, which lies over the main trunk of the facial nerve (originating in the pons), and also over the great auricular nerve (which originates at C2–C3), can affect both BP and cerebral blood flow, although it is mentioned surprisingly little in clinical studies on cardiovascular disorders.

Of the body points, the most commonly used appear to be P-6, LI-4, LI-11 and ST-36, followed by GB-20, GB-34, GB-39, LIP-3 and others. Paraspinal points, whether on the upper thorax, over the adrenals, or selected according to TCM principles, are also used. Thus, in a number of Russian studies, ear points, with their direct neural link to cardiovascular regulatory centres in the medulla, were alternated with BL-11–BL-15 to reduce sympathetic tone. Another combination is HE-7, P-6 and LIV-3 (LIV-2 in acute episodes), with auricular Heart, Hypertension point (in the triangular fossa) and Blood-pressure-reducing groove (on the medial surface of the ear).

For hypertension, 'homeostatic' points such as GB-34, LI-11, ST-36 and SP-6 may be used with the auricular Heart and *shenmen* points (perhaps adding BL-62, BL-18, LIV-3, ST-9 or Du-20 when using LA). One manufacturer has recommended KI-3, GB-20, LIV-3 and LI-11 – strangely, with high-frequency (HF) DD, as well as the more usual 'moderate-to-strong' LF. Whichever basic formula is adopted,

| Table 9.6.1 Some manufacturers' protocols for high blood pressure |||
| Device | Points | Parameters |
|---|---|---|
| G6805 | KI-1, ST-36, SP-6 | No details |
| Helio EA-2 | KI-3, GB-20, LIV-3, LI-11 | HF DD (e.g. 90/30 Hz) or LF CW moderate–strong |
| Likon | GB-20, LIV-3, LI-11 | 100 Hz, modulated at 2 Hz |
| WQ-6F | KI-3, GB-20, LIV-3, LI-11 | DD, intermittent, or LF (< 8 Hz) |

Abbreviations: LF = low frequency; HF = high frequency; CW = continuous wave; DD = dense-disperse.

other points may need to be added, depending on the patient's overall state or TCM diagnosis.

Table 9.6.1 lists some manufacturers' protocols for high BP.

## HYPOTENSION

Hypotension may be primary, secondary to other conditions, and/or postural. Moxibustion is generally recommended, rather than potentially 'reducing' treatments such as EA. However, MA at P-6 may elevate reduced systolic pressure, even when the mean of systolic and diastolic is normal.

**Points used** The auricular Adrenal point has been suggested for raising low BP and experimentally EA at LI-4 has been found to have a pressor effect with various stimulation parameters.

LF EA, LA or ultrasound at major homeostatic acupoints (LI-11, ST-36, SP-6, Du-20) may be used to increase BP. This may be tried daily for 3–4 days, with further stimulation at KI-1, P-6, Du-25 and Du-26, if not effective.

## TREATING BLOOD PRESSURE DISORDERS

**Parameters used** In general, it seems that *non*-stressful LF EA or TENS (up to about 10 Hz) has a sympatholytic effect, and HF TENS a sympathomimetic effect on circulation and BP, particularly if intense. Yoshiaki Omura, for instance, emphasised that motor level stimulation frequency should be 'about the same as heart rate' for optimum effects on circulation, believing that higher frequencies could slow microcirculation and curtail the after-effect of treatment. Intermittent EA at a frequency around the heart rate (HR) is sometimes recommended on courses in China for the same reason. Furthermore, whereas EA to ST-36 generally lowers BP, intense MA to this point, or even brief intense EA elsewhere, may raise it. Indeed, muscle contraction may be unnecessary for peripheral stimulation to reduce BP.

**Points to be used with caution** In cases of hypotension, ST-36 EA should be used with caution, as should ST-9, located close to the carotid baroreceptors, lest a sudden drop in BP is induced. In hypertensives, points such as P-6, Du-26 or scalp points should not be strongly stimulated.

**Other precautions when treating blood pressure disorders** Acupuncture (MA at points such as GB-20, for example) can result in hypotension. As a general rule, those receiving EA for the first time should not be left unattended, and EA should only be used cautiously in hypotensives. In such patients, generalised heating (for instance, with infrared) is contraindicated, although localised acupoint heating could well be useful in some cases.

In hypertensives, strong (especially HF) electrostimulation should be avoided,

In patients with spinal cord injury (at or above T8), autonomic 'dysreflexia' may include an abnormal tendency to raised blood pressure in response to stimulation, particularly in those who are already hypertensive. Such patients should be monitored during treatment.

## Peripheral vascular disorders

Peripheral venous disorders include varicose veins and venous thrombosis and endarteritis (inflammation of the innermost layer of the artery). Both can result in ulceration. In Raynaud's phenomenon (syndrome), (arteriolar) spasm brought on by cold or emotion results in pain, with pallor or cyanosis of hands or feet, or both, and sometimes of nose and ears.

MA has been employed for obstructive artery disease, and also for Raynaud's syndrome (Box 9.6.1). It has also effectively reactivated arteriovenous blood flow in rheumatoid arthritis with associated capillary angiopathy. Both acupuncture and TENS have been utilised in management of the painful diabetic foot. EA has been used for peripheral vascular disorders of the lower limbs. Birger Kaada's protocol for LF TENS at LI-4/~SI-3 may produce widespread and prolonged increases in skin temperature in patients with peripheral vascular insufficiency, owing to improved microcirculation. This method has been used for Buerger's disease, vibration disease and diabetic angiopathy.

LF EMS also improves lower extremity circulation in peripheral vascular disease. In general, TENS is considered as indicated in conditions involving peripheral circulatory impairment. Thus it has been used clinically for the ischaemic leg pain that can occur even when at rest in severe cases. However, given the reduced skin and muscle sensitivity in some peripheral arteriopathies, both TENS and acupuncture may need to be used with caution.

TENS has also been used for less serious but still distressing problems such as 'restless legs' syndrome.

Combining local LILT and LF intermittent TENS has been proposed as an effective method for dealing with a variety of peripheral vascular disorders, even when severe. As might be expected, although LA was found helpful for functional lower-limb angiopathy in diabetics, improving pain, peripheral circulation and thermographic readings, it was

---

**BOX 9.6.1**

**Haemodynamics and thermal effects: the background**

Peripheral circulation is clearly affected by acupuncture, with concomitant changes in temperature. Such changes may be partially responsible for the benefits of acupuncture in many conditions, including myofascial and complex regional pain disorders. Locally, MA has been considered to lead to an initial vasoconstriction (for up to 20 minutes), followed by a longer (2–3-hour) phase of vasodilation. Thus, with MA, pain relief in musculoskeletal conditions is associated with reduced sympathetic vasomotor activity (increased finger temperature).

EA, like MA, may also induce local short-term cooling and reduced blood flow before recovery and generalised warming. In one study of haemoptysis in lung disorders, for example, unilateral low-intensity LF EA at P-6 and LU-6 reduced peripheral blood flow during treatment and stemmed bleeding, with a rebound effect following treatment, whereas the opposite effects were found with P-3 and LU-5 (i.e. greater initial peripheral blood flow and exacerbation of bleeding).

In one study comparing the use of MA, handheld probe TENS (pTENS) and LA after injury, skin temperature increased both in the affected area when treated locally, and also, to a lesser extent, on the contralateral, untreated side. Temperature remained relatively unchanged in healthy controls. In contrast, in a study of angina pectoris, although MA increased skin temperature in the target area, it did not do so peripherally.

---

less effective when the condition had progressed to obliterating atherosclerosis.

Ultrasound 'focused' within the tissues at ST-36 and ST-41 (*yangming* points) has been used to improve microcirculation in the leg. Ultrasound has also been combined with MA for nocturnal leg pains, at points such as BL-60, KI-7, GB-34 and tender regions between BL-60 and KI-7, together with light bandaging of the affected leg. However, only *athermal* (pulsed) ultrasound should be applied in areas of impaired circulation (occlusive vascular disease), as for other electrotherapy modalities.

## TREATMENT TO BENEFIT CIRCULATION

**Points for general stimulation** In experimental studies, general points such as ST-36, ST-41 and SP-6 have been used to improve circulation, and also to enhance tissue repair.

Clinically, BL-40 and BL-57, P-6, LI-4, ST-36, ST-40, SP-6 and SP-9 have been used for peripheral ischaemia and related conditions, as has Kaada's protocol. Other points have been added according to the area treated (e.g. further Bladder, Stomach or Spleen meridian points for the leg, and Heart, *sanjiao* or Lung points for the arms).

KI-3 appears in a number of protocols for a variety of circulation problems using very different treatment modalities; SJ-8 EA has been used to induce vasodilatation in patients undergoing cardiac surgery.

**Points for local stimulation** Points such as *baxie* and *bafeng* have been used in EA treatment of gangrene.

**Points for central stimulation** Stimulating dorsal nerve roots leads to peripheral vasodilation. Thus paraspinal points may be used according to innervation of the affected area, one possible rationale being that stimulation of the paraspinal sympathetic ganglia may enhance arterial blood flow. Instead of implanted electrodes (as in spinal cord stimulation, SCS), electrodes can be positioned directly over the spine too, at ~Du-11/Du-7, for instance. In clinical studies, points such as BL-21–BL-24, or other paraspinal points, both thoracic and lumbar, have been employed, as well as stimulation over the stellate ganglion. Thus LILT directed at Erb's point (level with C6 and posterior to the belly of the sternocleidomastoid muscle) or cervical nerve roots has been used to treat experimental ischaemic pain. MA in this area should not be undertaken by the inexperienced.

**Points for autonomic stimulation** Virtually all aspects of circulation are governed by the autonomic nervous system. From experimental research, ST-36 in particular appears to have sympatholytic effects. By contrast, Du-26, and sometimes P-6 or LI-4, have sympathomimetic effects on circulation, with MA at Du-26, for instance, raising the heart rate. Curiously, though, some researchers have concluded that, although the cardiovascular effects of P-4 and BL-21 may be sympathetically mediated, those of P-6 are mediated by the vagus nerve.

In one study by Thomas Lundeberg's group, SJ-5 and LI-11 are suggested as upper-extremity points evoking general sympathetic responses, with BL-60 and GB-34 as lower-extremity points segmentally related to the somatovisceral innervation of the sympathetic nerves regulating peripheral blood flow.

Joseph Wong, on the other hand, in his system of neuroanatomical acupuncture, proposes that Du-20, Du-26 and *yintang* may be useful for their direct effect on central autonomic control, Du-14 for sympathetic dysfunction in the head and neck region, SI-17, ST-10 and ST-11 for disorders associated with the cervical sympathetic and stellate ganglia, Du-4 and BL-23 for control of sympathetic activity in the lower extremities, and Du-1 for the coccygeal ganglion. In his approach, the most commonly used 'sympathetic switches' for control of sympathetic/arterial function are LI-4 and LI-11 in the upper extremity, LIV-3 and ST-36 in the lower extremity. His 'parasympathetic switches' include HE-7 and P-6 in the upper extremity and SP-6 and SP-9 in the lower one. He considers that these may facilitate venous and lymphatic return flow.

**Parameters used** Clinically LF, HF, intermittent and DD peripheral electrostimulation have all been used to improve peripheral circulation. Of these, the first three have some experimental or theoretical justification. One standard electrotherapy recommendation for improving venous insufficiency is 10–20 minutes of HF *interrupted* (5–10 seconds on, 10–20 seconds off) biphasic or monophasic electrostimulation at motor level, but not so strong as to induce muscle spasm (overstimulation in general may induce vasoconstriction). On the other hand, for neurovascular disorders, mild sensory level *continuous* stimulation is recommended at slightly higher frequencies.

Very-low-frequency stimulation (~0.1 Hz) may increase vascular smooth muscle contraction and so *reduce* local skin blood flow and temperature. Muscle blood flow and lymphatic circulation may be more effectively *enhanced* by frequencies similar to those of physiological tremor (~10 Hz) rather than higher (tetanic) or lower (twitch) frequency stimulation, particularly if this is interrupted rather than continuous. However, in some studies on muscle stimulation, bursts of higher tetanic frequencies did give better results.

## Peripheral vascular obstruction

### VERTEBROGENIC VASCULAR SYNDROMES

Some painful conditions due to structural compression at the spine can be associated with circulatory changes in the periphery. If the cervical vertebrae are involved, arterial compression can contribute to cerebral ischaemia. Symptoms of occlusion or stenosis (compression) of the vertebral arteries may include headache, dizziness, blurred vision, tinnitus or even ataxia (reduced muscular coordination). Arterial spasm due to sympathetic irritation can lead to the same symptoms.

This 'vertebrobasilar insufficiency' has been treated with acupuncture. MA has been used to improve blood supply, using shoulder and distal points such as SJ-15, LI-4, LI-11 and LI-16. Cervical spondylopathy with vertebral artery involvement has also been treated with MA and moxibustion ('warm needling'), with acupoint injection, or MA together with interferential current therapy. LF EA has been applied at segmental TrPs (combined with heat), or at local and distal points, at local points alone, or at local points in combination with Du-20 moxibustion.

## Arteriosclerosis and atheroma

Arteriosclerosis, the hardening of the arteries due to calcium deposition, results in impaired arterial vasodilation. Atherosclerosis, the furring up of the arteries due to deposition of fats, goes hand in hand with arteriosclerosis, which involves calcium entry into the smooth muscle cells of the arterial wall. It is the prime cause of heart disorders such as angina pectoris, coronary thrombosis and coronary insufficiency, and is also responsible for many strokes.

In Russian studies, acupuncture, alone or in combination with diet and fasting, or with medication, appeared to contribute to lower cholesterol levels. In one small French clinical pilot study, weekly MA at BL-18, BL-19, LIV-2 and LIV-6 reduced blood cholesterol and triglyceride levels, but did not affect high-density lipoprotein (HDL) cholesterol or blood sugar levels. In a more robust RCT, MA did not appear to reduce cholesterol level or alter the ratio between different lipoprotein fractions in any significant manner.

In comparison with the French study mentioned above, it appears from one German report that EA at body points may more effectively lower blood cholesterol and triglycerides than MA, although this has not yet been tested in a properly structured study. Auricular EA has also been used for its effects on blood lipids, while DD EA at various body points was found to reduce serum triglycerides more than standard medication in one Chinese study of ischaemic stroke (effects on cholesterol were similar).

## Thrombosis and phlebitis

In one uncontrolled Romanian study, MA was successfully used in the treatment of thrombophlebitis. However, there is also a report in the literature of deep-vein thrombophlebitis occurring after MA, although whether MA might 'cause' thrombosis in the absence of other precipitating factors is another question. Non-charge-balanced EA could certainly lead to blood clotting, given needles inserted sufficiently close together.

For recurrent thrombosis or phlebitis, Voll used what he called 'transverse shock therapy' (transcutaneous electrodes foot-to-foot, in LF 'tonification' mode), emphasising that the positive electrode should always be used locally, not the negative, to reduce risk of thrombolysis and embolism. However, this approach should be used only with caution, given that local treatment of thrombophlebitis is sometimes contraindicated in electrotherapy. In particular, strong motor level stimulation could dislodge a deep-vein thrombus, leading to embolism, and may also disrupt clotting. Thus some authorities consider EA to be contraindicated in severe arterial disease. None the less, motor level stimulation of the calf muscle has been used both during surgery and postoperatively to *prevent* thrombosis

Experimental studies on rabbits have shown that acupuncture, at P-6, for example, can reduce blood viscosity. Clinically too, EA at BL-14, BL-15, BL-17, P-6 and the auricular Heart point may reduce viscosity. HF EA has been found to lower platelet aggregation rate and thromboxane levels in patients with vascular headache, and also following stroke.

Some authors have suggested LILT should be avoided in phlebitis, yet it has been used locally for thrombophlebitis, with Endre Mester's standard dose of 4 J/cm$^2$.

**Points used** KI-3, P-6, and back *shu* points such as BL-14, BL-15 and BL-17 have been used to reduce blood viscosity.

**Parameters used** For prevention of venous stasis and postoperative thrombosis, brief tetanic LF trains of HF impulses were found to be more effective than single LF impulses. None the less, Voll recommended 2.5 Hz for oedema associated with varicose veins (but 10 Hz for phlebitis), and the manufacturers of one Chinese EA device similarly advise that LF sawtooth stimulation will enhance absorption of tissue fluid.

## Haemorrhage, bruises and haematomas

Unusual bleeding should always be investigated, although it is not always pathological in itself, and may sometimes be a way of restoring balance.

In haemophilia, however, there is a predisposition to intramuscular or intra-articular bleeding, with possible long-term consequences, such as haemarthrosis. Although MA has been used for the pain this causes, it has been suggested that needling in this condition should be undertaken only with proper safeguards, which are unlikely to be available to non-medical acupuncturists. Otherwise, EA is no more contraindicated than MA for haemophilia. Both TENS and acupoint EHF have been used for joint haemorrhage in haemophiliacs. TENS has also been used for traumatic haemarthrosis.

LILT is particularly indicated for haematoma; if this occurs as a result of injury, LILT should be started at the earliest opportunity. However, in some injuries early treatment could aggravate a tendency to bleeding, so, although LILT may be applied even within 48 hours after injury, it should be used locally with caution.

## Oedema and inflammation

Oedema and inflammation, when part of the picture in musculoskeletal conditions, tend to respond well to electro-stimulation, although results with chronic oedema, even when applying motor level stimulation, can be disappointing.

LF intermittent TENS may be useful as an adjuvant home treatment for patients with inflammation and oedema, in addition to clinical use of EA or LA. Judicious use of an electrical roller may also be helpful. High-voltage pulsed galvanic treatment (HVPG) is frequently used in North America for acute oedema following trauma or surgery. Other forms of monophasic stimulation, such as ryodoraku (in its 'dragon chasing' variant) and microcurrent TENS (MENS) are also used, and even piezoelectric stimulators.

LILT has often been used locally for oedema and inflammation. It has a potentially important role in dentistry. For oedema following radiotherapy, LA was found to be superior to both MA and medication alone, in one study. In part due to its ability to increase lymphatic and venous drainage, LILT is also often considered helpful for prostatitis.

### LYMPHATIC STASIS
MA has been used in the treatment of both *luo li* (swollen lymph glands) and lymphoedema. In one study, in which MA was combined with moxibustion following lymph node dissection for malignant gynaecological tumours, an increase in deep body temperature in response to treatment was found to be essential for successful prevention or treatment of lymphoedema.

Although results with chronic oedema may be disappointing, lymphoedema may respond to electrical treatment: Reinhold Voll, for example, used his non-local LF biphasic 'transverse shock therapy' for lymphatic swelling and oedema, with one electrode in the armpit or groin, and the other applied to the palm or sole. EA has even been used for lymphoedema following radical mastectomy (but see below for a cautionary note in favour of using contralateral acupoints in this condition).

For localised lymphatic swelling (lymphadenopathy) in the head and neck area, as in tonsillitis, pharyngitis and glandular fever (infectious mononucleosis), MA and LA have been used at points along Voll's 'lymphatic meridian,' together with LI-4. Another approach has been to use sonopuncture and vitamin B12 injection at ST-21, Ren-4, Ren-6 and Ren-12, for localised lymphadenopathy in glandular fever, with acupoint injection at ST-36 and SP-6 for generalised lymphatic congestion.

**Points used** Contralateral needling is advised when treating an oedematous limb. For generalised oedema, John Amaro has suggested using a piezolelectric stimulator or HeNe LA at BL-23, KI-2, KI-3, KI-6, KI-16, KI-27, GB-25, SP-6, SP-9 and Ren-9, stating that he 'saw a patient lose 18 lbs of water weight in seven days with this formula'. This is rather a sledgehammer treatment for stimulating kidney function, but useful *in extremis*, if it works.

**Local stimulation** For localised oedema, it has been suggested that MENS pads are applied in 'parallel' (across the affected area) or in 'crossfire' mode (four pads, with currents crisscrossing the area). In general, both bipolar and monopolar electrode placement may be effective for elec-trotherapy of acute oedema, bipolar being favoured for chronic oedema, with both electrodes in the affected area.

**Parameters used** For acute oedema, a standard electrotherapy recommendation is to use 80–100 Hz at sensory level, CW (continuous rather than burst), for as long as 2–4 hours daily (in combination with cold applications), and for chronic oedema a lower frequency (40–50 Hz) to induce tetanic contractions at motor level, interrupted (5–10 seconds on, 15–120 seconds off).

Experimentally, LF (5 Hz) low-intensity EA reduced neurogenic inflammatory oedema more than MA, although 10 Hz and 100 Hz were also effective. On the other hand, very strong EA could induce inflammation and oedema.

## Varicose veins and haemorrhoids

MA has been used in the traditional treatment of haemorrhoids, as have bleeding with cupping, local herbal injection, and point injection at Du-28. Reinhold Voll used his LF biphasic 'transverse shock therapy' for varicosities. Haemorrhoids have also been considered to be amenable to auricular or body acupoint TENS or pTENS.

HeNe LILT has been used for mild to moderate haemorrhoids, with pain alleviation following the first session. This method has been considered harmless in pregnancy.

Combining ultrasound with mild electrostimulation may be helpful for varicose veins, massaging over the veins towards the heart with the soundhead. Daily treatment for 6–8 weeks may be required, in addition to oral vitamin C. Ultrasound can also be applied at GB-34, LU-9, ST-36 and where veins are particularly prominent (over thread veins, for instance). LA is another option.

**Points used** Various points along the Bladder meridian and Governor Vessel, either local, such as Du-1, or on the head, at Du-20 or Du-28, are generally suggested for MA treatment of haemorrhoids, with others depending on the practitioner's favoured approach. In one microcurrent protocol, points around Du-20 are used, as well as Du-20 itself.

# CIRCULATION AND HEALING

In soft tissue injury and wound healing, an initial inflammatory stage is followed by a proliferative/repair stage proper. A final remodelling stage then starts after about 3 weeks. Poor healing may result if microcirculation is impaired, as with early atherosclerosis or diabetic angiopathy (disease of the blood vessels), or with gross impairment, as with varicose veins, thrombosis or paralysis. Thus any method of improving local circulation may well encourage healing, as will enhancement of immune function.

## Treatment of wounds and injuries

Simple needling, which itself results in microinjury that may not heal for several days, can restart a stalled tissue repair process. This in itself may explain some of the benefits of EA for tissue repair. On the other hand, low-intensity TENS may also enhance wound healing, although overvigorous motor level stimulation may aggravate existing tissue damage.

LILT affects various cellular processes that in turn result in vasodilation and eventual vascularisation. Wound healing has even been considered 'the cardinal indication' for LILT in physical therapy, with results superior to those of ultrasound.

## Ulcers: dermal, varicose and decubitus (pressure sores)

Ulcers may be due to poor microcirculation and nutrition of the area ('trophic' ulcers), gross structural problems (as with varicose ulcers or fracture), or mechanical factors ('decubitus' ulcers from being bedbound, or pressure sores from other causes, such as wearing an artificial limb). Trophic ulcers frequently occur following phlebitis as a result of circulatory stasis. Poor nutrition and lack of exercise are major contributory factors to ulcers, and stress may inhibit healing.

Local motor level electrical stimulation can act as a decompression 'pump' when venous flow is reduced, and thus has often been used for non-healing ulcers. LF EA is no exception. Reinhold Voll, for example, recommended his 'transverse shock therapy' for varicose ulcers (electrodes foot-to-foot, in LF 'tonification' mode), and Yoshiaki Omura both LF EA and TENS for lower-extremity circulatory disturbances with pain, intermittent claudication and ulceration. However, it was in Italy during the 1970s that most research on EA for ulcers was carried out. There were experimental animal studies, including RCTs, investigations into morphological and histochemical changes and a number of clinical MA and EA studies.

LF motor level TENS stimulation unilaterally at LI-4 and ~SI-3 was advocated by the Norwegian Birger Kaada for many conditions in which poor peripheral circulation is a factor, from atopic eczema to peritendinitis of the shoulder, and including ulcers. Any resultant improvement in microcirculation is probably due to sympathoinhibition. EA too has been proposed for trophic ulcer, using points on meridians that traverse the affected area and frequent but short treatments to avoid fatiguing the denervated muscle. Both methods could also be considered for other types of neurogenic ulcer, such as those that appear in the late stages of complex regional pain disorder or diabetes.

Another option for dermal ulcers and wounds is monophasic current, either applied at low ('microcurrent') intensity within or at points around the lesion, or in the form of HVPG, with one electrode placed directly over the wound.

Whereas local heating has been used in the prophylaxis of pressure sores, athermal pulsed shortwave ('Diapulse') has been used to treat them.

LILT has frequently been used for non-healing ulcers, with effects on both immune function and microcirculation. One of Endre Mester's early findings was that irradiation resulted in enhanced vascularisation of the ulcer. Even fistulas (deep ulcers) have been treated with HeNe LILT, and long-standing leg and malignant ulcers adjunctively with mixed-wavelength LILT. LILT is not infrequently combined with LA in the treatment of trophic ulcers, with LA giving more convincing results with chronic ulcers and indolent wounds than for musculoskeletal pain.

## Frostbite and chilblains, burns and scalds

In one small uncontrolled study ($N = 10$), MA, 'warming needle' and EA were compared for their effects on nail microcirculation in patients with frostbite. Warm needling gave the best results, with MA and EA producing less local warming. Results were not related to whether treatment was experienced as uncomfortable.

Acupuncture has been used both experimentally and in patients with thermal injury, and also for ulceration following burns. EA is best combined with other interventions as part of a programme of therapy, rather than employed in isolation. Low-intensity EA at either the back *shu* or auricular points reduces vascular permeability in experimental thermal injuries, probably owing to suppression of histamine release from the injured tissue. LILT has been used for minor skin burns, and with LA for scald injury.

## Soft tissue injury

Muscle, ligament and tendon injuries are frequently the result of sporting or domestic accidents. The ensuing oedema and inflammation, if prolonged, can themselves interfere with the healing process. Enhancing circulation is just as important in this kind of soft tissue injury as in overt wound repair.

Body and auricular MA have been used for soft tissue injury, as has EA. TENS has been used for haemarthrosis (bleeding into a joint) following severe ankle and knee injuries. There have also been a number of experimental studies on the use of low-intensity DC and MENS to accelerate healing of ligaments and tendons.

LILT is frequently used in traumatology for soft tissue injuries. Muscle tears, haematomas and tendinopathies respond particularly well, although with variable results for conditions such as bursitis and muscle spasm where improving the circulation is not such a contributory factor. Higher dosages are required than when dealing with superficial wounds, which may account for some less positive findings in severe tendon strains. However, as mentioned above, caution should be observed if using LILT within 48 hours after injury, lest any bleeding is aggravated. On the other hand, as with most of the modalities mentioned here, early treatment gives the best response.

## Blood flow, joints and other skeletal structures

Vasoconstriction and reduced synovial blood flow within the joint may contribute to cartilage degeneration and inflammation in joint disease. Electrical stimulation parameters should be carefully selected with this in mind.

LF EA was found to improve local circulation and contribute to recovery in cases of lumbar disc prolapse. LILT has been shown to reduce joint swelling in rheumatoid arthritis, but possibly not sufficiently to be clinically useful.

**Combinations and comparisons** A number of combination treatments have been used for ulcers: EA with ultrasound, LILT with pulsed electromagnetic fields (PEMF), static magnetic fields with electrophoresis, LILT with TENS, and LILT with infrared light. Mixed-wavelength *non*-coherent light, combined with hyperbaric oxygen, has been investigated as a means of enhancing wound repair during NASA space missions. Given the different effects of modalities such as EA and PEMF or LA, these too could also be combined for wound healing. TENS and ultrasound have been combined as a therapy for suppurative wounds.

As a general protocol for slowly healing wounds, ulcers, and peripheral vascular disorders, Pekka Pöntinen has proposed a combined treatment: TENS three times daily for 30–45 minutes for the first 2–3 weeks, then less frequently, according to patient response, with successful treatment being marked not only by a reduction in pain but also by an increase in skin temperature, generally within 24–48 hours. LILT (4–8 J/cm$^2$) or non-coherent red or near-infrared light can be applied directly to wounds or ulcers once or twice weekly simultaneously with TENS. Blood pressure should be monitored, in case improved microcirculation and lower peripheral resistance cause it to drop.

**Points used for tissue repair** General points such as ST-36, ST-41 and SP-6 have been used to improve circulation and enhance tissue repair in experimental EA studies. Kaada's LI-4/~SI-3 combination has been widely utilised, if not always supported by rigorous clinical trials. Even auricular points have been used. On one laser manufacturer's website, LA at points such as BL-40, KI-8, P-7, LI-4, LI-11, ST-36 and SP-10 is recommended, in addition to local LILT.

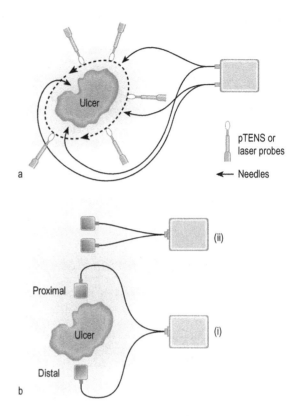

**Figure 9.6.1** Local treatment for ulcers. (a) Surrounding the lesion, using EA, probes (pTENS) or LILT. (b) TENS can be applied (i) with electrodes proximal and distal, or (ii) both proximal to the lesion.

A straightforward approach would be to use local treatment in conjunction with major points along meridians that pass through the area of injury, or are likely to improve circulation in the affected limb.

**Local stimulation** (Fig. 9.6.1) Local stimulation can play an important role in tissue repair, whether 'surrounding the dragon' with EA or LA, or treating injured tissue directly. Thus, for non-healing ulcers EA can be applied with four needles around the lesion, as well as direct ultrasound for a few seconds daily applied through gauze soaked in sterile saline. The same technique has been used successfully for burn healing.

TENS electrodes can be positioned as close to the ulcer as possible without compromising sterility, 'bracketing' it (proximally and distally). If sensitivity is impaired distally, both electrodes can be positioned proximally. Microcurrent (probes or pads) can be positioned around the ulcer. Stimulation through sterile gauze directly over the ulcer is clearly not so practical as TENS or MENS, and has the added disadvantage of possible mechanical damage to newly formed tissue.

This is not a problem with non-contact LILT, and although the non-contact method may lead to reduced penetration depth over intact skin, this can be discounted when treating open skin wounds. Several authors have noted that LILT may

---

**BOX 9.6.2**

Kaada's protocol for TENS

This protocol employs 2 Hz pulses or 2–5 Hz trains with 100 Hz internal frequency, at an intensity sufficient to cause local pain-free muscle contraction (up to 50 mA in some cases), with the active (negative) electrode at LI-4 and the return (positive) electrode at ~SI-3, for 30–40 minutes once to three times daily (longer individual treatments are not required).

---

have *contralateral* effects on tissue repair. The same is true for acupuncture in general, with clear benefits if a lesion is inaccessible under dressings, or within a cast, for instance.

**Parameters used to benefit tissue repair** For pressure sores, 2 Hz motor level charge-balanced TENS twice daily for 20–30 minutes has been recommended, with sensory to motor level 50 Hz for other forms of ulcer (for up to an hour each time). However, if muscle pumping is intended, clearly this should be interrupted. Thus EMS for 30 minutes every 2 hours, strong enough to induce *slight* muscle contractions, was used early on for non-healing wounds, and for 30 minutes three times daily in one report on facial ulcers. In some of the Italian studies on ulcer healing, 25 Hz EA was continued for up to 7 hours daily.

Some authorities have suggested that different currents may be required for different types of wound, and that a minimum current of 4 mA is required to enhance ulcer healing when using surface electrodes. It has also been suggested that 40–60 minutes daily for 5–7 days each week is the *minimum* required to produce a clinical response when treating diabetic ulcers. For postoperative ischaemic flaps, 80 Hz TENS twice daily for 2 hours may be appropriate.

On the other hand, microcurrent clearly has a role, and has been recommended for ulcer treatment. One possible advantage of using monophasic stimulation is that the negative electrode can be used over the ulcer when its bactericidal effect is required, and then the positive electrode to reduce scar tissue formation.

Box 9.6.2 details Kaada's protocol for TENS.

# THE HEART

## Coronary heart disease (CHD) and angina pectoris

Atherosclerosis of the coronary arteries is the main cause of angina (chest pain), coronary thrombosis and coronary insufficiency (heart failure).

There is considerable experimental evidence that acupuncture may be effective for angina, if not too severe. In TCM terms, angina may be induced by stagnant Heart *qi*, stagnation of *qi* and Blood, or obstruction of the Heart Orifices due to Blood stasis or turbid Phlegm. Because it blocks sympathetic activation, MA may be therapeutic for patients with heart

failure in whom sympathetic nerve activity may be two to three times higher than normal.

EA appears to regulate coronary microcirculation following acute myocardial ischaemia (AMI), redistributing and improving blood flow and possibly relieving microvascular spasm. Thus it may regulate blood pressure, strengthen cardiovascular contraction, improve metabolism (glycolysis) and recovery rate, and protect against myocardial damage. Interestingly, timely analgesia (whether with drugs or acupuncture) immediately following cardiac infarction may have benefits on haemodynamic and respiratory function, not just on pain.

Experimentally, MA has been used to improve revascularisation of the ischaemic heart muscle. Clinically, MA to P-4 has been found to elicit immediate changes in cardiovascular function in patients with coronary heart disease or angina. MA can also improve microcirculation in cases of acute myocardial infarction.

Like MA, EA has frequently been used for CHD, chiefly to control angina, the main symptom of cardiac ischaemia. Apart from fewer and less severe angina attacks and improved exercise tolerance, some studies indicate associated improvements in angiography, ECG and other objective measures of heart function, as well as in BP, HR, various haematological measures and medication intake.

The authors of one textbook on auricular therapy suggest LF EA for angina, at points such as Chest, Excitation and Liver (for *qi* and *yin xu*), *mingmen*, Brain and Excitation (for *qi* and *yang xu*), or *sanjiao*, Lung, Spleen and Chest (for stagnation of Phlegm) for 30–60 minutes, once every other day for 12 sessions (courses being repeated after an interval of 3 days). Brief moxibustion can be used once needles are withdrawn, in cases of *yang* deficiency. This treatment, which induces only minor ECG changes, is probably appropriate only for those in the early stages of heart disease.

TENS too has been found to be helpful for angina, even for patients with the refractory angina of end-stage CHD (i.e. no longer responsive to medication, or unsuitable for further revascularisation). It now appears clear that this is due to a direct effect on sympathetic activity rather than a consequence of pain inhibition. Thus there is no risk of a 'silent', pain-free ischaemia continuing unnoticed.

Moxibustion has been used for CHD: applied at BL-15, P-6 and Ren-17, it was found superior to MA in one study. In line with this, several Russian authors have reported benefits in applying infrared LILT over regions segmentally related to the heart and associated organs (their 'projection zones'). For example, LILT may reduce atherogenesis and strengthen myocardial contractions. LA at P-4 has been used in experimental studies on myocardial ischaemia, as well as clinically.

**Combinations and comparisons** TENS together with LILT/LA has been used for chronic chest pain following myocardial infarction. LILT has been used with magnetic field stimulation for ischaemic heart disease. There are also Soviet patents for a device to treat acute myocardial infarction or angina using brief combined LILT, continuous infrared and a static magnetic field over the precordial area.

**Points used** In one experimental study of CHD patients, MA at P-2, P-3, P-4 and P-6, as well as at 'non-points' along the same meridian, resulted in greater changes in eight different cardiac measures than MA at off-meridian points or GB-37. In experimental studies on acute myocardial infarction, of all the Pericardium and Heart meridian points, P-6 is the most frequently used. EA at ST-36 has less effect on ischaemia than EA at P-6. Although low-back extrasegmental points are unlikely to have any effect on cardiac blood flow associated with angina, distal points on the KI-meridian may be useful in CHD.

Clinically, P-6 appears to be the most used point for CHD, in line with the experimental research on acute myocardial ischaemia. The auricular Heart point is also popular, while various points on the Heart meridian are used too. EA, TENS, LILT and magnetic fields have been applied locally, at points on the back in the C4–T7 dermatomes, as well as on the chest over the heart. In the acupuncture-based studies, these are usually the standard acupoints, while the focus tends to be on zones of referred pain (or *ashi* points) in physiologically based trials.

Points such as P-5, P-6, ST-36, SP-6 and Ren-17 are often recommended for acupuncture treatment of angina. P-4 and P-6 may be combined with back *shu* points BL-14 and BL-15. In one manufacturer's manual, EA at distal points (HE-5 and P-6) is combined with chest points (ST-18, Ren-14 and Ren-17) and dorsal points (BL-15). For diffuse myocarditis, EA at P-3 and P-7 has been suggested, together with vitamin B12 acupoint injection at Ren-17.

TENS is usually applied on the chest wall, bracketing or over the area where most angina pain is experienced. Anterior–posterior electrode placement should be avoided if cardiac pacing is not the aim of treatment.

**Parameters used** A variety of parameters have been used in experiments on acute myocardial infarction, both LF and HF, at high and low intensities. Cao Qingshu has been the main researcher in this area, and studies from his laboratory have employed 50 or 60 Hz several times. Clinically, LF EA appears to be more common than HF EA, although one author on EA has suggested that 150 Hz may be appropriate, while one manufacturer recommends mild-to-moderate DD in a protocol not employing chest points.

HF TENS is most often used for cardiac ischaemic pain (angina), preferably at around 70 Hz according to some authors, although for only 1 hour 2–3 times daily, at a level just below the pain threshold. If MA, EA or TENS are too strong and experienced as stressful, then they are unlikely to attenuate anginal pain.

## Cardiomyopathy and valvular heart disease

MA, EA and LA have been used for these conditions, generally applied at Heart meridian points, P-6 or ST-36, BL-15 (the back *shu* point for the Heart), or the auricular Heart point, although some have used a more varied selection of points, based in part on TCM considerations. MA at P-4, for example, has been explored for its effects on the ECG in patients with chronic coronary insufficiency. From the few studies available, it seems that LF EA is preferred, at either low or high intensity.

## Heart rate (HR) and arrhythmias

MA may affect HR, with beneficial effects on erratic tachycardia and the capacity for physical activity. Reductions in HR may accompany decreases in BP with MA. In experimental studies, EA tends to increase or decrease HR to maintain cardiovascular homeostasis, with more studies reporting that HR slows with stimulation. The effects of LF EA on HR may also depend on time of day of treatment– something that could be important when treating coronary heart disease patients. Both MA and EA are used clinically for the treatment of some arrhythmias.

MA has been known to result in immediate restoration of a normal heartbeat following surgically induced atrial fibrillation. Auricular EA may prevent stress-induced lowering of the threshold for fibrillation. On the other hand, the presence of atrial fibrillation in stroke patients may indicate that only a poor response to EA or TENS is likely, although DD TEAS may both lower heart rate and reduce the incidence of palpitations during drug withdrawal.

**Points used** From one experimental HR study, albeit on healthy volunteers or non-cardiac patients, it would seem that EA at HE-7 and P-4 may activate *both* sympathetic and vagal mechanisms simultaneously. Other experimental studies, again on healthy people, indicate that EA at points along the Pericardium meridian, such as P-4 and P-6, may have more influence on HR or other aspects of heart function than EA at points such as ST-36. However, P-4, P-6 and ST-36 EA, as well as auricular EA, have all been found helpful for experimental arrhythmias, with auricular or P-6 EA having a useful antifibrillation effect.

Thus one manufacturer recommends EA (moderate DD) at P-4, P-6 and ST-36 for tachycardia, and is followed by another in suggesting EA (again, moderate DD) at P-6 and ST-36 together for bradycardia. From the few available studies on arrhythmia, P-6 would seem to be the point most used.

**Parameters used** In experimental studies 2 Hz TENS trains resulted in long-lasting local vaso*constriction*, whereas HF TENS produced inconsistent short-lasting responses. Similarly, it appears that both LF and HF EA at ST-36 can reduce HR, but this effect lasts only after treatment with the former, as with so many effects of EA. Thus HF P-6 EA was used in one clinical study for patients liable to arrhythmia under epidural anaesthesia when a long-lasting effect was not required. As already mentioned, if ST-36 EA is strong it may potentiate sympathetic arrhythmia, whereas if gentle it will calm. Overly strong stimulation may increase HR, just as it does BP.

## Shock

Shock, or collapse of circulation, results from major trauma (surgery or severe haemorrhage, for instance), dehydration,

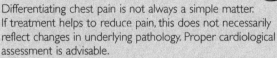

## Cardiac cautions

Differentiating chest pain is not always a simple matter. If treatment helps to reduce pain, this does not necessarily reflect changes in underlying pathology. Proper cardiological assessment is advisable.

Scalp EA has been known to induce angina pectoris in susceptible patients. There are also occasional reports of acupuncture inducing arrhythmia, so EA should be used only with care in patients in whom this could be problematic, particularly those who have recently suffered a heart attack. In such cases, ECG monitoring is advisable. Adverse effects of EA on patients with pacemakers have been reported, and both EA and TENS should only be used in these circumstances according to very strict guidelines, if at all.

TENS has been used to stimulate diaphragmatic breathing in patients with chronic respiratory problems. If the heart is already struggling to maintain adequate circulation in such cases, TENS may in fact worsen this 'decompensation,' with deterioration of right ventricular function but no change in pulmonary hypertension and arteriolar tone. Furthermore, TENS for angina has been known to induce temporary tetany in the intercostal muscles, resulting in impaired respiration.

Local EA, with both needles inserted directly over the heart, or using electrodes that 'sandwich' the heart front to back, is probably best avoided, particularly in those with a serious or unstable cardiac condition.

LILT should be used with caution over sympathetic ganglia, the vagus or the cardiac region in patients with heart disease.

infection, or toxic or allergic reactions. It is quite different from syncope (fainting), and unless promptly dealt with is life threatening.

Many EA studies on shock (allergic or haemorrhagic) make use of Du-26 and Ren-24, or P-6.

# SURGERY AND CIRCULATION

## Blood pressure changes during surgery and anaesthesia

The stress of surgery and some of the associated procedures may increase BP, whereas many anaesthetic agents depress the cardiovascular system and lower BP with potentially serious complications.

There are many reports that AA, and EAA in particular, has a stabilising effect on BP during surgery. So, for example, mean arterial pressure in patients undergoing cranial surgery with EAA increased only slightly (by 3.6 mmHg) compared with a drop of 13.9 mmHg with conventional anaesthesia, while it fell below 90 mmHg in only 2.4% of patients undergoing lung resection with EAA but in 14% of those receiving general anaesthesia. There have been similar

results in other studies of AA or EAA or EAA combined with low-dose epidural.

In a more recent study, MA was used (at GB-34) in patients undergoing thyroid surgery with EAA, in order to lower BP that had become raised. Conversely, auricular MA at the Occiput point was shown in one RCT to increase BP significantly when it dropped following i.v. administration of the barbiturate anaesthetic thiopental for abdominal surgery.

Thus when controlled hypotension was required during neurosurgery, a lower dosage of the hypotensive anaesthetic isoflurane was needed when the HANS device (TEAS) was used in addition to standard anaesthetics, and the same device reduced BP, although not significantly, in another study, with 2/100 Hz DD applied bilaterally at ST-36 and GB-34. HANS also reduced BP during thyroid surgery with or without sympathetic inhibition by means of cervical plexus block, with mean arterial pressure (MAP) depressed more following the combined treatment than with HANS alone.

Neither auricular EA nor segmental TENS appeared to inhibit the BP increase that accompanies laryngoscopy or intubation for abdominal surgery. However, in a RCT of LF TEAS at LI-4 and ST-36 combined with general anaesthesia for endoscopic laryngeal surgery, although systolic BP was higher in controls and TEAS patients *before* laryngoscopy, diastolic BP was significantly lower in TEAS than control patients, and postoperative increases in both diastolic and mean arterial pressures were significantly less in TEAS than control patients, with a lower requirement for antihypertensive medication.

## Heart rate during surgery and anaesthesia

There are many reports that HR changes relatively little during surgical AA or EAA, even in response to mobilisation of internal organs or in anxious patients. Because of this apparent stability of HR under EAA, it has been used when there is a risk of atrial fibrillation. In other studies, little difference was found between HR with MAA and general anaesthesia, or between combined EAA and epidural anaesthesia alone. Such different results might in part be due to variability in the effectiveness of the EAA itself. As indicated above, better analgesia correlates with less cardiovascular disturbance, and worse analgesia with greater changes in HR, ECG or stroke volume/cardiac output.

HF EA at P-6 has been used to regulate arrhythmia during gynaecological operations performed under epidural anaesthesia.

## The physical trauma of surgery

### PREOPERATIVE TREATMENT

With premeditated injury, it is possible to treat before a wound is inflicted. If skin temperature and blood flow increase in response to presurgical EA, this is usually, although not always, associated with more effective AA or EAA. Thus 1°C skin temperature increases in response to a preoperative test of AA have been associated with less pain during surgery, an 80% success rate as compared with only 35% if the temperature falls or remains unchanged.

## INTRAOPERATIVE TREATMENT (CHANGES OTHER THAN THOSE IN BP AND HR)

Cardiovascular changes during EAA for surgery have frequently been described, with claims that AA either interferes little or not at all with circulation, or that AA, and particularly EAA, has a regulatory or stabilising action both perioperatively and postoperatively. As with BP and HR, changes in central blood flow in the brain, as well as peripherally, may correlate with the degree of analgesia achieved. TENS may have similar effects.

Because of these effects, AA and EAA have often been used for patients with cardiovascular pathology. AA has also been considered to be appropriate for Caesarean section, as the blood supply to the fetus is regulated as well as that of the mother. Interestingly, there are reports of lessened bleeding during labour assisted by EAA.

During lengthy surgery under conventional anaesthesia, electrostimulation is sometimes used to prevent venous stasis. In patients with a high risk of thrombotic complications, EAA, combined with endotracheal nitrous oxide, has even been used instead of more conventional methods. As another variant, EA at SJ-8 has been used with the intention of inducing vasodilatation in patients undergoing cardiac surgery.

It has frequently been observed that AA, and EAA in particular, appears to reduce bleeding during many types of surgery compared with conventional anaesthesia, that EAA has fewer associated risks than conventional anaesthesia (aspiration of blood in tonsillectomy, for example), and that it regulates blood coagulation postoperatively.

In a number of reports, EAA is described as contributing to postoperative wound healing, even accelerating it. Others have suggested that healing occurs normally, but that less scar tissue is formed, or is formed more rapidly (with MAA). Wound healing was further improved by combining EAA with HeNe LA in one study of hysterectomy.

## Postoperative treatment

This is dealt with more fully in Chapter 9.14.

## SUMMARY

Some key points in this chapter are:

- EA and TENS/TEAS can be helpful for blood pressure disorders when used in combination with other interventions
- Although beneficial, they should not replace basic preventive measures
- They are less likely to be helpful if vascular structure is impaired
- They may be important in some heart conditions, such as angina and possibly some arrhythmias
- They may have a regulatory effect on cardiac activity and other aspects of circulation both during and after surgery.

### Additional material in the CD-ROM resource

In the CD-ROM resource, in addition to more information on the topics presented here, the following are also discussed:

- Circulation and its general effects:
  —Effects on the blood (anaemia, the haematoporphyrias); haemoirradiation
- Peripheral circulatory disorders:
  —Thoracic outlet syndrome
- The heart:
  —Circulation in other organs of the body, including the brain
- Circulation and healing:
  —Other types of wounds: anal fissures, Behçet's syndrome, non-healing spider bite, gangrene and tissue necrosis, gunshot wounds
  —The use of cold in soft tissue injury
  —Nerve and bone healing
- Surgery and the cardiovascular system:
  —The use of EAA in venous surgery.

**9.6** Summary of relevant studies in the electronic clinical studies database (number of studies)

| Condition | EA | Other |
|---|---|---|
| **BP – cholesterol – blood** | | |
| Hypertension | 24 | 114 |
| Hypotension | 1 | 8 |
| Cholesterol and other blood lipids | 3 | 5 |
| Anaemia | 2 | 3 |
| Haematoporphyria | 1 | 1 |
| Other | 1 | 4 |
| **Coronary disease (angina)** | | |
| Angina | 24 | 79 |
| **Other cardiac conditions** | | |
| Cardiomyopathy and valvular heart disease | 5 | 10 |
| Arrhythmia | 8 | 10 |
| Other | 3 | 7 |
| **Cerebral circulation** | 5 | 23 |
| **Peripheral circulation** | | |
| Ulceration | 6 | 43 |
| Peripheral ischaemia | 12 | 51 |
| Scleroderma (systemic or localised) | 7 | 6 |
| Varicose veins and haemorrhoids | 0 | 7 |
| Peripheral circulation: other studies | 6 | 9 |
| Neurocirculatory dystonia | 4 | 3 |
| Postoperative circulatory problems | 1 | 7 |
| **Tissue repair (other)** | | |
| Tissue repair for burns, scalds and other conditions | 4 | 9 |
| Haemorrhage, bruises and haematomas | 0 | 1 |

# RECOMMENDED READING

*A general review:*
Smith FWK Jr Acupuncture for cardiovascular disorders. Problems in Veterinary Medicine. 1992 March; 4(1): 125–31

*Something a little more technical:*
Lundeberg T 1999 Effects of sensory stimulation (acupuncture) on circulatory and immune systems. In: Ernst E, White AR (eds) Acupuncture: a scientific appraisal. Butterworth-Heinemann, Oxford, 93–106

*Two unusual applications:*
Wang WC, George SL, Wilimas JA Transcutaneous electrical nerve stimulation treatment of sickle cell pain crises. Acta Haematologica. 1988; 80(2): 99–102
Kaada B, Emru M Promoted healing of leprous ulcers by transcutaneous nerve stimulation. Acupuncture and Electro-therapeutics Research. 1988; 13(4): 165–76

*A different approach again:*
Sumano H, Mateos G The use of acupuncture-like electrical stimulation for wound healing of lesions unresponsive to conventional treatment. American Journal of Acupuncture. 1999; 27(1–2): 5–14

*A useful discussion of this condition and its treatment with acupuncture:*
Raut C Successful treatment of thrombophlebitis by acupuncture. American Journal of Acupuncture. 1984 July–Sept; 12(3): 245–9

# 9.7 THE RESPIRATORY SYSTEM

*Josephine Cerqua and David F Mayor*

In this subchapter, respiratory diseases are discussed under the headings of asthma, upper respiratory tract infection, acute bronchitis, pneumonia and pleurisy, chronic obstructive pulmonary disease (COPD), tuberculosis, hyperventilation and lung cancer. Lung surgery and the respiratory effects of surgery in general are considered in brief. Sinusitis, rhinitis, tonsillitis and laryngitis are covered elsewhere.

## ASTHMA

Asthma is characterised by airway hyperresponsiveness, with periodic attacks of wheezing, dyspnoea and a productive cough. Atopic (extrinsic) asthma, common in children, is mediated by immunoglobulins (IgE) and is exacerbated by a variety of environmental agents including foods, house dust mites, cockroaches, animal dander, mould and pollens. Non-atopic asthma does not appear to be immunologically mediated and is associated with an inflammatory response to endotoxins produced by bacteria in the upper or lower respiratory tract, with symptoms mostly occurring in the fourth decade of life. Non-atopic (intrinsic) asthma is almost always chronic, tends to be more severe, and usually needs more aggressive treatment.

Factors that trigger an episode of asthma, which can also include cold, exercise and emotional stress, do so by causing obstruction to the air flow through bronchospasm (autonomically mediated) and an inflammatory reaction (vascular), with oedema of the bronchi and mucous exudation. In an acute attack, air flow decreases and airway resistance increases, but inspiration will be close to total lung capacity.

Western medical treatment of asthma is targeted at prevention (avoiding allergens, if known) and controlling symptoms with bronchodilators and anti-inflammatory medication. New classes of drugs, such as leukotriene receptor antagonists, may be effective against exercise- and allergen-induced bronchoconstriction, and aspirin-sensitive asthma. Side-effects of bronchodilators include nausea, abdominal pain, headache, tremor, insomnia, palpitations, convulsions and cardiac arrhythmias.

In traditional Chinese medicine (TCM), asthma has traditionally been treated with acupuncture and is symptomatically divided into wheezing (*xiao*) and dyspnoea (*chuan*). *Xiao* refers to the sound, whereas *chuan* refers to the difficulty in breathing. Both of these occur simultaneously and arise from the same mechanism so they may be jointly described as one disease entity: asthma (*xiao chuan*). This is the result of 'hidden Phlegm' stored in the Lungs. Accumulation of Phlegm and body fluids blocks the passage of *qi* in the Lungs.

The Liver is believed to be particularly involved in the development of intrinsic asthma. The upward movement of Phlegm propelled by rebellious *qi* narrows the airways and causes wheezing. At root, the condition may be Empty, despite the symptoms of Fullness.

A number of systematic reviews of acupuncture have included studies on asthma, although the general opinion is that trials to date are commonly of poor quality and give contradictory results, or that, although there may be significant improvement subjectively, changes in objective measures are only moderate. Clinical studies on asthma have reported the use of manual acupuncture (MA), electroacupuncture (EA), transcutaneous electrical acupoint stimulation (TEAS), laser acupuncture (LA) and various other acupuncture modalities.

MA was shown to have a weak and short-lived bronchodilatory effect in one brief uncontrolled study of bronchial asthma. A single session of MA did apparently provide better protection than placebo MA against exercise-induced asthma, and single-session MA also decreased total respiratory resistance more than placebo in a study of acute asthma. However, MA had no effect on response to cold air challenge in a further controlled trial on patients with mild asthma.

EA has been less frequently used for asthma than MA, but there is still a considerable literature on the subject, although most studies are small and uncontrolled. In one such study, for example, spirographic indicators improved along with clinical improvement in 90% of study participants. In another uncontrolled study, extrinsic asthma responded better to EA than intrinsic asthma, with poorer results in cortisone-dependent patients. In an uncontrolled TCM-based report, immediate improvement was found to be more likely in Cold-type (chronic, allergic) bronchial asthma than in Heat-type (acute, infectious) asthma. Auricular EA may be more effective for mild than severe bronchial asthma. However, EA alone, simply at bilateral auricular Lung points, can sometimes be of benefit for status asthmaticus.

As with MA, some of the studies giving positive results have used extended courses of EA. In one, maximum response was not attained until patients had received ~17.5 sessions.

**Combinations and comparisons** Acupuncture and its variants are best combined with other interventions when treating asthma. In one study, MA at body or ear points greatly increased the effectiveness of desensitisation treatment, whereas a combination of MA at body points, desensitisation and the use of sodium cromoglicate gave even better results.

EA was only marginally superior to superficial MA in one Western randomised controlled trial (RCT). However, experimental research indicates that combining EA, but not MA, with a bronchodilator may be useful.

**Points used** Specific acupuncture points may be used for their ability to provide bronchodilation and improve the body's immunity. In EA studies, the most commonly used points for asthma include BL-13, LI-4, LI-11, ST-36, Ren-17, Ren-22, Du-20, *dingchuan* (M-BW-1) and the auricular Lung points. The manual for one popular EA device shortens this list to BL-13, Ren-22 and Du-14, with the addition of BL-17. Other manuals suggest LU-5 and ST-40 as well. In MA studies, BL-17, LU-7 and Du-14 are also greatly used, but LI-11, Ren-17 and Ren-22 less so. KI-3, which has been claimed to be useful for inspiratory dyspnoea, is sometimes employed, but rarely with EA. EA at LU-6 and LU-10 has been investigated for acute asthma.

Some reviewers consider that use of standard formulae for treating asthma may give suboptimal results. From a TCM point of view, different points will of course be appropriate at different times – points with very specific actions during a full-blown acute asthmatic episode, points with a more general action between attacks, when treating a background deficiency condition is more likely.

In one interesting report on patients with both soreness in the neck and shortness of breath, MA inactivation of trigger points in the levator scapulae muscles (between C4 and the vertebral border of the scapula) led to immediate improvements in both symptoms. Subjective shortness of breath may not be symptomatic of bronchial asthma, but a concomitant of myofascial pain.

**Parameters used** Both low-frequency (LF) and high-frequency (HF) EA, as well as LF/HF dense-disperse (DD) EA, have been used in the treatment of asthma, with a possible preponderance of HF stimulation. Intermittent HF (10–50 Hz) stimulation has also been recommended, with 3 Hz (at body points) or 100–150 Hz (at ear points) in between attacks. Others have suggested 10–20 Hz for auricular stimulation. Although some studies clearly used strong stimulation ('to tolerance'), in others only low motor level intensity was employed.

Studies with more positive outcomes appear to have involved longer periods of therapy, or at least repeated 10-session courses. One reviewer, for example, considers 15 sessions 'essential', preferably followed by monthly maintenance treatments. As a rule of thumb, brief intensive treatment may be appropriate for acute, recent onset asthma, and long-term and more gentle interventions when this has become chronic. As for the length of individual sessions, 40 minutes of EA may improve small airway function more than either 20 or 60 minute treatments.

## UPPER RESPIRATORY TRACT INFECTION

Upper respiratory tract infections include infectious rhinitis (the common cold) and influenza. Incubation period is 48–72 hours, with infectivity to others peaking with symptoms at 3-5 days. Symptoms are sneezing, nasal congestion and discharge, sore throat, burning watery eyes, dry cough, muscle aches, fever and malaise. Many variants of acupuncture, including EA and LA, have been used for upper respiratory tract infections.

**Points used** Traditionally, moxibustion is applied at points such as BL-12, LI-4 and Du-14 as prophylaxis against upper respiratory tract infections. Back *shu* points in general have been used with mild moxibustion to improve resistance to recurrent respiratory tract infections in children, and also with sliding cupping during the infection itself (also over Governor Vessel points). More specifically, BL-17 EA has been recommended for colds and infections.

## ACUTE BRONCHITIS, PNEUMONIA AND PLEURISY

Acute bronchitis is usually marked by fever, dyspnoea and coughing (with chest pain). It may be due to infection, inhalation of dust or fumes, or exposure to cold. There are surprisingly few studies on the treatment of acute bronchitis with EA and MA, although MA has been used for dust bronchitis.

Pneumonia, or inflammation of the lungs, comes in many forms. As with acute bronchitis, MA and EA seem to have been less used than LA for pneumonia.

In pleurisy, the pleura, or linings surrounding the lungs, become inflamed, with exudation into the cavity between them. EA has been investigated for its effects on experimental pleurisy. In studies exploring the effects of different parameters and points, local (dermatome or myotome) stimulation gave best results, with auricular points also being useful, especially at 10/60 Hz DD EA.

## CHRONIC COUGH

Chronic or persistent cough, even if not associated with infection, can be irritating and debilitating. MA at Ren-17, with LU-7 and LI-4, has been used for this problem.

Dryness of the upper respiratory tract has been considered to be a sign of electrical hypersensitivity. If this is so, EA or other such treatments should be considered cautiously.

## CHRONIC OBSTRUCTIVE PULMONARY DISEASE (COPD)

COPD is defined as pulmonary disease (emphysema or chronic bronchitis) characterised by chronic typically irreversible airway obstruction resulting in a slowed rate of exhalation. Risk factors include smoking and exposure to smoke, occupational pollutants, family history, low social class, recurrent respiratory infections, and protease deficiencies. Childhood bronchial hyperreactivity may be a predisposing factor.

Prevalence, incidence and mortality rates of COPD increase with age. The most common form of COPD is a combination of chronic bronchitis and emphysema that causes loss of lung function. It occurs mostly after the age of 40 years and affects twice as many men as women. COPD causes pulmonary hypertension, with a resultant strain on and enlargement of the right heart (*cor pulmonale*), pulmonary hypertension and swelling of the legs and ankles (oedema).

Acupuncture appears to be used rather more frequently for chronic bronchitis than for acute pulmonary problems. Thus, in one review of 10 years of research, there were over 60 studies on the acupuncture treatment of chronic bronchitis. Methods included MA, EA, moxibustion, point pressure and point injection; 18 400 cases were included, with a reported effective cure rate of 70–97%. Steroid-dependent patients were noted to improve less.

MA has been reported to have an immunoregulatory influence in patients suffering from chronic bronchitis and undergoing long-term treatment with corticosteroids. In one small RCT for COPD, subjective clinical response was better in the real MA than sham MA group, although objective measures remained unchanged. In another small placebo-controlled RCT, this time with a no-treatment control group, results on some measures were better with MA than sham, comparable to those reported with inhaled steroids, and superior to results in other studies using drastic surgical measures. Treatment had a large impact on quality of life, with both MA and sham groups wanting to continue despite initial scepticism.

In one controlled study ($N = 1493$), EA gave better results than medication. Uncontrolled studies are fairly positive, with improvements in some immune parameters, and in both large and small airway function, for example.

**Points used** For acute bronchitis and pneumonia, the most used points are BL-13, Ren-17, Ren-22, Du-14 and *dingchuan* (M-BW-1), with points such as BL-12, Lung meridian points, ST-36 and others often as adjuncts. LU-5, LU-7, LI-4 and *dingchuan* (M-BW-1) with moderate to strong DD are recommended in one EA device manual.

For chronic bronchitis, BL-13, LI-4, ST-36, Ren-17, Ren-22, Du-13, Du-14, *huatuojiaji* points and *dingchuan* are most commonly used, with further points such as BL-17, LU-9, LI-11, ST-40 and Ren-1 added according to TCM principles.

**Parameters used** Most EA studies appear to use HF (~80Hz) stimulation, and low frequencies less commonly. However, the authors of one case report found DD and intermittent stimulation to be most suitable for emphysema. As for intensity, these same authors followed traditional guidelines in using gentler stimulation for older or weaker patients. One manufacturer recommends moderate to strong DD for acute bronchitis, but only moderate DD when this is chronic.

# PULMONARY TUBERCULOSIS (TB)

The airborne tubercle bacillus that causes tuberculosis (TB) mostly affects the lungs, but may spread to other areas (such as the kidney or spinal column) from local lesions or by way of the lymph or blood vessels. Symptoms are variable, but include cough with shortness of breath (particularly on effort), bloody sputum (haemoptysis), severe fatigue and loss of appetite, sometimes with fever and drenching night sweats. The infection leads to inflammation in the lungs, with the formation of readily spreading caseous (cheese-like) necrosis and areas of fibrosis. The most commonly used 'first-line' drugs for the treatment of TB in developed countries are rifampicin, isoniazid, pyrazinamide and ethambutol.

MA in combination with medication has been used for supraventricular tachycardia and other problems when associated with TB. Haemoptysis in patients with TB appears to respond to EA.

**Points used** EA at LU-6 and P-6 (but not LU-5 and P-3) reduces haemoptysis due to TB.

# BREATHING AND CONSCIOUSNESS: HYPERVENTILATION AND HYPOXIA

In hyperventilation ('respiratory neurosis'), breathing rate and depth increase, reducing the carbon dioxide content of inhaled air and blood (hypocapnia). Symptoms include a feeling of panic, suffocation and tightness of the chest. The heart rate speeds up, and things begin to feel unreal. Blood pressure falls, and fainting is not uncommon. The usual solution is to ask the patient to breathe into a brown paper bag, both to restore carbon dioxide levels in lungs and blood and to demonstrate that the symptoms are reversible.

MA has been found helpful for hyperventilation, with normalising effects on the EEG as well as respiratory parameters and subjective symptoms.

At high altitudes, oxygen intake is reduced and hypoxia can occur. In those who are not acclimatised, symptoms can include shortness of breath on exertion, headache, dizziness, difficulty in concentrating, sometimes euphoria or delirium, palpitations and nausea (hence 'mountain sickness').

Experimentally, MA at points such as ST-9 and Du-26 has been used to counter such symptoms in animals under general anaesthesia. Du-26 EA also increases oxygen perfusion in the brain. Auricular EA has been investigated for its effects on cardiac arrhythmias at mid-altitudes (2100 metres). EA at ST-36 with P-6 may marginally decrease oxygen consumption and carbon dioxide production.

# LUNG CANCER

Atmospheric pollution and industrial exposure to dusts, particularly asbestos, have increased the incidence of lung cancer, but the dominant cause is tobacco smoke. Symptoms include cough, haemoptysis, breathlessness, wheezing, chest pain, persistent respiratory infection and stridor (a high-pitched breathing sound, also found in laryngeal obstruction).

MA has been used for cancer-related breathlessness. DC stimulation of needles directly inserted into pulmonary tumours has also been used for middle and late stage lung cancer unresponsive to conventional methods. Combining this approach with TCHM gave better results than either modality separately.

# SURGERY AND RESPIRATION

Acupuncture for surgical analgesia (acupuncture analgesia, AA) is most effective for head, neck and chest surgery. Thus it has often been used for cardiothoracic surgery, even without endotracheal intubation.

Nowadays, AA is commonly combined with medication (in 'acupuncture balanced analgesia'), and so intubation is more likely, enabling control of respiratory rate by the anaesthetist. Thus EAA has often been combined with endotracheal anaesthesia, usually with artificial respiration. Using this combined method, extubation can be carried out much sooner than with general anaesthesia alone, and respiratory parameters recover more rapidly. For longer operations such as pulmonary resection, some anaesthetists prefer MAA, believing that electrical stimulation over a long period may result in tolerance and reduced effectiveness.

In one controlled study, bronchoscopy was easier to carry out under AA than conventional anaesthesia, enabling a more accurate diagnosis. In keeping with this, EEG monitoring during AA for lung lobectomy indicated that patients were awake but relaxed during all but the most painful phases of the operation, and that recovery was more rapid than with the deep unconsiousness induced by conventional anaesthesia. EAA may also reduce the likelihood of adverse haemodynamic reactions and respiratory effects during surgery.

**Points used** In one review of AA for pulmonary resection, points such as SI-3, BL-65, KI-3, P-4, P-6, SJ-6, GB-41, LIV-3, LU-10, LI-4, ST-43 and SP-3 were used, bilaterally if the operation crossed the midline, and unilaterally if not. In a comprehensive European 1978 textbook on AA, KI-22, P-6, GB-24, LU-1, LU-2, ST-36 and SP-6 were recommended for thoracic surgery. Simpler protocols were developed in China, using just one or two points, such as P-4 through to SJ-8 alone for thoracotomy, or just LI-14 or the scalp thoracic area for pulmonary resection. The most commonly employed body points are P-4, P-6, SJ-8 and LI-4 (others include LI-10, LI-18, SP-20 and *xiayifeng*, 2 *fen* below SJ-17). Lung and *shenmen* are the most used auricular points for thoracic surgery, with others such as Heart, Kidney and Trachea also in evidence.

**Parameters used** A wide range of EAA frequencies has been used in thoracic surgery, with clusters around 15 and 50 Hz, as well as higher and lower frequencies. In one study, HF was used prior to the initial incision, then reduced. Amplitudes also vary (from around 10 to 50 mA).

In one report, higher currents (up to 28 mA) were used for adults and lower ones (10 mA) for children. Given the possibility of tolerance during long operations, EAA during pulmonary resection would probably best be applied with non-constant parameters (such as DD, or other combinations of different frequencies and/or amplitudes).

## Postoperative respiration

Pain following thoracic or abdominal surgery can inhibit respiration and lead to further complications. Many conventional analgesic methods are employed in this situation, although a number of drugs, particularly opiates, may themselves depress respiratory function. MA and EA have been explored too, with EA superior to standard care in two studies. As with AA during operations, MA may be more helpful for pain following thoracic than abdominal surgery. Interestingly, while EA (at ST-36 and SP-6) was found experimentally to improve intestinal peristalsis inhibited by intrathecally injected morphine, it did not appear to improve respiration depressed by the drug.

**Precautions when treating respiratory conditions**

One of the commonest adverse effects of acupuncture is pneumothorax: puncture of the pleural cavity so that air can enter it. Signs may include sudden or delayed respiratory distress, tachycardia, hypotension, tracheal deviation to the contralateral side, and neck vein distension. Pneumothorax is more likely in those whose build is slight, in the elderly and in those with a long history of respiratory illness. Best practice is to avoid deep near-perpendicular needling at any point where pneumothorax is at all possible.

# SUMMARY

Some key points from this chapter are:

- Many studies report positive results for respiratory conditions, particularly asthma, with MA being used more frequently than EA
- Acupuncture and its variants appear to be most effective for asthma when combined with other forms of treatment
- Better outcomes for the acupuncture treatment of asthma are almost always associated with extended periods of treatment
- Acupuncture is used more for the treatment of chronic than acute bronchitis
- Rigorous research is ambivalent on whether EA and associated modalities have more than a peripheral role to play in the treatment of respiratory disorders.

## Additional material in the CD-ROM resource

In the CD-ROM resource, in addition to further information on many of the topics presented here, the following conditions are mentioned:

- Complementary and alternative medicine (CAM) and asthma
- Immunoregulatory and neurochemical effects of acupuncture for asthma
- Heart and lung: pulmonary heart disease
- Cystic fibrosis
- Respiratory arrest, asphyxia, sleep apnoea and snoring.

**9.7** Summary of relevant studies in the electronic clinical studies database (number of studies)

| Condition | EA | Other |
|---|---|---|
| **Asthma** | 15 | 114 |
| **Other lung conditions** | | |
| Tuberculosis | 3 | 8 |
| Acute bronchitis and other acute respiratory conditions | 3 | 30 |
| Chronic obstructive pulmonary disease (COPD) | 10 | 36 |
| Cancer and other chronic disorders | 1 | 7 |
| Respiratory arrest, sleep apnoea, hyperventilation | 9 | 2 |
| Mixed respiratory conditions | 0 | 4 |

# RECOMMENDED READING

*Two very different reviews of acupuncture for asthma:*

Jobst KA Acupuncture in asthma and pulmonary disease: an analysis of efficacy and safety. Journal of Alternative and Complementary Medicine. 1996 Spring; 2(1): 179–206

Martin J, Donaldson AN, Villarroel R, Parmar MK, Ernst E, Higginson IJ Efficacy of acupuncture in asthma: systematic review and meta-analysis of published data from 11 randomised controlled trials. European Respiratory Journal. 2002 Oct; 20(4): 846–52

*Three very different studies:*

*This MA study demonstrates short-term effectiveness when stimulating non-acupoints:*

Luu M, Maillard D, Pradalier A, Boureau F [Spirometric monitoring of the effects of puncturing thoracic pain points in asthmatic disease]. Respiration. 1985; 48(4): 340–5

*The use of auricular EA for severe asthma:*

Wen HL, Chau K. Status asthmaticus treated by acupuncture and electro-stimulation. Asian Journal of Medicine. 1973; 9: 191–5

*An unusual form of modified EA involving a family member in treatment:*

Zhu SS Successful treatment of sleep apnea syndrome by transfusion of "vital energy". Chinese Medical Journal. 1980 April; 93(4): 279–80

# 9.8 THE GASTROINTESTINAL SYSTEM, LIVER, GALL BLADDER AND PANCREAS

*David F Mayor and Lyndsey A Taylor*

Electroacupuncture (EA) and other non-traditional acupuncture modalities have been used for many gastrointestinal (GI), liver and gall bladder conditions, particularly peptic ulcer, nausea and vomiting.

## THE OESOPHAGUS

### Reflux oesophagitis

Reflux oesophagitis is caused by frequent regurgitation of stomach acid and peptic juices. The main symptoms are heartburn, regurgitation of bitter fluids and occasional difficulty with swallowing. Western medical (WM) treatment includes antacid medication, reduction of smoking and coffee intake, weight loss and oesophageal dilatation or surgery.

In traditional Chinese medicine (TCM), reflux oesophagitis may involve the Stomach, Spleen and Liver. Typical disharmonies are Liver *qi* invading the Stomach, Stomach and Liver heat, Stomach and Liver *yin* deficiency, and Spleen deficiency, often associated with Phlegm.

In addition to EA, methods such as small-diameter probe stimulation of acupoints (pTENS), LA (laser acupuncture) and microwave resonance therapy (MRT) have been used for this condition.

**Points used** Points such as P-6, SJ-5, LI-4, ST-36 and SP-6 (EA) and P-5, ST-25, Ren-13, Ren-14 and Ren-21 (LA) have been used for gastro-oesophageal reflux.

### Nausea and vomiting

There is substantial evidence that acupuncture is an effective treatment for nausea and vomiting. It has been used for postoperative nausea and vomiting (PONV), morning sickness during pregnancy, motion sickness and in chemotherapy. WM treatment for nausea and emesis is based on antiemetic medication, although this is not always effective.

In TCM, nausea and emesis are related to rebellious Stomach *qi* and may be due to a number of disharmonies, such as invasion by pathogenic factors (Cold, Damp, Heat, Wind), or deficiency of Stomach and Spleen *qi*, *yin* and *yang*.

#### POSTOPERATIVE NAUSEA AND VOMITING
The most common and distressing symptoms following general anaesthesia and surgery are pain and emesis.

Standard treatment for PONV is drug based, and many anaesthetists routinely administer antiemetics to all patients. However, these drugs themselves often have central nervous system (CNS) side-effects, so that any way of reducing their dosage can contribute to postoperative recovery.

There are more randomised controlled trials (RCTs) on PONV than for any other application of acupuncture except stroke. Both manual acupuncture (MA) and EA have been compared with standard antiemetic medication. In at least two P-6 EA studies, effects were equivalent, and in a further one, P-6 EA appeared to give better results than ondansetron at an early stage in the trial. With no side-effects, P-6 MA, LA and acupressure may thus represent good alternatives to the pharmacological prophylaxis and treatment of PONV.

P-6 TEAS (transcutaneous electrical acupoint stimulation) has frequently been used for postoperative emesis after many different types of surgery. For *established* PONV, combining TEAS with antiemetic medication may be more effective than TEAS alone.

**The timing of treatment** Some local and general anaesthetics may reduce the effectiveness of electrostimulation and MA. AA, acupuncture analgesia *during* surgery, has been found to reduce postoperative vomiting, presumably in part because it significantly reduces requirements for opioids. P-6 EA, started before the induction of anaesthesia and continued through surgery, may reduce postoperative pain. In contrast, if P-6 stimulation is started during drug anaesthesia, it may well not be effective. Thus John Dundee's group recommended that P-6 EA be started even before premedication, not just before induction of anaesthesia (60–90 minutes later), particularly if opioid preanaesthetic medication is used.

However, effects may vary, depending on the type of anaesthetic employed. In one study, MA was still effective when given after induction of anaesthesia, but before the start of surgery or administration of morphine. Dundee's group concluded that P-6 EA is prophylactic rather than a means of treating established sickness.

The effect of a single session of P-6 electrostimulation on PONV appears to last about 6–8 hours. Thus treatment needs to be repeated, or effects prolonged by, for example, the use of P-6 acupressure.

#### CHEMOTHERAPY-INDUCED NAUSEA AND VOMITING
A well-known side-effect of chemotherapy is constant nausea and emesis. This chemotherapy-induced nausea and vomiting (CINV) has been treated with acupuncture-based methods. Although MA has been used, there are probably

more studies on EA for this problem, most being from John Dundee's group. In a more recent report, by Joannie Shen and colleagues, low-frequency (LF) EA was applied at ST-36 in addition to P-6, with no difference between true EA and minimal stimulation (no EA) in terms of the total number of emesis episodes experienced over 5 days. However, all patients were already on an antiemetic cocktail, which may have lessened intergroup differences.

P-6 TEAS, as a non-invasive alternative to EA, has been explored by John Dundee's group as well as others (using the ReliefBand® device). The overall conclusion appears to be that P-6 electrostimulation is useful, especially as an adjunct to conventional drug therapy.

### MOTION SICKNESS

Acupressure (usually 'Sea Bands') on P-6 has frequently been used prophylactically for motion sickness. P-6 TEAS, however, may be more effective, at least in suppressing nausea. TEAS has also been tested, with positive results, in a small crossover study of subjects in a small boat on the open sea. The watch-like 'ReliefBand®' device used incorporates two small surface electrodes that are positioned at P-6. The 32 Hz biphasic output current can be increased up to 60 mA.

**Comparisons and combinations** MA and EA at P-6 are both effective for PONV. Similarly, both EA and TEAS at P-6 appear effective, although the benefits of the invasive treatment may be greater, and last longer. For cancer chemotherapy, EA is more effective than minimal MA, and also more effective than TEAS.

**Points used** Traditionally, points such as BL-20, BL-21, P-6, LIV-3, LI-4, ST-21, ST-25, ST-36, SP-4 (for dyspepsia) and Ren-12 or Ren-13 (for gastric fullness) have been used for nausea and vomiting, with additional points such as HE-7 for anxiety, or Du-20. The auricular points Liver, Stomach, Sympathetic and *shenmen* have also been suggested. Other points have included KI-20, KI-21, ST-19, ST-20, ST-40, Ren-10, Ren-11 and Ren-14 (MA for morning sickness), and BL-18 to BL-24 or BL-20 to BL-26 (intradermal needling for upper and lower abdominal surgery, respectively). Experimentally, ST-36 EA has been found to reduce both duration and frequency of induced vomiting.

Further points used include KI-5, ST-37 (EA for PONV), LIV-13, LI-1, LI-11, SP-5, SP-6, SP-10 and SP-16 (LA for chemotherapy-induced nausea), or BL-10, BL-11 and GB-34 (acuplaster application following strabismus surgery). In ryodoraku, reactive electropermeable points (REPP) on the back have been used for nausea, without reference to particular meridians.

However, by far and away the most frequently used point used for antiemesis is P-6. John Dundee's group found that P-6 EA was superior to sham point EA for nausea, and also that results with P-6 stimulation may be marginally better if this is carried out on the subject's dominant arm. As George Lewith has pointed out several times, P-6 antiemesis

appears to be acupoint specific. ST-36 and then LI-4 are the next most frequently used points.

**Parameters used** One manufacturer (CEFAR Medical) has provided a programme specifically for nausea treatment (10 Hz, 180 μs) in some of their EA and transcutaneous electrical nerve stimulation (TENS) products. Dundee's group suggests that comfortable LF stimulation (10–15 Hz, usually 10 Hz) may be more effective than high frequency (HF, 100 or 1000 Hz), but this is not unequivocally supported by other studies. Thus the author of one pocketbook on TENS, although aware of Dundee's protocol of 10–15 Hz TEAS for 5 minutes every 2 hours, prefers 100 Hz 200 μs burst TEAS for up to an hour every 2 hours (cathode to P-6, anode to return).

However, 'inappropriately high' (or long) levels of P-6 stimulation may actually increase nausea and vomiting. Dundee's group found, for instance, that 5 minutes of 10 Hz EA gave a better result than EA for 15 minutes (or even 1 kHz for 5 minutes). For PONV, others have treated for the duration of surgery (starting prior to premedication or induction of anaesthesia, and often continuing after waking), or continuously for 7 days for CINV (in one TENS study beginning 2 hours before chemotherapy).

It is possible that different parameters may be helpful for different types of nausea. The TEAS ReliefBand® has been set at around 8 Hz for chemotherapy-induced nausea, but at 32 Hz for motion sickness, for example.

In one EA device manual, moderate to strong dense-disperse (DD) stimulation is recommended for vomiting (at P-6, LIV-3, ST-36, Ren-12); 2/100 Hz DD EA at P-6 (at a 'comfortably tolerated' level, instigated 20 minutes before induction of anaesthesia) was found not only to reduce PONV but also appeared to reduce pain following major breast surgery. Conversely, DD EA (at a wider selection of points) for postoperative pain was reported to have beneficial effects on PONV.

## THE STOMACH

### Gastric pain

Gastric pain (gastralgia) is frequently treated with acupuncture, both MA and EA.

**Points used** BL-21, P-6, LI-4, ST-36, SP-6 and Ren-12 have been suggested when using EA for gastric pain. GB-34 was combined with BL-21 in one MA study.

**Parameters used** Moderate HF or DD is suggested in one EA device manual.

### Gastric function and electrical activity

Acupuncture, both MA and EA, is well known as having a regulatory effect on stomach function. In healthy volunteers, for example, 2 Hz ST-36 EA may normalise gastric activity, whereas 8 Hz ST-36 EA tends to do so in peptic ulcer patients. ST-36 TEAS may enhance gastric myoelectrical regularity in healthy subjects.

Clinically, EA has been used as part of a comprehensive approach to stimulate (regulate) gastric motility in patients with pyloroduodenal stenosis.

Gastroelectrical activity is also affected by moxibustion, LA and 'magnetic needling'.

**Comparisons** Both ST-36 EA and TEAS similarly enhance gastric myoelectrical regularity in healthy subjects.

**Points used** The main acupoint utilised in studies on gastric motility and electrical activity is ST-36. Points such as ST-2 and ST-44 have also been studied. The 'Hunger' point on the tragus of the ear can also slow gastric peristalsis. Even electrostimulation of points on the Small Intestine, Liver and Spleen meridians will affect the electrogastrogram (EGG).

**Parameters used** Simple but elegant research has shown that 2 Hz but not 100 Hz EA at ST-36 can normalise the EGG in healthy subjects. However, gastrointestinal electrical activity is affected by stimulation at both 1 Hz and 28 GHz.

## Gastric acidity

Experimentally, and in patients with peptic ulcers or chronic superficial gastritis, acupuncture has been found to regulate or reduce stomach acidity. In one MA study, points on the Stomach and Spleen meridians inhibited gastric acid output more than points on other meridians.

ST-34 EA reduced acidity in obese patients in one study. EA at P-6, SP-6 and Ren-12 reduced stomach acidity and serum gastrin levels in patients with gastritis.

## Gastritis

Gastritis, or inflammation of the gastric mucosa, can be acute or chronic. In acute gastritis, there is superficial erosion of the surface epithelium, generally due to drugs, chemicals or *Helicobacter pylori* bacteria leading to epigastric tenderness and haematemesis. Chronic or atrophic gastritis generally occurs more with age and increased thinning and degeneration of the mucosal wall. Symptoms may include anorexia, nausea and vomiting, fullness and epigastric pain.

In TCM, gastritis may be viewed in terms of a number of disharmonies of the Stomach, Spleen and Liver, involving Cold, Heat, Phlegm, Damp and Blood, with deficiency of *qi*, *yang* or *yin*.

MA and EA have been used in the treatment of gastritis, and 'electrical heat acupuncture' for chronic superficial gastritis associated with Spleen *yang* deficiency.

**Comparisons** In experimental studies, LILT and MA were found to be less effective than both 3 Hz EA (at BL-21, ST-36, Ren-12) and 5 Hz TENS in reducing gastric acidity levels.

**Points used** In one controlled study, ST-36, Ren-12 and Ren-13 gave good results for gastritis. In another, P-6 and SP-6 were used in chronic superficial gastritis (with a better effect on gastroelectric activity when used together). Experimentally, the combination of ST-36 and ST-37 has been utilised, while clinically ST-36 alone has been used to protect gastrointestinal function against the adverse effects of chemotherapy. BL-20, BL-21 and LI-4 have been used in other gastritis studies. Other suggested points for EA include LI-11, ST-25, SP-9 and Ren-4, depending on TCM differentiation.

**Parameters used** In one controlled study, strong 10–20 Hz EA gave good results for gastritis. Low-frequency, high-intensity EA (conventional EA, CEA) has also been used. One manufacturer recommends 'continuous' stimulation (frequency unspecified). Experimentally, 2/15 Hz DD was found to have a protective action on gastric mucosa.

## Peptic ulcer disease

Ulceration in the stomach (gastric ulcer) or duodenum (duodenal ulcer) is known as peptic ulcer. In gastric ulcer hyperacidity may not be a factor, whereas it often is in duodenal ulcer. WM treatment includes antacids, antibiotics and anticholinergic medication, or surgery.

TCM syndromes for peptic ulcer involve the Stomach, Spleen and Liver, with disharmonies of *qi*, Blood, *yin*, *yang*, Heat, Cold, Damp and Phlegm.

Acupuncture has long been considered helpful for the control of ulcer pain. It clearly also has a healing effect, and has been used even when the ulcer has perforated the gut wall. Clinical studies on EA and other forms of acupuncture have shown benefits for peptic ulcer. EA has also been used as part of a comprehensive approach to pyloroduodenal stenosis, the commonest complication of peptic ulceration.

There are many positive studies on the use of non-invasive acupoint MRT to accelerate ulcer repair, as well as reports on its use *pre-* and postoperatively in peptic ulcer patients, in whom immune function is enhanced as a result.

LA and LILT have also been used in treating peptic ulcer.

**Cautions**
- Local stimulation may not be appropriate if there is internal bleeding. Even distal stimulation (at points such as ST-36 and Du-26) may affect visceral circulation.
- Local heating can affect visceral circulation. Thus warmth applied to the epigastrium may cause a previously unsuspected ulcer to bleed.

**Points used** The main points for peptic ulcer disease include P-6, ST-21, ST-25, ST-36 and Ren-12. BL-20 and BL-21 (at the level of the sympathetic ganglia innervating the stomach) are also frequently used. Points for 'general adaptation' such as BL-10, GB-20 and Du-14 are sometimes employed, along with points such as BL-18, GB-34 and LIV-3, ST-20 and ST-44.

The auricular Stomach point is another possibility, with a greater effect on gastroelectric activity in ulcer patients than the auricular Heart point, for example.

**Parameters used** For EA treatment of peptic ulcer, strong stimulation tends to be used, at either LF or HF.

With MRT, frequencies are often selected individually from the 53.6–78.3 GHz range, on the basis of the patient's 'sensor response', with intensity in the region of 3 mW/cm². If a sensory reaction cannot be obtained, a fixed frequency may be used. Treatment is for 20–30 minutes (6–12 daily sessions).

## Gastroptosis

Downward displacement of the stomach in the abdomen was a diagnosis previously used in WM to explain various abdominal complaints. The main symptom is chronic regurgitation of undigested food.

In TCM, gastroptosis is associated with Spleen and Stomach *qi* or *yang* deficiency. EA has been used for gastroptosis, in one study giving better results than MA with intermittent needle manipulation.

**Points used** In EA studies, abdominal points such as KI-21, ST-23, Ren-6, Ren-12, *tiwei* (N-CA-10) and *weishangxue* (N-CA-18) have been used, with distal points such as P-6 or ST-36. An alternative approach could be to combine ST-36 EA with through needling from ST-21 to Ren-8.

In conjunction with ST-36 TEAS, local stimulation has also been suggested, over the upper and lower parts of the stomach.

**Parameters used** DD EA to tolerable intensity has been used. In line with this, one manufacturer recommends 'moderate' DD EA, both at abdominal points and at ST-36.

## Endoscopy and gastroscopy

Endoscopy can be both uncomfortable and distressing. Both MA and EA have been used clinically for gastroscopy, with EA in some studies giving results as good as those with sedative drugs. TENS has also been found experimentally to reduce the discomfort of gastric or duodenal distension.

**Points used** Points such as P-6, LI-4, ST-36, SP-5 and points on the Conception Vessel overlying the oesophagus (Ren-12, Ren-17, Ren-23, Ren-24) have been used.

**Parameters used** In one EA study, body points were stimulated at 12 Hz. In another, when ear points were used, stimulation was at 3–4 Hz.

## THE INTESTINES

Lower abdominal gastrointestinal pain may accompany adhesions or intestinal obstruction, appendicitis, dysentery and other infective disorders, and functional or inflammatory bowel conditions.

## Intestinal adhesions

WM treatment for adhesions is usually surgical, although adhesions are themselves frequently the result of poor healing following earlier operations.

In TCM, intestinal adhesion may be classified as due to Blood stagnation in the Intestines.

EA and audiofrequency TEAS have been used in the treatment of intestinal adhesions.

**Points used** Local points, at either end of visible scars, or either side of tender abdominal areas, have been used, together with points such as BL-21, P-6, LIV-3, ST-25, Ren-12 and Du-1, and different groups of auricular points.

**Parameters used** HF EA and audiofrequency TEAS have both been used for local scar tissue treatment.

## Paralytic ileus

MA, EA, TENS and ultrasound have been employed for paralytic ileus, a form of intestinal obstruction, following surgery.

**Points used** One authority has suggested that ST-36 and SP-6 are the main acupoints to use for paralytic ileus. Locally, ST-25 and Ren-6 have been used, and also the back *shu* point for the colon, BL-25, but in general distal points are stimulated, such as LIV-3, LI-4 and ST-37 in addition to ST-36 and SP-6, and sometimes P-6 or other points.

**Parameters used** Experimental research indicates that forceful stimulation may inhibit intestinal smooth muscle activity. Thus, for paralytic ileus, high intensities may be counterproductive.

## Appendicitis

Acute appendicitis presents with a discomfort around the umbilicus at first that then develops into more severe lower right quadrant pain.

In TCM, appendicitis may be diagnosed as Damp or toxic Heat of the Intestines and may also involve stagnation of *qi* and Blood.

Acupuncture has a long history in the treatment of acute appendicitis, with MA and EA being used, particularly for pain relief, but also to benefit immune function. Thus ryodoraku has been claimed to relieve appendicitis pain more effectively than conventional analgesics.

EA is often used for postoperative pain relief following appendectomy and TENS too has been used, although not always successfully.

**Points used** Local points such as ST-25 (~McBurney's point on the right, or Munro's point on the left) and SP-14 have been recommended.

Distal points such as ST-37 and *lanweixue* (M-LE-13) are also suggested.

*Lanweixue* has been used in LA and point injection studies, as well as EA.

Other points used include ST-36, with additional points for fever such as LI-4 and LI-11.

**Parameters used** In one EA device manual, moderate to strong DD is recommended, at both local and distal points.

## Constipation

Constipation can be symptomatic of many different conditions. WM treatment is related to the nature of the constipation and may include bulk supplements, stool softeners, laxatives, enemas and bowel retraining. Historically, there is also a tradition of electrotherapy being used for chronic constipation in the West.

In TCM, constipation may be classified into Excess and Deficiency types. Excess patterns are caused by the presence of the pathogens Heat or Phlegm and stagnation of *qi*. Deficiency patterns include *qi* and *yang xu*, leading to lack of digestive motility. Deficiency patterns such as deficiency of Liver and Kidney *yin*, *qi* and *yin* deficiency, and Blood deficiency, may be particularly evident in the elderly.

Acupuncture (MA and EA) may help constipation. There are many MA studies on the condition, including several on neurogenic constipation.

**Points used** In one Hong Kong textbook, DD EA at ST-29 and SP-15, alternating with Ren-5 and SJ-6, is recommended. Other local points for EA include ST-23, ST-25, SP-14, Ren-1 and Du-1.

Further points include BL-25, BL-32, P-6, ST-40 and SP-6, with others according to TCM differentiation. Additional points from MA studies include ST-28, ST-29 and ST-36.

It should not be forgotten that trigger points in paraspinal and abdominal muscles can contribute to constipation. Auricular points should also be considered.

**Parameters used** Willem Khoe used LF EA (at distal points GB-34 and LIV-1) for constipation. Other authors have suggested DD EA (at local and distal points). Intermittent, 10 Hz and HF stimulation have all been used.

## Diarrhoea

Causes of acute diarrhoea include infection, food poisoning or medication. Chronic diarrhoea may be symptomatic of many problems. WM treatment is dependent on the cause and includes medication and dietary review.

Excess patterns include Damp-Cold, Damp-Heat and Summer Heat, whereas deficiency patterns include Spleen *qi xu* and Kidney *yang xu*. A mixed pattern of Liver *qi* stagnation invading the Spleen is also common.

Clinically, acupuncture is frequently used for diarrhoea. Most studies appear to be on infantile diarrhoea or enteritis. Apart from MA (sometimes combined with moxibustion) and pTENS, LA and magnetic needling (or 'magnetic ball' needling) have been used, as have simple magnets, locally over the abdomen, and other methods.

**Points used** In MA studies, ST-25 and ST-36 are the main points used, with additional points such as SP-6, Ren-6 and Ren-12. In one EA device manual, BL-20, ST-25 and ST-36 are recommended for chronic diarrhoea. One EA study on neurogenic diarrhoea used BL-20, BL-25, P-6, ST-25, ST-37, ST-39, Ren-4 and Du-1, according to the TCM syndrome involved. In LA studies, again P-6, BL-20, ST-25, ST-36, ST-37, SP-6, Ren-4 and Ren-6 are used, but also Ren-8 and the extra 'enteritis' point *zhixie* (N-CA-3).

pTENS at ear points has been used for acute diarrhoea.

**Parameters used** Gut motility is decreased if sympathetic activity is increased. Thus strong brief local stimulation may be helpful for some diarrhoea, although DD at 'moderate' intensity has been recommended for chronic diarrhoea (locally, at ST-25, as well as at BL-25 and ST-36).

Strong LF auricular pTENS was beneficial in one report.

## Irritable bowel syndrome and intestinal spasm

Irritable bowel syndrome (IBS) is the commonest functional disorder of the digestive system in the West. Symptoms are classically those of altered bowel movements, pain and abdominal distension, but may include many other intestinal and abdominal disturbances. Pharmaceutical treatment is symptomatic and includes prokinetic medication, antidiarrhoeal and antispasmodic drugs, laxatives and antidepressants.

IBS has been treated with MA, EA, TENS/TEAS and LA.

**Points and parameters for IBS** The points for IBS are similar to those used for diarrhoea in general. Thus EA at ST-25, Ren-6 and Ren-9 was combined with MA in one IBS study. And low-frequency, high-intensity TEAS (ALTEAS) has been applied in 'chronic colitis' with anodes at ST-25, ST-36, ST-37, SP-6, SP-9 and Ren-12, and a single cathode over the most problematic area. Gordon Gadsby recommends BL-25 or ST-25/SP-15 as points of choice for TEAS.

## Inflammatory bowel disorder: ulcerative colitis and Crohn's disease

Non-specific ulcerative colitis is a chronic disease characterised by diarrhoea, abdominal pain and the presence of bloody pus and mucus in the stool. It is often limited to the rectum (proctitis) and sigmoid (left) colon (distal colitis), but may extend throughout the large intestine. WM treatment is with anti-inflammatory drugs, locally administered in mild to moderate distal colitis, or orally if it is more diffuse. Surgery may be necessary if medication fails.

Crohn's disease is a chronic condition in which segments of the bowel become inflamed, thickened and ulcerated. It generally affects the ileum and may lead to partial obstruction of the intestine and other complications such as anal fistulas and malabsorption. WM treatment is via anti-inflammatory drugs, antibiotics, dietary modification and surgery.

In TCM, Crohn's disease and ulcerative colitis are considered together in terms of syndromes such as Damp-Heat, Cold-Damp, Summer Heat, Liver *qi* stagnation, Liver *qi* invading the Spleen, Blood stagnation, or *yin* and *yang* deficiency affecting the Stomach, Spleen or Kidney.

MA may be helpful, particularly for diarrhoea and mucus in the stool, with Spleen and Stomach *xu* cases responding better than more chronic ones with Kidney *yang xu*. Frequent, even daily, treatment is often needed during an acute phase, and must be maintained until this has ended completely.

EA, LA and 'magnet frequency acupuncture' have been used for ulcerative colitis.

**Points used** The points for Crohn's and ulcerative colitis are very similar to those already listed above for diarrhoea and IBS. Ventral or dorsal segmentally related points may be particularly appropriate.

**Parameters used** EA and TEAS have both been applied at low frequency, whether at abdominal and distal points (EA) or back *shu* points (TEAS). LF stimulation has been used at other points too.

## Faecal incontinence

Faecal incontinence, or failure to control the anal sphincter, can result from spinal injury (traumatic or congenital), CNS degeneration in old age, stretch injury during childbirth, or even excessive straining at defaecation.

MA, EA and TENS have been used for faecal incontinence. In general, electrotherapy is considered appropriate for faecal incontinence, but not if this is completely uncontrolled, with no residual nerve function.

**Points used** EA has been used at Ren-1, Du-1 and perianal points for anal incontinence in spina bifida, and at local points for rectal paralysis.

In spinal cord injury, EA at paravertebral Bladder meridian points has been used, or at points such as BL40, GB-30, GB-34, SP-12, Ren-3, Ren-4 and *weibao* (M-CA-16), together with EA at either end of the damaged spinal cord region. In this latter study, additional points were HE-3, LI-11 and LI-18.

## Anal/rectal prolapse

Prolapse of the rectum is generally due to weakness of supporting tissues. It occurs most commonly in the elderly, multiparous women, and those with certain bowel conditions, both acute and chronic. WM treatment is surgical repair.

In TCM, prolapse is due to *qi* and Blood *xu*, with Spleen *qi* sinking.

**Points used** Traditionally, points such as BL-20, BL-25, ST-36, Ren-6, Du-1 and Du-20 might be used, with SP-9 and LI-11 added in acute cases. Auricular points have also been suggested.

## Colonoscopy

MA, EA and TENS have been used before and during colonoscopy. In one EA study, for instance, although pain level was not significantly reduced, patient requests for rescue medication were much reduced, possibly because EA lessened discomfort and anxiety.

**Points used** For EAA in the anal region, ST-36, SP-6 and Du-1, or BL-57, Ren-1 and Du-1 have been recommended. P-6, LI-4, ST-36 and SP-4 were used in one report, while in a British TEAS study electrodes were applied at ST-25.

**Parameters used** HF stimulation was used with both EA and TEAS. EA treatment was started 30 minutes before colonoscopy, while TEAS was only begun 5 minutes before the procedures, and ended 5 minutes afterwards.

# THE LIVER

## Jaundice and hepatitis

Jaundice is caused by hyperbilirubinaemia – high levels of plasma bilirubin – and is recognised by a yellow/green pigmentation to the skin and the sclera of the eyes. WM treatment is dependent on the type and aetiology of the jaundice.

TCM treatment of jaundice particularly emphasises the role of Damp and the difference between *yang* and *yin* types of jaundice.

Acupuncture (MA) has been used in the treatment of hepatitis, both acute and chronic. Liver function tests have been used in some studies to confirm clinical improvement. EA too has been used to treat hepatitis, and TENS for jaundice and acute hepatic failure due to mechanical obstruction.

MA and moxibustion have been used to strengthen immune function in asymptomatic hepatitis B carriers, as has EA.

**Points used** From the little information available, it would seem that LIV-3 and ST-36 are appropriate points to use for hepatitis. Other points, suggested by Willem Khoe, include BL-18, BL-19, BL-21, GB-34, LIV-13, LIV-14, ST-21, SP-6, Ren-9 and Ren-12.

Auricular points used include Liver, Pancreas, Gall Bladder, Spleen, Stomach, *sanjiao*, *erzhong* and *jiawozhang*. Khoe also used EA between the Hepatitis point (in the triangular fossa) and a needle through Liver *yang* 1, Helix 1 and Liver *yang* 2 (at Darwin's tubercle).

# THE GALL BLADDER

Cholelithiasis and cholecystitis are the two main gall bladder problems encountered. In TCM, these are commonly considered together under hypochondriac, costal or gastric pain and jaundice. Cholecystitis has long been treated with acupuncture. However, focus on acupuncture treatment of cholelithiasis is more recent, and in many cases exemplifies the integration of WM and TCM methods.

## Cholelithiasis

Cholelithiasis (gallstones) is common wherever people are exposed to a modern Western diet. Stones formed in the gall bladder can remain dormant (cholecystolithiasis) or travel and become lodged in the cystic or common bile ducts. Such obstruction results in pain and cholecystitis – distension and inflammation of the gall bladder. WM treatments for cholelithiasis include drug therapy to dissolve the stones, lithotripsy (shockwave therapy, usually applied from outside the body) or removal of the gall bladder (cholecystectomy).

In TCM cholelithiasis is associated with several disharmonies – long-term Liver and Gall bladder *qi* stagnation, complicated by the presence of Heat, Damp and Spleen deficiency.

EA (at BL-18 and LIV-14) promotes bile secretion and so reduces cholelithiasis. The earlier EA is used, the lower is the rate of lithogenesis. EA at the auricular Liver and Gall Bladder points can also induce contraction of the gall bladder and encourage the passage of stones. MA at *dannangxue* (M-LE-23), 1–2 *cun* below GB-34, also results in contraction of the gall bladder, while with GB-40 MA it relaxes. Further, auricular EA (20 Hz EA at the *left* auricular Gall Bladder/Pancreas point) can relax smooth muscle spasm in the common bile duct, while GB-34 EA can rapidly relax the sphincter of Oddi, just proximal to where the common bile duct meets the duodenum. This relaxation could encourage the expulsion of gallstones, and also occurs in response to LI-4 TEAS in patients with biliary dyskinesia.

There are a number of studies on EA for cholelithiasis. EA has been combined with MA and plum blossom needling for cholecystolithiasis. EA has been shown to be better than oral magnesium sulphate (Epsom salts) for promoting the expulsion of gallstones.

**Points used** Points found useful in experimental research include BL-18, GB-24, GB-34 and LIV-14.

Points such as BL-19, SJ-6, GB-24, GB-34, LIV-13 and LIV-14 are recommended for both cholelithiasis and cholecystitis in one EA device manual.

Similar points are used in many clinical EA studies, particularly the combination of local anterior points such as GB-24 and LIV-14 (sometimes LIV-13), with or without back *shu* (BL-18, BL-19) and other Bladder meridian points. Distal points are less in evidence, except for *dannangxue* (M-LE-23), connected with Ren-12 in one study, and sometimes GB-34,

GB-39 or LIV-3. P-6 and SJ-6 have also been used, though less commonly.

**Parameters used** LF or DD EA has been recommended in one overview of acupuncture for cholelithiasis. In one EA device manual, it is suggested that DD be applied at moderate to strong intensity. In general, strong LF or DD stimulation is used (although in one Western study 8–20 Hz was employed).

Although 2/15 DD EA may take around 8 minutes to increase bile flow, the effect of EA on Oddi's sphincter occurs in just over a minute.

## Cholecystitis

Cholecystitis, or inflammation and distension of the gall bladder, is generally caused by obstruction due to gallstones lodging in the cystic duct. WM treatment consists of antibiotic and analgesic therapy, with cholecystectomy if necessary.

In TCM, cholecystitis may be due to Damp-Heat in the Liver and Gall Bladder, potentially progressing to toxic Heat. Atrophic cholecystitis, in which there is marked shrinkage in the size of the gall bladder despite being filled with sand-like stones, may respond better to treatment aimed at tonifying Stomach and Spleen.

Biliary colic, the pain associated with cholecystitis, has been treated both with MA and EA. Chronic cholecystitis, with or without cholelithiasis, may respond well to EA and associated methods.

**Points used** Similar points are often recommended for both cholecystitis and cholelithiasis. Thus BL-19, GB-24 and the auricular Gall Bladder points are recommended for cholecystitis and biliary colic in one EA device manual. Other points for EA include BL-18, BL-20, BL-21 (or *jiaji* points), LIV-13, LIV-14, Ren-12 or Ren-13, together with distal points such as GB-34 or *dannangxue*, LIV-3, ST-36 and SP-9.

For biliary colic, ST-19, ST-36 and Ren-14 have been used. In one study on tender point injection, the most tender point in the triangular region defined by GB-24, LIV-14 and Ren-14 was selected.

**Parameters used** In one EA device manual, moderate to strong DD is recommended. Voll suggested 3.5 Hz as an appropriate frequency for biliary colic. However, there appears to be little consistency in the parameters used for cholecystitis, with some authors using HF, others DD, and Labarthe 8–20 Hz.

## Biliary ascariasis

Biliary ascariasis is infestation of the biliary tree by the large roundworm *Ascaris lumbricoides*. About 25% of the world's population is infected, particularly where environmental hygiene is poor. The main presenting symptoms are colicky pain and obstructive jaundice. WM and TCHM treatment is with anthelmintics (worming agents).

Both MA and EA have been used in the treatment of biliary ascariasis.

**Points used** ST-36 alone was used in one MA study. In the single EA study located, BL-18, BL-19 and Du-9 were the main points used, with supplementary points GB-34 and ST-36.

## Cholecystectomy and lithotripsy

Cholecystectomy, surgical removal of the gall bladder, is a standard treatment for cholelithiasis and cholecystitis.

EAA combined with epidural anaesthesia has been used, with a reduction in the need for other anaesthetic agents, and epidural anaesthesia in particular.

TEAS has been used for cholecystectomy and bile duct surgery.

MA, EA, TENS and LILT have been investigated for postoperative pain relief following cholecystectomy. MA, EA and EHF may all speed recovery, but TENS appears to offer no major advantages over conventional treatment.

EAA has been used for extracorporeal shockwave lithotripsy (ESWL, treatment to break up the stones so they can be passed), with favourable results and fewer side-effects than conventional medication in uncontrolled trials. Results with TENS/TEAS for ESWL are conflicting.

**Points used** For cholecystectomy, points such as GB-27, LIV-14, LI-4, ST-36 and SP-6, or GB-25, LIV-5, LIV-13 and LIV-14, have been recommended. P-6, paraspinal and auricular points have also been used.

For postcholecystectomy pain, points such as GB-26, LIV-2, LIV-3, LIV-13, LI-4, ST-36 and SP-4 were used in one Russian report. In a TENS study, no differences were found whether electrodes were positioned paraincisionally or at distal acupoints (TEAS).

In his studies on ESWL, Emil Iliev used points such as BL-18, BL-19, GB-34, LIV-3, LI-4, ear *shenmen*, Gall Bladder, Liver and Subcortex.

**Parameters used** Both LF (body) and HF (auricular) EA have been used for postcholecystectomy pain. Neither the latter nor paraincisional HF TENS were considered effective in some studies.

In his work on ESWL, Iliev combined LF EAA at auricular and distal points with HF EAA at body points.

## THE PANCREAS

### Pancreatitis

WM treatment of both acute and chronic pancreatitis is based on drug therapy and surgical intervention. EA and TENS have been used for pain associated with chronic pancreatitis.

**Points used** In a much-cited study by Søren Ballegaard's group with mediocre results, distal, auricular and local (segmental) points were used. Although the latter were logically selected, there are probably better points to use than SJ-18, SP-4 and the auricular Lung point.

Of note are two studies in which local stimulation of the coeliac plexus was helpful.

**Parameters used** A combination of LF EA, CTENS and intermittent TENS was used in the study by Søren Ballegaard and colleagues, but was not found that beneficial for acute pancreatitis pain. CTENS, however, does appear to be useful for the pain of chronic pancreatitis.

## SUMMARY

Some key points in this chapter are:

- EA and other non-traditional acupuncture modalities have been used for a wide spectrum of gastrointestinal, liver, gall bladder and pancreatic disorders
- There is good evidence that they can be helpful in a number of these, particularly nausea and vomiting, gastritis, peptic ulcer disease and cholecystitis
- The use of P-6 has become a standard treatment for post-operative nausea and vomiting, with best results obtained if used *before* premedication
- EA may successfully reduce the problems associated with endoscopy
- EA has a regulatory effect on stomach function.

Additional material in the
CD-ROM resource

In the CD-ROM resource, in addition to further information on many of the topics presented here, the following conditions are mentioned:

- dysphagia, achalasia, PONV in children, nausea as a result of acupuncture-related treatment, the gag reflex
- abdominal pain, functional dyspepsia, gastric carcinoma, other stomach disorders, gastrectomy and other stomach surgery
- intestinal obstruction, hernia
- cholera and dysentery
- haemorrhoids, anal fissure
- liver toxicity, liver function and non-specific liver disorders, cirrhosis of the liver, cancer and the liver, surgery and the liver.

**9.8** Summary of relevant studies in the electronic clinical studies database (number of studies)

| Condition | EA | Other | Condition | EA | Other |
|---|---|---|---|---|---|
| **Nausea and vomiting** | | | **Colon – rectum** | | |
| Antiemesis (general) | 0 | 3 | Faecal incontinence | 9 | 3 |
| Postoperative nausea and vomiting | | | Constipation | 8 | 6 |
| (PONV) | 15 | 45 | Diarrhoea and irritable bowel syndrome | | |
| Chemotherapy induced emesis | 15 | 13 | *Infantile diarrhoea* | 0 | 22 |
| Morning sickness etc. | 0 | 15 | *Acute diarrhoea* | 3 | 7 |
| Motion sickness | 0 | 7 | *Irritable bowel syndrome (IBS)* | 2 | 10 |
| Other nausea and vomiting | 3 | 6 | *Inflammatory bowel disorders* | 3 | 16 |
| **Gastritis – ulceration** | | | *Other chronic diarrhoea* | 3 | 5 |
| Peptic ulcer | 19 | 87 | The rectum and anus | 0 | 2 |
| Gastritis | 6 | 15 | **Ileus (postoperative, other)** | | |
| **Oesophagus – stomach** | | | Ileus (postoperative) | 7 | 7 |
| The oesophagus | 1 | 13 | Ileus (due to other causes) | 6 | 4 |
| The stomach | | | **Spleen/pancreas** | | |
| *Gastric motility and emptying* | 4 | 4 | The pancreas | 4 | 11 |
| *Gastric tone: gastroptosis and gastric* | | | **Gall bladder and liver** | | |
| *spasm* | 9 | 8 | The gall bladder | | |
| *Other/mixed gastric disorders* | 1 | 3 | *Cholecystitis and cholangitis* | 1 | 14 |
| General digestive problems | 1 | 5 | *Gallstones: cholelithiasis and cholecystolithiasis* | 15 | 17 |
| Abdominal pain | 13 | 8 | *Biliary ascariasis* | 3 | 2 |
| **Small intestine – appendix** | | | *Biliary dyskinesia* | 1 | 3 |
| The small intestine | | | *Other aspects of biliary function* | 2 | 0 |
| *Intestinal adhesions* | 4 | 2 | *Mixed/other gall bladder conditions* | 1 | 3 |
| *Duodenal stasis and other conditions* | 0 | 3 | The liver | | |
| *Ascariasis (intestinal)* | 0 | 4 | *Hepatitis and jaundice* | 6 | 20 |
| The appendix | 5 | 7 | *Mixed/other liver conditions* | 1 | 10 |

# RECOMMENDED READING

*A useful review of the field:*
Diehl DL Acupuncture for gastrointestinal and hepatobiliary disorders. Journal of Alternative and Complementary Medicine. 1999 Feb; 5(1): 27–45

*An excellent discussion of one of the most researched applications of acupuncture:*
McMillan CM 1998 Acupuncture for nausea and vomiting. In: Filshie J, White A (eds) Medical Acupuncture: a western scientific approach. Churchill Livingstone, Edinburgh, 295–317

*Two applications of Kaada's protocol:*
Kaada B Successful treatment of oesophageal dysmotility and Raynaud's phenomenon in systemic sclerosis and achalasia by transcutaneous nerve stimulation. Scandanavian Journal of Gastrenterology. 1987 Nov; 22(9): 1137–46

Guelrud M, Rossiter A, Souney PF, Mendoza S, Mujicia V The effect of transcutaneous nerve stimulation on the sphincter of oddi in patients with biliary dyskinesia. American Journal of Gastroenterology. 1992 May; 86(5): 581–5

*A useful if cautious summary:*
Li Y, Tougas G, Chiverton SG, Hunt RH The effect of acupuncture on gastrointestinal function and disorders. American Journal of Gastroenterology. 1992 Oct; 87(10): 1372–81

*Not acupuncture, but a fascinating insight into gut neuroscience:*
Gershon MD 1998 The Second Brain: The scientific basis of gut instinct and a groundbreaking new understanding of nervous disorders of the stomach and intestine. Harper Collins, New York

# 9.9  THE GENITOURINARY TRACT

*Josephine Cerqua and David F Mayor*

---

This chapter covers sexual problems (mainly those of men), male infertility and prostate conditions, and then urinary tract disorders such as incontinence, enuresis, urine retention, urinary tract infections and kidney conditions, including the formation of urinary stones.

## ERECTILE DYSFUNCTION AND IMPOTENCE IN MEN

Erectile dysfunction (ED), the repeated inability to get or keep an erection firm enough for sexual intercourse, is mainly caused by vascular and neurological disease. Other contributory factors include medication and drug use, psychological factors, hormonal problems, heavy smoking, high cholesterol, diseases affecting the erectile tissue of the penis and severe chronic diseases such as kidney and liver failure.

The term 'impotence', often used interchangeably with ED, is commonly used to describe other problems that interfere with sexual intercourse and reproduction, including lack of sexual desire and problems with ejaculation or orgasm, such as premature ejaculation, retarded ejaculation, counterflow ejaculation (into the bladder), and orgasmic failure.

TCM diagnoses of ED and impotence include decline of *mingmen* Fire, exhaustion of Essence and Blood (*jing* and *xue*), damage to the Kidney, Heart and Spleen, damage to the Stomach and Penetrating (*chong*) meridians and downward flow of Damp-Heat. Failure to ejaculate is commonly diagnosed as Liver *qi* stagnation with obstruction in the meridians, whereas disharmony of the Liver and Gall Bladder may frequently be involved in ED.

Treatments for ED have included manual acupuncture (MA), electroacupuncture (EA) and transcutaneous electrical nerve stimulation (TENS).

EA was used in a number of studies to treat male sexual dysfunction, including ED, diminished libido and ejaculation disorders. Transcutaneous electrical acupoint stimulation (TEAS) has also been used.

TENS successfully increased penile rigidity when used to stimulate striated ischiocavernous muscle. Electrical stimulation of smooth muscle of the penile corpus cavernosum gave better results in one report.

Other treatments have included cranial electrotherapy stimulation (CES), microwave resonance therapy (MRT) and acupoint injection.

Moxibustion has been used for functional non-ejaculation associated with a deficiency of Kidney *yang*.

Pelvic floor muscle exercises, which are non-invasive, easy to perform, painless, cost effective and free from drug side-effects, should be considered an important adjunct to any of the treatments mentioned above.

In part because of traditional associations between Essence (*jing*) and semen, and the importance in Daoist psychospiritual practice of preserving *jing*, there is considerable emphasis on moderation of sexual activity and methods of curtailing nocturnal emission of semen ('wet dreams') in TCM. MA, alone or in combination with auricular acupressure, has been used for the latter. According to Bob Flaws, spermatorrhoea (involuntary loss of semen) in young Westerners may often be associated with an excess condition (Damp-Heat in the Lower *jiao* or Burner) rather than deficiency.

## Acupuncture, neuropathy and sexual function

ED can be caused by neuropathy, in which nerve function is impaired as a result of diabetes, multiple sclerosis (MS), prostate surgery or damage to the spinal cord. In a controlled trial of diabetic patients with ED, ejaculation disorders or diminished libido it was shown to be useful for ED and diminished libido, although ineffective for ejaculation disorders.

Lumbar pain may accompany sexual disorders, associated either with general debility or with neurovascular reflex problems. Local EA, together with MA at traditionally appropriate points, was found to improve sexual function in men with lumbar but not radicular symptoms.

## Psychogenic sexual dysfunction in men

Psychological factors such as depression, anxiety, guilt and fear were once thought to be the major cause of sexual dysfunction. It is now believed, however, that physical factors are present in most men with such difficulties, with embarrassment or 'performance anxiety' often making the physical problem worse. ED from psychological causes is found most commonly in young men.

In one controlled study, EA was found to be slightly less effective than hypnosis, but more effective than a vitamin regimen, as a treatment for non-organic male impotence.

## Peyronie's disease

One physical cause of ED is Peyronie's disease, an autoimmune condition where a fibrous, inelastic plaque is formed that does not expand with erection, causing curvature of the penis and pain. Over the years many treatments have been used, including medication and surgery, with in some cases a prosthesis if the condition is serious.

While there are no reports on the use of acupuncture for this condition, non-invasive low-intensity laser therapy (LILT) has been recommended, particularly when combined with ultrasound. A rather more vigorous approach is the use of extracorporeal shortwave therapy (ESWT), in which high-energy shock waves are used to break up the plaque.

Given possible parallels with scleroderma, Kaada's protocol (low-frequency high-intensity or acupuncture-like TEAS, ALTEAS, at LI-4/~SI-3) may be worth exploring as an adjunctive or preventive treatment for Peyronie's disease.

## Testicular pain and other conditions

Orchitis (inflammation of the testes), often viral in origin (mumps), has been treated with body or auricular MA, as well as with EA or acupoint injection (at KI-11, Ren-8, SP-6 and Ren-2). Late stage painful orchitis due to trauma has been treated with MA.

There is one interesting study on a condition that is not often reported, here called 'epididymal stasis,' following ligation as a method of birth control. Large TEAS electrodes were positioned over acupoints, above and below, or either side of the genital area. Ten out of eleven patients were cured.

EA has been used to treat hot flushes in men castrated to retard progression of prostate cancer.

**Points used**  Daoist treatises document Ren-6 as the primary acupuncture point for treatment of male impotence. Joseph Wong reports that BL-18 stimulates the adrenal cortex and releases testosterone. ST-36 may also increase production of adrenal steroid hormones (and so, indirectly, of testosterone). Ren-6 and BL-18 are both included in Norman Shealy's 'ring of fire' point protocol (BL-22, KI-3, P-6, LI-18, Ren-2, Ren-6, Ren-18 and Du-20). In TCM, BL-18 is utilised for impotence due to stagnation of Liver $qi$.

In clinical studies, commonly used points include BL-23, BL-32, SP-6, Ren-3, Ren-4, Ren-6 and Du-4. Kidney points are also used, people suffering from impotence in ancient China being diagnosed with 'Kidney failure'. Some points, such as BL-28, KI-1, KI-3, HE-7, P-6, ST-30, Ren-1, Ren-2 and Du-1, have been suggested on the basis of their anatomical location and possible physiological function. In particular, segmental patterns of innervation must be considered when treating different functional or painful conditions. Various authors have stated that needling of the abdominal points should induce a sensation radiating to the penis.

Ear points for impotence include Uterus (*jing* palace), Seminal vesicle, External genitalia, Testis and Adrenal (or 'internal tragic apex').

**Parameters used**  Experimental studies indicate that high-frequency (HF) stimulation may be more appropriate than high-intensity, low-frequency (LF) EA or TENS/TEAS when it comes to sexual performance. Thus, in one study of 106 patients experiencing ED, HF EA (>100 Hz) was used in combination with moxibustion. However, 1 Hz EA was shown to be highly effective in one Chinese clinical audit of 46 men with inability to ejaculate, while in a study of sexual dysfunction in diabetic patients, tonification at 0.5–5 Hz and sedation at 15–50 Hz were used, for 2–5 and 20 minutes respectively.

## SEXUAL DIFFICULTIES IN WOMEN

Many factors contribute to female sexual problems, some psychological and others physical. Physical causes include changes in contraception, pain on intercourse (dyspareunia), hormonal changes at different times in the menstrual cycle, medication, childbirth, approaching menopause, thyroid disorders, or changes in brain chemistry. Psychological factors may involve anxiety, past traumatic experiences or negative attitudes about sex.

There is little information on the use of acupuncture in the treatment of female sexual dysfunction. Stephen Aung reports one case of female sexual dysfunction due to a history of traumatic early sexual experience being treated with a combination of MA and EA. In another briefly reported case, a woman complaining of 'frigidity' was treated with MA and TENS, and after the third treatment experienced vaginal secretion and normal sexual activity.

Aung has also created what he calls 'conjoint sexual alignment therapy' to treat partners' mutual loss of sexual interest and libido. In this method, reminiscent of Eeman's 'circuits', low-intensity LF EA is used. The couple touch hands or other parts of their body so that the electrical stimulation flows through both of them in a complete circuit. Use of P-8 in the palm of the hand is optimal. Furthermore, the man's Ren-6 is wired to the woman's Du-4 and the woman's Ren-6 to the man's Du-4. Bilaterally, the man's LIV-8 is wired to the woman's SP-6 and both partners' KI-10 points are interconnected.

## MALE INFERTILITY

In at least one-third of couples presenting with infertility, the condition is attributable largely or entirely to abnormalities in the male, leading to no sperm in the semen (azoospermia), a low sperm count (oligospermia) or abnormal sperm (the most commonly observed cause).

Impaired production or delivery of sperm may result from hormonal dysfunction, trauma or defect in the reproductive system, or illness. Other causes include inflammation, obstruction (due to repeated infection, inflammation or developmental defect), retrograde ejaculation, testicular trauma, certain drugs and varicoceles.

According to TCM theory, production of sperm is related to Kidney *yin* and sperm activity to Kidney *yang*. MA, EA and LILT have been used in the treatment of male infertility due to sperm abnormalities.

MA, for example, may improve sperm count or quality. In one study, all 28 subfertile men given 10 sessions of MA over 3 weeks exhibited an improvement in sperm quality.

Such improvements did not correlate with psychological changes, suggesting that they were not the result of placebo. In another study of subfertility, MA was shown to improve total functional sperm fraction, percentage viability, total mobile sperm count per ejaculate and integrity of the axonema (linking the body of the sperm to its tail). Patients with prostatitis may respond less well.

In one randomised study of sterile men, best results were obtained with a combination of acupuncture, acupoint injection and herbal medicine, particularly in younger men (aged 25–30). Satisfactory clinical results were also reported through the use of Chinese herbs in the treatment of semen abnormalities. LF EA, combined with moxibustion containing specific herbal ingredients, has been used for infertility due to abnormal semen.

**Points used** Most commonly used points are those on the Kidney meridian and Conception Vessel, including KI-2, KI-6, Ren-2, Ren-3 and Ren-4.

**Parameters used** Little concrete information is available on appropriate stimulation parameters for treating infertility. LF EA has been used to good effect in uncontrolled studies. In some MA studies, radiation of *deqi* down to the penis and testis is emphasised. However, strong local electrical stimulation should probably be avoided in case of adverse effects on the sperm themselves.

# PROSTATE CONDITIONS

## Prostatitis

Chronic prostatitis is an inflammation of the prostate gland that develops gradually, continues for a prolonged period, and typically has subtle symptoms. These can include low back pain, testicular pain, pain/burning on urination, perineal or pelvic floor pain, pain on ejaculation, pain with bowel movement, recurrent low-grade fever, pain on urination, decreased urinary stream, urinary hesitancy, frequent urination, blood in the urine and incontinence. Chronic prostatitis is usually caused, at least initially, by a bacterial infection, the most common being *Escherichia coli*, *Proteus*, *Enterobacter* and *Klebsiella* bacteria.

In TCM, chronic prostatitis is often assigned to the categories of '*Lin* syndrome' or retention of urine, being differentiated into Damp-Heat type, Blood stasis type and Kidney deficiency type. These three types are often mixed. It may also fall into the categories of incontinence, turbid urine and blood in the urine.

Treatments for chronic prostatitis include MA, EA and laser acupuncture (LA). In one study, invasive LA (through needles) was shown to be more effective than MA alone, with longer-lasting results. LA has also been combined with moxa, and with injection of *shuang huanglian* into the gland, MA with microwave therapy, and EA with magnetic plasters. LILT has been applied via endorectal or endourethral probe. In one study, more than 200 patients with chronic prostatitis were treated with a GaAs diode laser; 65% obtained relief from some symptoms for up to 6 months after treatment.

## Prostate enlargement

Benign prostate enlargement (prostatic hyperplasia or adenomatous hypertrophy) results from a cumulative androgen effect. Increasing with age, it begins in the fifth decade of life. It commonly causes urethral obstruction and is usually treated by transurethral resection (TURP) and open prostatectomy. Transurethral incision of the prostate (TUIP) is another approach, comparable to TURP in long-term efficacy.

EA has been used for prostatic hypertrophy, alone or in combination with LA or Chinese herbal medication. EA anaesthesia (EAA) has been used during both open and transvesical prostatectomy, for instance epidurally at Du-4 and a more caudal point. TENS has been incorporated into treatment for postoperative prostatectomy pain.

A number of combination devices for home treatment of prostate conditions are marketed in China.

**Points used** In studies on invasive LA for prostate conditions, Ren-1 or a special prostate point located 1–2 cm anterior to the anus may be used, the latter being needled laterally towards both sides to a depth of 5 cm in one report.

**Parameters used** Most EA studies for prostatitis or prostatic hyperplasia appear to use LF or dense-disperse (DD) stimulation. With LILT/LA, helium–neon (HeNe) lasers have been used primarily for prostate conditions.

# URINARY TRACT CONDITIONS

## Types of incontinence

### GENUINE STRESS INCONTINENCE
Genuine stress incontinence is defined as the involuntary passage of urine when intra-abdominal pressure is raised through, for example, coughing or lifting. This can result from a urethra that is not properly held in place, which is often associated with laxity of the pelvic floor muscles resulting from pregnancy and childbirth. Closure of the bladder outlet is compromised, but there is no neurological defect.

Depending on the severity of stress incontinence, conservative or surgical methods can be used. Pelvic floor exercises are most commonly recommended. Adjunctive treatments may include biofeedback, mechanical devices such as vaginal cones, pharmacological treatment and electrostimulation.

### URGE INCONTINENCE
Micturition (urination) results from contraction of the detrusor ('pushing down') smooth muscle of the bladder, together with simultaneous relaxation of the bladder outlet. In urge incontinence, often with detrusor overactivity or instability, the perception of the desire to void is followed within seconds or minutes by voiding, even though the individual attempts to delay it. Voiding is usually complete.

Urge incontinence is more common in women and the elderly. In men, the detrusor (pubovesical) muscle is closely associated with the prostate. Urge incontinence may be due to secondary bladder injuries caused by benign prostatic hypertrophy (BPH), or bladder outlet obstruction from an enlarged prostate.

Urge incontinence may reflect local disease, neurological injury (such as spinal cord injury or stroke), neurological diseases (such as multiple sclerosis, MS), infection, bladder cancer, bladder stones, bladder inflammation, or bladder outlet obstruction. The majority of cases are classified as idiopathic, without underlying neurological abnormalities.

### REFLEX INCONTINENCE

Reflex incontinence is sometimes considered a subtype of urge incontinence. Voiding occurs periodically without advance warning. The most important causes are spinal lesions, either complete or incomplete, above the level of the sacral efferent nerves that govern bladder activity.

### MIXED STRESS AND URGE INCONTINENCE

Mixed forms of stress and urge incontinence are common. As treatment of the two conditions is different, it is important to decide which symptom is the relevant one. Failure of incontinence therapy can often be ascribed to failures in pretreatment evaluation.

### OVERFLOW INCONTINENCE

Overflow incontinence usually manifests itself with leakage of small amounts of urine, initially often at night only, and is most often seen in men with prostatic hypertrophy. Other cases result from neurological lesions.

### SENILE URINARY INCONTINENCE

This form of incontinence is often multifactorial, particularly neuropathic. It has been suggested that this may result from dysfunction of the brainstem micturition centre due to arteriosclerosis and insufficient blood supply.

In TCM diagnosis, the Kidneys and Lungs are commonly indicated when incontinence occurs. A deficiency of Lung *qi* leads to the Lungs not controlling the water passages and if Lung *qi* is deficient it will fail to support the Bladder in its function of *qi* transformation (common in elderly people). Kidney *yang xu* is the most common cause of incontinence according to TCM theory.

## Acupuncture and incontinence

Acupuncture has been found clinically useful in the treatment of bladder dysfunction, with the suggestion that it may have an effect on the micturition centre in the pons, and so in turn on the bladder. Treatments have included MA, EA, LA and TENS, with numerous studies on TENS for detrusor instability.

Both MA and EA have been used for the treatment of urinary bladder neural dysfunction ('neurogenic' bladder) in diabetic patients, and in the treatment of frequency,

urgency and dysuria in women. Scalp acupuncture with electrical stimulation was combined with MA (body points) in one study for the treatment of senile urinary incontinence.

HeNe LA (at SJ-4, GB-20 and Ren-3, stimulating both the medulla and locally) gave better results than MA in one small study of incontinence. LA has also been used for detrusor instability in women, and for 'neural polyuria' (HeNe, GaAs).

## Urinary function, stroke and spinal cord or peripheral nerve damage

Neurological damage can lead to both retention of urine and incontinence, as well as to incomplete bladder emptying. Treatments for urinary incontinence due to spinal cord injury (SCI) have included MA, EA and TENS, as well as their combinations. MA has been investigated experimentally for urinary disorders due to sacral vertebral laceration, and clinically for neurogenic bladder following cerebral infarction or embolism. MA with herbal medication has been used for paralysis of the bladder with urinary retention due to injury to the parasympathetic nerves following surgery for early or intermediate uterine carcinoma. MA has also been helpful for urinary incontinence caused by detrusor hyperreflexia in SCI patients. In one study they experienced a significant increase in average maximum bladder capacity, with incontinence being completely controlled in three of the eight patients in the study.

EA has been used to treat urinary and faecal dysfunction due to spina bifida.

Box 9.9.1 details the use of mainstream Western electrotherapy in urinary dysfunction.

**Points used** Experimentally, EA at BL-23, BL-28, auricular points or distal points such as LI-4 all affect bladder function in different ways.

Clinically, EA at BL-23, sacral points (BL-28, BL-31–34), SP-6, Ren-3 and Ren-4 is frequently used for incontinence associated with SCI. EA applied at Governor Vessel points has also been used to improve lower urethral function in traumatic paraplegic patients (Du-3, Du-4 and Du-20, for example). BL-54, KI-11 and the lumbar *huatuojiaji* points are among many other points used in this situation. Points used for other forms of incontinence are very similar, including BL-23, BL-28, KI-11, ST-28, SP-6 (and SP-9) and Ren-3 (as well as Ren-4 and Ren-6).

However, in one MA study comparing the effects of different point combinations on dysuria and residual urine in the bladder in patients with incomplete paraplegia, clear improvements were found with local points such as BL-28, BL-32 and Ren-3 (with *deqi* spreading to the perineum), but not with distal points such as KI-10, SP-6 and SP-9.

Correspondingly, in a number of Western electrotherapy (TENS or interferential) studies, points on the thigh segmentally related to the bladder have been used following SCI, as well as for bladder dysfunction in multiple sclerosis. Perianal, suprapubic and third sacral foramen locations have also been tried, corresponding to Ren-1/Du-1, Ren-3 and

Even before acupuncture became well known in the West in the early 1970s, electrical stimulation methods were being used for urinary incontinence. A particular TENS method that has been explored is interferential therapy (IT), which has been successfully combined with pelvic floor exercises in the treatment of urinary stress incontinence. However, one RCT that compared weighted vaginal cones and interferential therapy for stress incontinence found that there was no significant difference in improvement in the two groups. Cones required less supervision and so were more suitable for home use.

TENS and 'sacral neuromodulation' via implanted electrodes function through the same central nervous pathways. Thus, in one study of S3 segmental neuromodulation and S2–S3 segmental TENS for the treatment of idiopathic detrusor instability, no statistically significant differences were found between the two treatments. When quality of life is severely impaired, as is often the case with refractory voiding dysfunction due to SCI, the whole device ('neuroprosthesis') may be implanted, with benefits both for incontinence and urinary retention, as well as chronic pelvic pain.

Another approach is spinal cord stimulation (SCS), an invasive procedure used for bladder problems in multiple sclerosis, for example. Improvements in conduction characteristics of the innervation of both urethral and perineal sphincter musculature with *transcutaneous* SCS would support the use of TEAS or EA at Governor Vessel and *huatuojiaji* points (see previous page) for both urinary and faecal incontinence.

A semi-invasive method is to use intravaginal or intra-anal electrodes. In one such study, 10 Hz 'maximal' stimulation was used by patients with either idiopathic detrusor instability or an uninhibited overactive bladder. In some cases additional stimulation was administered via a single-needle bipolar electrode inserted directly into the pudendal nerve. All patients showed a significant increase in functional bladder capacity and 11 reported a 30% decrease in frequency of micturition.

BL-33, respectively, points used with EA as well. TENS has also been applied distally over the common peroneal or posterior tibial nerves, sometimes at acupoints.

In LA studies on incontinence, both local (BL-23, BL-28, Ren-2, Ren-3) and distal points (BL-64, BL-65, SP-6, SP-9) have been used, with GB-20 stimulated in one report, possibly with a view to affecting the pontine micturition centre.

**Parameters used** Neurogenic bladder due to SCI has been treated with EA at 20–30 Hz (at 'local' points BL-32, Ren-3, Ren-4), while in diabetic patients with impaired bladder function 0.5–5 Hz was used for tonification and 15–50 Hz for sedation, whether at local or distal points.

In one study of stress incontinence low-intensity 8 Hz EA was used at both local (KI-11, Ren-6) and distal points (BL-57, ST-36), resulting in a significant increase in 'closing pressure' of the urethra. Senile urinary incontinence has been treated with MA at body points in combination with strong scalp EA at around 33 Hz. LF stimulation (distally with TENS, locally with IT, and in some EA studies), has also been used.

## Enuresis

Enuresis, defined as bedwetting in, or beginning in, childhood, is more common in children with psychological problems or organic diseases of the kidney or urinary tract, or both. In 85% of affected children, bedwetting is not accompanied by other voiding disorders or daytime incontinence.

Primary enuresis is due to insufficient maturity of the reflex controlling voluntary micturition, whereas secondary enuresis may have an organic cause, such as obstructive lesion of the urinary tract or lumbosacral lesion. Treatments include psychotherapy, bladder training, biofeedback, use of an electric alarm, or medication.

According to TCM theory, normal urination depends mainly on functional activity of the Kidney and Bladder. In TCM, enuresis is differentiated into Kidney *yang xu*, Spleen and Lung *qi xu* types.

Treatments for nocturnal enuresis have included MA, (sometimes with moxibustion), EA (again in combination with moxibustion, or acupoint injection), LA and TEAS.

A number of the MA studies emphasise that needling manipulation should be strong, or that the sensation of *deqi* should be made to spread to the genitals. Less uncomfortable alternatives to needling may be important when treating children. In one study of scalp MA, a massive 41% dropped out because they found needling too painful. For the remaining stalwarts, better results were obtained in older children, with longer needle retention (up to 8 hours), and when treatment was given in the afternoon rather than morning.

**Points used** The most commonly used points for enuresis include BL-23, BL-28 and other sacral Bladder meridian points, KI-3, ST-36, SP-6, Ren-3 and Ren-4. Not surprisingly, these are much the same points as are used for incontinence. In one informal report, HE-7, P-6 and LIV-3 were also suggested, with home treatment by parents at SP-6 and Ren-4 emphasised (these two are traditionally recommended for enuresis).

**Parameters used** LF, HF and DD EA have all been used. LA studies have mostly used HeNe lasers, or other red light lasers.

## Retention of urine

The causes of urinary retention in TCM can be in the Upper, Middle or Lower *jiao*, but the roles of the Bladder and *sanjiao* (Triple Burner) are all important. The Bladder has the function of transforming *qi*, and the *sanjiao* governs the free passage of water in the

Lower *jiao*. Other possible pathologies include internal Heat, and insufficiency of Kidney *qi* in the elderly.

In WM terms, the physiology of urinary retention (uroschesis) involves both central and peripheral neural pathways. Urine retention not infrequently occurs following childbirth, surgery (such as hysterectomy) or other Lower *jiao* trauma, but may also be symptomatic of serious illness, usually of the urinary tract itself.

Although acupuncture may have an adjunctive role in the treatment of such internal disorders, it may be unsatisfactory in cases of organic changes in the urinary system and is most often used for urine retention following childbirth or surgery. Treatment includes MA and EA. When compared with drug anaesthesia, EA anaesthesia (EAA) may even enhance diuresis *during* surgery. Beneficial effects on restoring micturition are also sometimes reported as an aside in studies of acupuncture for postoperative pain.

When using MA for urine retention, strong stimulation is generally emphasised, used on its own (at SP-6, or SP-6 and Ren-4, for example), or in combination with EA. Other treatments for urinary retention have included warm needle moxibustion, auriculomagnetic therapy and Ren-3 acupoint injection. Cooling the navel is a traditional approach to urine retention in the presence of internal Heat. Lancing points such as BL-31–34, Du-4 and *yaoqi* (M-BW-29) has been used for urine retention due to prostatomegaly.

**Points used** The points most commonly used for urinary retention include BL-23, sacral Bladder points, LIV-3, ST-36, SP-6, SP-9, Ren-3, Ren-4 and Ren-6. Of these, SP-6, SP-9 and Ren-3 are traditionally recommended. In one report, BL-35 (*huiyang*) was used as a single point for MA treatment of postpartum-inhibited urination, a condition caused by prolonged compression of the perineal nerve by the head of the fetus. Auricular points such as Bladder, Kidney, Ureter, Urethra and External and Internal genitals have been used. MA at *shenmen*, Sympathetic and the centre of the triangular fossa was found helpful in one short report on urine retention due to postoperative anal pain.

**Parameters used** LF, HF, DD and intermittent stimulation have all been used for EA treatment of urine retention.

## Urinary tract infections and cystitis

Cystitis, or inflammation of the bladder, is usually the result of infection. Symptoms include painful or difficult urination (dysuria), frequency, urgency and strangury (slow, painful urination), with pus or bacteria in the urine (pyuria, bacteriuria), in which case it is normally cloudy and may be foul smelling. Cystitis is usually accompanied by a degree of constitutional disturbance.

Interstitial cystitis (IC) is suggested when there are bladder symptoms such as urinary urgency, frequency and bladder pain, but urine tests show no evidence of infection or other obvious pathology, and antibiotics fail to resolve the symptoms. Whereas cystitis due to infection is common in younger women, the median age of IC onset is 40 years.

Possible causes of interstitial cystitis include autoimmune dysfunction, inflammatory processes and abnormal structure or neuromuscular function of the bladder.

TCM Diagnosis of cystitis overlaps that of prostatitis and urinary stone disease. 'Painful urination' or *Lin* syndrome is usually considered under six headings: Heat, Stone, Qi, Blood, Damp and Fatigue. The most common patterns in recurrent cystitis are Spleen/Kidney *yang/qi xu* (54%), and Liver *qi* stagnation (36%), with less than 10% having other TCM patterns.

Treatment for cystitis has included MA, EA and TENS. For example, the authors of one MA study ($N = 180$) reported that symptom severity scores reduced by over two-thirds in more than 50% of those treated with MA and moxibustion, with urinary frequency (both day- and nighttime) reduced by about half on average. More formally, MA has been shown in Scandinavian studies to be significantly more effective than sham acupuncture or no treatment for frequently recurring urinary tract infections in women.

TENS has been used in a number of studies for interstitial cystitis, with positive results, although its mode of action in this condition is not altogether clear. LA has been used for the treatment of various types of cystalgia. In particular, LA following 'thermopuncture' preheating of acupoints (of the nasal mucosa, in this case) has been used for the stress of bladder tuberculosis.

**Points used** As mentioned above, EA at points such as BL-23 and BL-28 has been shown experimentally to affect bladder function, while LI-4 EA may also decrease urine excretion and bladder contraction. Deep puncture at BL-29 or BL-35 may directly activate relevant nerve pathways. Clinically, as for most lower urinary tract problems, BL-23, BL-28 and sacral Bladder meridian points, KI-3, KI-11, ST-36, SP-6, SP-9, Ren-3 and Ren-4 are commonly used points. Du-20 (MA) is sometimes added. BL-29 has been suggested as appropriate for impotence, enuresis and urinary retention, as well as prostate pain and sciatica.

Given a possible link between IC and myofascial pain, trigger point treatment should not be overlooked, either locally, as in the pelvic floor or piriformis, but also in muscles in remote parts of the body.

**Parameters used** LF EA and TENS/TEAS have been used in treating cystitis. However, optimal parameters for TENS (and EA) as a treatment for IC remain unclear.

## Urinary stones (urolithiasis)

Urinary stones usually present with renal or ureteral colic, resulting from partial or complete obstruction to the flow of urine. Pain is intense and nearly always accompanied with blood in the urine (haematuria). Less dramatic presentations may involve passing tiny stones or gravel, with associated discomfort or dull backache.

Conventional treatment includes analgesia with opiates and generous fluid intake to encourage passage of the stone. If a stone is large, intervention may be in the form of open surgery, endoscopic snaring from below or percutaneous removal from above. Many stones in the kidneys or ureter can be fragmented in situ by external shock wave lithotripsy (ESWL). In this method, focused ultrasound is used to shatter renal or ureteral stones in vivo, allowing spontaneous passage of the fragments. MA and EA have been used to reduce the discomfort of ESWL.

In China, there is a long tradition of treating urinary stones with acupuncture and Chinese herbs. In TCM terms, stone formation is due to a combination of Kidney *qi xu* and retention of Heat in the Lower *jiao*. Therapeutic effects are better in strong than in weak patients, worse in patients with pronounced Kidney *xu* syndromes, elevated nitrogen and proteinuria (as in nephritis), and poor in those who have undergone several ESWL treatments. In general, stones in the lower ureter appear to be more easily expelled, and those in the kidney itself the hardest.

Treatment in the acute phase is focused on reducing pain and expelling stones. In several studies, MA was combined with other interventions such as anaesthetic blockade of tender points or Chinese herbs. In one 'general attack' method, EA was combined with drinking plenty of water, as well as Chinese herbal decoctions, exercise and drugs.

In several controlled studies and RCTs, EA gave superior results when compared with medication or herbs. In one, however, EA gave less pain relief than medication, but reduced short-term recurrence of pain more effectively.

Special purpose acupuncture-based devices for treating both kidney and gallstones are available in China.

**Points used** Commonly used points used include BL-51, BL-52 and GB-25 (the front *mu* point of the Kidney). In one study, points were also chosen according to the location of the stone and, in an MA trial, limb points with low electrical skin resistance were selected. Strong and deep needling at ST-36 alone has been used for renal colic, while LIV-3 (again alone) was utilised in a single case report of MA in combination with a herbal remedy.

Deep needling of the T12–L2 *huatuojiaji* points, which is safer than at points such as BL-23, can enhance peristalsis in the renal pelvis and ureter. Furthermore, this treatment raises blood pressure in the glomeruli of the kidney, so increasing urine production. Both these factors facilitate stone discharge. In addition, stones larger than 1 cm in diameter may actually break up under the influence of strong DD EA at *huatuojiaji* points. Thus EA at L1–L2 *huatuojiaji* points (with some other back and distal points) was more effective than a combination of commonly used points in one study.

**Parameters used** Most studies of acupuncture for urolithiasis emphasise strong treatment, so that EA (particularly DD) is commonly used, although in one experimental investigation of MA intensity, greater ureteral peristalsis was observed with weak rather than strong stimulation at BL-60 and SP-6. However, although this may be the case in healthy subjects, the situation may be very different in patients with actual stones Kidney *xu* patients may not respond well to strong treatment.

# THE KIDNEYS

In both WM and TCM, the kidneys are fundamental to maintaining bodily functions and health. Kidney conditions include nephritis (Bright's disease, affecting the blood vessels in the organ), infection (pyelonephritis or pyelitis), nephrosis (degeneration of the kidney tubules, leading to dropsy), kidney tumour, uraemia and renal failure, often associated with polycystic kidney disease.

Nephritis, or non-bacterial inflammation of the kidneys, can occur in response to streptococcal respiratory infection, but may be idiopathic. Protein in the urine is an invariable sign. More common in children and adolescents than adults, it affects the blood vessels of the kidney rather than the tubules. Chronic nephritis can lead to hypertension and uraemia.

MA, with Chinese herbs, has been used for nephritis proteinuria associated with the autoimmune disorder systemic lupus erythematosus. Both acupuncture and CES have been used for renal hypertension. LA has been used for nephritis, both acute and chronic, with beneficial results in one controlled study. It has also been used, as has transcranial electrotherapy (TCET), to treat kidney disease during pregnancy. 'Freezing acupuncture' has also been used in the treatment of Kidney *xu* patients with chronic nephritis.

Acute kidney infection usually results from infection lower in the urinary tract and may be preceded by cystitis. Symptoms include fever, rigors (muscle rigidity), renal pain and tenderness. Patients with chronic pyelonephritis may present with symptoms and signs of chronic renal failure or hypertension. Severe reflux may give rise to renal pain or predispose to attacks of acute pyelonephritis. In management, attention must be given to electrolyte balance and control of blood pressure (BP).

MA, alone or in conjunction with local infrared heat, has been used for pyelonephritis, producing better urodynamic changes than WM control treatment in one study. Chronic calculous pyelonephritis has been treated with LA, together with modulated sinusoidal currents. LA and LILT have also been used as part of a comprehensive treatment strategy for pyelonephritis in pregnancy.

**Points used** Stimulation of points over the sciatic nerve (such as GB-30) or the deep peroneal nerve (ST-36 or ST-38) can increase kidney filtration (patients have been known to interrupt treatment rather hurriedly when ST-38 is needled, for example!).

Clinically, points such as BL-23, BL-28, KI-3, ST-28, SP-6 and Ren-3 have been used. Ear points too may enhance diuresis. Ren-4 and Du-4 have been used with MA and moxibustion for Kidney *xu* conditions. However, there are too few relevant studies to draw any meaningful conclusions on optimum point selection or stimulation parameters for kidney conditions.

Experimentally, MA at BL-21 has been shown to increase excretion of urine, sodium and chlorine. Renal function may also be enhanced by EA at BL-23 (and Ren-3), but inhibited by the same treatment if subjects are 'loaded' with water, or with saline plus diuretics. Thus the effects of stimulation at one and the same point will vary, depending in particular on whether or not patients are on diuretic medication.

# UROLOGICAL SURGERY AND OTHER INTERVENTIONS

EA has been used for intra- and postoperative analgesia in renal surgery. When used in conjunction with medication for kidney transplant operations, not only were heart rate and BP reported as more stable with EAA, but also urination started over 3 minutes sooner.

Auricular EA and magnetic stimulation have been used for the discomfort of cystoscopy, with better results claimed for EA than for conventional local anaesthesia. TENS ('percutaneous electrical stimulation') has also been used to provide analgesia in patients undergoing urological endoscopy.

# SUMMARY

Some key points in this chapter are:

- Acupuncture has been used for centuries in China as a primary treatment for urological disorders
- Modern methods such as EA and TEAS continue to have a role in the therapy of male erectile dysfunction
- For Peyronie's disease, combinations of LILT, ultrasound and possibly TEAS may be useful
- MA and EA have been used for male infertility
- For urinary incontinence and retention, it is helpful to consider EA as a variant of electrotherapy which has been investigated in some detail for these problems
- Non-traditional acupuncture methods have been used for urinary tract infections and cystitis, but are more likely to be considered appropriate for urinary stones

Additional material in the CD-ROM resource

In the CD-ROM resource, in addition to further information on many of the topics presented here, the following are also mentioned:

- Male sex hormones, the effects of drugs on sexual function, cryptorchidism, other prostate conditions, urethral syndrome.

**9.9** Summary of relevant studies in the electronic clinical studies database (number of studies)

| Condition | EA | Other |
|---|---|---|
| **Kidney** | | |
| Kidney stones | 6 | 5 |
| Other kidney conditions | 3 | 11 |
| **Bladder dysfunction** | | |
| Incontinence | | |
| *Incontinence due to spinal injury or other neurological deficit* | 21 | 16 |
| *Urge incontinence (detrusor instability)* | 2 | 18 |
| *Stress incontinence* | 2 | 2 |
| *Nocturnal enuresis (infantile enuresis)* | 8 | 31 |
| *Senile incontinence* | 3 | 0 |
| *Enuresis of uncertain type* | 1 | 5 |
| *Mixed incontinence* | 0 | 4 |
| Urinary retention | 5 | 5 |
| *Postoperative/postpartum urinary retention* | 15 | 6 |
| **Other urinary tract conditions** | | |
| Urinary tract stones | 11 | 14 |
| Urinary tract infection and cystitis | 2 | 16 |
| Other urinary tract conditions | 0 | 2 |
| **Prostate** | 14 | 33 |
| **Male genital – andrology** | | |
| Erectile dysfunction | 15 | 14 |
| Infertility | 2 | 8 |
| Other pathology | 0 | 2 |
| Andrology | 1 | 1 |

# RECOMMENDED READING

*Two thought-provoking articles on sexual dysfunction:*

Aung SKH Sexual dysfunction: a modern medical acupuncture approach. Medical Acupuncture. 2002; 13(2): 7–9

Wong J Male sexual impotence, sildenafil citrate and acupuncture. Medical Acupuncture. 2002; 13(1): 33–6

*A novel approach for Peyronie's disease that deserves to be better known:*

Koci K, Procházka M Combined therapy of Morbus Peyronie (induratio penis plastica) with non-invasive laser and ultrasound. Online. Available: www.laserpartner.org/en/laserpartner6.htm [accessed 2004 July 7]

*Combination treatment for chronic prostatitis – example of an increasingly common approach:*

Ma RH, Ji P, Wang Y, Wang SM, Cong H, Wang J, Liu QX, Zang YW [Clinical study on treatment of chronic bacterial prostatitis by combination of laser acupuncture with injection of shuang huanglian into the gland]. Chinese Acupuncture and Moxibustion. 1996 Aug; 16(8): 8–10

*Essential reading for an understanding of urinary incontinence in terms of Western electrotherapy:*

Fall M, Lindstrom S Electrical stimulation. A physiologic approach to the treatment of urinary incontinence. Evaluation and treatment of urinary incontinence. Urologic Clinics of North America. 1991 May; 18(2): 393–405

*An invaluable internet resource is the review of genitourinary problems by Phil Rogers:*

Rogers P Acupuncture in genitourinary & related conditions. Online. Available: http://homepage.eircom.net/~progers/gu1.htm [accessed 2004 August 20]

# 9.10  PAIN AND ITS TREATMENT

*With a contribution by Mike Cummings*

This chapter introduces different types of pain and their treatment with electroacupuncture (EA) and associated methods. General guidelines for treatment are given, with a focus on selecting which intervention parameters to use in the concluding sections of the chapter.

## PAIN

Pain can be defined as 'an unpleasant sensory and emotional experience associated with actual or potential tissue damage, or described in terms of such damage'. We sense pain, we respond emotionally to it, we give it meaning. If we 'kill' the sensation of pain, or deal with our feelings about it, or conceptualise it differently, sometimes we can bear it more. Understanding can lead to a sense of control for both practitioner and patient.

Pain may be acute, or chronic, or even 'acute on chronic' (an acute episode of one pain on a background of another, chronic pain). It may originate in the body (somatogenic pain), or in the mind (psychogenic pain). Somatogenic pain may further be differentiated into nociceptive and neurogenic pain, as well as 'idiopathic' pain, or diffuse pain that does not conform to any of these categories.

### Acute pain

Acute pain, by definition, is short lived and has a purpose, signalling actual or likely tissue damage. An initial inflammatory phase (lasting 1–3 days) is followed by a phase of 'subacute' pain that often lasts longer. Acute and subacute pain are usually characterised by clear, well-focused sensory characteristics. However, such pain is not a purely sensory experience. Sympathetic activation and generalised arousal are very much part of acute pain, so that it is frequently associated with anxiety. Sometimes the degree of anxiety experienced, or the patient's conviction that acute pain is symptomatic of more disturbing underlying disease, can signal the likely transformation of acute into chronic pain.

### Chronic pain

Arbitrarily, pain is usually considered chronic if it has lasted at least 3 months. However, the difference between acute and chronic pain is qualitative and not just one of duration. When pain becomes chronic, whatever its original cause, it very often has no ongoing known pathological basis in physiology, or anatomy, or nociceptive input. Thus, although some chronic pain may be maintained by myofascial trigger points, or by radiculopathy, it is often considered to be maintained primarily by *central* mechanisms, such as sensitisation or kindling, whereas acute pain has both peripheral and central components. Unlike acute pain, which warns of possible damage, chronic pain may well have no biological function.

Chronic pain itself may be periodic, sometimes with intermittent attacks of acute pain. It is not necessarily continuous. The sensory characteristics of chronic pain are often multifocal and vague, and sometimes inappropriate for the organic pathology evident. The affective dimension of pain is more evident than with acute pain, often leading to chronic pain being unfairly dismissed as psychogenic.

Chronic pain can be immensely difficult to treat – without apparent cause, without biological function, purpose or meaning, bewilderingly uncontrollable, and often totally disruptive of work, social and family life. Chronic pain patients may be demoralised, or frankly depressed, and can in turn demoralise even the most rational practitioner.

Sufferers from chronic pain often come to depend on medication for relief. Such reliance can in turn have iatrogenic consequences, such as gastric irritation, bronchospasm, increased bleeding time or skin reactions from non-steroidal anti-inflammatory drugs (NSAIDs). Reliance on medication can also distort the experience of pain, compounding problems of depression and sleep disturbance. It not infrequently leads to addiction, particularly to benzodiazepines and hypnotics, and more recently to opioids.

Given the multifactorial nature of chronic pain, therapeutic goals of management and rehabilitation may be as important as pain relief in some cases, especially in the elderly. Some authors, for instance, have suggested a threefold approach, striving for a 50% decrease in pain (intensity or duration, or both), a 50% increase in function and mobility, and a 50% decrease in medication with the elimination of potentially addictive agents. Given the potential side-effects of many conventional treatments, acupuncture and related treatments may have benefits for chronic pain patients in all of these areas.

### Nociceptive pain

'Nociceptors' are nerve terminals receptive to pain sensation. Nociceptive pain generally occurs as a result of damage to non-nervous tissue, occurring as a result of activation of specific peripheral nociceptors in musculoskeletal tissue, in supportive bony–cartilaginous tissue, or in the viscera. It is localised, may be present at rest, but typically increases with loading (e.g. weight bearing). If somatic in origin it is generally aching or throbbing, if visceral more a dull aching or cramping, the latter poorly localised. Even though nociceptive signals may not themselves reach consciousness, quite often motor or sympathetic spinal reflexes may become involved, with muscle splinting or blood vessel constriction around the actual site of injury.

Nociceptors are activated by peptides and prostaglandins released when tissue is damaged. Thus local inflammation is often evident, if not outright physical damage, with distinct and localised muscle tenderness or painful joint movement, but without other sensory disturbance. Nociceptive pain generally responds to analgesics.

## Neurogenic pain

Neurogenic or neuropathic pain includes the neuralgias, pain due to peripheral nerve injury, and that resulting from neuropathy. It originates from trauma or injury to the nervous system itself, including the peripheral nerves, spinal roots, spinal cord and supraspinal structures. Nerve endings are not involved, although it may feel as if tissue damage is present. Neurogenic pain may continue long after the original injury is past, and can be very severe. It tends to occur in older age groups.

In contrast to the local signs usually found with nociceptive pain, neurogenic pain often radiates along the path of the damaged neuronal structure. Sensory, and sometimes motor, deficits will also occur in neuroanatomically related areas. However, it is not always easy to differentiate clinically between nociceptive and neurogenic pain, and they may occur together. Reversible pain resulting from nerve root entrapment, for example, may follow a 'neurogenic' distribution, but should be distinguished from established nerve damage.

## Myofascial pain

Chronic myofascial pain has been defined as musculoskeletal pain without an obvious cause. It is almost always associated with muscle shortening (contracture rather than spasm), leading in turn to nerve entrapment and neuropathic (sensory, motor or autonomic) manifestations. These may be particularly evident if shortened paraspinal muscles lead to compression of nerve roots.

Within shortened muscle trigger points (TrPs) occur, small, localised and extremely tender points where sustained pressure reproduces chronic pain in areas where it occurs spontaneously. While chronic pain is generally considered centrally maintained, many who work with chronic myofascial pain believe it is sustained because of continuing nociceptive peripheral input from trigger points.

## Idiopathic and psychogenic pain

Pain is considered idiopathic, or sometimes psychogenic, when it is neither clearly nociceptive nor neurogenic in origin. Like neurogenic pain, however, it tends not to respond to opioid medication.

Pyschogenic pain has some characteristics in common with chronic pain. Thus it is not easy to differentiate between pains that stem primarily from the mind or from the body, although psychogenic pain may appear exaggerated, as well as spatially diffuse and variable in time – throbbing, as opposed to constant, in the case of headaches, for example. Those with psychogenic pain tend to complain more about it, with elaborate descriptions and an emphasis on affective discomfort rather than just sensation.

# PAIN AND ACUPUNCTURE

Acupuncture, and EA in particular, is generally considered as a treatment for both pain and functional disorders. However, although traditionally the prevention of disease was considered a priority, with disease treatment secondary and dealing with pain a subsidiary objective, there are now more acupuncture consultations for pain, particularly musculoskeletal pain, than for any other problem.

There is a vast literature on acupuncture for pain. Sun Peilin's magnificent tome is the single most useful reference work on the traditional Chinese medicine (TCM) treatment of pain, analysing many sorts of pain in traditional terms. There are also several reviews of acupuncture for pain from various Western perspectives, although unfortunately none of these link TCM syndrome differentiation to Western labels for differentiating pain, such as acute/chronic or nociceptive/neurogenic.

Box 9.10.1 details the causes of pain in TCM terms.

---

**BOX 9.10.1**

**Causes of pain in TCM**

In TCM terms pain can be due to stagnation of qi and/or xue (Blood), or deficiency of either or both. It can result from invasion of external factors such as Wind, Cold, Heat or Damp, or from internal causes.

Excess conditions associated with invasion of external factors are more likely to be acute (short-lived, fixed in location, constant and strong), and deficient pain conditions are more likely to be chronic (gradual in onset, moving, intermittent).

Blood stagnation pain tends to be fixed and stabbing, associated with hardness of the affected area and to occur at night. Qi stagnation pain is more moving, spreading, associated with softness of the painful area and occurring more in the day.

Pain due to predominance of Wind can be severe, coming and going, and paroxysmal. Cold pain, on the other hand, is more likely to be fixed, with restriction of movement and improvement with warmth. Heat pain may resemble that due to inflammation in Western medicine (WM), with heat, redness and swelling. Damp pain is deep, heavy, dull, fixed, difficult to move and often accompanied by numbness or swelling.

In Chinese clinical studies of EA, treatment effects are often explained only in vague and general TCM terms. EA is considered, for example, to 'regulate *qi* and *ying*, dredge the channels, create analgesia and promote body resistance'. Little attention is paid to syndrome differentiation, or whether different forms of treatment might be appropriate when conditions are analysed according to a traditional approach. TCM is also virtually ignored in almost all Western studies of EA for pain, in keeping with the perception of acupuncture, historically, as an easy-to-learn method of *locus dolendi* stimulation.

However, as stated earlier, acupuncture is a treatment for *both* pain *and* functional disorders. For best results, these two aspects of acupuncture, as 'local treatment' for pain (segmental 'reflexotherapy') and root cause therapy (homeodynamic regulation) should both be taken into account. The focus will vary between treating the pain itself, what are considered its underlying causes, or both of these, depending on the severity of pain experienced.

In this context, it is as well to remember that acupuncture, and EA in particular, appears to have more effect on the affective than the sensory dimension of pain. This can be important when considering how to assess responses to treatment. Effects of electrostimulation on general mood may also occur independently of changes in pain intensity. If pain is relieved, then muscles will tend to relax, movement will become more possible and circulation will improve, with benefits for local tissue repair, as well as on other levels as well.

EA was developed originally in the 1950s as a means of treating pain, first postoperative and intraoperative, and then other forms of acute and chronic pain. It was reintroduced to the West in the early 1970s just as transcutaneous electrical nerve stimulation (TENS) was being explored for its effects on pain following the 1965 publication of the Gate Control Theory of pain (GCT) by Ronald Melzack and Patrick Wall. The focus on pain and EA intensified during the 1990s, as EA became a standard tool of research into the mechanisms of pain and pain control. However, one should always remember that responses to clinical and experimental pain can be very different.

Clinically, EA is indicated for pain that is unresponsive to MA, or for severe and chronic pain conditions, particularly those involving nerve damage. TENS has been considered suitable for many types of pain, and according to one authority, 'an important axiom is that no pain should be considered untreatable by TENS unless proved otherwise'. However, high-frequency (HF) TENS may be more effective for chronic pain in the extremities than midline pain.

Most Chinese traditional acupuncture practitioners consider EA more likely to be successful if the sensation of *deqi* can be obtained, and the *qi* directed towards the affected area. Correspondingly, the paraesthesiae elicited by TENS should be 'directed into the painful area' for best results.

Auricular acupressure, generally with ear 'pellets' or seeds, is commonly used for pain. Pain is also one of the main indications for microcurrent treatment.

**Comparisons and combinations** In many experimental studies on pain, the effect of EA is superior to that of MA. However, if stimulation intensity is strong in both instances, effects may be comparable, and the combination of EA with periodic needle manipulation may be more effective than EA alone. There are few clinical trials that compare EA and MA, and the choice between them is often a matter of personal preference and experience.

Experimentally, there is little difference between EA and TENS in terms of their antinociceptive effects or the neural mechanisms involved. The same is very possibly the case with clinical pain, although some individuals may respond better to one or the other.

From experimental studies, it seems that probe TENS (pTENS) may be slightly less effective than EA for pain, although there are too few comparative clinical reports to be able to generalise this to patients.

Acupuncture and related techniques should never be employed in isolation. Adjunctive methods such as cold or hot packs, massage, exercise and diet may all be usefully combined with EA, TENS and the other approaches described here.

## Painful conditions commonly treated with acupuncture

A glance through the clinical studies database 💿 shows that EA and related methods have been used for a wide variety of painful conditions.

A survey of pain clinics in the USA found that cervical and low back pain were the commonest conditions treated, whether with TENS or with other methods, and in a survey of pain clinics in Scotland and the North of England, lower back and buttock or leg pains were those most frequently reported. However, in a corresponding Japanese survey, herpes zoster and postherpetic neuralgia presented for treatment more frequently than lumbar and neck–shoulder pain.

Leading indications for TENS in the elderly are probably chronic neuropathy and postfracture recovery.

## Acupuncture and acute pain

Of four systematic reviews of acupuncture for acute pain published by early 2001, only one, on acute dental pain, was positive in its findings. However, a less formal review concluded that EA is of great value in both acute and subacute pain. Some authors clearly consider EA to be more useful for acute than chronic pain, although in one such study the acute pain was predominantly nociceptive in origin, and the chronic pain neurogenic, which complicates the comparison.

In one retrospective (uncontrolled) review, pTENS was found beneficial for two-thirds of patients with acute pain. As for TENS, the authors of one review of its use for musculoskeletal pain concluded that, although there was little evidence that TENS could be useful if such pain were chronic, it could be helpful for acute pain. Other authors too have considered TENS more effective for acute than chronic pain. Although outcomes for acute pain are not infrequently positive in non-randomised studies, there are more negative randomised controlled trials (RCTs) than positive acute pain. In one RCT, however, high-frequency, low-intensity TENS (conventional TENS or CTENS) was found about as effective as acetaminophen (paracetamol) with codeine for acute traumatic pain, but without the side-effects of medication.

**Comparisons** For acute sprains, EA gave better results than MA in one RCT.

**Points used for acute pain** In TCM, the *luo* (junction, connecting) and *xi* cleft points are considered appropriate for acute pain, as well as 'corresponding' points (for instance, a shoulder point such as SJ-14 for a hip problem at around GB-30).

For acute pain using electrostimulation, Heydenreich suggested that the front *mu* points, *huatuojiaji* points and auricular points could be particularly useful. Strong stimulation at local points may be too uncomfortable for the patient, or even aggravate their pain, since local segmental circuits are already fully activated by the pain. Thus distal or contralateral treatment may be called for, and at fewer points.

## Acupuncture and chronic pain

Chronic pain is not a simple thing, and to do battle with it a familiarity with different approaches is a necessity. EA can be a useful addition for those who only use manual needling, but acupuncture alone is often not enough, particularly when the pain has proved resistant to other forms of treatment. The multifactorial nature of pain and the need for a correspondingly multidisciplinary treatment programme are emphasised repeatedly throughout the pain literature. In the West, this has led to a movement to set up specialist chronic pain clinics. Acupuncture treatment, like TENS, has become more and more an accepted part of what they have to offer.

Although short-term pain relief is achieved with acupuncture for around 50–70% of sufferers, long-term results are less promising, with some reviewers questioning whether they are in fact due more to psychological factors than to needling. Thus, although acupuncture was considered as 'possibly beneficial' for chronic low-back or head and neck pain in one 1989 meta-analysis, other reviewers have not been so sanguine, commenting that even the better studies were of poor quality. It is tempting to speculate whether the 1989 review was more positive because it included quite a high proportion of EA RCTs (6/14, or 42.9%). However, whereas EA in other early reviews of acupuncture was considered of great value for acute and subacute pain, its usefulness for chronic pain was not so clear.

As so often in clinical research, the poor quality of studies available for analysis precludes definite conclusions. Thus the authors of one systematic review of acupuncture for chronic pain could conclude only that there is insufficient evidence to compare the effectiveness of acupuncture with that of placebo, sham acupuncture or standard care. However, trials in which patients received six or more acupuncture treatment sessions were found to be significantly associated with positive outcomes.

In one retrospective (uncontrolled) review, pTENS was found to be effective in around 63–66% of chronic pain (amputation pain, neuralgia and degenerative joint disorders), but only in 50% of a further, heterogeneous group of conditions. Ronald Melzack and Joel Katz, in contrast, in a controlled crossover study of auricular pTENS for chronic pain, did not find it reduced pain scores at all.

TENS has often been used for chronic pain. Donlin Long, an early protagonist of TENS, wrote in one standard electrotherapy textbook: 'It is probable that transcutaneous electrical stimulation represents the single most effective physical entity yet produced in the management of chronic pain.' While it is true that TENS has more frequently been investigated for its effects on chronic than acute pain, results of recent reviews of TENS for chronic pain are still inconclusive. As with acupuncture, short-term benefits of TENS tend not to last, dropping off rapidly over the first year, particularly during the first month. Even so, clinicians still claim that TENS can be of significant long-term benefit to around 40% of chronic pain sufferers. It is worth noting, however, that caffeine, sometimes used in pain treatment, reduces the effectiveness of HF TENS.

Cranial electrotherapy stimulation (CES) has been used to treat chronic pain, although benefits in at least some instances may well be due to a placebo effect.

LA has been used for chronic pain. TrP infrared LA, for example, was found in one small double-blind study to accelerate chronic pain rehabilitation in professional athletes. LILT has also been used for chronic pain in a number of larger, retrospective (uncontrolled) studies, with an overall reduction in pain levels of some 60–70%. It has been argued that the long-term effects evident here would indicate that benefits are unlikely to be due to placebo. Some clinicians have even found LILT comparable, if not actually superior, to interferential therapy or shortwave diathermy in treating pain. However, despite some positive results in LILT controlled trials from Japan, the authors of one 1997 review of physical therapy modalities for chronic musculoskeletal pain concluded that there was little evidence that LILT, TENS or ultrasound had any long-term efficacy.

Box 9.10.2 details some other factors in the treatment of chronic pain.

**Comparisons** Adrian White, reviewing the clinical applications of EA, has concluded that it results in long-term benefits in around 25% of chronic pain patients, including those with musculoskeletal pain. Hyodo Masayoshi, in a retrospective review of ryodoraku for chronic pain, found that this form of EA was more effective for musculoskeletal conditions than for neurogenic pain, which was more responsive to nerve block. Other authors have also found EA in general to be more suitable for musculoskeletal pain.

**BOX 9.10.2**

**Some factors in the treatment of chronic pain**

Omura Yoshiaki considers that much chronic pain has become intractable because of coexisting localised microcirculatory dysfunction. He believes that this may be due to factors such as chronic infection, heavy metal toxicity or harmful environmental electromagnetic fields, and that physical treatments that enhance circulation, such as MA, LF EA or TENS, LA, heat, certain electromagnetic fields, *qigong* energy, and some drugs or herbal medicines, may as a consequence benefit chronic pain.

Chronic pain is also often associated with depression. Moderate to severe depression is associated with significantly less pain relief from EA, regardless of the pain intensity experienced. TENS too may become less effective.

EA was found to be more effective than MA for both pain reduction and restoration of autonomic and trophic functions in patients with chronic post-traumatic pain. EA also appears to be more effective than simple retained needling for chronic pain, and gave more effective short-term pain relief than MA in one study of mixed chronic pain types.

Richard Cheng and Bruce Pomeranz, comparing EA and acupuncture-like TENS (ALTENS) applied at acupoints for chronic musculoskeletal pain, found little difference between them. Stephen Abram and colleagues, in a small crossover study on chronic pain, concluded that LF EA, TENS and placebo EA all had comparable effects on mean pain ratings. However, in a large retrospective study of pain clinic patients, whereas MA, HF EA and TENS gave similar results in the short term, long-term benefits were greater with TENS. Comparable results were obtained in TEAS (transcutaneous electrical acupoint stimulation) studies with the Codetron device.

Ronald Melzack's group found little difference between MA and TENS in the treatment of chronic pain. In contrast, Gabriel Stux has suggested that LA is less effective than MA for acute pain, and a number of studies appear to support this.

**Points used for chronic pain**   In TCM terms chronic pain is likely to be associated with underlying deficiency. Treatment will therefore need to be directed at that, in addition to local stimulation for the pain itself. An elaborate discussion of constitutional treatment for pain is included in Sun Peilin's book. He suggests that the *yuan* and *xi* Cleft points may be used together for chronic pain, and that fewer needles should be used for a deficient patient, but more for a chronic, complicated pain picture.

When using electrostimulation methods (as well as LA or moxibustion), Alf Heydenreich suggested that the back *shu* points, *yuan* and *luo* points, as well as entry–exit points,

may be particularly useful for chronic pain, whereas Sun favours the *luo* points for acute pain. At least one review of acupuncture for chronic pain found that studies where the acupoints used varied from treatment to treatment produced more positive outcomes than 'formula acupuncture' applied at fixed points. However, in one briefly reported study of MA for chronic pain, there was no difference in either short- or long-term benefit between patients treated with TCM and those treated with modern 'Western acupuncture' protocols. Similar results were reported in one RCT of EA for chronic pain, distal meridian points being compared with local tender points, in this case.

George Lewith and Charles Vincent have suggested that, particularly in chronic pain, both endorphinergic and autonomic mechanisms are involved, so that both general and specific points may need to be used. In contrast, practitioners from such different backgrounds as Boris Sommer and Alexander Macdonald consider that local points should be used preferentially for chronic pain, a view supported by Thomas Lundeberg, who adds that more points may be stimulated than when treating acute pain. Trigger points are frequently mentioned, as indeed are auricular points.

LILT has been applied over the stellate ganglion for chronic musculoskeletal pain.

**When to use what – parameters for chronic and acute pain**
Scanning through the studies in the electronic database, it seems that DD modulation is far less common than simple continuous stimulation in the treatment of chronic pain, that HF tends to be used more than LF stimulation, with a number of studies making use of a middle range, around 8–16 Hz, and that strong treatment is less common than comfortable or gentle treatment. From the little information available on acute pain it seems that low frequencies (< 10 Hz) appear to be used less commonly than those above 10 Hz, while intensity may be 'to tolerance' or at motor level.

However, given the variety and complexity of painful disorders, it is difficult to make useful generalisations, and this is reflected in the literature. Thomas Lundeberg and Tim Watson have suggested, partly on theoretical grounds, that stronger stimulation can be used for chronic pain and milder stimulation for acute pain. From reviewing clinical studies, Adrian White has concluded that LF EA appears to be more effective than HF EA for patients with chronic pain. Together, these would indicate that LF, high-intensity acupuncture-like stimulation (ALS) is more suited to chronic pain treatment, and HF, low-intensity TENS-like stimulation (TLS) to acute pain – an approach considered standard by many physical therapists. Taking the opposite view, however, Clifford Woolf and John Thompson have proposed that TLS is more appropriate for chronic pain than ALS – a position also taken by John Low and Ann Reed in their textbook on electrotherapy.

Conventionally in electrotherapy, electrical or ultrasound treatment is given at lower intensity in 'irritable' acute conditions, and higher in chronic ones, where, for example, muscle may be lacking in tone or subject to fatigue. However, chronic pain can sometimes be exacerbated by strong electrostimulation, which is therefore best avoided at least initially if the pain is severe. Thus several authors have recommended sensory level LF for chronic pain, but motor level HF for acute pain. In ryodoraku, strong but brief EA tends to be used for acute pain, and mild but longer stimulation for chronic pain.

When using microcurrent therapy for acute conditions, it has been suggested by one author that high-voltage steep incident 'waveslope' stimulation should be avoided. However, the author of a different microcurrent textbook states that a rapid rise time and relatively 'high' current (100–200 μA) at 30 Hz may well be used for acute pain, but that a slow rise time, lower current (40 μA) and lower frequency (0.3 Hz) should be used for chronic pain.

One British advocate of LA has found that pulsing a 10 mW 660 nm diode laser at lower frequencies (5–20 Hz) is effective for many acute disorders, whereas 150 Hz is better for chronic conditions. In general, LILT pulsed at low frequencies may be more appropriate for acute or subacute conditions, and at higher frequencies for chronic ones. As for dosage, some authors have recommended lower doses for the former, and higher for the latter.

## Acupuncture and nociceptive pain

General points on nociceptive pain and its treatment can be found elsewhere in this chapter. For information on treating specific conditions, see Subchapter 9.12, by Pekka Pöntinen.

## Acupuncture and neurogenic pain

Since there are many types of neurogenic pain, and many methods of treatment, only a brief overview is given here. The treatment of specific conditions is covered in more detail in the next subchapter.

Pains due to nerve injury, neuritis or neuralgia are often considered as indications for LF electrotherapy, neuritis and the neuralgias for galvanotherapy, and an even wider spectrum of neurogenic pains for TENS, including stump and phantom pain, pain arising from a neurinoma (nerve fibroma) or neuroma, and complex regional pain disorder (CRPD). From a Western medical point of view, methods of peripheral stimulation (MA, EA or TENS), or of central stimulation (spinal cord or brain stimulation) all depend on the targeted neurological structures being able to respond. If they have been totally destroyed, this is no longer possible. Peripherally, although TENS and acupuncture may be effective for a neurological condition if there is associated superficial tenderness, they may be less so if there is reduced sensation (hypoaesthesia) in the area treated. Thus acupuncture (MA and EA) was considered to be less effective for pain associated with nerve damage in one early, uncontrolled American study. Correspondingly, in another retrospective review TENS was found to be less effective for pain associated with metabolic

peripheral neuropathy, or central pain secondary to injury of the central nervous system (CNS).

EA, like other forms of LF electrotherapy, is used for various neurogenic pains and paraesthesiae, as well as neurological conditions where the motor system is particularly affected. However, despite the view that TENS is more effective for neurogenic than nociceptive pain, some authors consider that long-term pain relief with MA and EA is far more likely for nociceptive than neurogenic pain. For example, periosteal HF EA (not the most comfortable of procedures) was more effective for the pain of osteoarthritis than for that associated with phantom limb or disc problems. Correspondingly, in one retrospective study of silver spike point (SSP) therapy, results were better for nociceptive than neurogenic pain.

LA and LILT are quite often used for neurogenic pain. Similarly, neurological indications for EHF include neuritis, neuralgia and vertebrogenic radiculopathy (disease of the nerve roots, the nerve fibres as they arise from the spinal cord).

Peripherally, improving circulation in a region of nerve injury or degeneration may well help restore nerve function and reduce pain, just as it can for nociceptive pain. The influence of methods such as MA/EA, TENS, LA/LILT, PEMF and EHF on local circulation may contribute to any effects they have on neurogenic pain.

**Comparisons** There is some agreement that TENS or EA is more effective than manual needling in the management of chronic neurogenic pain.

**Points used for nociceptive and neurogenic pain** Nociceptive pain is generally treated with segmental stimulation. Combination with extrasegmental stimulation may well prolong the duration of pain relief, and also enhance it, particularly if the extrasegmental TENS or EA is at a high intensity.

An interesting hint on points to use for neurogenic pain is given by Sun Peilin, who observes that the *luo* points may be used when superficial pain is accompanied by paraesthesiae and loss of sensation.

Alexander Macdonald cautions against needling areas where there is marked allodynia, as this may be exacerbated. He suggests that it is better to treat such regions with TLS, in the same segment but well proximal to the abnormal region. Keith Tippey similarly cautions against using TENS directly over a region of nerve compression, preferring to stimulate within the segment in which referred pain is perceived. However, he is also an advocate of stimulation over the spinal nerve roots for neurogenic pain, and employs motor points (MPs) and TrPs too. In the event that segmental stimulation exacerbates neurogenic pain, extrasegmental stimulation (in non-hyperalgesic areas) should be used. In particular, contralateral treatment may be appropriate.

CTENS requires intact *cutaneous* afferent nerves to be effective, whereas ALS depends on properly functioning *muscle* afferents. If there is 'denervation' of muscle, with cutaneous sensory nerves affected as well, progress will be difficult. On the other hand, if afferents are affected only on the dermatome level, for instance, stimulation can still be directed to points in the involved myotome.

When using LILT for chronic neurogenic pain within a Western model, David Baxter has recommended stimulating all relevant nerve roots, plexuses and trunks, as well as TrPs.

**When to use what – parameters for nociceptive and neurogenic pain** Neurogenic pain is very often chronic. Thus when Luther Kloth recommends ALTENS for chronic pain, he includes not only the chronic pain associated with degenerative joint disease and chronic inflammatory disorders, but also neurogenic pain. In keeping with this, when using TENS or EA, a number of authorities have suggested that nociceptive pain responds better to TLS, and neurogenic pain, especially with hyperaesthesia, to ALS, or to interrupted TENS/EA, although this recommendation is by no means universally accepted. Although strong stimulation has been shown experimentally to be appropriate for nociceptive pain, it may well exacerbate neurogenic pain.

Keith Tippey differentiates neuropathic pain (for which he recommends CTENS) and radiating or referred neurogenic pain, as in sciatica or cervical rhizopathy, for which he finds interrupted TENS more helpful. Thus he will use a combination of CTENS and interrupted TENS paraspinally for neurogenic pain. Mark Johnson suggests that ALTENS may be appropriate for radiating neurogenic pain, and similarly uses CTENS over the nerve root, with ALTENS over the main muscle mass through which pain appears to radiate. In neurogenic pain, where there is frequently cutaneous sensory deficit or hyperaesthesia, it clearly makes sense to use ALTENS rather than CTENS over the affected area.

When using LILT or LA for neurogenic pain, a low dose has been recommended initially, in case pain is exacerbated, although David Baxter proposes a mid-range dosage of around 10–12 J/cm² at first.

## Acupuncture and myofascial pain

For myofacial pain, the literature is enormous on MA and 'dry needling', as well as interventions such as TrP injection or cryotherapy. TENS is also used for myofascial pain, EA less so. See Subchapter 9.12 for further details, and Case study 9.10.1 on EA in the treatment of chronic myofacial pain in athletes.

Because of the association of muscle shortening with myofascial pain, stretching can be a very important part of any treatment. In Chinese acupuncture literature, the patient's movement during needling is repeatedly emphasised.

**When to use what – parameters for myofascial pain** Interrupted TENS has been recommended for deep myofascial pain, and modulated TENS to exercise shortened muscle, as well as to improve circulation within and around it.

Gad Alon has suggested that TrP motor level stimulation may be helpful for chronic musculoskeletal pain (15–200 Hz,

20–100 µs, 1–5 min/pt). Another interesting approach to treating myofascial TrPs transcutaneously is to use frequencies of 1–5 kHz and very short pulses in either continuous or interrupted mode. Stimulation should not be too intense, as this can aggravate myofascial pain, and treatment may need to be continued for long periods for maximum benefits.

## Acupuncture and psychogenic pain

Although acupuncture has been used in the treatment of psychogenic pain, particularly by Italian medical acupuncturists with a psychoanalytic background, it is sometimes considered that this form of pain is less amenable than other forms to peripheral stimulation techniques. In particular, after only one course of treatment, long-term benefits are less likely for psychogenic than nociceptive pain. Some authors consider that psychogenic pain responds better to EA than MA, although psychogenic pain is frequently exacerbated by electrical stimulation methods.

## Some conclusions on which intervention to use

MA, EA and TENS may all be appropriate interventions for pain, in different circumstances. When comparing acupuncture and TENS, for example, one important difference is the practitioner–patient relationship: whereas this is central to acupuncture, TENS can be used more independently. Economic factors, intelligence and dependency issues may determine whether one modality or a combination is optimal for a particular patient. When treating chronic pain, for example, the depression and weakening of inner resourcefulness often associated with it may contribute significantly to a decline in home use and effectiveness of TENS.

TENS is frequently used for pain in the elderly, its leading indications probably being chronic neuropathy and postfracture recovery.

LA (and LILT) may be particularly suited to treating children, the elderly or those for whom electrical or invasive stimulation may not be appropriate.

**Points for pain** Traditionally, *bi* (painful obstruction) syndrome, which roughly corresponds to the Western category of musculoskeletal pain, is treated using points local or adjacent to the painful area, together with distal points along the involved meridians (e.g. SI-3, SJ-5, LI-4 or LI-11 on the arm, or BL-40, BL-60, GB-34 or ST-44 on the leg). Treatment is also directed at expelling the external factors held to be responsible, using combinations of points spatially unrelated to where the pain is.

In TCM, the *luo* (junction or connecting) points and *shu* stream points are also important, the former for superficial (acute) muscle pain, perhaps diffuse and accompanied by paraesthesiae and sensory loss, and the latter for joint pain. Furthermore, the *yuan* (source) points may be helpful for deeper pain more clearly located along a meridian pathway. Other points such as the *xi* Cleft and eight *hui* meeting

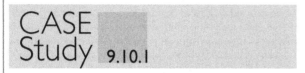

# CASE Study 9.10.1

## EA in the treatment of chronic myofascial pain in athletes
### Mike Cummings

Like many Western-trained medical acupuncturists, my use of acupuncture or dry needling targets the treatment of myofascial pain and dysfunction (Fig. 9.10.1). In most subjects my preference is for direct needling of the primary MTrP, and in the majority of cases the condition resolves after one to three sessions of brief direct needling. In chronic cases the pain may have been present for years at varying degrees of severity, or may have followed a relapsing course, and under these circumstances I often introduce EA early in the treatment course. In painful conditions where complete resolution is unlikely I use EA because it appears to have a more prolonged effect than manual needling alone.

The following cases are representative of my use of EA in the treatment of chronic myofascial pain from a single primary myofascial trigger point (MTrP). The cases are very similar, and in many ways commonplace, but they are unusual in that the subjects are elite athletes.

### Initial assessment and diagnosis

Both subjects presented to my private clinic in 1997. The first was a 45-year-old marathon canoeist preparing for a gruelling 125-mile race in which the serious competitors paddle non-stop, day and night to complete the distance in around 24 hours. She complained of a 10- to 12-year history of right shoulder girdle pain that came on after 1 to 5 miles of paddling or 3 miles of running. She described the pain as sharp and burning in nature, and commented that it was constant whilst she was paddling. The pain was exacerbated by carrying heavy bags and relieved by massaging with a rubefacient.

On physical examination I noted that she was a particularly muscular athlete with a normal range of movement of the shoulder girdles and cervical spine. Soft tissue palpation revealed a firm band of skeletal muscle within the right rhomboid minor, which was tender near its insertion into the scapula. Pressure over this tender point mimicked the subject's symptoms. This was clearly a chronic, primary MTrP of the right rhomboid minor. The major aetiological factor appears to have been overuse, as

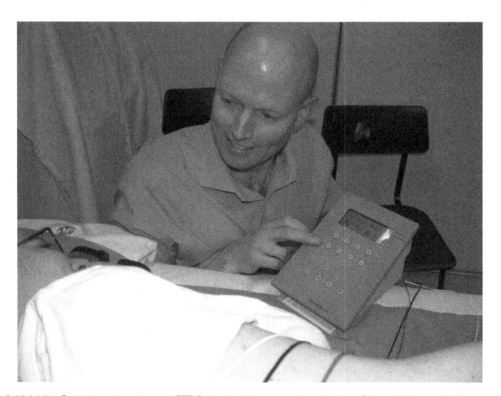

**Figure 9.10.1** Mike Cummings with patient and CEFAR Acus II electroacupuncture stimulator. Patient is being treated for chronic myofascial pain in the neck and shoulder girdle muscles.

the symptoms first appeared during a previous long distance race. Other contributory factors may have been paddle technique and a minor thoracic scoliosis.

The second subject was a 37-year-old champion butterfly swimmer. She complained of a 17-month history of intermittent 'right rhomboid pain', and commented that she had gained some relief from acupuncture for this condition in the past. The pain was clearly related to her intense swimming training and, whilst it did not always disturb her during swimming, she suffered considerable aching discomfort for hours or even days after a strenuous pool session. Physical examination revealed a particularly tender area in the lower border of her right rhomboid major, close to its insertion into the scapula. The associated taut band within the muscle was not as prominent or as firm as in the first, more chronic case. So this appeared to be a chronic, primary MTrP of the lower border of rhomboid major.

In both cases I felt the problems arose from overuse, which equates to repetitive microtrauma. Support for this contention can be derived from analysis of the biomechanics of the two different disciplines. The power stroke of the lower arm in forward paddling involves retraction and elevation of the scapula from a position of less than 45% of scapulothoracic rotation at maximum reach, thus the rhomboid minor is more stressed in this manoeuvre. In contrast, the butterfly stroke involves circumduction of the shoulder, which includes full scapulothoracic rotation, so it is the lower border of rhomboid major that is subject to the greatest dynamic range and therefore the most biomechanical stress.

## Treatment

The two subjects were seeking an understanding of their respective complaints, and hoping for sufficient symptom relief to allow optimal performance. It is important to recognise that athletes have considerable psychological investment in their physical abilities, and a thorough explanation of the nature and aetiology of the problem is an essential part of therapy. Furthermore, it is naive to expect to entreat an athlete to rest, especially in the run-up to an event.

My treatment goals were similar in both cases: to facilitate the subjects' understanding of the problem, to encourage appropriate rehabilitative activity, and to reduce the symptom load from their MTrPs in order to allow continued training.

I generally start acupuncture treatment of MTrPs with direct manual needling. However, I occasionally use EA at the first session if the subject has had acupuncture previously with no adverse effects or signs of great sensitivity,

as in the case of the swimmer here. In treating chronic MTrPs with EA, I directly needle the primary MTrP and place a second needle a short distance (2 to 4 cm) along the associated taut band. If there is a second MTrP or simply a tender spot nearby in the same muscle, I would choose this site for the second needle in preference to the taut band of the primary MTrP.

I use a DD pattern of LF and HF stimulation, from 2 to 4 Hz at the lower end to approximately 100 Hz at the upper end. I encourage the individual under treatment to adjust the power of the stimulus so that the sensation is strong but just below the threshold of aversive pain, and in most cases visible muscle contraction is apparent at the sites of needle insertion. The EA is generally applied for 10 to 20 minutes, but occasionally for up to half an hour.

In both cases the EA was applied at weekly intervals, and between sessions the subjects performed specified stretching manoeuvres with or without prior ischaemic compression. Stretching and ischaemic compression can be safely taught to subjects for the treatment of MTrPs at home.

After two sessions, one manual needling and one EA, the canoeist paddled 42 miles over a training weekend. She reported some stiffness after 17 miles but suffered no significant pain. The symptoms from her MTrP reduced considerably in spite of her continued training, and after four further sessions of EA the MTrP in her right rhomboid minor was no longer palpable, and she was symptom free.

The butterfly swimmer improved considerably after a single session of EA. She began performing specific stretching exercises enthusiastically, having understood the importance of this activity in countering the muscle-shortening effect of an active MTrP and maintaining the healthy functioning of the muscles. After three sessions she had her right rhomboid pain under control, and has continued to manage the problem herself without requiring further treatment. Unfortunately, her training schedule had been sufficiently disturbed that she could not attain peak form in time to defend her title; however, she subsequently went on to beat her own national record.

## Discussion

EA is a very useful therapy in the management of chronic or relapsing myofascial pain. Unfortunately there is no research evidence as yet to support this contention. In my opinion the principal advantage of EA over manual TrP needling is that the maximum tolerable stimulus can be given with a minimum of needling-induced tissue damage, although tissue damage from acupuncture needles is rarely a significant factor. However, in the above cases there would have been a considerably higher risk of pneumothorax if manual needling had been applied with sufficient vigour to produce a similar level of sensory stimulus to that produced by the EA.

points may also play a role, depending on how an individual practitioner likes to design a treatment.

From the numerous studies on EA for experimental pain, segmental stimulation based predominantly on spinal rather than supraspinal pathways seems clearly important ('local treatment'), but general points such as LI-4 and ST-36 may also be effective through their activation of supraspinal mechanisms. Many authors argue that, for endorphin-mediated analgesia, usually associated with stronger stimulation, it really does not matter too much which points are used. Combining segmental and extrasegmental stimulation, with their involvement of different and complementary pathways, may thus prolong pain relief.

Clinically too, EA at points like LI-4 has been found to reduce pain throughout the body. George Ulett, for example, simply recommended electrostimulation at LI-4 for upper body pain, and at ST-36 for the lower body. There are also points such as *luoling* on the back of the hand, or the region of the philtrum, which have been singled out as being particularly useful for pain.

When treating the root cause of the problem, whether you are more comfortable with TCM syndrome differentiation or think in terms of the autonomic system and particular patterns of innervation, carefully selecting combinations of specific AcPs becomes far more important. From a Western perspective, George Lewith and Charles Vincent have suggested that, particularly in chronic pain, both endorphinergic and autonomic mechanisms are involved, so that both general and specific points may need to be used.

Nerve block is commonly used for pain, and parallels have been drawn between the sites used for this and acupoints, with some authors emphasising proximal stimulation as a result. The use of the paraspinal *huatuojiaji* points, for the most part located close to the sympathetic ganglia, could also be viewed in this light, although stimulation here in cases of sympathetically maintained pain may sometimes exacerbate it. An alternative approach, used by Saul Liss with his HF stimulator, would be to position one electrode over the spine at or above the level of pain and the other directly over the pain site.

Other authors emphasise peripheral stimulation. Thus, using the 'Bicom' device described in Chapter 10, an electrode at the site of pain could be paired with one at the terminal point on the digit of the corresponding meridian. In particular, distal points within the segment could be used if treatment local to the complaint is too painful, or increases the risk of infection. In general, for severe (or acute) pain, it may well be better to use distal rather than local points, although *gentle* stimulation may still be appropriate locally. However, repeated strong local stimulation may exacerbate pain, possibly through some of the same mechanisms that lead to chronic pain.

Thomas Lundeberg, in a review of electrical stimulation for pain relief, states that, when using CTENS, electrodes should be applied directly over the painful area (*locus dolendi*), or either side of it. Lundeberg's research group has also pointed out that analgesia will be greatest if both electrodes are positioned within the same segment or along the same meridian, as nerve fibres are excited by lower currents when these are longitudinal rather than transverse to the nerve. This could be taken to indicate that low-intensity stimulation, whatever the frequency, may best be applied segmentally. Thus, for EA, points along meridians or nerves from the affected area have been used, sometimes proximal and distal to it, or across (straddling) it. In contrast, for systemic or underlying conditions, it has been proposed that linked bilateral acupoints should be stimulated with EA.

In line with Lundeberg's comments, Richard Sternbach, another very experienced clinician, has recommended that TENS electrodes are best applied at local points of low electrical skin resistance (SR). Sternberg's recommendation may be a clue to why in one study of EA for experimental pain, pain threshold (PT) increased more when true acupoints (LI-4, ST-36) were stimulated than non-acupoints in the same dermatomes. However, in the presence of inflammation, regions of low SR may be areas rather than points, so that precise electrode location may be less of an issue.

Which stimulation parameters to use at which points should also be taken into account (Fig. 9.10.2). As a general rule of thumb, the effects of TLS are primarily segmental, whereas those of ALS are both segmental and non-segmental, allowing for greater flexibility in its use. In particular, extrasegmental ALTEAS may extend the duration of segmentally induced analgesia. Some devices allow for

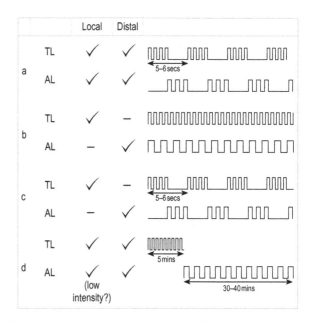

**Figure 9.10.2** Some strategies when using different parameters. (a) DD at all points. (b) TL locally, AL distally (simultaneous). (c) TL locally, AL distally (alternating). (d) TL (5 min) preceding AL (30–40 min) (DD = dense-disperse; TL = TENS-like, or high frequency, low intensity; AL = acupuncture-like, or low frequency, high intensity.)

simultaneous treatment with different frequencies at different points.

**Trigger points and ashi points** Palpating for tender points and along meridians is very much a part of traditional acupuncture. When locating points in this manner, however, remember that they may vary in sensitivity, both in different parts of the body and over time. In the short term, for example, sensitivity may vary in different phases of the menstrual cycle, while the incidence of tender points increases with age, at least in women. Points may also become more electrically active in emotionally stressed patients, or more tender with the patient in one position than in another. Thus, in ryodoraku, *ashi* points are deliberately sought when the patient is in the most painful position for them rather than when they are relaxed.

Precision is a key to successful TrP treatment for myofascial pain. However, if treatment is directed solely at tender points, although these may become less tender to pressure, other *ashi* points may then appear. It is important to treat both at root and branch levels, or at least to check for other tender points once those initially found have been inactivated. The more very tender points there are, the more likely it becomes that the condition will be difficult to treat. An abnormally low tolerance to pressure pain in muscle tissue, as often found in fibromyalgia for example, may signal a poor prognosis for physical therapies. In contrast, a large difference between pain threshold and pain tolerance may indicate that treatments such as needle acupuncture or LA/LILT could be helpful.

**The microacupuncture systems** Auricular acupuncture is frequently used for painful conditions. There are many anecdotal reports that the combination of auricular and body points may be more effective than either alone. Another less well-known approach is to use points in the philtrum region below the nose, which are reported as having a rapid analgesic effect.

**A note on laterality** Stimulation on one side of the body affects both sides of the body, particularly with ALS (via supraspinal descending pain inhibitory pathways) rather than TLS. Thus pain may be treated ipsilaterally, contralaterally, or bilaterally. For experimental pain, bilateral EA/TENS may be more effective than ipsilateral EA/TENS, and contralateral stimulation the least effective. Clinically, ipsilateral and contralateral EA (HF, followed by LF) may sometimes be similar in effect. However, what is appropriate for clinical pain may depend on the severity of the pain and the sensitivity of the patient, as well as the stimulation parameters used and the location of the pain.

There are also systems of acupuncture where not only contralateral points but points in opposite 'quadrants' of the body are used, and sometimes points on the back of the body are used to treat pain more towards the front (EA at Governor Vessel points for abdominal pain, for example).

Contralateral stimulation can be used if skin conditions (e.g. irritation, infection or injury) preclude local treatment. It may be more relevant if there is impaired motor function rather than just pain per se.

**Parameters used** It is important to remember that there is no one right way of using EA or TENS for pain. Different approaches have developed in different cultures: lighter treatment techniques are used in urbanised countries, whereas strong stimulation is more common in Chinese treatments. It may also be important to consider a person's condition in TCM terms. Excess and Deficiency conditions will need to be treated differently. For example, Chinese researchers compared HF, LF, increasing and decreasing frequencies in one RCT on painful conditions. They found that changing the frequency gave better results than fixed HF or LF, increasing frequency better for Deficiency, decreasing frequency for Excess.

To recapitulate what has been covered in previous chapters, EA/TENS may be applied at high frequency and low intensity (TLS, conventional TENS, CTENS, or TENS-like EA, TLEA), or low frequency and high intensity (ALS, conventional EA, CEA, or acupuncture-like TENS, ALTENS). A higher frequency may also be interrupted regularly at a low frequency, resulting in trains of stimuli (interrupted EA or TENS), or high and low frequencies may alternate (DD). Various other forms of modulation of a basic constant frequency output are also possible.

In China continuous or DD stimulation tends to be used for pain, and interrupted (or LF) stimulation for muscular conditions (e.g. paralysis, muscle weakness). In the West, CTENS has been recommended for arthritis, back and neck pain, postoperative pain, neuralgia and pain due to CNS injury, whereas intermittent TENS has been recommended for radiculopathy (with radiating limb pain), deep muscle pain or when tactile sensitivity is altered or reduced. An alternative view is that high-intensity HF TENS may increase tolerance and endurance of moderate pain, with low-intensity interrupted TENS more appropriate for low-level pain.

The general consensus appears to be that, when treating pain, the sensation elicited by electrostimulation should be 'strong but *comfortable*', although the intensity a patient considers comfortable may vary, increasing with familiarity but sometimes decreasing with changes in the condition being treated. ALS should evoke visible muscle twitching, whereas TLS should not. Intermittent EA/TENS may or may not.

Pulse duration should be adjusted (or preset) so that motor fibres, but not nociceptive C fibres, are stimulated. This is not always straightforward in practice, however. The general consensus is that, for HF, shorter pulse durations should be used, around 80–100 µs, and longer pulse durations, around 200–250 µs, at LF. In the end, however, it may be more important to adjust pulse duration for comfort rather than on theoretical grounds.

Issues of comfort can also be a problem with DD. The low frequency used may not be strong enough to evoke a motor response if the higher frequency at the same amplitude is already painful.

There are, in fact, a number of reports of continuous HF TENS aggravating pain, although whether this was because it was applied locally at high intensity and was uncomfortable because it induced muscle spasm, or was inappropriate to the type of pain being treated, is not always clear. It may be as well to avoid strong stimulation local to the source of pain or if pain is chronic and severe, at least in initial treatments. Overly strong stimulation may temporarily aggravate pain (particularly if applied around head and neck), may also lead to 'DOMS' (delayed onset muscular soreness), and can have other adverse effects. Localised *brief* intense stimulation, however, in the form of a few rapidly repeated short bursts of tetanic HF TENS, may have a useful analgesic effect.

At the other end of the spectrum, low-intensity stimulation may also have analgesic effects, as is often claimed by proponents of minimal needling or microcurrent techniques. Reviewers, however, have found little evidence that microcurrent has any useful effects in pain management, and experimental research into TENS and EA for nociceptive pain seems to indicate that strong stimulation is necessary for best results.

An alternative to varying output intensity can be to vary electrode size. With SSP, for example, larger-diameter (13 mm) electrodes may be more effective for pain, and smaller ones (10 mm) for other conditions.

In general, lasting after-effects are found with more intense EA/TENS stimulation, particularly at low frequencies and with longer pulse durations. The duration of analgesia may be increased by extrasegmental ALTEAS. In contrast, the effects of TLS are usually coincident with the stimulation itself, with a rapid onset and only a brief after-effect.

Surprisingly, in one study of experimental pain, LILT pulsed at a higher frequency (70 Hz) resulted in a slower onset and longer-lasting hypoalgesia than LILT pulsed at 16 Hz. In Paul Nogier's system, frequency 'E' (4672 Hz) is supposedly indicated for pain control.

When using LILT or LA, it has been suggested that stronger stimulation (6–8 J/point) be used in the first three sessions to inhibit pain, followed by a lower dosage (3–4 J/point) in subsequent sessions to enhance tissue repair, in line with the Arndt–Schulz law.

**Treatment duration** Most researchers consider that, to achieve widespread pain relief involving supraspinal opioid pathways, longer stimulation (30–40 minutes) is required than for local, segmental analgesia (short-term local analgesia may result even from 5–10 minutes of CTENS). In general, 20–30 minutes of EA is recommended, with little advantage if the treatment is prolonged to 40 minutes. TENS, too, is often used for just 30 minutes, although 40 minutes, or even 60, may give a better response. With SSP, treatment may also need to be longer than with EA to obtain similar effects. Results from experimental research with handheld pTENS are not altogether consistent. In some studies, best results were obtained with stimulation for about 10 minutes, which is clearly not very practical.

Although pain relief is likely to occur during a treatment of the appropriate duration, one that is too long may become stressful. With overlong CTENS treatment, for example (more than 30 minutes if used several times daily, or more than 60 minutes if just once daily), tolerance can develop. Modulating the output was originally introduced to counter this, but really has little significant benefit for a treatment lasting only 30–60 minutes. Nor, as a general rule, does it suppress pain to any greater extent than CTENS or intermittent TENS. However, it may well be experienced as more comfortable (and comforting) than LF stimulation.

For auricular stimulation, Terrence Oleson recommends stimulating for around 8–24 seconds per point in general, but up to 2 minutes for chronic conditions.

**How often to treat** Traditionally, acute painful conditions are treated more frequently (even more than once daily) than chronic pain. In modern TCM, the standard recommendation is to give a course of daily treatments, generally 7–10, followed by a break of a few days to rest the body, and then further courses as required. In the West, where chronic pain is more common, it may be more difficult to balance what is best for patients with what they can afford to pay, as well as dealing with the practicalities of attending for frequent treatments. Also, tolerance can develop if treatment is repeated too often.

TENS is generally used on a daily basis, if not several times daily, sometimes for extended periods. Single treatments are unlikely to give any indication as to whether it will be helpful in the long term, at least for chronic pain. Again, tolerance can develop if treatment is repeated too often.

For acute conditions, it has been suggested that microcurrent therapy be used daily, reducing treatment frequency to every 2–3 days when subacute.

**How many treatments** According to one large-scale survey of acupuncture for pain, about 51% of patients experienced some relief within four treatments, although a small proportion needed more than 10 sessions before feeling relief. A good initial response, however, may not be maintained unless patients received booster treatments at intervals.

Studies of chronic pain patients treated with EA have demonstrated that evoked potentials in the brain change little with a single treatment, but show a tendency to normalisation by the fifth, and more so by the tenth. Acute painful conditions, on the other hand, will generally respond more rapidly, sometimes even during the initial treatment. If a condition is going to respond, it will generally start to do so within 6–8 sessions. If there is no change within 8–10 sessions, the condition is unlikely to respond to the modality used.

With TENS, a single treatment is less effective than longer-term use. Acute conditions should begin to respond within the first 1–2 days of regular treatment; if they do not, alternative parameters should be utilised. With chronic pain, on the other hand, it may take as long as a month of daily treatment before any improvement is noticed, and there may be little purpose in testing alternative treatment parameters before then.

**What to use where** As a general rule, TLS results in rapid if short-lived pain relief, and is more appropriately applied segmentally, with less effect if used extrasegmentally, whereas ALS requires a longer induction period, but also has a longer-lasting effect, and may be used segmentally or extrasegmentally. So, for example, John Low and Ann Read recommend using CTENS at the site of pain and ALTENS in the related dermatome, myotome or sclerotome (with DD or interrupted CTENS at acupoints, MPs or TrPs, and DD or modulated output over peripheral nerves).

Thus CTENS might be used initially, and then the potentially more uncomfortable LF, high intensity EA (conventional EA, CEA) could be added. Alternatively, if the equipment used allows it, TLEA can be applied locally, with simultaneous CEA on distal meridian points or points with general effect (Fig. 9.10.2). In contrast, several groups of researchers have started with LF EA, than progressing to higher frequencies (sometimes increasing intensity concurrently) during the treatment session.

With all these various findings and recommendations, whether based on theoretical considerations, personal experience or literature review, it is salutary that the final conclusion has to be that there are no patterns of treatment parameters that emerge as universally helpful for specific conditions or types of pain. A certain amount of trial and error cannot be avoided when trying to decide what are the optimal parameters to use for a particular patient, starting with the best indicated, and then switching to different ones only if there is no benefit with these after two to three sessions. It is always advisable to err on the side of caution, especially early on in treatment, so it is probably best not to use strong stimulation initially, until you have a feel for how a particular patient is likely to respond. A failure to improve may signal the need to use stronger or longer treatments. When it comes to home use of TENS or other forms of self-treatment, it seems that patients do tend to stick with those parameters they find comfortable, and these may have little relationship to the cause or site of pain.

## SUMMARY

Some key points in this chapter are:

- Pain can be considered as acute or chronic, nociceptive or neurogenic
- EA and related techniques are useful for many types of pain when used within a comprehensive treatment programme
- Long-term relief of chronic nociceptive pain with EA may be more likely than for neurogenic pain
- Strong local stimulation is best avoided in cases of neurogenic pain
- General guidelines can be given, but the final conclusion has to be that there are no patterns of treatment parameters that emerge as universally helpful for specific conditions or types of pain.

 Additional material in the CD-ROM resource

In the CD-ROM resource, in addition to a much more detailed discussion on many of the topics presented here, the following are also mentioned:

- Pain in young and old
- Visceral pain
- Procedural pain (burn debridement)
- Parameters used: polarity.

Charts summarising the icon database studies on localised nociceptive (musculoskeletal) and neurogenic pain can be found in the chapters on these topics. Studies on the many other painful conditions for which EA is used are listed in other chapters too. Those remaining are summarised here.

**9.10** Summary of relevant studies in the electronic clinical studies database (number of studies)

| Condition | EA | Other |
|---|---|---|
| **Chronic pain** | 52 | 71 |
| **Acute pain** | 0 | 6 |
| **Mixed conditions (pain)** | 30 | 64 |
| **Arthritis – ankylosing spondylosis – gout (bi zheng)** | | |
| Fibromyalgia and myofascial pain | 14 | 35 |

## RECOMMENDED READING

*An overview of chronic pain:*
Mayor DF Understanding chronic pain and its consequences. European Journal of Oriental Medicine. 1997 Winter; 2(4): 4–10, 60–1

*Three textbooks on the acupuncture treatment of pain, with very different approaches:*
Baldry PE 1993 Acupuncture, Trigger Points and Musculoskeletal Pain. Churchill Livingstone, Edinburgh (2nd edn)
Gunn CC 1996 The Gunn Approach to the Treatment of Chronic Pain: Intramuscular stimulation for myofascial pain of radiculopathic origin. Churchill Livingstone, New York (2nd edn)

Sun PL 2002 (ed) The Treatment of Pain with Chinese Herbs and Acupuncture. Churchill Livingstone, Edinburgh

*A book with much useful information on EA and TENS, for both practitioners and patients:*
Berger P 2003 The Journey to Pain Relief. P Berger, Sandton, South Africa

*A useful review of acupuncture for pain in general:*
Birch S, Hammerschlag R, Berman BM Acupuncture in the treatment of pain. Journal of Alternative and Complementary Medicine. 1996 Spring; 2(1): 101–24

*The effects of acupuncture on different pain types:*
Carlsson CPO, Sjölund BH Acupuncture and subtypes of chronic pain: assessment of long-term results. Clinical Journal of Pain. 1994; 10(4): 290–5

# 9.11 NEUROGENIC PAIN – HEAD AND FACIAL PAIN – NECK PAIN

*With contributions by Jennifer Chu, Stuart Ferraris, Maureen Lovesey, Juliette Lowe and Ron Sharp*

In this chapter, treatments for neurogenic pain, head and facial pain, and neck pain are described. The focus is on electrical stimulation, but some information is also included on laser acupuncture (LA) and low-intensity laser therapy (LILT).

## NEUROGENIC PAIN

Neurogenic pain may be due to nerve injury, neuritis or degenerative neuropathy, and be either peripheral or central in origin. It can take the form of neuralgia, paroxysmal or fulminating pain along the course of one or more nerves, or be less severe but prolonged, sometimes with a correspondingly increased or decreased excitability to electrical methods of stimulation. Neurogenic paraesthesiae (distorted sensations) may include burning, 'pins and needles', or numbness.

### The neuralgias

#### POSTHERPETIC NEURALGIA

Following the acute stage of herpes zoster, postherpetic neuralgia (PHN) can develop if the virus has not been adequately contained. PHN tends to be more of a problem in older people, and once chronic can be very difficult to treat. Conventional treatment usually includes sympathetic blockade, antidepressant medication or the anticonvulsant carbamazepine.

PHN most commonly affects the ophthalmic division of the trigeminal nerve and midthoracic dermatomes. The pain may be both steady and paroxysmal. Sensory loss, allodynia and dysaesthesia (disturbances of sensation) are also common, while hyperalgesia (pain of abnormal severity following noxious stimulation) is less so. There may be a better chance of recovery if allodynia or sensory deficit is absent.

In one observational study, manual acupuncture (MA) was not found to be useful for PHN patients older than 65 years with severe pain for over 6 months. However, MA was useful in other patients, especially if treated early in the course of the disease. Nevertheless, results are not always good, and the authors of one RCT found MA no more helpful than placebo for PHN.

Electroacupuncture (EA) has been used in a number of studies for PHN, although in one retrospective review of low-frequency (LF) EA, it was not considered particularly helpful. As with MA, the more chronic PHN becomes the less amenable it is to treatment.

Peter Nathan and Patrick Wall found that 12 hours or more of HF, low-intensity transcutaneous electrical nerve stimulation (conventional TENS, or CTENS) alleviated PHN. However, one Italian group found good results with TENS only if used within 3 months after onset, and another researcher observed no additional benefits with TENS when patients were already taking tricyclic and neuroleptic medication. In one report, facial PHN responded better to TENS than PHN on the trunk. Long-term results with CTENS are not as impressive as short-term benefits.

Low-intensity laser therapy (LILT) has been used for PHN, as well as laser acupuncture (LA) together with focal irradiation. LA reduced local hyperaesthesia in one study.

**Comparisons and combinations** Although MA is probably not very effective for PHN, TENS, and particularly CTENS, has often been considered to be helpful. However, in one small randomised controlled trial (RCT), EA (5/60 Hz dense-disperse, DD) for 6 weeks gave better results than CTENS. Pain in the EA group worsened again after treatment was terminated, suggesting that the increased attention received by these patients may have been a factor in their improvement. In another study in which both EA ('muscle stimulation' with needles) and TENS were used, EA was often helpful in patients with dermatomal lack of sensation where CTENS was not appropriate. Again, continued treatment was necessary for extended pain relief.

EA has been combined with cupping for PHN. The results of this study are fascinating, if difficult to interpret: 100% of the 25 Chinese patients treated were reported as cured, but only 6.2% of German patients, whereas 20% of the latter did not respond at all!

**Points used** Keith Glennie-Smith has suggested that segmental acupuncture may not be effective because myelinated afferents have been destroyed by the virus, and that points rostral or contralateral to the affected dermatome or auricular points should be treated instead. For the same reason, deep muscle stimulation may be more effective than superficial dermatomal treatment.

Paravertebral (or *huatuojiaji*) points at the level of the lesion are recommended by some authors, appearing several times in the CD-ROM resource database 💿 alongside auricular and contralateral points, GB-34, LIV-3, LI-4, ST-36 and SP-6. The most common approach is to use some form of local treatment, although ST-36 has been described as the most frequently selected point for PHN in Chinese studies.

Electrode placements in the TENS studies of PHN include trigger points, selected dermatomes, low-electrical-resistance acupuncture points, over the painful area and proximal to the pain. John Thompson and Jacqueline Filshie suggest electrodes close to, but not directly over, the affected area, in the same or adjacent dermatomes, possibly straddling the affected dermatome. Contralateral TENS may be an alternative.

Glennie-Smith also uses LILT locally, as well as over intervertebral points, directed at the posterior root ganglion and dorsal horn at the affected spinal level as well as in dermatomes immediately above and below it.

**When to use what – parameters for postherpetic neuralgia**
PHN did not respond well to LF EA in one retrospective study. However, LF EA did give good results in another uncontrolled trial. 5/60 Hz DD EA also gave better results, at least in the short term, than CTENS.

In the PHN TENS studies, parameters varied widely: stimulation frequency from 10–180 Hz, intensities from 'low' to comfortable to the maximum tolerated, with duration from 20 minutes daily to 'prolonged'. Even with this limited data, there does appear to be some evidence that high-intensity 100 Hz stimulation, long term, may be of benefit. Margareta Eriksson and colleagues considered that HF or burst TENS gave better results for PHN than LF, high-intensity TENS (acupuncture-like TENS, or ALTENS) and HF transcutaneous acupoint stimulation (HF TEAS) gave good results in one uncontrolled trial. However, Mark Johnson suggests that when there is hyperaesthesia ALTENS should be used, perhaps contralaterally, rather than CTENS over the affected area.

Keith Glennie-Smith has used red LILT (660 nm) for local superficial irradiation, with the same dose of infrared LILT (820–840 nm, 50 mW, 60–70 Hz) for deeper penetration at intervertebral points. Higher output power (150 mW rather than 60 mW) may be more effective still. He suggests twice weekly treatments initially. Boris Sommer, writing more recently, recommends a more intensive approach, with five to six daily sessions initially, slowly reducing treatment frequency to once weekly.

## ACUTE HERPETIC NEURALGIA
It is important to treat herpetic pain early if it is not to become chronic. MA and EA have been used for acute herpetic pain, with a reduced incidence of PHN with the latter in two studies.

TENS (over the stellate ganglion) is another treatment that has been investigated for acute shingles pain.

LA and LILT are frequently used for acute zoster pain.

**Points used** Local lesions are often the focus of treatment, using the 'surround the dragon' technique, for example (see Figs 9.6.1 and 10.1c on pages 162 and 282). Posterior nerve roots or *huatuojiaji* points in the same segment can be used, and in one report anterior segmental points were also employed. A similar approach was used in the 'PENS' (EA) study by Hesham Ahmed and colleagues, but with stimulation limited to neighbouring dermatomes. Of the traditional acupoints, GB-43, LIV-3 and LI-4 have been used in more than one study.

**Parameters used** LF, HF and 10 Hz stimulation have been used for acute herpes zoster pain. In one interesting report,

HF EA was used first (for analgesia), followed by LF EA for its neurotrophic effect.

## INTERCOSTAL NEURALGIA
EA and ryodoraku have been used for intercostal neuralgia.

David Ottoson and Thomas Lundeberg have recommended HF or burst TENS at just below pain threshold, with electrodes positioned above/below and anterior/posterior to the painful region.

**Points used** George Ulett recommends using paravertebral points at the level of the lesion involved, as with PHN. Apart from the *huatuojiaji* or back *shu* points (BL-17, BL-18), others such as GB-34, LIV-3 and LIV-14 have also been suggested, or LIV-3 and LIV-14 with other distal points such as SJ-6 and SP-9 or ST-40, when the condition is considered as due to stagnation of Liver *qi*. P-6 has been used for acute intercostal neuralgia.

**Parameters used** In one EA device manual, HF or DD is recommended for intercostal neuralgia, at a moderate to strong intensity. Another manual just favours DD.

# Peripheral nerve injury and compression syndromes

Nerve damage may vary from total transection, through disruption of the axon with the myelin sheath still intact, to mild contusion of the nerve. It is sometimes difficult to differentiate between nerve damage and reversible nerve compression.

MA has been used successfully in a case of peroneal neuropathy that was probably due to peripheral nerve injury sustained during surgery. It has also been used for injury of the superior clunial nerve.

When using EA in nerve regeneration, strong stimulation may be counterproductive: in one experimental study of experimental neuralgia due to nerve compression, weaker EA (1–1.5 mA) was found to be more effective than stronger EA (3–4 mA). It is also clearly important that stimulation be started as early as possible after injury. EA may well hasten the resumption of nerve conduction and reduces the incidence of complications.

Donlin Long has claimed that peripheral nerve injury responds well to TENS in over 70% of cases, with similar results in TEAS studies by Ronald Melzack and Bruce Pomeranz's group. Thus TENS, together with analgesics and infrared treatment, was helpful for burning pain and allodynia in a case of crush injury, although neither analgesics alone nor continuous epidural analgesia had been effective. However, Paolo Procacci's Italian group found that TENS was only briefly helpful for peripheral nerve injury pain when the nerve had been extensively damaged. Steven Wolf and colleagues consider that CTENS is less effective for peripheral nerve injury than for peripheral neuropathy.

The role of LILT in regeneration of sciatic nerve injury has been explored in experimental studies by Semion Rochkind's research group. LILT has been used both *during* surgery for peripheral nerve disorders and for peripheral nerve injury pain *following* dentistry.

**Comparisons** In general, nerve damage may respond better to EA than to MA, although Bruce Pomeranz has suggested on theoretical grounds that the opposite may be true.

**Points used** Peripheral nerve injury can result in pain if large-diameter myelinated afferents are damaged. If this is the case, then use of CTENS peripherally is rather pointless, but positioning of electrodes proximal to the site of injury can result in dramatic improvements. When using TENS for traumatic and compressive mononeuropathies, therefore, electrodes should be positioned proximal to the lesion, avoiding regions of abnormal (low or increased) sensitivity. When using TENS or acupuncture it may not be possible to elicit paraesthesia or *deqi* in the affected area if there is deafferentation and loss of sensation. However, there are reports of electroanalgesia without the development of paraesthesia in the precise area of pain and deafferentation, and it may be possible to select treatment locations from which paraesthesia can be obtained that *surround* an area of deafferentation in order to obtain pain relief. For acupuncture, points are usually selected near both ends of the injured nerve trunk, with local points and 'big' points on the Large Intestine and Stomach (*yangming*) meridians.

**Parameters used** Selective stimulation of large-diameter myelinated afferents using CTENS is quite often recommended to relieve the burning pain caused by peripheral nerve injury, on the basis that large-fibre loss may well be responsible for some of the pain of traumatic neuropathy. Steven Wolf and colleagues observed that results improved with higher-intensity stimulation.

However, from the study data, it would seem that LF or interrupted EA and TENS is more commonly used than CTENS.

## THE HEAD AND NECK
Cervical pain following nerve injury during surgery has been treated with EA and MA.

Post-traumatic neuralgia of the infraorbital nerve unresponsive to local anaesthetic nerve block has been treated with TENS or tricyclic antidepressant drugs, or a combination of these. Results were less good when prior surgery had been attempted.

## THE SHOULDER AND UPPER LIMB
The treatment of neurogenic arm pain can be problematic, especially if complicated by the presence of chronic regional pain disorder (CRPD). A number of work-related conditions are sometimes considered under the umbrella terms cumulative trauma disorder (CTD) or repetitive strain injury (RSI), sometimes also known as repetitive motion disorder (RMD). These include thoracic outlet and carpal tunnel syndromes. Ergonomic aspects of the workplace need to be considered in any treatment programme for CTD.

## THORACIC OUTLET SYNDROME
Symptoms of thoracic outlet syndrome include pain and paraesthesia in the arm and scapula, with the ulnar nerve affected in 90% of cases. Ulnar somatosensory evoked potentials (SEPs) are usually abnormal, and the middle, fourth and little fingers tend to be most affected. Vascular compression can lead to ischaemia, atheroma or thrombosis, and sometimes dilation of the subclavian artery.

EA has been used for thoracic outlet syndrome. Although the authors of one study noted relatively long-term benefits, they also commented that treatment itself may need to be prolonged.

CTENS was found to be helpful for thoracic outlet syndrome in one uncontrolled study.

**Points used** In one study, local points such as SJ-14 and LI-15 were combined with LI-4, LI-11 and ST-38 distally. Joseph Wong suggests using points in the C3–C4 segment for the scalene muscle, HE-1, LU-2 or ST-12 for the brachial plexus, and appropriate distal points on the arm. Katz applies microcurrent to P-6 and/or SI-3 (negative) connected with anterior scalene muscle trigger points, TrPs (positive), with LIV-4 and/or ST-41 as secondary points (usually contralateral). He uses surface electrodes positioned over inserted needles.

## CARPAL TUNNEL SYNDROME
Pressure on the median nerve within the carpal tunnel can lead to paraesthesia in the wrist and hand, with muscle wasting and functional impairment if the condition is severe or longstanding. Carpal tunnel syndrome (CTS) is not uncommon in pregnancy, menopause, or in association with rheumatoid arthritis.

Good results have been reported in uncontrolled studies of EA for CTS.

LILT and LA have been used for CTS. Some benefits were reported, for example, in a RCT of LA for patients awaiting surgery for CTS (but not postoperatively). However, in one small placebo-controlled study, no subjective or objective difference was found between LILT and placebo for median nerve compression.

The *Qi Gong* machine (QGM) has been used to treat CTS, applied paraspinally at C7–T1, at the elbow (if painful) and locally, for 10–15 minutes at low intensity. (If pain increases, the applicator is moved a short distance away from the area treated for about 5 minutes and then reapplied.)

Case study 9.11.1 details the treatment of a woman with bilateral carpal tunnel syndrome.

**Points used** Several authors have emphasised treating points in the neck region for CTS, in addition to limb points. However, in the single detailed EA study on CTS found in the database, P-6 and P-7 were the points employed.

Margaret Naeser uses LA at Heart meridian points near the wrist, P-7 and LU-9 (as well as *jing* and *baxie* points when treating peripheral neuropathy), whereas Alejandro Katz applies microcurrent to ~P-6 (positive) locally, with contralateral ST-41 and/or LIV-4 (negative). Whether or not symptoms are reproduced with palpation of ~P-6 after treatment will indicate which of the two contralateral points is likely to give better results. He uses surface electrodes, positioned over inserted needles if the patient is not too sensitive for this.

# CASE Study 9.11.1

## Bilateral carpal tunnel syndrome
### Ron Sharp

This diagnosis had been confirmed by nerve conduction tests, and the patient was on the waiting list for decompression surgery. She complained of bilateral arm and hand pain, with frequent pins and needles. The hands ached following the simplest of activities and became very hot and swollen, especially at night. These symptoms had been going on for over 18 months and had been getting worse over the last 6 months.

There was no history of neck, shoulder, arm or wrist injury. Her heart was fine, but there was an alteration to circulation in the arms with some slight general swelling. Aggravating factors were holding and gripping, driving any long distance and repetitive lifting, which was inevitable at times in her work as a book dealer. Previous treatments included heat, neuromobilisations and manipulation, none of which had helped. Relief was gained only by rest and anti-inflammatory medication.

On examination she had poor neck posture, with a poker neck. Gripping caused pain, reflexes were dull and equal and she had increased sensation on the left forearm. Both arms were cold to the touch, with tenderness to deep pressure. There was full range of movement at her shoulders, elbows and wrists, although there was some weakness on resisted wrist extension bilaterally, with pain. There was some slight restriction to neck rotation (down 10%), which was equal on both sides. Extension, side flexion and flexion were normal. The neural tension test was positive at the end of range on the median nerve complex bilaterally and Tinel's sign was positive bilaterally. The pulse was slow but even, and the tongue pale and dry, with a thin, white coating with good root.

The treatment plan was to move the energy in the arms, mobilise the neck and address any posture problems at her work. Acupuncture seemed to be the best approach for the arms, with mobilisations of the neck and postural exercises. The first treatment was the needling of LI-10 and SJ-5, bilaterally with even method, agitating the needles every 5 minutes for a period of 15 minutes. The patient was also given wrist splints to use at night and during the day if a heavy workload was scheduled, supplemented with neck posture advice and exercise.

There was a slight healing crisis with discomfort of the neck for only a few hours. The previous treatment was repeated, with needle retention for 20 minutes using the even method, followed by cervical manual traction in flexion for 3 × 30 seconds. Although she benefited from treatment and regained her full range of neck movement, the discomfort had not changed appreciably. The next few treatment sessions used the same points but with a strong drainage treatment at SJ-5 for 5 minutes, followed by even technique at SJ-5 and LI-4, with needle agitation every 5 minutes over a 20-minute period.

This strategy seemed to work well; the patient had good pain relief for about 5 days, with slight occasional discomfort depending on her workload. The right side had responded more effectively than the left, and the discomfort on the left had become more focused in the hand. The strategy now had to address the left-hand discomfort, so the points for acupuncture were changed to right LI-10, left LI-4, and *luozhen* (extra point). These were needled with the even method, with needles left in place for 20 minutes. This worked quite well, but again the effect lasted for no more than 5 days.

To try to lengthen the treatment effect I added electroacupuncture to the treatment regimen. The treatment consisted of right LI-10, left LI-4, and *luozhen* (extra point). Right LI-10 and left *luozhen* were connected to the electrodes and left LI-4 was needled with even method, all for 20 minutes. The treatment rate was 10 Hz, with an intensity that was just within the comfortable range, checked every 5 minutes to maintain the intensity and to counteract accommodation.

This strategy succeeded and the patient was totally asymptomatic after another three sessions. When she had to be out of the area for several months, we decided she should use a piezoelectric wand stimulator while away to maintain her pain control. I prescribed two weekly treatments of three charges at LI-10 bilaterally.

On review, her consultant decided to hold back on surgery for the time being, as acupuncture seemed to control her condition. The patient contacted me after being away for 5 months to say that she had no problems with her arms and hands. The consultant had discharged her and she would not require surgery. The piezoelectric wand had been used no more than a couple of times and that was only after a heavy session of stock taking.

---

**Parameters used** When using microcurrent, Margaret Naeser starts treatment with 292 Hz, following this with 0.3 Hz. LF EA, 'to tolerance', was used in one study.

With a low-power (5 mW) HeNe or 670 nm diode laser suitable for self-treatment at home, lengthy treatments are necessary (3–20 minutes per point). With a higher-power (15 mW) clinical laser, such long exposure times are not needed.

Kenneth Branco and Margaret Naeser recommend at least 15 sessions for CTS with their low/microcurrent protocol, or 4–8 weeks for the home treatment version.

## PLEXUS LESIONS

Traction lesions of the brachial plexus can involve avulsion of nerve roots from the spinal cord, particularly in motorcycle accidents, and may result both in total and irreversible paralysis and in paroxysmal pain that continues indefinitely and responds poorly to medication.

Brachial plexus injury and neuralgia have been treated with EA. Treatment was useless in patients with a complete plexus lesion or where nerves had been ligated, with better results in those whose injury was less severe, due to compression, contusion or traction, or relatively recent. The points used are generally selected according to where pain is experienced and the distribution of nerves or meridians passing through these areas.

TENS has been used for the severe pain of brachial plexus lesions, including avulsion injury, with one electrode positioned over C5–C7 and the other just proximal to the site of pain in an area where there is afferent input.

## CLUNIAL NERVE INJURY

The clunial (cluneal, clunical) nerve, which innervates the skin of the buttock, has three divisions: the superior, middle and inferior. The former originates from L1–L3, and the latter two from S1–S3. Following back surgery, superior clunial nerve (SCN) entrapment can cause low-back and buttock pain, often extending into the leg. It may be severe enough to make sitting, walking or standing possible for only short periods. Conventionally, this neuropathy has been treated with steroid injection, thermal ablation or surgery.

MA has been used for injury of the SCN, as have EA and TEAS. EA was found to be more effective than MA in one RCT.

**Points used** Stimulation of trigger points lateral to L1–L2 may relieve clunial nerve pain. Thus *huatuojiaji* and *ashi* points have been used for SCN in conjunction with points such as GB-34 and other distal points.

**Parameters used** LF EA or TEAS appears to be used more commonly than HF stimulation.

## PIRIFORMIS SYNDROME

The peroneal division of the sciatic nerve passes through the piriformis muscle, rather than under it, in some 10–20% of the population (Fig. 9.11.1). Spasm, contracture or injury of the muscle then compresses the sciatic nerve, leading to symptoms that mimic those of discogenic sciatica, as well as buttock tenderness and pain that sometimes radiates to the lower abdomen and genitals. Pain may be diffuse and, if the problem is chronic, atrophy of the lateral muscles of the calf may develop. Conventional treatment includes physical therapy, steroid injection or surgery.

Piriformis syndrome has been treated using MA, EA and a 'biofrequency spectrum' device. LA has been used for piriformis muscle injury.

**Comparisons and combinations** For sciatic pain presumed due to piriformis muscle spasm, ultrasound acupuncture (1 W for 60 seconds) at acupoints such as BL-27–BL-29 and LIV-12, at the greater trochanter and rectally, has been

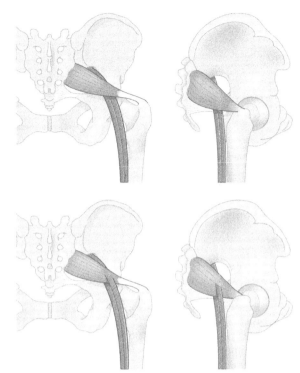

**Figure 9.11.1** Piriformis syndrome. This set of diagrams (rear and side views) illustrates the close proximity of the sciatic nerve and the piriformis muscle at the pelvic outlet. The lower pair of diagrams show a common anatomical variation in which the peroneal part of the sciatic nerve traverses the muscle fibres of piriformis – this occurs in approximately 10% of people. (Reproduced with permission of Dr Mike Cummings, Medical Director, British Medical Acupuncture Society.)

combined with 2 Hz EA at the L5 *huatuojiaji* points (15–20 minutes, to tolerance), and vitamin B12 point injection at auricular and hand points for the low back. Other authors have combined EA and acupoint injection for piriformis syndrome. EA has also been combined with far-infrared lamp (TDP) irradiation.

**Points used** For non-radicular compression lesions of the sciatic nerve, John Thompson has recommended that TENS electrodes are applied segmentally and proximal to the lesion.

## MERALGIA PARAESTHETICA

Nerve compression or injury in the groin can sometimes lead to neuritis in the lateral cutaneous nerve of the thigh, with symptoms in the lower two-thirds of the anterolateral thigh. It may occur during or following pregnancy, in obese individuals, or even as a result of wearing overly tight clothes ('jeans disease').

This condition has been treated with MA together with acupoint injection, with EA together with cupping, with electric plum blossom needling combined with moxibustion, and also with TENS. Local stimulation was emphasised in the EA (HF) and plum blossom (LF) studies.

# Amputation pain

Chronic postamputation pain is common, with both central and peripheral mechanisms responsible for its initiation and maintenance. Pain may be experienced in the stump or as phantom pain, and may be burning, tingling or cramping. The former tends to be associated with decreased blood flow in the residual limb, and the latter with muscle spasm.

One retrospective review of probe TENS (pTENS) for chronic pain reported useful effects in 65.8% of cases of pain due to amputation.

## STUMP PAIN

Stump pain is sometimes caused by 'ectopic' sensory nerve discharges from a neuroma.

Donlin Long reported good initial results for stump pain with TENS, although effectiveness dropped off considerably over time. TENS may also result in more rapid stump healing if used postoperatively.

MRT has been found to be beneficial for stump pain, muscle spasm and oedema.

**Points used** John Thompson recommends that TENS electrodes are positioned paraspinally in the same dermatome and actually on the stump.

**Parameters used** From the few studies available, it appears that HF stimulation is attempted more frequently than LF EA or TENS. Indeed, it seems that stump pain can respond well to CTENS. However, for burning pain and paraesthesia, parameters likely to improve blood circulation should be used, whereas for cramping pain parameters for muscle spasm would be preferable.

## PHANTOM PAIN

'Phantom pain' occurs in many patients after amputation; it can be very severe and, surprisingly, can be congenital as well as acquired. It can occur after removal of a limb, the bladder, the breast or even tonsils and, like stump pain, can be burning or tingling or, possibly more often, cramp-like. It should not be confused with non-painful phantom sensation, which may be tactile, kinetic (as if a leg is moving, for example) or even kinaesthetic (a limb may feel as if it is 'telescoping' over time).

Complete relief of pain may not be a realistic objective, although pain reduction may well be possible. The level of pain experienced may be related to stress, anxiety, exhaustion or depression, and treatment regimens may need to take these factors into account.

Acupuncture, both MA and EA, has been used for phantom limb pain. In one EA study, results were better on the upper than lower limb, and better in women than in men. The author of a small study on phantom limb pain in which MA, EA and moxibustion were all used commented that stump pain is more difficult to treat.

TEAS and TENS can give useful results in phantom limb pain, particularly if the pain is mild. Although sham TENS had a considerable effect on phantom pain in one study,

in another TEAS (Codetron) was only helpful in 25% of patients. TENS tends to lose its effectiveness for phantom pain slowly over time.

In addition to phantom limb pain, TENS has also been used for phantom bladder and phantom breast pain. In the latter case, when tolerance developed to treatment (that also incorporated auricular acupuncture and medication), metastases were subsequently detected.

Vigorous acupuncture and TENS have been reported as eliciting or exaggerating phantom limb pain, and TENS applied to the stump could also revive a phantom that had been successfully suppressed. Microcurrent TENS (MENS), on the other hand, may relieve phantom limb pain.

**Comparisons and combinations** In one case report, the patient's preference was for MA over both EA and TENS. In another, the combination of acupuncture and TENS was the only treatment that enabled the patient to wear his forearm prosthesis with a degree of comfort.

In an uncontrolled study, EA gave better results than TENS; best results were found with their combination. EA at scalp points has also been combined with MA and moxibustion for phantom pain.

**Points used** Given that local stimulation may exaggerate phantom pain, contralateral treatment should perhaps be attempted first. Auricular treatment may be another useful starting point. Scalp points, GB-20, Du-16, Du-24 and *sishencong* (M-HN-1) have also been used, together with major points on the limbs and *huatuojiaji* points.

Phantom limb pain is liable to be more severe if the stump itself is colder. Jacqueline Filshie has suggested the use of acupoints likely to block sympathetic activation. In the case of phantom breast she has employed both paraspinal (T1/T2) and suprascapular TrPs to good effect, the latter to reduce muscle spasm.

With conventional TENS, the peripheral nerve trunks are usually stimulated. However, if these are absent, as in the phantom limb, other strategies have to be adopted. David Bowsher, for example, suggested that the spinal cord itself should be stimulated at the segmental level involved. Other TENS electrode placements have included trigger points, acupoints, segmentally or contralaterally, over related peripheral nerves (particularly those supplying the extensor muscles of the phantom), or the stump itself. Laitinen and others obtained good results with contralateral stimulation.

**When to use what – parameters for phantom pain** EA studies have predominantly employed LF stimulation, 'to tolerance', or at 'bearable' intensity.

In TENS studies, a wide range of parameters has been used. CTENS is sometimes recommended, but is not always helpful. LF burst TENS is another possibility, although less effective than CTENS in one study where electrodes were positioned to stimulate phantom extensor muscle efferents. ALTENS has been used contralaterally. MA and low-intensity, HF stimulation (TENS-like stimulation, or TLS) have been suggested as appropriate parameters to use both preoperatively and following amputation. As with stump pain, parameters should be selected in accordance with whether the phantom pain is more burning or cramping.

# Peripheral neuropathy

Peripheral sensory neuropathy may accompany endocrine conditions such as diabetes or hypothyroidism, or may result from infectious diseases such as leprosy, Lyme disease or HIV, some nutritional deficiencies, or ingestion of toxic chemicals. Mixed sensory and motor neuropathies occur in uraemia and Guillain–Barré syndrome, as well as in most types of Charcot–Marie–Tooth syndrome, the commonest inherited peripheral polyneuropathy. In TCM terms, peripheral neuropathy is usually considered under the heading of *wei bi*, or *wei* syndrome.

Encouraging results have been reported in uncontrolled studies of EA for both drug-induced neuropathy and Guillain–Barré syndrome.

Whereas Donlin Long did not consider TENS to be particularly useful for peripheral neuropathy (with parameters selected according to patient preference), Steven Wolf and colleagues did find CTENS helpful, although their definition of 'peripheral neuropathy' included some neuralgias. Thus TENS has been used for painful neuropathy in Guillain–Barré syndrome. The Codetron ALTENS device was also helpful for a small cohort of peripheral neuropathy sufferers in one uncontrolled study.

Microcurrent TEAS was found to be helpful for peripheral neuropathy induced by antiretroviral medication in HIV patients.

MRT (58.57–69.6 GHz, 3 mW, 4–7 min daily at acupoints) has been used for alcohol-induced polyneuropathy, radiation sickness and infection, with better results in non-medicated patients. EHF acupoint stimulation has been found helpful for 'peripheral neuritis' (neuralgias, optic and auditory neuritis) in other reports.

**Points used** For drug-induced neuropathy, the most commonly used points appear to be ST-36 for the lower limb and LI-11 for the upper limb.

Electrode placements in the TENS/TEAS studies of peripheral neuropathy include acupoints proximal to or over painful areas.

With a two-output TENS machine, Gordon Gadsby and Michael Flowerdew suggest that one pair of electrodes can be positioned at the site of neuropathic pain, and the other pair bilaterally at ST-36.

One interesting approach tried for peripheral neuropathy combined acupuncture with home use of cathodal TEAS at ST-36 for the leg, or LI-11 for the arm, the return electrode (anode) being placed in a waterbath in which the affected foot or hand was also immersed. A similar approach with conventional EA has also been suggested for polyneuropathy: LI-11 in conjunction with the interdigital *baxie* points for the upper limb, or ST-36 and SP-6 with the corresponding *bafeng* points for the leg.

For peripheral neuropathy in the feet, Margaret Naeser has suggested a home treatment protocol for LA with local points such as BL-60, KI-3, KI-6, GB-40, LIV-4, ST-41 and SP-5, *jing* Well and *bafeng* points.

**When to use what – parameters for peripheral neuropathy** TLS, especially if not charge balanced, may not be suited to peripheral neuropathy with hyperaesthesia or serious sensory loss. Local treatment may serve only to exacerbate pain, while skin damage could occur without the patient's awareness.

Stimulation at >50 Hz may not be appropriate for peripheral neuropathy if denervation is a factor. In contrast, experimental research indicates that HF may more effectively reduce neuronal hyperexcitability than LF stimulation. Furthermore, increased blood supply to the nerve may occur only in response to HF, not LF EA.

Clinically, moderate intensity DD or LF EA has been recommended for polyneuropathy, although some practitioners prefer to use TLS.

## DIABETIC NEUROPATHY

Peripheral neuropathy is the most common complication of diabetes mellitus. In older diabetics, peripheral neuropathy can also be associated with peripheral ischaemia due to vascular disease. In what is termed the 'diabetic foot', the combination of neuropathy and ischaemia can have serious consequences: a trivial lesion can lead to rapid necrosis with the need for extensive surgery. Most drugs used for diabetic neuropathy are associated with significant side-effects.

Diabetic *autonomic* neuropathy can also cause dysfunction or actual damage in internal organ systems – cardiovascular (tachycardia), gastrointestinal (gastroparesis, diarrhoea), genitourinary (neurogenic bladder), adrenal and ocular (pupillary abnormalities). With reduced afferent input from limbs affected by peripheral neuropathy, neuropathic changes can occur centrally as well. Thus afferent stimulation can be an essential part of treatment. Acupuncture has been used for both autonomic and peripheral diabetic neuropathy.

Experimentally, EA has been found to compensate for neurochemical changes in peripheral nerves that may be associated with the development of neuropathy, and also to protect nerve function. EA at BL-23 and ST-36 appeared more protective against sensory neuropathy than TENS at the same points.

For peripheral diabetic neuropathy, results with EA were superior to those of MA (mock EA) in one crossover RCT. EA was also superior to medication in other controlled studies. Improvement was found by Romanian researchers to peak after about six to eight sessions.

Kaada's TEAS protocol was found to improve symptoms of diabetic neuropathy even more than those of Raynaud's disease in one very small, uncontrolled study.

There are several other uncontrolled TENS studies on diabetic neuropathy, usually with positive outcomes. In one RCT, the combination of TENS with amitriptyline resulted in significantly greater pain relief than use of sham TENS with the medication. Treatment may be less effective if there is gross sensory loss and poor distal vascular perfusion. However, as well as for 'pure' neuropathy, TENS has been used in the treatment of the diabetic foot.

**Comparisons and combinations** Norman Shealy reports good results for diabetic neuropathy by combining cranial electrotherapy stimulation (CES, 1 mA for 1 hour daily, using the Liss device) with MRT using the experimental GigaTENS. Each of the 12 acupoints in his 'ring of fire' protocol was irradiated for 3 minutes daily, using 52–78 GHz at 1 μW, for two 5-day courses separated by an interval of 2 days, and then 10 once-weekly treatments. Progesterone cream was also applied.

**Points used** The most frequently used point is probably ST-36. Other Stomach and Gall Bladder meridian points are often used as well, and less commonly with points on the Bladder, Liver, Large Intestine and Spleen meridians.

TENS studies usually focus on treating the leg and foot directly, perhaps with paraspinal lumbar electrodes in addition.

**Parameters used** LF stimulation is used more frequently than HF in the treatment of diabetic neuropathy. DD EA and HF TENS have also been utilised. There is little information available on the current intensities employed.

### HIV-RELATED PERIPHERAL NEUROPATHY
Neither MA nor amitriptyline was superior to placebo in one study on HIV-related peripheral neuropathy. However, both EA and pTENS were helpful in single case reports on this condition.

## Restless legs syndrome

'Restless legs syndrome', comprising unpleasant but not usually painful sensations in the legs, often disturbing sleep and relieved by movement, has been treated with MA, EA and TENS. In one very painful case the combination of TENS and vibration was more effective than either separately. Combined treatment with EA and a multifrequency lamp is another possible approach.

BL-56, ST-36 and SP-10 have been used for restless legs syndrome, as well as interrupted LF and HF stimulation.

## Radiculopathy-related pain

Radiculopathy-related pain is due to a combination of mechanical and biochemical events. Compression of the nerve root creates oedema, leading to intraneural inflammation (neuritis) and hypersensitivity. Symptoms may be sensory (hyperalgesia, allodynia), autonomic (vasoconstriction, excessive sweating on movement or needling, 'goose bumps', *peau d'orange*, dermatomal hair loss), or motor (muscle shortening, reduced range of movement, thickening of tendons where they attach to bone). Thus radiculopathy may alter both motor and sensory function. Here low-back pain and sciatica are considered.

### THE LOW BACK AND SCIATICA
Back pain can be considered under various headings, based on whether nerve compression or entrapment is an important factor. Papers on 'sciatica', without emphasis on assessment of aetiology have been listed separately in the CD-ROM database 💿 for this chapter. Here, studies on sciatica and lumbar pain with radicular involvement are considered together.

Sciatica is usually due to pressure on a nerve root and ensuing inflammation. A nerve root problem is most likely if flexion is not problematic, but extension and side bending towards the problem side increases pain in the affected extremity. L4–L5 and S1–S3 nerve roots are those usually affected. Thus L4–L5 lumbar disc herniation is one possible cause of sciatic pain. If L3–L4 nerve roots are affected, pain is likely to radiate to the sacroiliac joints, hips, posterolateral thighs and the fronts of the legs, with anteromedial numbness, weakness of knee extension and a decreased knee reflex. If L4–L5 nerve roots are involved, pain will radiate in much the same way but down the posterolateral rather than anterior lower leg. Numbness in this case will be lateral, perhaps extending into the dorsum of the foot and big toe, with weakened foot dorsiflexion but normal reflexes. L5–S1 and S1 nerve root involvement will result in a similar pattern of pain radiation, with numbness in the lateral leg, calf, foot and heel, as well as in the sole. Plantarflexion may be weak, and the ankle jerk reflex reduced or absent.

Conventional treatments for nerve root problems include disc surgery, radiofrequency ablation of the dorsal root ganglion of the implicated nerve and epidural steroids. Sciatica is generally considered amenable to electrostimulation, and pain due to disc herniation responds well to non-invasive treatment in many cases. In general, reversible radicular pain due to entrapment is more likely than established nerve damage (neuropathy) to respond to treatments such as acupuncture. Better results are likely, therefore, if treatment is started within 3 months of sciatic pain onset.

Sciatica is frequently treated with MA. In Russian studies, pain reduction was associated with improved alpha motoneuron reflexes and also with improved local and systemic circulation. MA also enhanced electrical excitability of muscle in patients with sensory and motor disturbance attributable to lumbosacral radiculitis. For acute exacerbation of long-term sciatica, MA together with antidepressant medication both extended short-term pain relief and reduced the number of days for which treatment was needed.

There are many studies on EA for sciatica. Severe sciatica may require lengthy treatment with EA.

Case study 9.11.2 is an example of the use of EA for acute back pain.

pTENS has been used on board fishing vessels for radiculopathy exacerbated by cold and overstrenuous activity. In one Japanese report, younger patients responded better to this modality.

TENS is often considered effective for low-back pain. In particular, it has been used for recurrent ischialgia due to conjoined nerve roots, and for pain associated with herniated lumbar discs, in both cases together with exercise. Although paraesthesia should be elicited by TENS in the affected area, the pain itself may be reproduced when TENS is applied. In one mixed study, CTENS was found to be less effective for radicular than for purely musculoskeletal pain.

# CASE Study 9.11.2

## Electroacupuncture for acute back pain: a case study

**Juliette Lowe**

Mrs B telephoned me with acute back pain: 'I am stuck on the floor and can hardly move, please can you help?'

Mrs B is a 68-year-old woman who is normally very fit and healthy, regularly taking her dogs for walks and leading an exemplary moderate life. She was in training to walk the West Highland Way and had been walking a little more than usual. There was no obvious cause for the back pain. She had moved a slightly heavy piece of furniture 2 days previously, but had felt no pain in doing so. She did, however, have a history of back trouble, but no recurrence after an operation 7 years ago to remove calcium from the fifth lumbar vertebra.

The pain was localised in the right sacrum and radiated down and around the right thigh into the medial knee (along the course of the dermatome associated with L2 and L3). The pain was of a deep ache in nature with sharp stabs on movement, and was slightly relieved by heat. The most comfortable position for treatment was prone with the right knee slightly bent and cushions under the stomach and right knee. On palpation, there was tenderness around the erector spinae muscles lateral to the right lumbar vertebrae, the right gluteus maximus and the right sacral foramen (all Bladder meridian points, from BL-23 to BL-34). The diagnosis was relatively straightforward, the type of pain indicating *qi* and Blood stagnation localised in the Bladder channel. This was probably due to a combination of the recent lifting and increased use on top of an old injury where there would be a tendency to stagnation from scar tissue formation.

The treatment principle was simple: to move *qi* and relieve Blood stagnation in the localised section of the Bladder channel using local, adjacent and distal points. I needled the local and adjacent points BL-23, BL-25, BL-28 to BL-34 and distal point BL-40 (on the right), using 3.75 cm (1½") needles in the lumbar area and 5 cm (2") needles in the sacral points. I used electroacupuncture in this case, as the pain was acute and seemed to be coming from muscle spasm, having found this method useful in the past. I paired up BL-23 and BL-25, BL-28 and BL-29, BL-30 and BL-31, BL-32 and BL-33 and used a DD wave with frequency settings on my AWQ104 stimulator of f1 = 25 and f2 = 50 (these readings were reached after adjustments to produce a sensation that dispersed the pain). The intensity required to achieve adequate stimulation was moderate

(2–3) on all points, and after 5 minutes I increased the intensity slightly (3–4) as Mrs B had got used to the level of stimulation. Initially she felt some relief from the pain and described a sensation as if the electroacupuncture were waving away the discomfort. However, after 15 minutes she began to find her position uncomfortable, so I turned off the machine and removed the needles. After she had moved I massaged her lower back, sacrum and buttock and gently stretched her legs.

I then gave Mrs B a few simple exercises based on the McKenzie 'Treat your own back ' series, involving lying on the floor and arching the back gently, slowly increasing as she was able to, followed by counterbalance stretching, lying on the back and pulling the knees into the chest. I advised her to do these for 10 minutes every 2 hours.

After the treatment Mrs B was still in a lot of pain and I didn't hold out much hope for my treatment. However, when I returned the following day, Mrs B was a transformed woman. She looked bright and alert, was walking with relative ease and even offered me a cup of tea! The pain was now only on certain movements and if she stayed in one position too long. It was localised in the right sacrum and no longer radiated down the leg. It was more of an ache, with only occasional stabs.

I repeated the treatment, but used fewer points: BL-23 to BL-29, BL-32 and BL-40 (on the right) and paired up points BL-23 and BL-24, BL-25 and BL-26, and BL-28 and BL-29 for electroacupuncture. I used the same DD wave as before, but found Mrs B required a higher intensity (4–5) on all points, increasing up to 6–7 after 10 minutes. This time I left the needles in for 20 minutes and followed the acupuncture with a deeper massage and fuller range of stretches and gentle manipulations. Mrs B found no major discomfort during the treatment and felt much better afterwards. She telephoned me the following week to say that she was fully recovered. I was surprised how effective the treatment was after the apparently poor initial reaction but, having treated many similar cases before and gaining predominantly good results, I should have been more confident.

On the whole, I use electroacupuncture for acute cases of pain and recent paralysis as I was taught to do at the London School of Acupuncture and the Railway Hospital, Nanjing. However, having worked in a hospital pain clinic for 5 years, I found that it could also be useful in many chronic conditions, often relieving pain rather than actually curing it. I therefore use it widely in my everyday practice, trying different methods (straight acupuncture, electroacupuncture, moxibustion, heat lamp and cupping, etc.) until I find a method that provides the best relief for the patient, regardless of the duration of the condition. I do, however, still find that in general electroacupuncture is more beneficial in acute conditions and moxibustion or heat lamp in chronic.

TENS, therefore, may be more useful when pain is relatively localised, and less so for sciatic or radiating pain, or when several nerve roots are involved. It will also be less effective if there are signs of denervation.

LILT has been used for radicular pain, which may respond well to trigger point (TrP) LA. In one uncontrolled study in which both MA and LA were used, patients with sciatica alone obtained a similar outcome to those with low-back and sciatic pain. Results were better in younger patients, more prolonged in recent cases, and slightly worse in those who had already had surgery. However, results with LILT may be short lived, and severe spinal pathology is likely to be unresponsive to LILT, which may therefore be more helpful in less chronic cases. Nevertheless, reduced protrusion of herniated lumbar discs has been documented following LILT.

**Comparisons and combinations** EA was better than MA for sciatic pain in several studies, and better than simple retained needling for intervertebral disc protrusion. However, in one controlled trial (CT), MA based on TCM syndrome differentiation gave better results than EA for sciatica. Pekka Pöntinen has warned that exacerbation due to hyperstimulation is more likely with EA.

EA and TEAS were both found to be effective for sciatica in one comparative study. However, in low-back pain due to degenerative disc disease, EA ('percutaneous electrical nerve stimulation', or PENS) at non-acupoints gave better results than paraspinal TENS. Following surgery for spinal osteochondrosis, EA was more helpful for pain than TENS with the same sinusoidal waveform and frequency, although both methods were effective for associated motor deficit.

MA was more effective than pTENS for sciatica in one comparative study.

In one RCT, LA gave better results than EA and ultrasound acupoint stimulation in discogenic lumbosacral radiculopathies.

EA for sciatica has been combined with various treatments, including TENS, the *shendeng* 'sacred lamp' or other multifrequency devices, massage, and acupoint injection. The latter combination was found to improve effectiveness, as was the addition of both acupoint injection and warm needling or a multifrequency lamp to simple EA. EA has also been combined with both infrared heat and point injection. EA with warm needling gave better results than just EA. Similarly, TDP irradiation with either MA or EA gives better results than MA alone.

The combination of EA and moxibustion with massage gave significantly better results than their combination with traction in one study where ultrasound scanning of prolapsed intervertebral discs was used to confirm these improvements objectively. When combined with EA and herbal 'steaming', the results of traction were improved. EA with medication applied to the skin, although perhaps more effective than EA alone, was not superior to combined massage and traction.

MA is often combined with massage for sciatica. In one report, it was combined with TENS, traction and HF electric field treatment.

**Points used** *Huatuojiaji* and *ashi* points can be important when treating radiculopathic pain such as sciatica, but strong local stimulation at hypersensitive points, or at many points, should be avoided, at least initially. Bladder meridian points (BL-11, BL-23, BL-36, BL-40, BL-54, BL-57, BL-60, BL-62), Kidney points (KI-3, KI-7), Gall Bladder points (GB-30, GB-34, GB-40) and other points such as ST-36, ST-44, SP-6, Du-2, Du-3, Du-4, Du-15 and Du-20 may all be relevant. From the studies in the database 🔘, the most used points for sciatica are those on the Bladder and Gall Bladder meridians: BL-23, BL-36, **BL-37**, BL-40, BL-54, BL-57, BL-60, and GB-31, GB-34, GB-39 and **GB-40**. Of the adjunctive points, only ST-36 appears frequently, while Governing Vessel points are well down the list, behind *huatuojiaji* and *ashi* points. Auricular points are rarely used.

For lumbar pain with a radicular component the points are very similar: BL-23, **BL-25**, BL-36, BL-40, BL-54, BL-57, BL-60; **GB-30**, GB-31, GB-34 and GB-39. (Points in bold type are those that occur in one or other of these lists but not both.) If anything, *huatuojiaji* and *ashi* points are even more emphasised, ST-36 appears somewhat less frequently than in the sciatica studies, auricular points are little used, but one of the most significant differences is the use of the local points Du-3 and Du-4.

With TENS, long electrodes can be positioned paraspinally to span several nerve roots (for instance, L1–L5 or L3–S2 for sciatica).

With LILT, Margaret Naeser and Xiu-Bing Wei suggest directing the beam at the nerve root site from three or four different directions, and then adding LA at points such as LI-4 (for cervical radiculopathy) or BL-60 or BL-67 (for lumbar radiculopathy).

**When to use what – parameters for radicular pain** DD mode has been recommended for muscle spasm in neurological conditions, and should be considered for radiculopathic pain. It has been used in a number of EA studies on sciatica and lumbar radicular pain.

In the main, although obtaining *deqi* is important, and the usual phrase 'to tolerance' appears frequently in the EA sciatica and low-back-pain studies, high-intensity stimulation is not emphasised unduly and some authors have emphasised that treatment should be gentle.

An interesting comment was made by Tian Deming, author of one uncontrolled study on sciatica, who states that HF EA can be used for patients in robust health, but that LF EA should be used if not. There are certainly more LF than HF EA studies in the database 🔘, as well as a few in which intermittent rather than continuous stimulation is employed. Sometimes LF EA has been used at body points, and HF EA at ear points. In an important Swedish study, 2 Hz EA resulted in longer-lasting improvements than HF EA for 'nociceptive' sciatica. Adrian White has suggested that LF EA may have been more 'convincing' as it involved muscle contraction rather than just a tingling sensation.

In an early trial comparing ALTENS and CTENS for chronic low-back and leg pain, analgesia was short lived with both modes. More patients found CTENS helpful, possibly because ALTENS was too strong for comfort. In a very small study comparing CTENS, burst and modulated TENS, three out of four sciatica patients responded best to burst TENS. At 2 months, two still benefited. In contrast, both motor level burst TENS and CTENS were found to give prolonged analgesia in one Russian study on lumbar and sciatic pain due to spinal osteochondritis.

In one EA ('PENS') study on degenerative disc disease, 30 minutes of stimulation gave better results than 15 minutes.

Needle depth may need to be adjusted according to whether sciatica is acute or chronic. A number of authors consider deep needling to be important.

Case study 9.11.3 details the use of automated methods of intramuscular stimulation in a case of low-back pathology.

## Complex regional pain disorder

Complex regional pain disorder (CRPD) may affect one or more extremities, may follow even slight injury and can be intense and disproportionate to the underlying pathology.

# CASE Study 9.11.3

**Automated twitch-obtaining intramuscular stimulation and electrical twitch-obtaining intramuscular stimulation**
**Jennifer Chu**

Clinically noticeable twitches do not occur with traditional acupuncture methods. Twitch elicitation, however, is inherent with electromyography (EMG) performed with the standard monopolar needle electrode. The presence of twitches in EMG, as opposed to acupuncture, relates to the slightly larger size of the Teflon-coated needle used in EMG and the intramuscular movements of this needle.

Movements during EMG at motor end-plate zones (MEPZs) cause electrophysiological and clinical level twitches to occur. The MEPZs that can twitch readily are clinically identified by the same tenderness at taut intramuscular bands, ropes or nodes as are found at trigger points. Additionally, the intramuscular or intermuscular grooves, along which many traditional acupuncture points lie, define motor lines. Stimulation of these yields linear twitches. Clinical experience suggests that MEPZs are the anatomical correlates of trigger and acupuncture points, and motor lines the correlates of acupuncture meridians.

Gunn hypothesized that spondylotic-radiculopathy-related myofascial pain syndrome arises from the traction effect of shortened muscle fibres on tendons, nerves, blood vessels, bones, intervertebral discs and joints, and achieved immediate muscle fibre contraction and relaxation through oscillating, twisting and turning motions of an intramuscularly inserted acupuncture needle. However, these effects are very limited compared with twitch-related muscle contraction and relaxation, especially if strong or elicited from deeper regions using thicker needles.

Long-term outcome studies using manually performed twitch-obtaining intramuscular stimulation (TOIMS) for the relief of cervical and lumbosacral radiculopathic pain gave promising results. However, the manual delivery of mechanical stimulation is relatively ineffective and the development of automation to help insert, oscillate and retract the needle from the muscle became medically necessary. This method, termed the automated twitch-obtaining intramuscular stimulation (ATOIMS), utilizes a handheld device that allows intensive treatments to multiple points in multiple myotomes of patients with diffuse nerve-related chronic muscle pain such as fibromyalgia. The ATOIMS device regulates and maintains only one smooth trajectory for the oscillating needle, thereby minimising tissue trauma, treatment pain and post-treatment pain. The device also removes the risk of cumulative and repetitive stress injuries to the treating physician.

Electrical excitation, however, is more powerful than mechanical stimulation for excitation of nerve and muscle tissues. The development of electrical twitch-obtaining intramuscular stimulation (ETOIMS) increased both the total number and force of elicited twitches. Their force is greater because submaximal microelectrical current stimulation of an intramuscular nerve trunk has a bias towards stimulation of large motor neurons due to their lower electrical threshold. Also, intramuscular electrical stimulation at the motor points elicits axon reflexes that not only activate the stimulated axon antidromically but also invade other branches of the same axon to stimulate the entire motor unit.

To stretch effectively muscle fibres shortened from partial denervation or neurapraxia, the stretch should ideally occur in the immediate vicinity of the affected muscle fibres. Such selective stimulation is possible with ETOIMS and ATOIMS. As a rule, the twitches occur immediately upon muscle penetration. The first in a series of twitches usually has the strongest force, or may be sustained as in a tetanic contraction. Not uncommonly, a single stimulus evokes multiple simultaneous twitches causing the muscle to flutter or go into a cramp.

Denervation-related muscle fibre shortening from spondylotic radiculopathy can recur or become progressive with further acute or chronic repetitive trauma to the

*(Continued)*

CASE Study 9.11.3 **Continued**

spinal nerve roots. ATOIMS and ETOIMS are both suitable for such conditions since these treatments, in skilled hands, are without side-effects and safe for repetitive use.

### A case history
### Chief complaint

Back and left-sided groin pain

### Current condition

A 36-year-old male came for management of left-sided back, buttock and groin pain dating back to his teens when he started developing pain over his low back at the age of 15 years. Since 1992 he also had groin pain associated with what was diagnosed as prostatitis. In 1997, he was evaluated by the author for an EMG. At that point, his left groin pain was attributed to spondylosis of the lumbosacral spine. It was recommended that he undergo ETOIMS/ATOIMS. He was lost to follow-up since then and his left leg and left buttock pain persisted.

He returned to the author in January 2000, his pain level rated at 6/10 on average, down to 2 or 3/10 on a good day, but as high as 9/10 on a bad day. The pain radiates from the left side of the low back to the left buttock and down the left posterior thigh, as well as involving the left groin. Associated symptoms are weakness and some numbness down to the left toes. Pain is better with lying down and weekly massage, worse with lifting, bending, driving and sexual activity. It is severe at night, but rarely wakes him. He falls asleep easily, does not wake unusually early and can sleep for 8 hours without medication. He has tried ultrasound therapy and physical therapy, as well as his weekly massage.

### Past medical history

In a car accident 5 years previously he sustained some left shoulder pain for which he received physical therapy for 3 months. His pre-existing low-back pain was aggravated. He lost his left index finger in a sawing accident.

### Review of systems

The patient has no blurring of vision, headaches or loss of consciousness, nor any chest pain or shortness of breath. He has no liver or kidney problems, but he does urinate about 10 times daily, as well as twice nightly. He has no erectile dysfunction, but some difficulty with ejaculation during intercourse.

### Physical examination

He has a full range of motion in neck flexion and extension. He has mild limitation of motion in neck lateral flexion, on neck rotation and on shoulder external rotation, with moderate limitation of motion in shoulder internal rotation. He has full range of motion on shoulder flexion, abduction and extension on the left, with mild limitation of motion on shoulder abduction on the right and with a full range of motion on shoulder flexion and extension on the right.

Shoulder and pelvis levels are elevated by 1 cm on the right. Spine flexion has a full range of motion. He has a full range of motion on spine lateral flexion and mild limitation of motion on extension. The supine straight leg raise test is 80° bilaterally. The sitting root sign is positive over both hamstrings with a grade II pain. There is negative Trendelenburg and the patient is able to do a full squat with no tight heel cords, as well as a full heel lift and toe lift bilaterally with alternate unilateral stance.

Examination of tender points shows mild tenderness over the L2 to S1 dermatomes as well as the C2 to C8 myotomes. There is grade 2+ paraspinal spasm at the T10 to S1 levels, with the left greater than the right. There is grade 2+ cervical paraspinal spasm with the left greater than the right and grade 2+ trapezius spasm on the left, greater than the right. Autonomic changes include skin thickness of +1 over the cervical, thoracic and lumbar spine. The pore size is +1 over the cervical and +2 over the thoracic and lumbar areas. Trophic neurogenic edema is noted to be +1 over the C2 to C8 dermatomes.

There are pilomotor changes of +1 over the C2 to S1 level, as well as vasomotor changes of +1 from C2 to C5 dermatomes.

### Neurological examination

The gait has good heel, toe and tandem walk. Reflexes are brisk and symmetrical bilaterally, with no Babinski, clonus or Hoffmann's sign elicited.

### Assessment

The patient was found to have nerve-related chronic low-back and groin pain, which was probably secondary to spondylotic radiculopathy over multiple levels.

### Recommendations

The patient was recommended to undergo weekly electrical ETOIMS/ATOIMS treatment over the lumbosacral paraspinal muscles as well as the muscles that wrap around the hip girdle, including the L2 to S1 myotomes.

### Treatment goals

These were to decrease the intensity of pain and frequency of painful exacerbations, increase the range of motion and maximise the overall level of performance as regards daily activities.

---

### CASE Study 9.11.3 Continued

#### Results

After the first treatment, his pain level decreased to 3–4/10, with most pain relief in his low-back region, but also a decrease in the burning painful sensation in his left groin. During treatment, all muscles treated in the L3 to S1 myotomes and the C4 to C7 myotomes showed difficulty in eliciting twitches owing to their tightness from chronic underlying nerve root involvement. After the fourth treatment, his pain level was as low as 2/10. The patient has continued with weekly treatments, was able to play golf for the first time since his pain was exacerbated in 1997 and has experienced improvement in his quality of life. He continues with treatment every 6–8 weeks to maintain his quality of life over a total follow-up period of 4 years since January 2000.

---

It may come in two guises. CRPD type I corresponds to what used to be called reflex sympathetic dystrophy (RSD), and is more likely to be diffuse, not following any dermatomal or other logical distribution. CRPD type II tends to have a more clearly somatic origin, and corresponds to causalgia (pain and hyperalgesia confined to the distribution of an injured peripheral nerve).

CRPD can accompany RSI, peripheral neuropathy or entrapment/compression syndromes, or follow burn or fracture injury, surgery or other insult to an organ. Not only sensory but also sympathetic nerves can be involved. In the first stage of CRPD type I, sympathetically maintained pain is accompanied by sensory changes, allodynia, hyperalgesia, non-pitting oedema and sudomotor and vasomotor changes. The affected extremity is likely to be warm, dry and red or slightly cyanotic. Stage 1 usually lasts for 1–3 months, but may persist indefinitely. In the second stage, the symptom picture widens and may include inflammatory changes in the skin, neurodermatitis, bruising, tremor, joint swelling, insomnia due to night pain, and emotional disturbances. The skin is likely to become shiny, pale, cool and clammy. Motor function can be impaired. In the third stage there may be spontaneous skin ulceration, infection, muscle atrophy, flexion deformities and osteoporosis, as well as the depression that may accompany any form of chronic pain.

Treatment for CRPD has to be intensive and is best started in the early stages of the condition. Response may be slow, and once the condition has become chronic it may become intractable. Even if it does respond, treatment may need to be repeated at intervals indefinitely. Spontaneous remission is rare.

MA has been used clinically for CRPD. In one very small trial, results appeared superior to those of sympathetic block, with better effects on circulation in the affected extremity as well as on pain in some cases. MA has been used for CRPD-like shoulder–arm pain following stroke.

Acupuncture, which can reduce both sympathetic overactivity and pain, should be helpful for CRPD. In experimental studies, both MA and EA have been shown to reduce some components of acute neurogenic inflammation, and thus may possibly be of benefit in the very early stages of CRPD. In general, however, clinical results with acupuncture for CRPD have been described as 'not very impressive'.

CTENS was not found very useful for CRPD in some early studies, becoming less effective with repeated treatment. In one small study comparing TENS and spinal cord stimulation (SCS), both gave better results than sympathetic block or sympathectomy. Although there were more 'excellent' outcomes with TENS, there were fewer total failures with SCS. Thus some authorities have considered TENS useful in general for the condition, particularly in combination with gentle exercises and relaxation.

The localised cooling that sometimes accompanies CRPD may be improved by TENS. In one quite large retrospective study, TENS (15–25 Hz, modulated) used for 22 hours each day made a considerable contribution to successful rehabilitation, not only in terms of pain control, but also for vasomotor symptoms. During the first 2 weeks of treatment, symptoms returned rapidly if TENS was discontinued, but after 2–4 months the unit could be dispensed with for several days before symptoms returned.

LA has been used for CRPD following surgery, with improvements in oedema, diffuse pain and extreme temperature fluctuations. MA had been unable to help this case. LA has also been combined with infrared in the treatment of CRPD.

**Points used** The studies in the CD-ROM database 💿 show that some authors emphasise local or *ashi* points, or both, although these should probably be used with caution initially. The most commonly used traditional acupoints are P-6, LI-4 and LI-11. Ear points have also been used.

For lower-limb CRPD, Alejandro Katz has used microcurrent at ST-36 and the *bafeng* points between the toes, ipsilaterally, or contralaterally for a few treatments if the condition is too painful initially. He positions surface electrodes over the needles. In a useful overview of CRPD treatment from a TCM perspective, John Stebbins recommends MA, followed with microcurrent stimulation, at points such as SJ-5, GB-34, LI-11, ST-36, ST-40, SP-6, SP-9, *baxie* and *bafeng*, together with points on the affected meridians both proximal and distal to the affected area.

However, when using TENS, Ronald Melzack and Patrick Wall found that stimulating proximal to an area of causalgia could markedly reduce hyperaesthesia, whereas stimulation distal to the area could aggravate it. Furthermore, TENS applied to the affected limb or area will probably feel stronger and be less well tolerated than if applied on the unaffected side, and may lead to uncomfortable spreading sensations that tend to outlast the stimulus. Contralateral treatment may thus be advisable. In contrast, ipsilateral paravertebral (C6–T3) and anterior neck electrode positioning to 'sandwich' the stellate ganglion was found to be helpful for upper-limb CRPD in one small Italian study.

**When to use what – parameters for CRPD** There seems to be little consistency in the parameters used to treat CRPD with EA and TENS. EA has been applied at both high and low frequencies, at 'maximum tolerable' intensity or 'maximum stimulation without discomfort'. Both CTENS and ALTENS have been employed. There are also several MENS studies, with varying protocols.

CRPD is a chronic neurogenic condition, and as such may well be exacerbated by strong treatment local or distal to the problem area. Thus Christer Carlsson advises against deep needling for CRPD. Katz similarly recommends superficial needle insertion and subthreshold stimulation only.

CTENS is sometimes recommended as appropriate for CRPD. TENS at 30 Hz, 'to tolerance', was used in the Italian study on stellate ganglion stimulation mentioned above. In a single case report of TENS for CRPD in a young child, 50 Hz (3.5 mA) was eventually found to give better pain relief than the 90 Hz (2.5 mA) used initially.

The overall message would appear to be that gentle stimulation is most appropriate for CRPD, that it should be started as early as possible and that treatment may need to be prolonged.

## Central pain

Central pain is defined as pain initiated or caused by a primary lesion or dysfunction in the central nervous system.

### PAIN FOLLOWING STROKE

Central poststroke pain is usually burning and accompanied by sensory deficit as well as by allodynia in around 50% of patients. It may be reduced by antidepressants such as amitriptyline, but treatment must be started early to take effect.

In one controlled study of EA for thalamic pain following stroke, 100 Hz stimulation of *huatuojiaji* points (M-BW-35), daily for 30 days, gave results statistically equivalent to those of carbamazepine.

TEAS (at LI-4 and ST-36), TENS and SCS have all been used for central poststroke pain. Indeed, the mechanism of EA at paraspinal points is probably similar to that of the more invasive method of SCS.

Both ipsi- and contralateral stimulation were used in the TEAS/TENS studies. In one of these, results were similar whichever side was stimulated. In the TEAS and other TENS study, emphasis was on treating the healthy side. In part this was because CTENS or TLEA becomes ineffective if there is sensory loss in the painful area to be stimulated.

However, 100 Hz was effective in the EA study (albeit at paraspinal points), whereas in one small TENS trial of those

patients that did respond (four, or ~27%), three (20%) appeared to respond similarly to both CTENS and ALTENS, with only two benefiting from contralateral treatment.

### PAIN FOLLOWING SPINAL CORD INJURY (SCI)

Persistent central neurogenic pain associated with SCI is characterised by burning, tingling or aching below the level of the lesion. Incomplete injury correlates with better prognosis, including motor improvement.

Conventional treatments considered most helpful in one survey were opioid medications, physical therapy and diazepam, whereas those rated least helpful were SCS, counselling and administration of paracetamol or amitriptyline. Alternative treatments reported as most helpful were massage therapy and use of marijuana, whereas acupuncture was tried by many but rated only moderately helpful.

In a careful but uncontrolled study of MA for chronic SCI pain (N = 22), nearly half the patients treated showed improvements in pain intensity. More than a quarter reported more pain, however, which was still present 3 months later. Results were poorer in those with central pain or complete transection of the spinal cord, and for pain below the level of injury.

EA was also found helpful for chronic SCI pain, although once treatment was terminated the pain started to return.

Auricular MA and TEAS (at SI-3 and BL-62) have been used together for acute SCI pain. Early treatment gave encouraging results in this CT.

TENS has been used for pain following SCI, with better results for localised than for radiating pain. Long-term TENS and TEAS treatment have been used with some benefit for sensory deficit in the legs following SCI, even though not started until 2 weeks after the initial trauma.

CES (SPES) has been used for chronic SCI pain, with very noticeable effects on patients' mood.

**When to use what – parameters for central pain** TLS is unlikely to benefit central pain, as it involves segmental rather than supraspinal mechanisms. Ottoson and Lundeberg, in their textbook on TENS, suggest that CTENS is most likely to benefit deafferentation pain, but it has also been suggested that burst TENS may give better results for central pain due to spinal cord or brainstem injury.

## HEAD AND FACIAL PAIN

Head and facial pain can arise from various neurological, musculoskeletal, dental or stomatological causes.

## Headache

Headaches can be subdivided as follows:

- *Tension-type headache*: steady, non-throbbing bilateral pain of the head, back of the neck and face. It may last up to several hours, and occur several times within a week, is usually episodic, but can become chronic.

Although the autonomic symptoms typical of migraine are absent or mild, both types of headache may occur in the same patient. In tension-type headache, tender or tight scalp points may be found predominantly along the Bladder meridian. In Western acupuncture terms, cervical myofascial trigger points are commonly implicated.

- *Cluster headache:* penetrating, non-throbbing and severe pain behind the eyes or in the temples, lasting for less than 2 hours, and continuing for 2–3 months at a time, often occurring at night.
- *Post-traumatic headache:* due to head or neck injury; it may be dull, aching, stabbing, sharp, or excruciating at the site of injury, sometimes starting years after the initial trauma.
- *Migraine headache:* unilateral intense head pain that may last several days, typically accompanied by nausea or vomiting, visual disturbances and extreme sensitivity to light. In migraine headache, tender or tight scalp points may, according to some authors, be found predominantly along the Gall Bladder meridian.

All of these types of headache may also be secondary to many other conditions, such as viral infections, dental, jaw or sinus problems, temporomandibular joint (TMJ) disorders, hypertension, stroke, intracranial aneurysm or tumour, functional hypoglycaemia or opiate withdrawal, all of which are dealt with elsewhere in this book.

Some reviewers have considered as equivocal the evidence that acupuncture has any effect beyond that of a placebo. Others have suggested that, whereas acupuncture may appear to benefit non-migraine headaches, this may be because tension headache sufferers tend to be more responsive to non-specific effects. It also appears from some MA studies that this form of acupuncture may reduce headache frequency and analgesic consumption, rather than headache duration or pain severity.

A Cochrane review of acupuncture for idiopathic headache concluded that 'patients should not be discouraged from trying acupuncture from a risk/benefit standpoint'. Critics of this review observed that no methodologically rigorous studies were included that assessed clinically relevant outcomes, and that the lower-quality trials reviewed resulted in more positive results. Nevertheless, some of the Cochrane authors went on to complete another systematic review of acupuncture, including EA and LA, this time for chronic headache (24 RCTs and 35 non-randomised studies). Here again, acupuncture appeared to have a positive effect, although better-quality studies produced lower response rates and it was clear that neither the patients nor the interventions in the RCTs were representative of routine acupuncture practice.

There are many heterogeneous studies on EA for different and mixed types of headache.

Headache has been considered to be a standard indication for TENS. Both TENS and pTENS have been used in a number of studies on mixed types of headache, with many reporting both significant improvement in symptoms and prophylaxis.

TCET (a more powerful version of CES) has been used for headaches of various aetiologies, as has the Liss CES device. In one study of cranial TENS, stimulation benefited patients whose headaches were of organic origin but was without effect in those whose headaches were psychogenic.

HeNe LA has been used for headache as well as TrP LA. MA, EA and LA were used in different combinations for various forms of post-traumatic headache (migraine, tension type and cluster) following an earthquake in Italy, with good results in a number of the patients, in some of whom symptoms began years after the original trauma.

**Comparisons and combinations (general)** The combination of EA with cupping was found to give better results than EA alone in one study on mixed headache types.

LA and MA for headache gave similar results in one report. However, in a small but more recent RCT, LA was not found to be superior to placebo for a mixed group of sufferers from migraine and tension-type headache.

In an unusual study comparing DC and more conventional TENS, 1 mA DC (between forehead and interscapular area) gave more prolonged benefits for chronic headache, although with adverse skin effects in a considerable proportion of patients.

**Points used for headache – general considerations** Peter Deadman and colleagues have prepared a useful synopsis of the main acupoints used in TCM treatment of headaches (17 local points, 21 adjacent and distal ones). Many other body points have also been used when treating headache with MA, as have microsystems such as Korean hand acupuncture. In the EA and other clinical studies for mixed headache types located here, the most commonly used points are GB-20, LIV-3 and LI-4, with others such as BL-10, GB-8, ST-36 and *taiyang* (M-HN-9) trailing behind, and a scattering of other points used even less frequently. A number of authors emphasise TCM differentiation; others stress that local treatment is best carried out at *ashi* points.

Indeed, in studies on experimental dental or other head pain, local points have sometimes proved more effective than distal ones such as LI-4. One Chinese reviewer noted that this seemed particularly the case for migraine, but less important when treating headache of neurogenic origin. In keeping with this approach, for instance, BL-2 and Du-23 were recommended for use with the Likon device, and points all around the crown of the head are stimulated in one LILT protocol. However, strong stimulation to head points can result in headaches.

Most formula approaches to treating headache make use of LI-4, either because it is traditionally indicated or because it lies within the C5 or C6 dermatome. Thus one EA device manual recommends GB-20 and *taiyang* (M-HN-9) with LI-4, whereas Dean Richards recommends LI-4 with *yintang* (M-HN-3) for pTENS. For CES using the Liss device, application at LI-4 as well as over the area of pain is suggested. Other recommendations are more sophisticated. George Ulett gives a combination of LI-4 with GB-20, Du-15, Du-20 and *taiyang*, for example.

In one Chinese EA device manual, points are grouped on the basis of headache location, although some of the points also have a TCM rationale:

| | |
|---|---|
| Frontal | GB-14, LI-4, ST-8, ST-44, Du-23, *yintang* |
| Temporal | SJ-5, GB-8, GB-41, *taiyang* |
| Occipital | SI-3, BL-10, BL-60, GB-20 |
| Vertex | BL-7, LIV-3, LI-4, Du-20 |

In another such manual, points are given on the basis of TCM syndrome differentiation:

| | |
|---|---|
| Exogenous (Cold) type | SJ-8, GB-20, LI-4, Du-14, *taiyang* |
| Upward disturbance of Liver-Fire | KI-3, GB-4, GB-5, LIV-3 |
| Phlegm blocking upper orifices | ST-40, Ren-12, Du-20, *yintang* |
| Hyperactivity of *yang* due to *yin xu* | KI-1, LI-4, SP-6, *yintang* |

**Parameters for headache – general considerations** In general, LF or DD EA was used more than HF EA in the clinical studies located. However, whereas DD EA has been suggested by the manufacturers of two different EA stimulators as appropriate for all forms of headache, one author recommended HF EA (15 minutes daily, on alternate days).

For those headaches that are triggered by stress or tension, treatment that fosters relaxation may be helpful; 0.5 Hz stimulation has been suggested as useful for this purpose when using photic/auditory stimulation, and could be considered for peripheral electrostimulation as well.

## TENSION-TYPE HEADACHE

This is usually muscular in origin, often with a stress-related component, but may also result from degenerative arthritis of the neck or be drug-induced, or both. There may be considerable overlap between tension-type headaches and myofascial pain or TMJ syndrome. Although antidepressant drugs are frequently prescribed initially, none of the currently available treatments demonstrates clear superiority. Additional methods such as acupuncture tailored to individual symptomatology may well be important, although some reviewers consider neither acupuncture nor TENS to be of proven benefit.

Some trials of acupuncture for tension-type headache indeed indicate that MA is only equivalent to placebo in effect, but others do suggest that MA may be more useful or as effective as standard treatment. Both MA and physiotherapy were found to be effective for myogenic headache in one Finnish study.

There are surprisingly few studies on EA for tension-type headache. In one mixed retrospective study, it gave good results, but in a series of controlled studies by Jane Carlsson and colleagues, standardised symptomatic EA appeared to be less helpful than individually adapted physiotherapy.

In one small crossover pTENS trial, a single pTENS treatment resulted in greater increases in pressure pain threshold at stimulated TrPs than sham stimulation.

TENS (both with and without physical therapy) was superior to biofeedback-enhanced neuromuscular reeducation in one CT of tension-type headache. TEAS/TENS was found helpful in several uncontrolled studies as well. In one interesting report of over 5000 patients suffering from headaches, of which 39.5% were cervicogenic in origin, manipulation of the cervical spine benefited 91% of those whose symptoms appeared to be due to vertebral displacement (67% of the cervicogenic group), whereas electrical nerve block using a variant of TENS benefited 80–90% of those whose symptoms were apparently caused by narrowing of the intervertebral foramina (33% of the cervicogenic group). TENS has also been found to be helpful for tension-type headache in children, alleviating symptoms in around 80% of sufferers.

**Comparisons and combinations** In one small study on chronic migraine, tension and post-traumatic headache, EA was found to be superior to MA for all three types.

**Points used** EA at SI-17 has been used for tension-type headache, although GB-20, GB-21 and LI-4 and TrPs are the most frequently used points.

Joseph Wong clearly differentiates the points that will be useful for this type of headache, primarily muscular in origin, from those he suggests for migraine or cluster headache: SI-15, GB-14, GB-20, GB-21, LI-18, Du-16, Du-18 and *taiyang* (M-HN-9).

**Parameters used** LF EA, pTENS and TENS appear to have been used in the various clinical studies more than HF stimulation, but data are sparse.

## CLUSTER HEADACHE

This is sometimes classified as a form of vascular headache, and can become chronic and unresponsive to medication. In some patients cluster headache can coexist with, or may even develop from, migraine.

MA has been attempted for cluster headaches but, although in one study it did significantly increase levels of met-enkephalin in the cerebrospinal fluid, it had little effect on the incidence of headaches.

**Points used** According to Joseph Wong, cluster headaches indicate a sympathetic dysfunction and are often associated with hypertension. He therefore recommends quite different points for treatment to those for migraine: SI-17, BL-23, LIV-3, LI-4, Du-1, Du-14, Du-20 and *yintang* (M-HN-3). Other points that have been used for cluster headache include GB-20, LI-11, ST-4, ST-7 and *taiyang* (M-HN-9).

## OTHER FORMS OF HEADACHE

Acupuncture has been used for postlumbar puncture headache, although this method was without success in one study. However, MA (at points such as BL-10, GB-11, LI-4, ST-8, Du-14 and Du-20) has been effective for postepidural headache. In another report, local Gall Bladder meridian points were selected according to headache location, together with LIV-3 and Felix Mann's 'cervical articular pillar' points.

EA was more effective than MA for persistent 'neurotic' headache in one small Chinese study. EA and LA have both been used for headache following trauma.

## HEAD AND FACIAL PAINS OF VASCULAR ORIGIN

Pain due to circulatory dysfunction can result from a restriction of blood flow, which is usually due to vascular constriction (ischaemia), or from excess blood flow to an area (hyperaemia). Both can lead to headache.

Vascular headache has been treated with MA, EA, pTENS, LA, magnetic stimulation and other methods.

Cephalic hypertension is often associated with muscle tension around the head and headache, even if blood pressure readings are normal in the arms. Yoshiaki Omura has found that light to moderate headache is experienced with systolic pressure over about 160 mmHg, and severe headache if it exceeds 220 mmHg. Reducing muscle tension with EA, TEAS or LA may reduce the raised blood pressure and accompanying headache.

## MIGRAINE

Migraine is usually classified as 'classical' (paroxysmal in quality, with a preceding aura) or 'common' (without the aura, more reactive in nature and generally longer lasting). The latter is found more frequently. In many cases, migraine runs in families. Conventionally it is generally understood as a form of vascular headache.

The vascular nature of migraine can be seen in those (the majority) who turn a deathly pale during an attack, shivering and cold (what Oliver Sacks calls 'white' migraine, or *yang* deficiency in TCM language), whereas others become flushed and hot ('red' migraine, perhaps *yin* deficiency or Liver *yang* rising). In some migraine sufferers, headache may mutate into neurogenic angina or laryngospasm.

Women are more liable to suffer from migraine than men. In many women migraine is associated with hormonal fluctuations, especially around the time of menstruation, possibly due to the effects of oestrogen on magnesium levels and vasodilation. After menopause, migraines often become less frequent, although migraines can actually begin or worsen perimenopausally. Menstrually related migraine is often associated with a disturbance of the basilar artery, in which case symptoms may include vertigo and poor muscular coordination.

Migraine is usually episodic, but in some patients becomes chronic. Such chronic migraine is associated with anxiety and depression, drug dependency and a generally reduced quality of life. Although disturbance, even hallucination, may occur in any sensory modality with migraine, in most people it is accompanied by cutaneous allodynia. Once this is established during an attack, neither the migraine nor the allodynia itself is likely to respond to tryptan medication such as sumatryptan (Imigran). Thus early treatment, while the migraine is still mild, would seem advisable.

Acupuncture and TENS have been used in migraine treatment. In one German hospital migraine was one of three conditions most frequently treated with acupuncture and TCHM.

Positive results have been reported in a number of uncontrolled MA studies. Bob Flaws, in his book on migraine from a TCM perspective, considers that acupuncture may help more than 50% of migraine sufferers. In one Scandinavian study, long-term results after one course of treatment (mixed MA and EA) were indeed better for migraine than for tension headache.

Nevertheless, evidence for acupuncture's efficacy is still unclear. In one migraine study, for example, MA was found to be useful prophylactically for the associated sickness, although not for the pain itself. MA has also been used for migraine-related vertigo as part of a comprehensive treatment programme. Others have found MA helpful for migraine pain, emphasising its prophylactic role during pain-free interludes.

George Lewith has observed that acupuncture can make patients more responsive to medication: 'someone with migraine may find that while powerful analgesics did not help at all, after acupuncture, one aspirin does the trick'. Hu Jisheng has observed that headaches from psychological pressures seemed less responsive to treatment, and others have concluded that those more extraverted patients with low scores for neuroticism tend to report better results with MA for migraine.

EA, like MA, has frequently been used for migraine, and some authors consider that it may be particularly helpful. However, in one American study, although good results were reported initially, a second course of EA treatment was less effective.

In an open study of 166 migraine sufferers treated with MA, EA or pTENS, a positive effect was claimed in 95.9% of the patients, results correlating with changes in electrophysiological and biochemical measures. Others have also found pTENS useful. Alf Heydenreich was the great protagonist of pTENS both for headache and for migraine, and his studies are some of the most convincing of its benefits for the latter condition, prophylactically as well as therapeutically.

Whereas TEAS for migraine has been investigated by various authors, TENS as such does not appear to have been used that frequently, although there are some positive reports on this application. It gave quite good results in one uncontrolled study, but was not found helpful if patients were also severely depressed. It has been utilised for children with migraine.

CES (SPES) has been used for migraine, with varying results depending on the type of migraine being treated. Good results have been claimed in unpublished double-blind and uncontrolled studies for the NET-I device. In one case report, CES was combined with MA.

Migraine has been considered an indication for LILT or LA at auricular points, although not all authors agree that LA is effective for migraine.

GHz (EHF) acupoint stimulation, combined with biofeedback and relaxation, was found to be helpful for migraine in one controlled study.

Blood magnesium levels tend to be low in migraine sufferers, but may be increased, even to above normal, by MA at SJ-5, GB-20, GB-34, GB-41, LIV-3, ST-36 and *taiyang*.

Use of oral magnesium supplementation in conjunction with acupuncture could potentially be a useful approach to treating migraine.

Although caffeine is used as a treatment for headache, in part because of its vascular and ANS effects, it should not be forgotten that overuse of caffeine, as well as withdrawal from it, can contribute to headache/migraine. Caffeine may also reduce the effectiveness of some forms of electrostimulation.

**Comparisons and combinations** Traditionally, MA has been combined with cupping in the treatment of migraine. EA and TEAS may be similarly efficacious for migraine.

In one RCT comparing MA and LA, the results were similar for each, although this study has been criticised on methodological grounds.

DC stimulation at 1 mA (between the forehead and inter-scapular area) gave more prolonged benefits than more conventional TENS for migraine, although with frequent adverse skin effects.

**Points used** Traditionally, acupoints for migraine treatment are selected according to TCM syndrome differentiation (*ben*), along with local or meridian points (*biao*). Thus, in one Chinese MA study, selection of acupoints according to TCM syndrome differentiation improved results. Ipsilateral cervical *huatuojiaji* points have also been used for migraine. In another Chinese author's report, *huatuojiaji* points were found useful in the ~10% of cases for whom an 'improper' sleeping position – prone with the head turned to one side – was considered partially responsible for their condition.

In general, MA at distal points such as SJ-5, GB-34, LI-11 and ST-36, with local points on the head and shoulders and auricular points such as *shenmen*, Subcortex and Sympathetic, has been used for migraine, together with additional auricular points depending on whether the patient is hypo- or hypertensive. Auricular EA has also been suggested for 'every type of vasomotor headache', together with EA at BL-17.

Because of parasympathetic involvement in migraine, Joseph Wong has suggested use of his system of 'parasympathetic switches', acupoints such as HE-7, BL-1, P-6, SJ-17, SP-6, Ren-22 and Ren-23, claiming that normalising parasympathetic function in this way can rapidly abort migraine symptoms.

MA at scalp and head points has also been utilised for vascular headache. Thus it is not surprising that GB-8 with GB-20 is one recommended EA combination for migraine, while EA at SJ-17 was found to improve cerebral blood flow in migraine sufferers, and EA at SI-17 has been used for vascular headache. From the EA studies, it appears that the most commonly used points are BL-10, SJ-23, GB-14, LIV-3, ST-8, ST-36, Du-20, *yintang* (M-HN-3) and *taiyang* (M-HN-9).

In the pTENS migraine studies, local points are selected according to the region affected, and stimulated in combination with distal/constitutional points such as HE-7, SI-3, SJ-5, LI-4 or ST-36. In one Russian report, once pain was stabilised using local stimulation, distal points were selected according to whether the patient's blood pressure was high (P-6, SP-6), low (GB-34, GB-41, Ren-14) or indifferent (LI-11, ST-36).

For acute migraine, TEAS has been recommended, at LI-4, Du-20 and *taiyang* (for unilateral pain, with positive polarity locally, negative at LI-4). Local points such as GB-5, GB-6, GB-14 and *taiyang*, with distal points like SJ-5, GB-41, LI-4, LI-11, ST-44 or SP-6, have also been suggested.

LA during an acute attack has been used, at SJ-20, GB-21, LI-4, ST-8, ST-44, Du-20, *taiyang* and *sishencong* (M-HN-1) every 5–10 minutes till the attack abates (904 nm, 2 mW, pulsed at 10 Hz; 15–20 seconds/pt, except for LI-4 and ST-44, on which 4 mW should be used for 20–30 seconds). Between attacks, courses of ten daily sessions can be given at the same points (all for 15–20 seconds/pt), along with HE-7, BL-2, LU-9, LI-11, SP-6, auricular Internal Secretion and *shenmen*.

**Parameters used** There is little consistency in the parameters used in migraine studies. LF, HF and DD have all been employed. Information on stimulation intensity is sparse.

Emad Tukmachi has suggested that LF EA should be used for acute migraine, and HF if it is chronic. For 'vasomotor' headaches, 10 EA sessions, daily or every other day, have been recommended, for 15–20 minutes at auricular points, and 30 minutes at points such as BL-17.

Hiranandani recommends TEAS at 12–30 Hz and high intensity during a migraine, at the points detailed above. However, given the increased photic driving to frequencies >18–20 Hz in migraine sufferers, at first sight it might seem that strong electrostimulation at such frequencies should be used with caution. Despite this, photic (flashing light) stimulation, to alternate eyes, has surprisingly been found to be beneficial for migraines, with the frequency selected for patient comfort at around 30 Hz, whereas stimulation at 8–12 Hz is more likely to provoke the scintillating visual scotoma and paraesthesia of migraine.

Both HF and LF CES have been used for migraine.

For LA, Hiranandani uses infrared (904 nm, 2 or 4 mW, pulsed at 10 Hz, for 15–20 or 20–30 seconds/pt), whether during or between attacks.

## Facial pain

When not idiopathic, the most frequent conditions leading to secondary facial pain include myofacial pain syndrome, sinusitis, cervical vertebral lesions, postherpetic neuralgia, malignant head and neck tumours and vascular lesions of the pain pathway within the skull. It may be chronic or acute, nociceptive or neurogenic in origin, and paroxysmal or persistent in nature. Chronic trigeminal neuralgia is the commonest example of paroxysmal neurogenic pain, while so-called 'atypical facial pain' is an example of persistent neurogenic pain.

Various types of chronic facial pain have been treated with acupuncture. However, although some reviewers have concluded that it can be effective for a variety of chronic facial pains, a number of authors suggest that it may be more effective when this is nociceptive (myogenic) in origin rather than neurogenic. Some authors have had disappointing results with MA for facial pain syndromes in general.

LF EA was used in one complex case of chronic continuous facial pain diagnosed as psychogenic, together with anxiolytic medication and *kanpo* herbal medicine. The pain gradually subsided, only to be replaced by a new, shooting pain, diagnosed as trigeminal neuralgia, that then responded to carbamazepine.

TENS has been used for facial pain, with some effect claimed even in supposedly hopeless cases. Some authors advise caution when using TENS on the face, particularly if the patient experiences hyperaesthesia.

TrP LA has been used for facial pain. However, there are a number of negative studies of LILT for chronic orofacial pain. Thus, although helpful for trigeminal neuralgia, HeNe LA was of no benefit for neuralgia of the pterygopalatine ganglion, for example.

**Comparisons and combinations – facial pain in general**
When TENS gave insufficient relief from facial pain, results were markedly improved by combining it with local iontophoresis of NSAIDs.

## TRIGEMINAL NEURALGIA, OR TIC DOULOUREUX

The trigeminal nerve is similar to spinal nerves in that it has two roots, one motor and one sensory. Two of the three branches of the nerve are purely sensory; the third is a compound nerve, and also supplies the muscles of mastication.

Trigeminal neuralgia (TN) is a chronic, severe, lancinating and burning pain on one side of the face. It is most commonly primary (idiopathic). Spontaneous remission can occur early on, but this happens less frequently as the condition progresses. Attacks are initiated by sensory irritation at trigger areas within the region innervated by the nerve.

The location of TN varies, depending which is the main branch involved: the first or ophthalmic (V1 or OB), second or maxillary (V2 or MxB), or third or mandibular (V3 or MnB) (Fig. 9.11.2). V2 neuralgia is the most common.

The causes of TN can be varied, even multiple. Dental, TMJ and sinus problems can all be contributory factors, as well as trauma and multiple sclerosis. Common treatments include carbamazepine, local neural block or stellate ganglion blockade, balloon compression of the Gasserian ganglion, or neurosurgery.

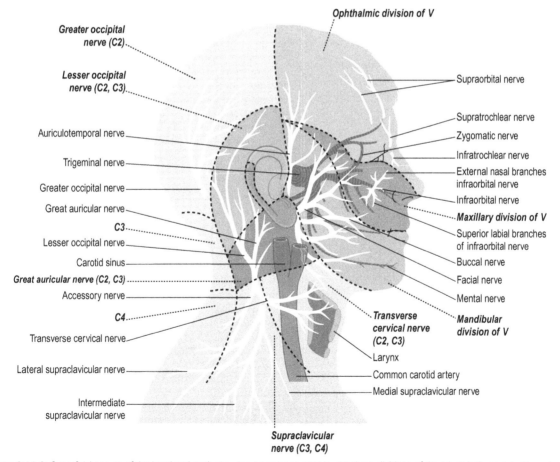

**Figure 9.11.2** Superficial nerves of the head and neck, showing areas innervated by the three divisions of the trigeminal nerve and branches of cervical nerves C2–C5. Note carotid sinus and larynx, where electrical stimulation should be avoided. (Adapted from Anderson 2000.)

Acupuncture has been used for cases of TN in a dental context. MA may not completely relieve TN, but it does help some patients. In one open study, for example, 30.8% claimed considerable improvement and 69.2% some overall benefit. A lengthy course of treatment may be necessary, with 'top-ups' once or twice a year, since although results may be good initially a high recurrence rate is also likely.

Some authorities consider that MA is sufficient, and that EA is not necessary when treating the condition. Others have used EA for neuralgia of the first and second branches of the trigeminal nerve, or for trigeminal paraesthesia following dental treatment. MA may be more useful for TN whose cause is peripheral rather than central. A very similar finding is that EA is likely to be effective in cases of secondary TN, but less helpful for primary TN of more than 1 year's duration, particularly if patients have received other medical treatment in the mean time.

TENS has been used for TN in children when other treatments have failed, although results are not always impressive. CES has also been used clinically for TN.

TN is generally considered to be an indication for LILT and can be useful in reducing dose requirements of patients on carbamazepine. LILT appears to be more effective for neuralgia of the maxillary or mandibular regions than for TN of the ophthalmic region. LA has been used for TN as well, although not always with good results.

**Comparisons and combinations** MA combined with conventional treatments such as carbamazepine appears to improve results more than the combination of carbamazepine with local ganglionic opioid analgesia.

EA combined with thread embedding at acupoints gave superior results to EA alone in one RCT. MA alone was not so effective as EA together with acupoint injection in another small study.

EA and TEAS were both found effective for TN in one comparative RCT.

LA, sometimes combined with infrared (just as MA is often used with moxibustion), has been used for trigeminal neuralgia.

**Points used** Most practitioners use different points, depending on the region of the face involved.

Joseph Wong recommends points as follows: for the ophthalmic division (V1, or OD): BL-1, BL-2 and *yintang*; for the maxillary division (V2, or MxD): SJ-23, LI-20 and ST-2; for the mandibular division (V3, or MnD): ST-7, Ren-24 and *taiyang* (M-HN-9); and for the Gasserian (semilunar) ganglion: GB-3.

Zheng Qiwei, in his discussion of acupoints to be used with EA, provides a simpler selection: BL-2 and GB-14 (V1), ST-2 and ST-7 (or SI-18) (V2), ST-7 and Ren-24 (V3).

Peter Deadman mentions an even more basic EA protocol in his account: *Taiyang* (V1), ST-2 (V2) and ST-4 (V3).

Wang Zongxue, again for EA, uses BL-2 to *yuyao* (M-HN-6) (V1), ST-3 to ST-2 (V2), and ST-4 and ST-7 to *foramen mentalis* (V3). Other local and distal points can be considered. For V1, for example, these might include GB-8 and ST-8, distal points SI-3, LI-4 and ST-41.

Wang Yanjie developed an interesting method, applying EA at ST-25 as a distal point first (after obtaining *deqi* at the point), and then using EA locally, provided the neuralgic pain had cleared temporarily, at points *taiyang* and *yuyao* (V1), ST-2 and ST-3 (V2), and ST-6, ST-7 or *jiachengjiang* (M-HN-18) (V3).

Given the traditional and neurological associations of LI-4 with facial pain, many studies have made use of this point. It forms part of the basic TCM-based point combination in the textbook by Gertrude Kubiena and Boris Sommer, for example, together with SJ-17, GB-20, ST-25 and ST-44, and is included in point lists in some EA stimulator manuals (in one, for example, with LIV-2, LI-10, ST-6 and ST-7, and in another with GB-8, ST-2 and ST-7 for V2 neuralgia).

George Ulett uses TEAS at BL-2, SJ-21 and *taiyang* (V1), at LI-4, LI-20, ST-1 and Du-26 (V2), and at SI-19, ST-4, ST-6 and ST-7 (V3). Other points such as ST-3 and Du-26 have been suggested for TEAS as well, with ST-44 as a distal point. For V1 TN, Phil Rogers has proposed using LI-4 as the main point, rotating the other electrode in turn between points such as SJ-17, GB-14, GB-20, GB-21, ST-7, ST-9, *taiyang* (M-HN-9) and the earlobe, or distal points (SJ-5, LIV-3, ST-36 and ST-44) if local points do not help.

Gabriel Stux recommends contralateral local treatment, but using bilateral distal points. Gordon Gadsby too prefers to use contralateral treatment locally, with the same points whichever trigeminal division is involved.

Various electrode locations have been used in TENS studies: local, where nerve branches emerge, proximal to the pain or directly over it, or distal. Mark Johnson suggests that ALTENS can be used either ipsi- or contralaterally. David Ottoson and Thomas Lundeberg position one electrode in front of the ear over the TMJ, with the other above the eye (V1), below and lateral to it (V2), or over the masseter (V3).

**Parameters used** Reinhold Voll employed pTENS at 7.5 Hz for TN (but 3.9 Hz for neuralgia in general). He derived these parameters from previous work by Oltrogge, but it is unclear how they were decided in the first place. It has also been suggested that with EA only LF (2–10 Hz) stimulation should be used initially in severe cases, and never higher than 50–60 Hz. Peter Deadman suggests 10 Hz for the basic point protocol mentioned above. Despite these recommendations, in the studies located, both LF and HF stimulation seem to have been used in about equal measure. In one Japanese study, frequency was increased from 3 Hz initially, to 40, 250 and finally 500 Hz as treatment progressed.

DD is recommended for TN in two EA device manuals. However, in the studies consulted, DD is far less common than either HF or LF EA.

Both high- and low-intensity stimulation have been used, with a predominance of studies describing intensity in terms of patient 'tolerance'. Strong or long stimulation has been emphasised as being superior to standard manipulation in at least one MA study. However, strong stimulation may well aggravate TN.

Phil Rogers has suggested ALTEAS to tolerance for TN. Mark Johnson also recommends ALTENS rather than CTENS, but only strong enough to elicit minor muscle twitching. David Ottoson and Thomas Lundeberg, however, suggest using burst TENS (high intensity, just below pain threshold) only if skin sensation is reduced, with HF TENS in all other cases.

When using LILT, it has been observed that a low dose can be much more effective than a high dose for TN (12–15 sessions, on alternate days).

## ATYPICAL FACIAL PAIN

Atypical facial pain may occur in the maxillary or mandibular region. It tends to be diffuse, and may be aching, throbbing, dull, burning, merely uncomfortable, or numb, persistent rather than overtly painful or shooting. It may not respond to antidepressant medication or carbamazepine. Onset may be gradual, and the pain may be accompanied by a variety of other symptoms indicating autonomic dysfunction.

LF EA has been used for atypical facial pain. In the ryodoraku system, electrical resistance readings at the representative measuring points are usually scattered, in keeping with the variety of symptoms that can accompany the condition.

TENS has been used for atypical facial pain, as part of a comprehensive programme of interventions.

**Combinations and comparisons** HF EA was combined with TDP, and MA with microwave stimulation, in one study of atypical facial pain.

In contrast to results with TN, ryodoraku was about as effective as nerve block for atypical facial pain.

**Points used** Joseph Wong uses his 'sympathetic switches' for atypical facial pain. Similarly, in ryodoraku the use of points with a general regulatory effect is recommended, starting with distal points, and only later carefully introducing facial points. *Ashi* points in tight neck and upper back muscles should also be considered.

**Parameters used** Treatment should be gentle initially. Strong stimulation at LI-4, for example, may have a marked vasodilatory effect on the face, and should be used cautiously. A cautious generalisation might be that EA is usually applied at low frequencies, possibly more at distal points like LI-4, and TENS at high frequencies locally.

## OCCIPITAL NEURALGIA

Occipital neuralgia involves the major or minor occipital nerves or the major auricular nerve, all of which originate from the spinal cord at C2–C3 level. It is generally paroxysmal, with unilateral pain radiating from behind the mastoid process to the occiput, ear and vertex, and is a common cause for persistent pain following whiplash injury. The neuralgia may be paroxysmal or continuous.

MA has been used for occipital neuralgia. In one such study, GB-20 together with *ashi* points gave significantly better results than MA at SJ-5, GB-20, GB-39 and *taiyang* (M-HN-9).

EA, both with and without TDP, has also been applied at local (BL-10, GB-20, etc) and distal (SI-3, SJ-5) points. Slightly better results were reported *without* the use of TDP irradiation. In one study, EA was applied at paraspinal, head and auricular points (40 Hz at body points, 90 Hz at ear points). Results were encouraging, although not fully satisfactory.

LILT has been found helpful for occipital neuralgia (GaAlAs 830 nm 60 mW; HeNe 10 mW 632.8 nm; local application at 15 seconds/point, 3–5 min total exposure). LA has also been used at local *ashi* points, in conjunction with MA at standard local and distal acupoints.

**Points used** Obvious points to use include BL-10, GB-8, GB-20 and distal points such as SJ-5. *Huatuojiaji* points are another possibility.

## TEMPOROMANDIBULAR JOINT DYSFUNCTION

The symptoms of chronic temporomandibular joint (TMJ) dysfunction are muscle pain, joint sounds during condylar movements and limitation in jaw opening. TMJ function can be affected by orthodontic and dental health, bruxism (tooth grinding), psychological stresses, physical trauma to the neck, jaw or head, diet, and even by the weather in some individuals. In many cases jaw movement may become limited or painful. Some jaw problems may be primarily biomechanical rather than muscular in origin, but surgery based on assumed joint pathology should be used only after less invasive methods have been tried, unless absolutely necessary. One standard treatment for myofascial jaw pain is the occlusal dental splint, which is designed to be worn for long periods to correct the bite and realign the jaw. TMJ dysfunction is often resistant to conventional interventions.

There are several acupuncture studies on TMJ dysfunction. In one systematic review of randomised trials, the authors noted that all the studies they considered were supportive of acupuncture's effectiveness in TMJ, although most came from one Swedish group. Other systematic reviews of acupuncture in dentistry have commented favourably on its use for TMJ dysfunction, when benefits are seen more rapidly than with an occlusal splint.

Acupuncture may be more effective for muscular TMJ problems and pain than for neurogenic craniofacial pain. In an open study, one medical acupuncturist found MA to be of considerable benefit for TMJ or muscular facial pain, sometimes to the extent that other treatments were not required. MA has been found helpful for TMJ in controlled studies as well.

Thomas List and colleagues in Sweden have carried out several careful acupuncture studies on craniomandibular disorders. EA was used in some, with the authors concluding that EA was superior to splint therapy for TMJ pain. In the many other EA studies on TMJ pain, some authors have concluded that EA may be more effective with functional than structural TMJ conditions, whereas others have found it helpful even when pain resulted from arthritic changes in the joint.

Ryodoraku has been used for TMJ, as has silver spike point (SSP) therapy, together with a splint. In one RCT comparing pTENS, occlusal splint and their combination, the best results were obtained with the combination, but pTENS alone was also more effective than just the splint.

TENS tends to increase free jaw movement, and so has been used for craniofacial pain and TMJ problems within the context of dentistry. It has been combined, for example, with amitriptyline and TrP injection, and with various other physical therapy modalities for pain, inflammation and reduced range of movement following TMJ arthroscopic surgery. Not all reports on TENS are enthusiastic, however.

Microcurrent has been used for TMJ problems. Once TrPs have been located electrically, smaller ones are treated with probe electrodes (0.3 Hz, 20 – 40 μA, 10–30 seconds/pt), and larger areas with pads, positive results being claimed within two to three treatments (14 or 48 hours apart). CES too has been used for TMJ.

TMJ is considered a standard indication for LILT. It may both reduce pain and increase jaw opening, when this is limited. However, there are a number of negative studies of LILT for chronic orofacial pain.

The QGM (at temple and jaw on the affected side, for 7 minutes in each position, together with concurrent QGM treatment of the top of the foot, over ~GB-41) has been used for TMJ, in conjunction with cervical manipulation.

**Comparisons and combinations**  In one rather unclear study of mixed facial pain types, MA and EA were found to be equally effective for TMJ problems.

TENS was found to be more effective than ultrasound in one RCT for TMJ dysfunction, improving the results obtained with medication only.

LILT was superior, although not significantly, to MENS for TMJ pain and mobility in one RCT.

EA has been combined with TDP, as well as with a different broad-spectrum irradiation treatment, results being better than with EA alone, though not significantly. Manipulation and massage techniques have been combined with EA and *qigong* for TMJ realignment, with changes reported as occurring within one to two treatments.

**Points used**  As with most *bi* syndrome problems, local and distal points are usually combined in the treatment of TMJ dysfunction. Local points most commonly used include SI-19, ST-6 and ST-7, and less commonly SJ-17, GB-20, ST-4 and *taiyang* (M-HN-9). By far the most used distal point is LI-4, although ST-36 also appears in some studies.

Joseph Wong recommends points such as GB-3, ST-5, ST-6, ST-7 and *taiyang*.

Even ST-36 MA alone was used for TMJ in one study, seemingly with good results after no more than six treatments.

In an EA study, ST-7 was the only local point used, emphasis being placed on deep needling (3–4 cm) and obtaining *deqi* before electrical stimulation. The importance of deep needling and obtaining *deqi* has been stressed by other researchers as well.

TrPs in the masticatory muscles are usually associated with TMJ-related pain, and are more tender than in non-sufferers. Their use is emphasised in a number of reports, and their correspondence with acupoints has been investigated.

George Ulett uses TEAS at SI-19, SJ-21 and LI-4 for TMJ. Points such as SI-19, ST-6, ST-7 and directly over the TMJ itself have been used with LA.

Pekka Pöntinen divides treatment into three phases, the first two not more than 4 weeks long: (a) phase one (one to two sessions per week), with treatment at local *ashi* points such as SI-18, SJ-21, GB-2, ST-6, ST-7 and TrPs of the masseter, temporalis and pterygoid muscles; (b) phase two, taking into account possible referred pain from other regions (neck, shoulder girdle), with more distal points, including SI-3, P-6, SJ-5, SJ-15, GB-21, LI-4, LI-10, LI-11, Du-14, with TrPs in muscles such as the trapezius, levator scapulae, supraspinatus, etc.; (c) phase three, taking into account any underlying problems (infection, fibromyalgia, scars, tumours, Sjögren's syndrome, etc.), together with an antistress treatment to include points such as GB-34 and LIV-3.

TrP stimulation is also frequently carried out with LA. Neighbouring muscles (e.g. trapezius, sternocleidomastoid, supra- and infraspinatus) may require treatment, as well as the jaw muscles themselves.

**Parameters used**  Because electrostimulation can relax muscles, ALTENS or 'ultralow-frequency' TENS may be particularly appropriate. Thus, in one study of mixed facial pain types, 30 minutes of 2 Hz EA was particularly effective when muscle tenderness or spasm was present, and also gave longer-lasting relief than either MA or TLEA. Indeed, LF EA is far more often used than HF EA, or indeed DD EA.

However, in one TENS CT, LI-4 ALTEAS surprisingly had less of a long-term effect than local CTENS. In another TENS CT, LF trigger point TENS was less effective altogether than CTENS or the Liss pain-suppressor device, but this comparison is probably invalid, as treatments were applied for only 10 minutes. In contrast, South African researchers did not find HF TENS useful for myofascial TMJ dysfunction.

Infrared LILT appears to have a better effect on TMJ than HeNe or red diode laser at a comparably intensity.

## DENTAL PAIN

Both electrical treatment methods and acupuncture have a long history of involvement in dentistry, a major application of acupuncture being for pain relief during or after dental procedures. Alan Bensoussan has systematically reviewed the role of acupuncture in dental pain, as have Ernst and Pittler for acute dental pain, concluding that acupuncture can alleviate it.

MA has been used for centuries in dentistry. EA, like MA, is usually considered as indicated for toothache.

Various TENS-based devices have been developed for procedural dental pain. TENS has also been used for the discomfort entailed in orthodontic movement of teeth. There are more studies on TENS than EA for acute pathological dental pain.

CES has been used for mild toothache, as well as for stress reduction in dental practice.

LILT and LA have a role in dentistry, although probably more for soft tissue conditions than dental problems as such. LILT has been used, however, for dental hypersensitivity.

100 Hz vibration can reduce toothache, although it may be less effective for the pain of dental interventions.

Case study 9.11.4 details the use of electroacupuncture and TENS in dentistry.

**Comparisons and combinations** Experimentally, TENS has been found to increase dental pain threshold (PT) more than EA, possibly because of the larger electrode/tissue interface involved. Again experimentally, MA that was familiar to subjects had a greater effect on PT than ALTENS that was not, with implications for both clinical trials and practice.

Some researchers have found that HF vibration is sometimes more effective than TENS for acute dental pain, and that the combination of the two modalities may improve results obtained with TENS alone.

**Points used** Experimentally, LI-4 EA has less effect on the sensory dimension of dental pain than LF EA at local points.

A number of studies have therefore emphasised the need to use local points in addition to or rather than LI-4, whether with EA or TENS. However, LI-4 EA may *prolong* analgesia induced by local stimulation. An experimental Italian study similarly showed that HF (300 Hz) EA was markedly effective for dental pain when applied to the lip, but not extrasegmentally.

Clearly, points should be selected according to which tooth is affected. Ursula Völkel has suggested:

- *upper jaw, front*: LI-20, Du-26
- *upper jaw, side*: SI-18, ST-2, ST-7, *taiyang* (M-HN-9)
- *lower jaw, front*: Ren-24
- *lower jaw, side*: SJ-17, ST-5, ST-6
- *molars*: SJ-23, GB-2
- *adjunctive distal points*: BL-60, LI-1, LI-4, ST-40.

# CASE Study 9.11.4

## The use of electroacupuncture and TENS in dentistry, with particular reference to the differential diagnosis of facial pain and its use in TMJ problems
### Stuart Ferraris

Electroacupressure differs from electroacupuncture in that no skin penetration occurs. The electrofrequency is applied through a probe to the skin point. After first being introduced to acupuncture, I favoured the use of electroacupressure (EAP), partly from my perception of patient needle phobia, and partly perhaps from my own lack of confidence at that early stage. Years of experience and further courses have changed that perception, and I now use needling and EAP to suit the individual case.

Early experiences with EAP convinced me that this technique has much to offer in the general dental practice environment. TENS technology has been well documented as a means of pain control. In the dental environment EAP frequencies can be used to reduce discomfort in muscle tension associated with TMJ dysfunction. This may be in the facial muscles directly affected, as well as indirectly involved muscles of the neck and back. Other uses include pain associated with other forms of headache and postoperative swelling after impacted tooth removal. The electrical stimulation is thought to ease pain in the usual way as well as by increasing tissue circulation and drainage, thus relieving the pain of turgid tissues.

I use two main pieces of apparatus. The first is the Stimul 3 (Tesla, Liberec, Czech Republic). This instrument is handheld. I generally use it with the one-probe application, but two-probe simultaneous application is available.

Neither application should be used across the midline. It uses two phases: the first is used to confirm the best point to stimulate; and the second phase stimulates to a maximum of 3 mA, while the detection current ranges from 1.5 to 20 mA. The Stimul 3 is powered by a standard replaceable battery, giving many hours of use.

I also use the Likon, a larger instrument that I usually place on the patient's lap if I am treating someone in the dental chair (Fig. 9.11.3). This allows the patient to control the level of stimulation. The Likon, a form of TENS, works on the method of modulation electrotherapy (MET), also known as pulse-modulated mid-frequency current therapy. This is a low-frequency wave that modulates a mid-frequency wave to produce stimulating pulses. The pulses produced are able to penetrate deep into the tissues of the body without causing discomfort to the skin. These pulses improve blood circulation and speed up metabolism, bringing about relaxation and relief.

The Likon electrodes use a pad application to the skin, much like the better-known TENS application instruments. The electrode pads are placed according to the directions on guide cards provided by the manufacturer, unless the operator feels experienced enough to modify locations to meet individual patient needs. For intraoral use, I have had electrodes made to accept the standard disposable electrode pads. The unit is fitted with a rechargeable battery pack that gives approximately 3 hours of treatment time before needing to be recharged.

Special intraoral pads can be used on the Likon leads delivering select frequencies for electroanaesthesia of segments of the jaws. This can reduce the need for local anaesthetic, adrenaline (epinephrine) and analgesics. The Stimul 3 or Pointer Plus probes are very useful for affecting an analgesic effect in dental neuralgia. This is particularly useful in cases where there is a need for differential diagnosis. A case history can illustrate this use more clearly.

*(Continued)*

CASE Study 9.11.4 **Continued**

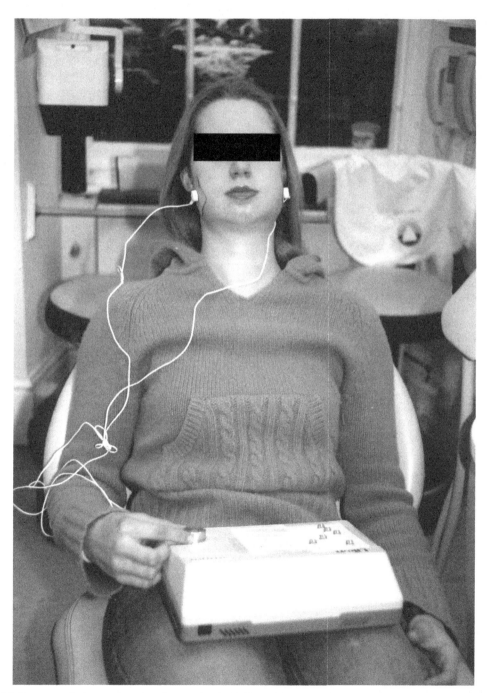

**Figure 9.11.3** Treatment of trismus, pain and swelling associated with bilateral surgical wisdom tooth removal, using Likon device.

### Case history

Mrs X presented with several teeth on her right, in both maxilla and mandible, giving symptoms of pulpitis. Neither clinical examination nor radiological findings could pinpoint any or all of them being the offending teeth, although I was sure one of the teeth was the culprit while the others were suffering referred symptoms. By applying EAP through the probe to several points on the right side of her face, as well as to points intraorally on the mucosa over the apical areas of the offending teeth, comfort was restored to the patient. The effect of the analgesia thus achieved lasted longer over the areas of referred pain while severe pain returned with very definite localisation over the upper second molar. This tooth was opened and treated endodontically, with total remission of all pain symptoms.

Another very useful benefit from EAP in the dental practice is the reduction of the gag reflex. This can be achieved very effectively by needling the 'anxiety' points just in front of the ear over the TMJ. EAP works just as effectively as needling, and offers a useful alternative if phobia of needles and needling is an issue (Fig. 9.11.4).

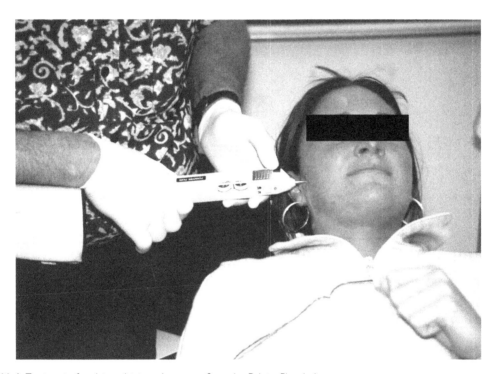

**Figure 9.11.4** Treatment of anxiety point to reduce gag reflex, using Pointer Plus device.

Variations of these points are usually recommended for EA treatment of toothache. For instance, ST-44 as a distal point, or LI-4, ST-6 and ST-44 for a Full-Heat condition, but KI-1, LI-4, ST-7 and SP-4 for Empty-Heat. Local and distal points can be stimulated from the same device output.

Other points that may be useful include ST-2 for toothache, with HE-7 or LIV-3 for relaxation.

George Ulett suggests ST-4, ST-5, ST-6 and/or ST-7 in conjunction with LI-4 when using TEAS for toothache.

TrPs should not be overlooked when treating dental pain. Pain in a tooth, and sensitivity of the tooth to percussion, which is usually assumed to be diagnostic of pulpal inflammation/necrosis, may be referred from TrPs in the masticatory muscles.

Treatment of locally tender areas, even if not acupoints or TrPs, may provide relief from toothache. With ryodoraku, needling directly into the gum near the affected tooth has been found to be the most effective method.

**Parameters used** When using extrasegmental EA at LI-4 experimentally, dental pain may be affected only at high intensities. Although LF (2 Hz) EA tends to give slow onset, generalised dental analgesia that lasts after stimulation ends, and 100 Hz EA results in more rapid but localised and relatively short-lived analgesia, 10 Hz EA in one report led to a rapid increase in PT, declining slowly during ongoing stimulation.

On the other hand, various frequencies of TENS all appeared to reduce dental pulp sensitivity by around the same amount.

In one experimental TENS study, 10 minutes of squarewave stimulation was found more effective against 'toothache' than both sine and sawtooth waveforms. There is little data to confirm the superiority of other commercially available waveforms.

Clinically, HF or DD at moderate to strong intensity have been suggested by EA device manufacturers. Strong 5–8 Hz EA has also been used (for 20–30 minutes).

Both LF and HF local TENS may result in similar relief of acute dental or periodontal pain. However, as in experimental studies, LF TENS gave relief for longer.

# NECK PAIN

Cervical disorders may be purely structural or may include nerve compression or a predominant vascular component. Soft tissue conditions or whiplash injury are other possibilities (see also Subchapter 9.12).

Structural spinal disorders include osteo- and rheumatoid arthritis, with spondylitis (vertebral inflammation) or spondylosis (reduced movement of the intervertebral joints). The associated pain is nociceptive in nature.

If spondylosis or a herniated disc causes irritation or compression of nerve roots, or both, then nociceptive pain may be accompanied by radicular pain in what is sometimes termed 'cervical syndrome'. Neck movement is frequently restricted, and pain can radiate as cervicobrachial neuralgia, sometimes with tingling extending to the fingers. Cervical spondylosis may also lead to pressure on sympathetic nerve fibres, resulting in a variety of autonomic symptoms, from vertigo and tinnitus to nausea or precordial pain.

Vertigo, headache and dizziness can also be caused by compression not of a nerve, but of the vertebral artery.

Soft tissue conditions can include acute torticollis, muscle sprain and fibromyalgia. Muscular tension in the neck is a frequent cause of headaches. Whiplash injury, which may involve structural, nerve or soft tissue components, can be a particularly unpleasant condition, and difficult to manage if not treated early.

Case study 9.11.5 is a study of interferential therapy (IFT) for neck pain.

MA has been used for cervical syndrome. There are also many studies of EA for cervical syndrome. In one retrospective Japanese study, it was claimed to give excellent results for 'neck–shoulder–hand syndrome' unresponsive to MA, alleviating both pain and numbness. Results in another report were better in patients without neurological deficit,

and also if the condition had not lasted for more than 5 years. EA has been found helpful for spinal cord pathology (myelopathy) by some authors, although in one study of EA and massage the results were better for cervicobrachialgia than for pain associated with myelopathy.

TENS has been used for cervicobrachialgia, in combination with mesotherapy (multiple local injections into the dermis and subcutaneous fatty tissue). However, in one mixed CTENS study, results with radicular pain were less good than for other types of neuropathic pain or musculoskeletal pain. CTENS did not benefit cervical nerve root compression pain in another such mixed study.

LA has been used for radicular cervical pain. Among physical therapists, LILT is often considered as indicated for chronic brachial neuralgia. 'Repetitive strain injury', associated with cervical radicular dysfunction rather than carpal tunnel syndrome, may improve with LILT as part of a comprehensive treatment programme. TrP LA has been used for myogenic neck pain.

**Combinations and comparisons** EA has frequently been combined with moxibustion for cervical syndrome. Indeed, EA with infrared was better than acupuncture alone, and the combination of EA with heated needles gave better effects than EA or heated needling alone, with EA used separately being slightly superior to heated needling. However, when heated needling was compared with EA 'as strong as the patient could bear', results were better with the traditional method. In another such study, specifically for 'cervical vertigo', heated needling gave a greater improvement both clinically and in vertebral artery blood flow.

EA has also been used together with ear point pressure, with massage, plum blossom needling and cupping, and with various multifrequency lamps, again sometimes with cupping. Such lamps have also been used together with moxibustion. EA with massage was more effective than massage alone in one report. In another study, results with the combination of EA and massage were further improved when a 'sacred lamp' (multifrequency irradiation) was added.

In one study, interferential therapy combined with MA improved vertebral artery circulation more than MA with LF TENS or MA with massage.

Ryodoraku was found to be more effective than nerve block for traumatic cervical syndrome (whiplash injury) in one retrospective review, the combined treatment being more effective still.

**Points used** The most used points for cervical syndrome (including cervicobrachial pain) include: SI-3, SI-11, BL-2, BL-10, P-6, SJ-5, GB-20, GB-21, LI-4, LI-11, LI-15, Du-14 and Du-20 (of these, SI-3, BL-2 and P-6 are used rather less). *Huatuojiaji* and *ashi* points are also emphasised.

Richard Umlauf has explored the potential of scalp EA (Yamamoto's new scalp acupuncture, YNSA) for cervicobrachial syndrome in an experimental study. Scalp points (including extra points such as *sishencong*, M-HN-1) are more used than auricular acupuncture.

# CASE Study 9.11.5

## Interferential therapy case study
**Maureen Lovesey**

Low-frequency currents occur in the body. Dr Nemec, an Austrian physicist, recognised that if problems were occurring in the body it might be possible to influence these conditions by beaming in other low-frequency currents. In order to overcome the problem of high skin resistance, Dr Nemec used two medium-frequency currents. The interaction of these two frequency currents produced a low-frequency modulation where they crossed (see Fig. 3.7 on page 31). This method is called interferential therapy, and has been used for more than 50 years.

With suitable placement of the four electrodes it became possible to introduce low-frequency currents to tissues at different depths between them. Some years later came the introduction of a rotating vector: by varying the relative strength of the two currents, the 'cloverleaf' interference pattern scanned the tissues and thus produced a more homogeneous field over a wider area (Fig. 9.11.5 on page 231). Other manufacturers, by superimposing the two alternating currents within the equipment, subsequently produced amplitude modulation within the machine, such that it was then possible to use a two-pole application.

The effects of IFT are an improvement in circulation, pain relief and mobilising of tissues and joints. All frequencies have beneficial effects on the circulation. If the main aim is to improve the circulation to aid healing, a frequency range of 0–100 Hz is usually used. For pain relief, the frequencies are the same as for electroacupuncture and TENS, namely range 2–15 Hz for long-acting relief of aching and around 100 Hz for quick-acting relief of sharper pain.

I have been using IFT since the mid 1970s. Prior to training in acupuncture in the early 1980s, I had been getting good results using IFT for treating pain, musculoskeletal, gynaecological and vascular conditions. I now use acupuncture a great deal in my physiotherapy practice, and would normally use it as a first-line modality in the treatment of someone with internal or multiple problems. However, many people do not like needles and I find that for simple musculoskeletal problems IFT and other forms of sensory stimulation produce good results.

## Case history

Mrs F: age: 52; occupation: housewife; hobbies: antiques, tennis, gardening, knitting.

## Assessment

Mrs F woke 2 days previously with acute left-sided neck pain, with constant aching and sharp pain at times on movement. The pain was radiating down into the left

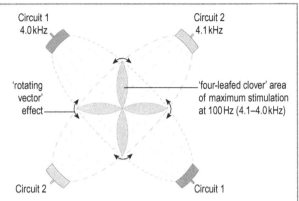

**Figure 9.11.5** Interferential therapy. Two sine wave currents of different frequencies, applied spatially at different angles (here at right angles), interfere at a beat frequency (see *Fig. 3.7*). If one is at 4 kHz and the other at 4.1 kHz, the area in which maximum stimulation occurs at 100 Hz is shaped like a four-leafed clover. Changing the relative amplitude of the two currents creates a 'rotating vector' effect, effectively increasing the treated area. (After Kitchen & Bazin 1998.)

scapula most of the time and intermittently down her arm as far as the radial side of her left wrist. Prior to this episode she had experienced only occasional slight neck stiffness. Her pain was aggravated by movement and driving. She was sleeping badly, waking about three times at night, and the pain was worse on rising.

## Neck movements

Flexion: Three finger-breadths loss (chin to chest)
Extension: Two and a half finger-breadths loss (occiput to nape)
Right rotation: 45°
Left rotation: 30°
Side flexion: 10° both sides.

On palpation, the whole of her neck was tender and there was some spasm. She was sore at left C5. She had no neurological deficit.

## Treatment

**Day 1:** after being assessed she was given IFT with the two-electrode method, using large flat electrodes. Electrode 1 was placed on the left side of her neck (this covers the nerve root and *huatuojiaji* points of the left side of the neck), held in place by a damp hot-pack. Electrode 2 was strapped to her left wrist, extending as far as LI-4. A further hot-pack was placed over her scapula. She was given IFT for 10 minutes at 100 Hz and for 10 minutes at 2.5 Hz. The treatment relieved the pain and left rotation improved to 45°.

**Day 2:** Mrs F reported that the pain relief had lasted about 3 hours and had then returned fairly fiercely. She had had a better night and had woken only once, but was bad on rising. Left rotation was 40°. Maitland

*(Continued)*

## CASE Study 9.11.5 **Continued**

posterior–anterior mobilisations grade II (gentle manual therapy) were given to left C5; left rotation increased to 50°. IFT was repeated as day 1. Gentle exercises were taught. Pain was eased, left rotation was 55–60°.

**Day 4**: pain eased about 6 hours after treatment, not quite so severe on return and only occasionally going below the elbow. Still waking once, was bad on rising. Treatment was as day 2. Pain had eased, rotation was 60°+.

**Day 6**: pain eased until the following day. Now some pain-free periods, pain to the elbow was less and rarely to the wrist. Exercises were checked. She was sleeping fairly well, but was still waking once. Mobilisations increased to grade II+. IFT given as day 2. Pain was eased, rotation was 70°.

**Day 9**: pain had eased about one and a half days. Pain-free periods were increasing. Pain much less severe, now only occasional, going down to the elbow but still quite bad at times in the neck and scapula. Mobilisations as day 6. IFT was neck to hand 2.5 Hz and 100 Hz, for 5 minutes each, then neck to left scapula 100 Hz for 7 minutes and 25 Hz for 8 minutes. She was pain free; the rotation was 75–80°.

**Day 12**: pain was now much less frequent and severe, mainly at the neck/scapula and over the top of the shoulder. Treatment was as day 9. She was pain free and rotation was 80°+.

### Review

Three weeks later she had only had occasional pain in the neck or scapula area. Neck movements were checked, rotation was 80°+. Mobilisations were III+ left C5, IFT was given neck to scapula for 20 minutes at 2/100 Hz (6 seconds at each frequency, alternating). Exercises were checked. Further advice was given on lifestyle.

### Discussion

When first using IFT, I used it on its own and found that it was particularly beneficial at reducing swelling and relieving spasm and pain. A few years later I started to combine treatments. Over the years I have found that combining modalities usually works better than using a single modality. This is not surprising as it appears that the way in which each modality produces its effect(s) is slightly different; therefore suitable combinations can enhance the overall effect. I often use interferential with laser acupuncture for injuries and musculoskeletal problems, and sometimes use acupuncture and IFT in combination for various conditions.

IFT, when directed at problem areas or tissues, also affects acupuncture channels or points. In the case of Mrs F, who was suffering from a severe nerve root irritation of the left C5, the electrodes placed to cover the left cervical nerve roots also covered the *huatuojiaji* points in the neck. The other electrode also covered LI-4 and LU-7. Another example of placement of electrodes that I sometimes use for supraspinatus tendonitis is with electrode 1 (large) on the base of the neck covering the C5–C7 nerve roots for shoulder/*huatuojiaji* points/origin of supraspinatus/ SI-14. Electrode 2 (medium or large) is placed over the supa-acromial space/LI-15.

### Conclusions

IFT is simple to use, is popular with patients and combines well with other modalities. It appears to be helpful for a range of conditions. A knowledge of acupuncture is helpful for the most beneficial placement of electrodes. Research is urgently needed to demonstrate the effectiveness of IFT, as very little has been carried out to date.

---

A very clear account of different MA point combinations useful for vertebral artery compression, radicular cervical spondylosis, spondylosis with sympathetic nerve involvement and cervical myelopathy has been given by Lü Shaojie. His recommendations are as follows: (a) with the points most commonly used in the EA studies consulted given below (b), in each case:

1. *vertebral artery compression syndrome:*
   (a) GB-8, GB-29, Du-16 and *taiyang* (M-HN-9)
   (b) BL-10, GB-20, GB-21, Du-14, Du-20, *sishencong* (M-HN-1) and *huatuojiaji*
2. *radicular cervical spondylosis:*
   (a) SI-9, SI-11, SI-17, LI-4, LI-10, LI-13 and LI-15
   (b) GB-21, LI-4, LI-11 and *huatuojiaji*
3. *cervical spondylosis with sympathetic nerve involvement:*
   (a) GB-20, *jingbailao* (M-HN-30) *and xueyadian* (2 *cun* lateral to midpoint between C6 and C7)
   (b) Du-14, *huatuojiaji*

4. *cervical spondylosis with myelopathy*
   (a) GB-20, GB-30, LI-11, Du-16, *jingbailao* (M-HN-30), *huatuojiaji* and scalp points
   (b) GB-34, ST-36, LI-11, Du-14 and *huatuojiaji*

**Parameters used** In general, continuous (CW) LF stimulation seems to be preferred, rather than HF or DD. In one instance, LF EA was specified for radicular cervical pain. LF EA is also common in studies when cervical syndrome involves vertebral artery compression, although here DD appears somewhat more frequently than in reports on other types of cervical problem. In some studies intermittent stimulation was used.

As for treatment intensity, only one paper stipulated that *deqi* was *not* to be obtained before beginning EA. Intensity is usually only described as 'to patient tolerance', and treatment as clearly moderate or gentle. Some authors, however, have used quite strong or motor level stimulation. Interestingly, in one study of acupoint microwave therapy, the strongest tolerable heat was used. Similarly, a 'strong' setting was used with the 'Zhoulin spectrum treatment instrument'.

# SUMMARY

Some key points in this chapter are:

- EA, TENS/TEAS and LILT/LA have been used for many types of neurogenic pain: neuralgias, peripheral nerve injury and compression syndromes
- EA and MA are often successfully used for migraine and other forms of headache
- There are several EA protocols for trigeminal neuralgia that offer possibilities for successful treatment when medication cannot control the symptoms

- Systematic reviews have confirmed the efficacy of EA as a treatment for dental pain.

 Additional material in the CD-ROM resource

In the CD-ROM resource, in addition to further information on many of the topics presented here, the following types of pain are also mentioned:

- Compression syndrome of the lateral cutaneous forearm nerve, ulnar nerve entrapment
- Cauda equina syndrome, spinal stenosis and arachnoiditis
- Horton's headache, Charlin's syndrome, Sluder's syndrome and Arnold's neuralgia.

**9.11** Summary of relevant studies in the electronic clinical studies database (number of studies)

| Condition | EA | Other | Condition | EA | Other |
|---|---|---|---|---|---|
| **Neurogenic pain I.** **Neuralgia, peripheral nerve injury and compression syndromes** | | | **Neurogenic pain III.** **CRPD and central pain** | | |
| Herpes zoster | | | Complex regional pain disorder (CRPD) | 7 | 32 |
| Postherpetic neuralgia | 12 | 34 | Central pain | 2 | 9 |
| Acute herpetic pain | 6 | 12 | Pain from spinal cord injury | 2 | 7 |
| Neurogenic pain by region | | | **Head and facial pain** **Migraine and headache** | | |
| The head and neck | 1 | 1 | Migraine | 27 | 74 |
| Thoracic outlet syndrome | 2 | 1 | Tension-type headache | 9 | 24 |
| Carpal/tarsal tunnel syndrome | 4 | 18 | Cluster headache | 0 | 6 |
| Plexus lesions | 3 | 3 | Other vascular headache | 6 | 10 |
| Other neurogenic upper limb pain | 1 | 4 | Occipital head pain | 6 | 4 |
| Clunial nerve injury | 3 | 1 | Trauma induced head pain | 1 | 3 |
| Meralgia paraesthetica | 2 | 4 | Headache associated with drug | | |
| Other neurogenic lower limb pain | 4 | 4 | withdrawal | 0 | 2 |
| Denervation/peripheral sensory nerve injury | 9 | 8 | Other headache | 3 | 10 |
| **Neurogenic pain II.** **Amputation pain and peripheral neuropathy** | | | Uncategorised/mixed headache | 28 | 45 |
| | | | **Orofacial pain** | | |
| Phantom limb pain | 9 | 25 | Temporomandibular joint (TMJ) disorder | 25 | 45 |
| Neuroma and stump pain | 0 | 9 | Trigeminal neuralgia | 51 | 66 |
| Peripheral neuropathy | | | Other (or undefined) chronic facial pain | 8 | 22 |
| Drug-induced neuropathy | 3 | 5 | Acute dental/jaw problems | 4 | 22 |
| Peripheral neuropathy and HIV | 2 | 2 | Other/mixed facial pain | 1 | 1 |
| Diabetic neuropathy | 7 | 13 | **Note:** Summary of database studies on neck pain and sciatica can be found in chapter 9.12, on musculoskeletal conditions. | | |
| Restless legs syndrome | 2 | 2 | | | |
| Neuropathic pain (mixed and other studies) | 8 | 36 | | | |

# RECOMMENDED READING

*Essential textbooks:*

Lü SJ 2002 Handbook of Acupuncture in the Treatment of Nervous System Disorders. Donica Publishing, London

Wong JY 2001 A Manual of Neuro-Anatomical Acupuncture. Volume II: Neurological disorders. Toronto Pain and Stress Clinic, Toronto

*The classic TENS study on postherpetic neuralgia (PHN):*

Nathan PW, Wall PD Treatment of post-herpetic neuralgia by prolonged electric stimulation. British Medical Journal. 1974 Sept 14; 3(5932): 645–7

*A comprehensive TCM analysis of some 40 types of headache:*

Scott J The diagnosis and treatment of headaches by acupuncture. Journal of Chinese Medicine (Hove, England). 1984 May; (15): 5–18

*pTENS for migraine:*

Heydenreich A, Thiessen M [Comparison of the effectiveness of drug therapy, invasive and non-invasive acupuncture in migraine]. Zeitschrift Ärtzliche Fortbildung. 1989; 83(17): 877–9

*Chen Kezheng on the different modalities of acupuncture for trigeminal neuralgia:*

Chen KZ Trigeminal neuralgia. International Journal of Clinical Acupuncture. 1994; 5(4): 429–34

*A positive systematic review!*

Ernst E, White AR Acupuncture as a treatment for temporo-mandibular joint dysfunction: a systematic review of randomized trials. Archives of Otolaryngology – Head and Neck Surgery. 1999 March; 125(3): 269–72

*Sources for figures*

Anderson DM, Novak PD, Keith J, Elliott MA 2000 (eds) Dorland's Illustrated Medical Dictionary. WB Saunders, Philadelphia (30th edn)

Martin D 1996 Interferential therapy. In: Kitchen S, Bazin S (eds) Clayton's Electrotherapy. WB Saunders, London (10th edn), 306–15

# 9.12 MUSCULOSKELETAL CONDITIONS: AN INTEGRATED APPROACH

*Pekka J Pöntinen, with a contribution by Steven KH Aung*

This subchapter focuses on joint and muscle problems and their treatment with electrical stimulation and low-energy laser. Integration of these methods with other treatment strategies is emphasised.

## OSTEOARTHRITIS

The most common of painful conditions affecting the joints is osteoarthritis (OA). Patients are typically older than 60 years of age, but more than 80% of people over the age of 50 already have radiological evidence of OA. The joints most commonly involved include knees, hips, feet, ankles, the distal interphalangeal (DIP) joints, proximal interphalangeal (PIP) joints, first carpometacarpal joints, the cervical spine, and the lower spine. Typical symptoms include morning stiffness lasting no longer than 20–30 minutes on waking or sitting over a prolonged period. Other problems arise from the limited range of motion (ROM) in the affected joint(s). The third, but no less important, diagnostic sign is early atrophy in the muscles supporting the affected joint. The management of OA is still far from optimal, with medications currently available providing limited symptomatic relief with a large number of side-effects.

Acupuncture, electrical stimulation (EA, TENS), and low-energy laser or LED (light-emitting diode) irradiation can relieve pain, reduce inflammation and restore sleep and movement. The great majority of OA patients have not only weak muscle force but also active and latent trigger points (TrPs) in the postural muscles. Aerobic exercise alone is not able to restore the muscle force and relieve muscle spasms from trigger activity. Electrical stimulation and light therapy are excellent additional tools for this purpose.

### Knee

In a recent RCT, idiopathic anterior knee pain benefited from both EA and placebo subcutaneous needling, with the pain-relieving effect remaining for at least 6 months. According to the authors, central pain inhibition, caused by either afferent stimulation or by non-specific therapeutic (placebo) effects, is a plausible explanation of these results. A Danish study group evaluated acupuncture treatment in patients with knee osteoarthritis waiting for a total knee replacement

and concluded that acupuncture could ease discomfort while waiting for an operation and perhaps even serve as an alternative to surgery.

TENS, EA (4 Hz, 0.1 ms) and ice massage were compared in a RCT with placebo in 100 knee arthritis patients. The points used were GB-34, ST-34, ST-35 and SP-9, with a treatment time of 20 minutes, repeated 10 times. Pain at rest, stiffness, 50-feet walking time, quadriceps femoris strength and knee flexion range were checked before and after treatment. All three treatment methods were effective and significantly better than placebo.

Two large reviews were more cautious in their conclusions. According to a Cochrane review, there was clear evidence that TENS was more effective than placebo in controlling the pain associated with osteoarthritis of the knee, if treatment persisted for 6 weeks. Another systematic review of seven trials representing 393 patients with knee OA, in which acupuncture therapy was based on TCM and only manual stimulation used, provided limited evidence that acupuncture is more effective than being on a waiting list for treatment or having treatment as usual.

A Turkish group conducted a prospective, double-blind RCT in patients with knee OA to evaluate the efficacy of infrared GaAs laser therapy, and compared two different LILT regimens in terms of such parameters as power output, stimulation time and pulsing frequency. In all groups, treatment was applied to two points at the anterolateral and anteromedial portals of the knee. The authors concluded that different dose and duration of exposure did not affect the results and that both therapy regimens were safe and effective in the treatment of knee OA.

Singh et al compared the efficacy of EA, diclofenac and their combination in symptomatic treatment of OA of the knee in a randomised, single-blind, placebo-controlled study using acupuncture points around the affected knee: ST-35 (*dubi*), extra point 32 (*xiyan*), LIV-8 (*ququan*), and the adjacent TrPs. Electrical stimulation (biphasic pulses at 2 Hz for 20 minutes) was applied simultaneously to each pair of needles until it reached the maximum level tolerable to the patient. Treatment was repeated three times a week for 4 weeks. EA alone was significantly more effective than placebo and diclofenac. The combination of EA and diclofenac offered no additional benefits.

### Hip

OA of the hip is commonly found in general medical practice. Typical symptoms include morning stiffness, aching deep pain at rest as well as when loaded, restricted ROM and early atrophy of anterior thigh muscles. The degree of the osteoarthritic changes seen in X-rays does not correlate directly with the symptoms, especially pain. The main origin of pain seems to be inflammation at the muscle insertion sites and trigger activity in the strained muscles supporting and moving the joint, not the joint capsule or the joint itself.

The efficacy of acupuncture has been tested in very few randomised controlled trials. In one trial using MA, six *ashi* points were needled within the hip area. In addition, regional meridian points BL-37, GB-30, GB-31 and the distal points ST-40 and BL-40 were chosen, as well as the master point for tendons and muscles, GB-34. *Deqi* sensation was obtained. Needles were left in situ for 20 minutes with intermittent twisting (two to three times per session). In the control group, needles were inserted at least 5 cm away from the classical acupuncture points and away from tender pressure points, and not manipulated. There was a significant improvement versus baseline in both groups following treatment, but no significant difference between the two treatment groups. The authors concluded that the improvement in symptoms was associated with needle placement in the area of the affected hip rather than with TCM principles.

Another study favourably compared acupuncture with advice and an exercise routine for patients with hip OA waiting for hip replacement surgery. The points used for the MA were GB-29 (*juliao*), GB-30 (*huantiao*), GB-34 (*yanglingquan*), GB-43 (*xiaxi*), ST-44 (*neiting*) and LI-4 (*hegu*) bilaterally and four *ashi* points around the greater trochanter, once a week for 6 weeks.

A neurophysiological approach is seen in the studies using non-habituating, burst-type, high-intensity, acupuncture-like transcutaneous electric nerve stimulation (ALTENS) with the Codetron®, a device created by Bruce Pomeranz and his study group for prolonged pain treatment. Treatment was 4 Hz, 125 ms trains with 200 Hz 1.0 ms internal frequency applied for 20 minutes per session. Hip and knee OA patients reacted with significant pain reduction and improved mobility after 2 months of treatment given twice daily upon the peripheral nerves and directed to BL-40 and BL-60, GB-30 and GB-34, LI-4, ST-36, SP-9 and SP-13, Du-4 and Du-14, plus three tender points around the joints.

Laser therapy has a beneficial effect for (1) pain relief and control of inflammation, and (2) restoring normal muscle activity and muscle mass and coordination of the partially atrophic thigh muscles in hip and knee. Pain relief is achieved with laser applied locally (tender points around the greater trochanter, 2–4 J/point), segmentally (muscle trigger points, 1–2 J/TrP) and through the meridian points (0.5 J/acupoint), one to two times a week (Lasotronic MED-130 IR < 50 mW). Electric stimulation of thigh muscles is then used to restore muscle tone.

## Osteoarthritis: summary and recommendations

A single acupuncture or LILT session may lead to rapid and nearly complete relief of pain, especially in the first stage of any OA. Therefore it is important to warn patients who have been more or less immobile for a longer time, and may have simultaneous osteoporosis, not to increase their daily physical exercise immediately. Overloading may lead to fractures, for instance of metatarsal bones, when a patient with hip or knee OA can walk again normally and without pain after a long interval. Muscle atrophy, typically in anterior thigh muscles (quadriceps femoris), is an early sign of hip and knee OA. In order to restore normal neuromuscular function in these muscles and to open the peripheral microcirculation, daily muscle care with electrical stimulation is recommended.

## OSTEOPOROSIS

Osteoporosis is a major risk factor for slowly healing fractures in elderly people around 60 years of age. Although osteoporosis is more common among women, fractures linked to osteoporosis are as common in men. The most common sites for fractures are the wrist, ankle, hip and spine (T10–T12). Vertebral fractures are quite often spontaneous or occur after a minimal trauma.

Immobilisation means progressive osteoporosis partially due to decreased microcirculation at the fracture site, partially owing to vasoconstriction as a response to pain. Therefore both increase of microcirculation and pain relief are essential for faster recovery. These can be achieved by local MA, EA, TENS or LILT, alone or in combination. Additional channel points (such as LI-4 and ST-36) complete the treatment, which should be repeated one to two times a week for 2–4 months. Home treatment with non-segmental LF (2 Hz burst), high-intensity TENS daily is recommended for peripheral vasodilation and improved microcirculation.

Vertebral fractures need special attention. They are often not seen immediately after the injury in plain X-ray pictures, but appear clearly 1–2 weeks later. The lower thoracic spine is the most common site (T10–T12). Needling sites include either *huatuojiaji* or back *shu* points bilaterally just cranially and distally to the fracture site. For further home treatment with local TENS, a pair of long electrodes (50 × 90 mm) is placed paraspinally on both sides of the fractured vertebra and either HF or LF (2 Hz burst preferred) stimulation, for 30 minutes, is repeated daily for 1–2 months, then two to three times weekly or as needed.

## SHOULDER PROBLEMS

Although tendinitis and fasciitis usually respond well to LILT, problems may arise when treating subacute or chronic shoulder pain, especially rotator cuff syndrome. Local therapy with MA, EA, TENS or LILT may induce a severe pain reaction lasting longer than 24 hours, sometimes even up to a fortnight. In these hyperreactive cases local therapy should be avoided and instead either the TrPs in the opposite, contralateral site should be stimulated segmentally, or remote channel points used, also preferably on the contralateral side. For shoulder treatment, ST-38 (*tiaokou*), GB-34 (*yanglingquan*) and SJ-5 (*waiguan*) are indicated.

Patients with poor pain relief and an exaggerated reaction to peripheral stimulation often have problems with peripheral microcirculation and trophic disorders in the affected extremity, including the whole body quadrant. This may lead to calcification at the injury site, too. LILT on *ashi* and trigger points in the painful quadrant can be combined with mobilisation exercises. In chronic cases with calcification, LILT combined with TENS (2 Hz burst) or local analgesic injection and MA, as well as ultrasound, are recommended.

Acupuncture treatment should be based on the patient's history and clinical findings. In simple myofascial pain restricted to overstrained muscles in the shoulder girdle, MA to typical muscle triggers according to manual palpation findings and completed with meridian points according to symptoms is often successful. An Italian RCT compared superficial and deep needling technique in shoulder myofascial pain. Deep needling to local tender TrPs and acupuncture points SI-3 and SI-9, SJ-14 and SJ-15, LI-11 and LI-15 and Du-14 (a cycle of eight sessions, the first four twice a week, then once weekly) gave significantly better results at the end of treatment and at 1- and 3-month follow-ups.

Results in the treatment of periarthritis humeroscapularis are related to the degree of injury and the time elapsed, with a favourable response to acupuncture in patients having no contracture, a shorter history and no microcirculatory disturbances in the affected extremity. A Japanese study has shown that MA is more effective on 'freezing' type patients than on those with a completely 'frozen' shoulder. In many freezing-type patients, the range of motion was expanded owing to pain relief. The authors concluded that acupuncture therapy is effective for relieving the pain of periarthritis humeroscapularis, particularly for patients having no spontaneous pain before they enter into the frozen phase. Other studies have concluded that the combination of acupuncture with shoulder exercise may offer effective treatment for frozen shoulder. However, excessive exercise on experiencing pain relief should be discouraged.

In sports medicine LILT has established a wide therapeutic spectrum in shoulder traumatology. Bringmann compared the therapeutic results of laser acupuncture (point treatment), laser irradiation (laser shower, scanner), and selected physiotherapeutic methods in the treatment of contused shoulder trauma, myogelosis, partial paresis of the circumflex nerve, humeroscapulary periarthritis and cervical syndrome. Both therapeutic forms of LILT showed sufficient to good dose-dependent results, in some cases better than physiotherapy alone.

Gonzáles Álvarez compared LA (HeNe) and MA in a prospective RCT in 62 patients with humeroscapular periarthritis. Conventional medical treatment was suspended during this 2-week trial. Both techniques were demonstrated to be effective for this condition, improving both clinical and radiological symptoms significantly when treatment sessions were concluded. Patients accepted LA better because of its painless character, shorter time of application and absence of bleeding and stress.

The combination of LA with TENS (Kaada's protocol, using burst-type, high-intensity stimulation) can be particularly useful.

Box 9.12.1 on page 238 describes the treatment of a shoulder dislocation– fracture.

Case study 9.12.1 on page 239 details the use of electroacupuncture in rotator cuff syndrome, or frozen shoulder.

# ELBOW AND HAND PROBLEMS

## Epicondylitis lateralis (tennis elbow)

Tennis elbow is a typical RSI (repetitive strain injury) or overuse syndrome inducing trigger activation in the extensors and inflammation at their tendon insertion area on the lateral epicondyle. Reduced muscle strength and limited function (ROM) in elbow and wrist complete the symptoms. Commonly used local steroid injections to the inflamed tendon site may give a temporary relief of pain and reduce inflammation.

In a RCT from Hanover Medical School the clinical efficacy of MA in the treatment of chronic lateral epicondylitis was evaluated against sham acupuncture, with significant reductions in pain intensity and improvements in the function of the arm and in maximal strength in both treatment groups, but significantly greater for all outcome parameters in the MA group at 2 weeks. At 2 months the function of the arm was still better in the MA group; however, the differences in pain intensity and maximal strength between the groups were no longer significant. A Cochrane review on acupuncture for lateral elbow pain, based on only four RCTs, however, has demonstrated needle acupuncture to be of short-term benefit (less than 24 hours).

Vasseljen et al demonstrated significant improvement of chronic lateral epicondylitis after eight IR LILT (904 nm, 3.5 J/cm²) sessions given three times a week. Other RCTs have shown that LILT is more effective than NSAIDs in subacute and chronic tendinopathies at the end of the treatment, and at 4 to 12 weeks thereafter. Our own experience with LILT in clinical trials confirms these results and shows a clear dose dependency; if the dose is below 1 J/point and LILT is applied only on local *ashi* or trigger points, clinically adequate improvement is unlikely. Optimal healing conditions for the injured tissues and inflamed tendon occur when the dose is increased to 2–4 J/point or 4–8 J/cm². Acupuncture points along the LI meridian (LI-4, LI-10 and LI-11), stimulated together with TrPs found in the shoulder girdle complete the treatment.

## Medial epicondylitis (golfer's elbow)

Medial epicondylitis is another painful dysfunction syndrome associated with overloading and misuse of flexor muscles in the arm. The same treatment principles as for lateral epicondylitis are valid here, too. The insertion sites of flexor muscles on the medial epicondyle are the main treatment

**BOX 9.12.1**

Shoulder dislocation–fracture: a case report on a first-time traumatic anterior dislocation–fracture of the left shoulder joint

A 67-year-old male physician fell directly on his left shoulder during an ice hockey training session. An anterior dislocation of the glenohumeral joint was blocked by fragments of the three-piece fracture of the tuberculum and caput of the humerus (Fig. 9.12.1a), and it was not possible to relocate it immediately. Further attempts were unsuccessful, too. Local laser irradiation (780 nm, < 50 mW) directly to local tender sites and around the shoulder girdle (trapezius, supra-, infraspinati and deltoideus muscles, 4–8 J/point) was started immediately and repeated as needed to maintain muscle relaxation and pain control (Fig. 9.12.1c). Instead of surgery, offered by the orthopaedic surgeon as the only choice to restore a functioning arm, relocation was easily and successfully carried out 36 hours after the injury, under propofol anaesthesia. No analgesics were necessary, and local tender

sites and segmental TrPs were irradiated one to three times daily the first week, then daily or every other day, together with TENS on the contralateral arm.

Further rehabilitation, in addition to normal daily activities, consisted of LILT + exercise for the first 3 weeks, with the arm supported in a sling for partial rest; finger exercises (piano playing); subliminal electrical stimulation with garment (glove) electrodes (Micro-Z, Prizm Medical, Inc, Duluth, GA) and contralateral TENS (2 Hz burst, high intensity).

The patient was back on the ice hockey rink in 4 weeks, with normal function and muscle force in 5 weeks. Some allodynia was present for about a year, causing no pain problem and treated with very-low-intensity or subliminal TENS (Micro-Z), or both. No redislocation occurred in 4 years, despite normal activities (Fig. 9.12.1b).

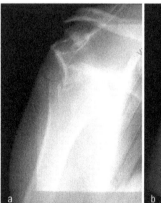 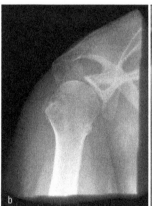 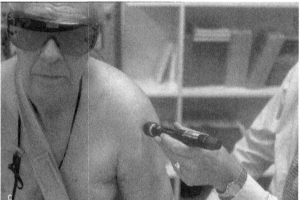

**Figure 9.12.1** Shoulder dislocation-fracture. (a) X-ray showing anterior dislocation of glenohumeral joint, with fracture of tuberculum and head of humerus. (b) X-ray after treatment, showing relocation of joint. (c) Treatment with LILT (note use of protective goggles). (Courtesy of Pekka J Pöntinen.)

areas for needles and LILT. Additional acupuncture points are to be located along the Lung meridian. In both lateral and medial epicondylitis the role of the cervical spine in therapy resistant cases should be considered.

### Dupuytren's contracture

Dupuytren's contracture, a typical connective tissue disorder, used to be a horseman's disease, but nowadays the majority of sufferers are women.

High-intensity, LF (2 Hz burst-type) TENS is an important adjunctive therapy to maintain adequate peripheral circulation. Static loading and poor microcirculation, as well as Raynaud symptoms, are underlying factors. Direct laser exposure is

indicated over the connective tissue hardening to reduce/eliminate inflammation and to induce pain relief.

## FIBROMYALGIA SYNDROME

The aetiology of fibromyalgia syndrome (FMS) is still unclear. The diagnostic criteria for FMS proposed by the American College of Rheumatology are a history of widespread pain for at least 3 months, and pain upon palpation of at least 11 of 18 designated 'tender points' over a minimum of three of the four body quadrants. Other typical symptoms include severe daytime fatigue, unrefreshed sleep, irritable bowel, chronic headache, morning stiffness, cognitive or memory

# CASE Study 9.12.1

## Electroacupuncture: an integrative clinical perspective II
**Steven K H Aung**

A 40-year-old man experienced a condition known as rotator cuff syndrome, or frozen shoulder. This painful, dysfunctional condition in his right shoulder was incurred playing golf. He was referred to me by his physician, since his prognosis with anti-inflammatory cortisone injections and physical therapy was not good.

In terms of traditional Chinese medicine, this patient was manifesting blockage of *qi* at the intermediate level along the Large Intestine, Small Intestine and *sanjiao* (Triple Burner) meridians on the right side of the body. A number of acupoints were indicated for treating this condition, including LI-4 (general pain control in the upper half of the body), LI-11 (anti-inflammatory), LI-15 (local pain control), SI-6 (soft tissue healing), SI-19 (neck and upper back pain), SJ-5 (arm and shoulder pain), SJ-14 (shoulder pain) and SJ-21 (neck and shoulder pain). Moreover, GB-34 (the Influential point of muscles/tendons, located on the Gall Bladder meridian) and BL-11 (the Influential point for bones/joints, located on the Bladder meridian) were prescribed.

The wires were connected and a pulse of low frequency (2 Hz) and intensity (continuous) was applied for 20 minutes. The wires were connected as follows along the right side of the body: LI-4 + LI-11, SI-6 + SI-19, SJ-5 + SJ-21 and LI-15 + SJ-14. GB-34 was connected to BL-11 bilaterally. After the first couple of treatments the patient reported improvement. Subsequent treatments over the course of several months returned the patient back to normal, and he was able to move his shoulder without pain or dysfunction.

impairment, reduced coordination and decreased physical endurance. FMS patients are hypersensitive to pain and their pain threshold is roughly one-half of the value for healthy pain-free controls. The autonomic nervous system is hyperactive in FMS, and many patients suffer from Raynaud's syndrome.

Although studies have consistently shown beneficial effects of acupuncture for fibromyalgia symptoms, the majority have been small, poorly controlled, non-randomised trials. Two excellently designed RCTs are the exception. In one, a 3-week RCT of electroacupuncture in 70 patients by Deluze and coworkers, EA at motor threshold level was given to 4–10 needles located at LI-4 (*hegu*), ST-36 (*zusanli*) and local tender TrPs in the active group. There were significant improvements in pain, sleep, global assessment scales and pain threshold in the real EA group. This study also revealed that strong stimulation may aggravate the symptoms. We have found that this occurs especially in sensitive patients and especially when local tender TrPs are repeatedly needled or given strong electrical stimulation.

Long-term follow-up is crucial, because FMS is a chronic illness and the analgesic effects of acupuncture may be transient, especially with brief treatment protocols. Maintenance therapy is of the utmost importance.

The use of pre-exercise high-intensity, LF or burst-type TENS, as well as low-intensity LED or laser treatment directed to trigger areas and muscles in spasm after exercise, may restore sleep and relieve muscle pain and aches. Gur et al have demonstrated the efficacy of GaAs laser therapy in the symptomatic treatment of FMS by improving the quality of life and decreasing pain more than placebo, either alone or in combination with low-dose amitriptyline.

According to Chinese medicine, rheumatoid arthritis and related diseases including FMS belong to the category of *bi* syndrome caused by a disturbance in the flow of energy (*qi*) and Blood. The factor causing pain can be Cold, in which case pain is relieved by heat. Typically FMS patients are sensitive to weather changes and especially to humidity and cold. Typical acupoints include Du-14 (*dazhui*) for the shoulder girdle, Du-4 (*mingmen*) for the pelvic girdle, LI-4 (*hegu*) and ST-36 (*zusanli*) as analgetic and immune-response-enhancing points, and the influential point for tendons and muscles, GB-34 (*yanglingquan*), as well as local tender *ashi* points and meridian points in areas of radiating pain.

## Recommendation

Although there is no consensus regarding optimal treatment for FMS, acupuncture (MA, EA, TENS, LILT) should be considered in conjunction with small doses of antidepressants, aerobic exercise and cognitive behavioral therapy. There are, however, no specific recommendations for the duration and frequency of treatment, or the degree of acupoint stimulation.

## RHEUMATOID ARTHRITIS

The analgesic and anti-inflammatory effects of acupuncture and LILT are ideal to complement conventional treatment of rheumatoid arthritis (RA). In particular, a number of experimental studies indicate that EA may affect pain and/or inflammation in animal models of RA. Clinically, pain relief and reduction of morning stiffness in interphalangeal (PIP) and metacarpophalangeal (MCP) joints were reported when laser irradiation was directed to the points over the joint space. Interestingly the corresponding joints in the other hand given placebo treatment reacted positively in the majority of cases. Heat sensation, erythema, swelling and tenderness were also significantly reduced with time in both hands.

Both HeNe and IR lasers have been effective for pain relief when applied to these small joints. However, improvements in morning stiffness and ROM have been reported only after IR laser application.

## Recommendation

Chronic pain and inflammation may turn RA patients hyperalgesic and very sensitive to needling. Therefore non-invasive methods, magnet therapy (MT) and LILT could be better choices for acute and maintenance therapy. Although small joints usually respond better to local therapy than large ones such as hips and knees, there is always a general whole body response to all peripheral stimulation modalities. Therefore it is advisable to start treating the neck and shoulder girdle first, to induce general pain reduction and muscle relaxation, often accompanied with better sleep. Analgetic points LI-4 and ST-36 should be combined with SJ-5 and Du-20. *Ashi* points combined with peripheral points on paired *yang* meridians (vertical axes) passing through the joint area form the basis of treatment for the larger joints.

## ANKYLOSING SPONDYLITIS

Only one small study was found in the literature, comparing EA with sham (superficial) acupuncture at true acupuncture points given once a week for 3 weeks, and then crossed over after a 3-week washout period. There was no difference in pain, stiffness improved in both groups, and a small improvement was seen in the neck ROM in the EA group.

Our clinical experience gained with MA, EA, TENS and LA over 30 years has shown very good response in stiffness and to some extent in pain reduction. The recommended treatment scheme is: LA paravertebrally at T1–T2, T12–L1, and L4–5 (2–4 J/point), additional points being LI-4, ST-36, LIV-3, and SI-3, BL-60 and GB-34 (MA or LA 0.5 J/point). Treatment is given one to two times a week for 3–8 weeks, then one to two times a month. Additional complementary home treatment with TENS at the same paraspinal sites is highly recommended.

## PSORIATIC ARTHRITIS

In principle, psoriatic arthritis responds like RA to acupuncture, with one exception. Psoriasis itself is a skin disease with joint involvement in some cases. New psoriatic skin eruptions may start from any skin lesion – so-called 'Koebner's phenomenon'. Therefore acupuncture needling may lead to a new itching eruption, which could be harmful, especially when located on the face, or on the earlobe after auriculotherapy. Non-invasive methods (TENS, LILT, MT) are to be recommended.

## GOUT

Gout is a form of monoarthritis caused by uric acid crystals and most often located in small joints, especially the first metatarsophalangeal joint. Inflammation, redness and extreme hyperalgesia are typical during the acute phase. LA applied locally to the affected joint is effective almost immediately, relieving pain and reducing swelling (2–4 J/joint space, *ashi* points, and additional points including LI-4, SJ-5, ST-36 and LI-V-3). MA and EA are also effective

## WHIPLASH INJURY

In typical whiplash injury, local tissue damage is often minimal and limited to the soft tissues. Neurological findings are inconsistent and not clearly limited to a specific segmental level. Infrared thermography (TG) is a useful method to verify the skin regions with abnormal microcirculation. The main injury site is often a 'hot spot', whereas temperature in the referral pain zone is lower than normal.

In acute cases it is possible to use acupuncture needling locally to *ashi* points, together with Du-20 (*baihui*), P-6 (*neiguan*) and LI-4. It is better to avoid strong stimulation and too many needles at the beginning. For LILT the pathological skin areas shown in TG reveal the proper irradiation sites (2–4 J/cm²). These skin temperature differences should be balanced in a few minutes after completed irradiation. If LILT is started during the first 2–4 days a permanent cure is possible.

Patients with chronic pain and autonomic symptoms after whiplash injury may display hyperalgesia and allodynia. They are also prone to exaggerated pain after any modality of sensory stimulation given locally or segmentally, even when there is no longer any apparent tissue damage. One choice is to try subliminal electrical stimulation with low-impedance, large-surface area garment electrodes (gloves, socks, etc.) to induce pain relief and improve microcirculation.

## CERVICOBRACHIALGIA

Local tender points (*ashi* points) and active muscle TrPs provide useful irradiation sites for effective LILT in cervicobrachialgias. Their exact location can be confirmed by pressure algometry or Omura's O-ring test. Tenderness is referred from deeper-sited injury, either in the muscles or at the nerve root level from a disc protrusion or spondylarthrosis, and so is reflected in decreased muscle force in the same segmental innervation zone. Using the O-ring test, we can use fingers to check relative changes in muscle force (Fig. 9.12.2). The first pair – index finger against thumb to form a closed ring – reflects changes above C5, the second pair – middle finger against thumb – reflecting those above C5–6, the third pair reflecting C6–7, and the fourth pair reflecting C7–8, all

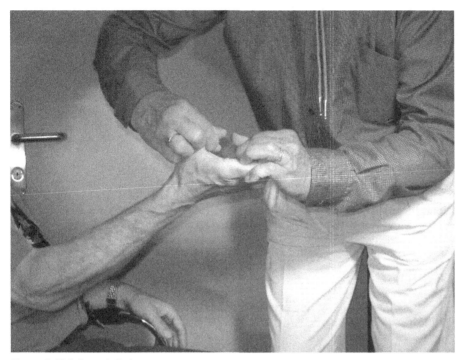

**Figure 9.12.2** Omura's O-ring test.

unilaterally reflecting changes only on the side of the tested hand. Normally there is a gradual decrease of muscle force towards the little finger.

In acute cases LILT at 4–6 J (760–830 nm) locally should relieve pain and muscle tension in 15–20 minutes (Fig. 9.12.3). If there is no improvement in finger force and only partial relief of symptoms, further diagnostic procedures are indicated and often surgical intervention is necessary. Subacute and chronic cases need a combination of local LILT and regional/segmental TrP and meridian acupuncture treatment, two to three in the first week and once weekly thereafter as necessary.

**Figure 9.12.3** Paraspinal LILT in cervicobrachialgia.

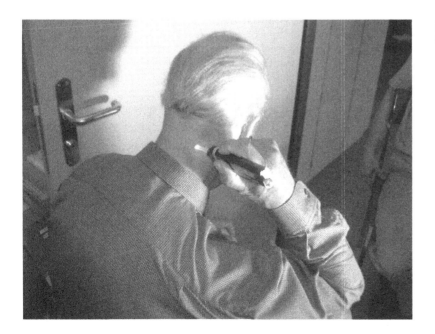

# LOW BACK PAIN AND SCIATICA

Lower-back pain (LBP) and sciatica are signs and symptoms of many different musculoskeletal disorders such as prolapsed intervertebral disc, spondylarthrosis, ankylosing spondylarthritis, various neurological disorders, lumbosacral insufficiency, simple lumbago, muscle spasms and trigger activation with referred pain due to weak postural muscles or ergonomically bad working positions, or both. Commonly used opioids and NSAIDs are of limited long-term benefit and often produce adverse effects.

An Italian double-blind RCT compared the efficacy of superficial and deep insertion of acupuncture needles in the treatment of patients with chronic lumbar myofascial pain for more than 3 months. Patients had at least one active TrP at the lumbar muscular level, and normal neurological findings. In both groups Du-6 and *shiqizhuixia* (M-BW-25) were needled as well as GB-34, BL-40 and BL-62 bilaterally, in eight sessions over 6 weeks. At 3 months, deep stimulation had a better analgesic effect than that of superficial stimulation. In a Chinese study on sciatica comparing needling (0.5–1 *cun*) to deep needling (2–3 *cun*) at GB-30 (*huantiao*), no difference was found between the groups, however.

Ghoname et al compared the effectiveness of percutaneous electrical nerve stimulation (PENS) with transcutaneous electrical nerve stimulation (TENS) and flexion–extension exercise therapies in patients with long-term LBP secondary to degenerative disc disease. Four therapeutic modalities (sham-PENS, PENS, TENS and exercise therapies) were each administered for a period of 30 minutes three times a week for 3 weeks. Results demonstrated that PENS, a variant of EA, was significantly more effective than the other therapies in decreasing pain score after each treatment. The average daily oral intake of non-opioid analgesics decreased significantly with PENS compared with other treatment modalities.

In their meta-analysis of RCT on acupuncture for back pain, Ernst and White concluded that acupuncture was shown to be superior to various control interventions, although there was insufficient evidence to state whether it is superior to placebo.

There are very few controlled studies on LILT in LBP. Soriano and Rios have analysed the efficacy of gallium arsenide (GaAs) laser therapy on chronic LBP patients in a prospective, double-blind RCT with a 6-month follow-up. They concluded that irradiation with GaAs laser relieves chronic LBP in a significant proportion of older patients without causing any adverse side-effects. In our experience, local irradiation at the nerve root level of the affected segment is often effective in acute cases, particularly if response is rapid to a first treatment.

MA may induce complete pain relief, even in cases with a total disc prolapse, but for only a few hours. During this pain-free period a thorough neurological examination is possible and reliable. In some chronic cases with a long history of unsuccessful conventional therapies, the anti-inflammatory and regenerative properties of LILT may lead to the restoration of normal neuromuscular function, as shown by Abe. A 40-year-old woman with a 2-year history of LBP radiating to the left hip and leg, diagnosed as being due to a ruptured disc between the fifth lumbar and first sacral vertebrae, was treated with a gallium aluminium arsenide (GaAlAs) diode laser in outpatient therapy. After 7 months, her condition had dramatically improved, as confirmed by MRI scans, which showed clearly the normal condition of the previously herniated L5/S1 disc.

Chronic pain associated with lower-back disorders may also have its origin in piriformis muscle spasm and trigger activity in other pelvic floor muscles. Khoe already demonstrated positive results with ultrasound acupuncture in the 1970s. He used rectal stimulation (1 W for 60 seconds), then around the greater trochanter and at LIV-12 and BL-27–BL-29 (1 W, 60 seconds/point), with needles at *huatuojiaji* L5 (EA 2 Hz, 15–20 min, maximum tolerable), combined with relevant ear and hand points.

## Recommendations

A combination of local/segmental tender points and areas with peripheral TrPs in the pain referral zone, and acupuncture points along the *yang* meridians (mainly Bladder and Gall Bladder) traversing the pain area can form the basis for a successful treatment. Special techniques such as Kinoshita's paraneural acupuncture or Gunn's intramuscular stimulation (IMS) may be indicated in some very resistant, chronic LBP cases.

The intensity of peripheral stimulation should be adjusted to avoid side-effects from overstimulation, such as a pain reaction, which may last several days or even for over a week, not uncommonly after a first session of EA.

The optimal frequency of needling sessions (MA) is about two to three times a week, and when using EA or PENS one to two sessions a week. TENS has no local long-term effect and for optimal pain relief and vasodilatory response it should be applied daily.

## STRESS FRACTURES

A sudden change or increase of activity may lead to a stress fracture, which is commonly seen in the foot and lower leg. The first symptoms are local pain and swelling, and sometimes bruising in the foot, marking inflammation (periostitis). First aid is normally ice packs, anti-inflammatory drugs and rest.

Local LILT (4–8 J to the fracture line) twice a week can relieve inflammation and pain as well as shorten recovery time. It is important to continue active muscle exercises and passive muscle care (electrical stimulation) during the first 3–4 weeks before a gradual increase of normal activities. Daily non-segmental, high-intensity, LF (burst-type) TENS is recommended, especially for FMS and Raynaud patients, to improve peripheral microcirculation and to hasten the healing process.

## Recommendations

### METATARSAL AND TIBIAL STRESS FRACTURES:
Local LILT (two to three per week) and non-segmental TENS (2 Hz burst, high-intensity) treatments are given daily or every other day. With no bed rest, lightened exercises, less walking, the patient should be back to normal in 3–4 weeks.

### VERTEBRAL FRACTURES:
Local LILT or TENS are given as above, for up to 3–4 months.

## ANKLE SPRAIN

Electrical probe stimulation (pTENS) has been shown to shorten rehabilitation time when added to standard physical therapy in the treatment of second-degree ankle inversion sprain, with more rapid recovery of ROM for plantar flexion–dorsiflexion, and inversion–eversion.

Kumar et al compared LILT and conventional physiotherapy for the treatment of acute inversion injuries of the ankle. The LILT group, treated every other day for 1 week with 830 nm, < 60 mW GaAlAs laser, showed more rapid resolution of symptoms and an earlier return to full weight bearing than the physiotherapy group. However, in a double-blind, placebo-controlled RCT ($N$ = 217) there was no statistically significant difference on primary outcome between placebo, high-dose (5 J/cm$^2$) LILT at skin level or low-dose (0.5 J/cm$^2$) LILT (GaAs 904 nm, 25 W) after 12 sessions in 4 weeks (only one local point was irradiated).

In acute inversion injuries LILT (IR, 780 or 830 nm) applied to the injury site (4–8 J/point) daily or every other day for the first week and twice weekly thereafter as needed, combined with application to TrPs in the calf muscles, can markedly shorten recovery time.

## PLANTAR FASCIITIS

Plantar fasciitis is a painful inflammation of the fascia between the heel and metatarsal heads. The most common causes include wearing high heels, gaining weight and an increase in running exercises.

Vrchota et al compared EA with sham acupuncture and conventional sports medicine therapy. All groups were instructed to do regular lower-leg stretching exercises, and had their sports shoes assessed and changed as necessary. All groups improved over the study period, but at the end of treatment and at follow-up the EA group experienced a

significantly greater decrease in subjective pain than the sports medicine group.

LILT given to the insertion sites of the plantar fascia at the calcaneus and at the metatarsals is an effective method to relieve pain and inflammation. In particular, it is effective in our experience for patients who have failed to respond to steroid injections and NSAIDs orally. It is important to check for TrPs in calf muscles and at the sides of the Achilles tendon, too.

## SHIN SPLINTS

Shin splints and compartment syndrome are related overuse disorders, either preceding a stress fracture or the sequelae of one that already exists. They are commonly seen in athletes. Pain, impaired circulation in tightly packed muscle compartments and an inflammatory reaction of the periosteum form the symptom triad.

The earlier that treatment is initiated, the better the response. Evidence gained from one acupuncture trial suggests that 100% pain relief is possible within 4 weeks when the following acupoints are needled: LIV-2, SP-5, SP-9 and KI-1. Our experience in sports medicine, particularly in those in their late sixties and early seventies, clearly supports this view. Needling LIV-3 (*taichong*), ST-36 (*zusanli*), ST-32 (femur *futu*), BL-60 (*kunlun*) and Du-20 (*baihui*) combined with some tender muscle triggers in the gastrocnemius and tibialis anterior muscles effectively restored normal ROM and muscle coordination, and relieved tension and spasms in the fatigued muscles after hectic ice hockey games. Athletes may be more receptive to TENS and LA than to needling.

## MUSCLE INJURIES

Muscle contusions and strains are common sports injuries. Normal first aid involves ice packs, rest and local LILT to relieve pain and to avoid an inflammatory reaction to muscle fibre tears. It is better to use non-invasive local therapy and apply needles to segmental and meridian points. Common analgesia points like LI-4 (*hegu*) and ST-36 (*zusanli*) may markedly elevate pain threshold and reduce inflammatory reaction at the injury site.

In a comparative RCT on old gastrocnemius muscle injuries EA (G6805, amplitude to tolerance) applied to LI-4 bilaterally for 30 minutes and combined with a Chinese herbal bath was more effective than the herbal bath alone after three series of 10 daily treatments. In another controlled trial, Yang favourably compared EA (15 min to tolerance) and moxa cones on main points (LIV-11, SP-9, Ren-2 and *ashi* point) every other day for 10 days with conventional care in a control group. Auxiliary points were BL-32, BL-36, GB-31 and LIV-10. The therapeutic effect was obviously better in the treatment group.

# SUMMARY

Some key points from this chapter are:

- Acupuncture can not only relieve pain, but also enhance circulation and tissue repair
- Recent studies have shown both EA and TENS to be effective in the treatment of osteoarthritis of the knee
- Acupuncture treatment of hip pain from OA has not been tested frequently in RCTs, and authors of one study suggest that treatment, where successful, owes more to local needling than general TCM principles
- Authors of a study of the treatment of frozen shoulder suggest that treatment of the 'freezing' rather than 'frozen' shoulder is more likely to be effective
- Two recent well-designed RCTs suggest that EA can be extremely effective in the treatment of fibromyalgia

- However, gentle methods are preferred to avoid aggravation of symptoms in this difficult condition
- Similarly, patients with rheumatoid arthritis can become hypersensitive, and non-invasive methods of treatment such as MT and LILT may be the best long-term maintenance options.

## Additional material in the CD-ROM resource

In the CD-ROM resource, in addition to further information on many of the topics presented here, LILT is introduced in more detail for those who are unfamiliar with it:

- Indications for LILT in traumatology
- Recommendations for effective treatment
- Contraindications and precautions.

**9.12** Summary of relevant studies in the electronic clinical studies database (number of studies)

| Condition | EA | Other | Condition | EA | Other |
|---|---|---|---|---|---|
| **Cervical** | | | **Lower limb** | | |
| Cervical spine disorders | 58 | 59 | Sciatica | 42 | 38 |
| *Cervical spine disorders with nerve compression* | 47 | 33 | Hip | 5 | 21 |
| | | | Knee | 37 | 62 |
| *Cervical spine disorders with a predominant vascular component* | 17 | 11 | Calf | 0 | 4 |
| | | | Foot | 11 | 14 |
| Soft tissue conditions and whiplash injury | 12 | 33 | Other lower limb pain | 5 | 3 |
| Mixed or nonspecific neck conditions | 4 | 4 | **Arthritis – ankylosing spondylosis – gout (*bi zheng*)** | | |
| **Shoulder and upper limb** | | | Arthritis (general) | 11 | 40 |
| Shoulder girdle | 53 | 80 | Osteoarthritis | 33 | 55 |
| Elbow and forearm | 16 | 48 | Osteochondrosis | 3 | 13 |
| Wrist and hand | 5 | 22 | Rheumatoid arthritis | 13 | 39 |
| Upper limb (general and mixed studies) | 2 | 6 | Ankylosing spondylitis | 2 | 4 |
| **Thoracic and low back** | | | Gout | 1 | 2 |
| Low back pain (general) | 37 | 66 | Other bone or joint conditions | 1 | 10 |
| *Low back pain with nerve entrapment* | 47 | 39 | Fibromyalgia and myofascial pain | 14 | 35 |
| Chronic back pain | 29 | 99 | Other conditions resembling fibromyalgia | 1 | 2 |
| *Chronic back pain with nerve entrapment* | 30 | 24 | Other conditions of tendon and muscle | 2 | 4 |
| Acute back pain | 9 | 22 | **Trauma management / soft tissue injury** | 10 | 44 |
| *Acute back pain with nerve entrapment* | 0 | 3 | **Fracture and bone repair** | 5 | 13 |
| Other thoracic pain | 3 | 13 | **Physical performance** | 1 | 6 |
| Coccygodynia and perineal pain | 0 | 2 | | | |

## RECOMMENDED READING

*Some articles by the author:*

Pöntinen PJ Acupuncture hyperstimulation syndrome. American Journal of Acupuncture 1979 April–June; 7(2): 161–5

Pöntinen PJ Omura's "Bi-Digital O-Ring test" as a guide to acupuncture treatment. Acupuncture and Electro-therapeutics Research. 1986; 11(3–4): 217–18

Pöntinen PJ, Airaksinen O Evaluation of myofascial pain and dysfunction syndromes and their response to low level laser therapy. Journal of Musculoskeletal Pain. 1995; 3(2): 149–54

*Two useful textbooks, on LILT and EA, respectively:*

Pöntinen PJ 2003 (ed) Laserfibel. Handbuch für Lasertherapie. Laser Therapy Institute, Baar, Switzerland

Yelizarov N 2003 Treatment for Muscle Strain Injuries (MSI), Repetitive Strain Injuries (RSI) and Other Related Health Conditions. Llumina Press, Coral Springs, FL

# 9.13 ACUPUNCTURE ANAESTHESIA

*Mark Bovey, with a contribution by Lynnae Schwartz*

Topics covered in this subchapter include the use of acupuncture anaesthesia (AA) for different operations, combining acupuncture with drug anaesthesia, the effectiveness of AA, how it works and how it may be improved, its advantages and disadvantages.

Complete anaesthesia comprises amnesia, unconsciousness, analgesia and total muscle relaxation. Strictly speaking, acupuncture provides little muscle relaxation, and certainly does not impair memory or consciousness. It should, therefore, be called acupuncture analgesia.

In this chapter acupuncture anaesthesia will be used as a blanket term to denote any type of acupuncture, laser, TENS or associated electrotherapeutic intervention to assist surgery. EAA refers to electroacupuncture analgesia.

## ACUPUNCTURE ANAESTHESIA IN CHINA AND THE WEST

AA first appeared in China in 1958, initially to relieve postoperative pain and later for providing analgesia during the operation itself. Its use peaked at over 5% of all operations in the late 1970s, although subsequently it has become restricted largely to head and neck, neurological and cardiothoracic sites, and mostly for selected patients rather than routine use. By the 1990s AA continued in only a few TCM hospitals in China, and the standard approach now combines (largely) EAA with adjuvant medications – 'acupuncture balanced/assisted/combined anaesthesia'.

## USE OF ACUPUNCTURE ANAESTHESIA FOR DIFFERENT OPERATIONS

AA works better near the midline and above the diaphragm. The most effective operative sites have been the brain and cranium, dental, neck and chest, with internal fixation of fractures and superficial operations in general.

### CRANIOCEREBRAL

Craniocerebral operations by AA were performed on more than 10 600 patients in China between 1965 and 1982. The majority were via the anterior fossa, where the most successful results have been obtained. Surgery in the posterior fossa is viewed as somewhat less successful, and parietal and occipital areas the least successful of all. Operations have included craniotomies for tumours of various kinds, arterial anastomoses, nerve root amputations, abscesses and lesions.

### OPHTHALMIC

Wang Benxian has recorded impressive numbers and success rates, especially for glaucoma operations. Other applications have included cataract, retinal damage and strabismus.

### DENTAL

Most dental surgery requires relatively little anaesthesia and is of short duration and predictable course – all aspects that favour AA. Thousands of tooth extractions have been reported from China and Japan, with cautions only if teeth are impacted or the area is acutely inflamed. AA has also been used in a wide variety of other dental operations, including fillings and periodontal and restorative work.

### OTHER FACIAL

AA has been used for sinus operations, various ear, nose and throat procedures, trigeminal neuralgia, cleft palate and other plastic surgery.

### NECK AND THROAT

Thyroid operations for cysts, tumours and hyperthyroidism continue to be one of the few routine areas for AA. Other popular operations have been laryngectomy and larynx reconstruction, tonsillectomy and cervical vertebrae surgery. Most of these are again short, superficial procedures.

### THORACIC, CARDIAC AND PULMONARY

AA for cardiac surgery in China has declined to more of a specialist service for patients at particular risk from conventional anaesthetics, although there are recent Chinese studies on EAA for open heart surgery. Lung resections are also regarded as suitable for AA, but its use has similarly declined.

### ABDOMINAL

The most reported operations have been gastrectomy, appendectomy, hysterectomy, Caesarian section, tubal ligation and hernia repair. Reported rates of success are comparable to AA use elsewhere, but there are particular problems with insufficient muscle relaxation and vasovagal reactions to visceral traction. However, when used as an adjuvant to drugs, EAA has consistently reduced the amount of medication required across a range of upper – and lower-abdominal operations.

### ORTHOPAEDIC

The limbs are thought to be the least-suited sites for AA. Adequate analgesia has been reported for orthopaedic surgery, limb amputation and replantation, muscle reconstruction and broken bones, but the most convincing accounts are for the use of electrostimulation in brachial or sciatic nerve plexus blocks for hand or foot surgery.

### OTHER

AA has also been used for skin surgery, operations for burns, varicose veins and wound drainage.

# COMBINED ACUPUNCTURE AND DRUG ANAESTHESIA

Since AA can be insufficient and variable, combined anaesthesia is nearly always better than AA alone, except perhaps in shorter and more superficial operations. Initially in China very little medication was used, often just a premed. Doses were kept to a minimum, nowhere near large enough to induce anaesthesia on their own. Subsequently more complex regimens were developed using opiate agonists, neuroleptic dopamine blockers and serotonin (5HT) releasers.

For major surgery, combination AA may incorporate a premed, induction anaesthesia, maintenance anaesthesia, a local anaesthetic at the incision, and a muscle relaxant. In the West the emphasis has been on AA being the adjuvant, used to reduce the requirements for anaesthetic drugs.

Although some anaesthetic medications reduce the effectiveness of AA experimentally, results in practice do not always follow expectations, and there may even be a synergistic action between them.

Case study 9.13.1. details the use of EAA in a paediatric patient.

# EFFECTIVENESS OF ACUPUNCTURE ANAESTHESIA

From 22 studies published in China in the late 1970s and early 1980s, the mean number of cases was 2250, the success rate averaged 95% and the superior rate 82%. In the majority

---

# CASE Study 9.13.1

### Electrical stimulation of acupuncture points and meridians in paediatric patients II
**Lynnae Schwartz**

A 10-year-old girl with neurofibromatosis type I was scheduled for 'awake' craniotomy resection of an enlarging, infiltrating left parietal astrocytoma, previously found to be inoperable under general anaesthesia because of significant risk of permanent aphasia. Preoperative preparation included left temporal craniotomy under general endotracheal anaesthesia for placement of a subdural grid for speech mapping, child life services daily for 5 days prior to the definitive surgery, careful teaching and assessment by the pediatric anaesthesia service. Pulses and appearance were consistent with sufficient *qi* for therapeutic manipulation with acupuncture.

Management was as follows:

- Monitored anaesthesia care with intravenous sedation and analgesia titrated to surgical stimulation and patient response.
- Local anesthetic infiltration of scalp prior to incision and wound closure.
- Continuous patient support and guidance by the child life specialist who remained at the patient's side throughout the entire procedure.
- 0.16 × 15 mm needle in *yintang*, retained 45 minutes as arterial, venous and urinary catheters were placed.
- 30 gauge 2.5 cm (1″) stainless steel needles placed with strong technique to obtain *qi* at LIV-3 (*taichong*), ST-43 (*xiangu*) bilaterally, GB-41 (*zulinqi*)

right foot only. An ITO-F3 acupuncture unit (see Fig. 9.3.1 on page 118), with lead wires to all foot needles, provided continuous stimulation with progressive increases in intensity as suggested by patient responses to direct questioning and surgical stimulation. Needles with electrical stimulation were retained 4.25 hours.

The patient remained fully cooperative, communicative and calm throughout the entire 5.5 hour procedure. She had no evidence of adverse neurological or neuropsychiatric effect in the immediate postoperative period, or upon sequential long-term follow-up.

### Discussion

1. Electroacupuncture augmentation of intravenous analgesia and sedation, along with local anaesthesia to the surgical field was successful in this case, illustrating the importance of preoperative patient selection, child life support, and prior responses to stressful diagnostic and surgical procedures when contemplating this modality.

2. Ample time was available prior to surgical care for the patient to be assessed, taught and brought to the point where she could accept guidance and coaching, especially from child life staff in the operating room.

3. Although English language full text material describing acupuncture anaesthesia for craniotomy exists, detailed descriptions of individual cases are not readily found. It is therefore not known whether our experience is consistent with that of others caring for children under these circumstances.

(Another case history by Lynnae Schwartz was presented in Subchapter 9.3, together with a general discussion on the issues involved.)

of studies patients routinely received small amounts of adjuvant medication, but where AA has definitely been the sole anaesthetic reported rates of success have been considerably lower (60–80%).

One difficulty with interpreting these results, however, is the lack of definition of outcomes. When outcomes were recalculated in Western terms, where patients expect no pain at all, the figures reduced from 80%+ down to around 30%, or even as low as 10%. Recent reviews in both East and West agree that AA alone usually provides insufficient analgesia for surgery, although it may still give significant postoperative pain relief.

There is overwhelming evidence that, combined with an appropriate type and dosage of medication, AA can augment the anaesthetic effect, leading to a reduced requirement for both intra- and postoperative drugs. This can have substantial benefits for patients' health, such as the avoidance of serious complications, faster recovery and less immunosuppression. Perhaps the most interesting comparative studies are of the type AA + drug X versus drug Y + drug X, where AA replaces one component of a standard multidrug anaesthetic approach. Drug X has often been the premedication, with AA being compared with the main anaesthetic drug, but many different combinations have appeared, and AA has usually been found to be as effective as drug Y.

## EFFECTS ON CARDIOPULMONARY AND OTHER VITAL FUNCTIONS

Most studies have observed a stabilisation of blood pressure and heart rate during EAA operations. Other possible benefits are less fluctuation in heart rhythm and various haemodynamic parameters, as well as no or reduced suppression of breathing or coughing. It has also been noted that EAA reduces the adverse effects of surgery and medication on gastrointestinal function.

### Muscle relaxation and visceral pain

It is generally agreed that AA does not, by itself, induce sufficient muscle relaxation or control of visceral pain. Hence there are problems with abdominal operations, especially those involving visceral traction, which often sets off nausea and other vasovagal reactions. Even when AA is combined with some premedication, additional sedation will be required if there is traction sensation.

### Stress and the immune system

AA has been found to inhibit increased sympathetic nervous system activity and overproduction of adrenal hormones, thus modifying the biochemical changes induced by surgical stress. However, in most trials comparing AA alone with drug regimens there have been no significant differences in respect of stress effects, and the antistress effects of AA revert to normal as fast as with drug anaesthesia, leading to the same stress hormone profiles postoperatively. Numerous authors, however, have attested to an improved immune status with lasting postoperative benefits following AA.

## HOW DOES ACUPUNCTURE ANAESTHESIA WORK?

### Brain activity

Several controlled trials have indicated that EAA produces EEG patterns at mostly awake/subvigilant/tired-but-alert frequencies (primarily $\alpha$ waves), whereas medically anaesthetised patients are deeply sedated ($\beta$, $\theta$, and $\delta$ waves, depending on the drugs used). Likewise EAA maintains a more aerobic pattern of brain tissue metabolism when compared with neuroleptic anaesthesia and leads to faster recovery of the preoperative state.

### Endorphins

Acupuncture analgesia has been demonstrated in unconscious (superficially anaesthetised) patients – measured as a decrease in the need for extra analgesic medication. However, the effects are apparently much smaller than when conscious, and are antagonised by naloxone. Other studies have found that the analgesia from EA or TENS in conscious patients is not significantly modified by opiate antagonists. This would suggest a small endorphin-mediated effect of acupuncture, present whether the patient is conscious or not, and a much greater effect, present only when conscious and largely not reliant on endorphin pathways.

### Other neurotransmitters

Other neurotransmitters have been implicated in the action of AA, including enkephalins, dynorphin, dopamine and acetylcholine. Successful EAA produces EEG changes similar to those from exogenous 5HT.

## IMPROVING THE EFFECTIVENESS OF ACUPUNCTURE ANAESTHESIA

### Patient selection

PREDICTING THE 'GOOD' REACTORS
Only a minority of patients obtain sufficient analgesia from AA alone (the 'strong reactors'). The Chinese have put considerable effort into developing predictive procedures, but the combination of sufficient accuracy and ease of use has proved elusive.

Stability of vital processes/autonomic nervous system
Indices with different combinations of parameters, anything from 2 to 20 in number, have commonly included pulse rate

and volume, tactile threshold, skin resistance and temperature and respiration rate. Most have proved too time consuming for routine use.

Yin and yang   *Yin* and *yang* deficiency patterns apparently respond differently to pain and to AA, with the latter showing decreased reflexes, respiration rate, skin resistance and blood flow, and the former the opposite. Analysis of the effectiveness of AA in thyroid operations was found to be 93% for *yang* deficiency patients but only 65% for *yin*. Similar correspondences with some other TCM diagnostic patterns have been reported, but even simple predictive models using y*in*/*yang* deficiency have been found impractical.

Deqi and pain tolerance   It is generally agreed that the best and most practical predictive approach comes from the existence, strength and direction of *deqi* sensations, possibly together with pain tolerance measurement.

Mental state   AA is more successful in patients who are not overly nervous or agitated.

Biochemical   A prediction equation derived from the radioimmunoassay of serum gastrin, endorphins, oestradiol and progesterone proved to be 80% correct – but this could hardly be used as a routine preoperative procedure.

## PATIENTS WHO ARE SUITED TO AA BECAUSE CONTRAINDICATED FOR DRUG ANAESTHESIA

These include:

- Those with severe heart or lung conditions.
- Those with debilitated states of other organs such as the liver or kidneys.
- Those in a generally poor condition, weak, or elderly.
- Those allergic/intolerant to anaesthetic medications.
- Those who refuse or resist drugs for whatever reason.
- Those who are afraid of needles in dental work.

## PATIENTS WHO MAY BE UNSUITED TO AA

These include:

- Children under 14 – because they may not be cooperative enough.
- Patients who are uncooperative, nervous, apprehensive, squeamish, sceptical, emotionally unstable or with psychological problems.
- Those due for long operations or complex cases with an uncertain course.
- Those with epilepsy, large meningiomas or aneurysms, coma or severe shock, severe blood loss or cardiac lesions.
- Those with pacemakers, heart arrhythmia, cerebral ictus or transient ischaemic arrest.

# Other procedures

## INFORMATION

Many studies of hospital patients in general and AA patients in particular have shown that they experience less pain and leave hospital sooner if given reasonable prior explanation, expectations and reassurance.

## COOPERATION

This may be strongly influenced by information provision, but also the rapport developed with the medical team.

## RELAXATION

For conscious patients with incomplete muscle relaxation, or with no premed sedative, it can be vital to coach them in relaxation techniques – verbally, by hypnosis or through breathing exercises.

## SURGICAL TEAM

The unit should maintain a stable and experienced team and use the best operating techniques.

## HERBS, MINERALS AND OTHER SUBSTANCES

The effect may be enhanced by use of the herb *Corydalis*, oestradiol and the amino acid D-phenylalanine, as well as by increased magnesium levels

# The intervention

## INSTRUMENTS

Although MA has been observed to work as well as EA, most clinicians have favoured the latter, as it requires less effort, can be adjusted more easily and produces stronger stimulation and more effective analgesia. MA may be useful in long operations to avoid tolerance developing, but equally there are alternative strategies for using EA.

A variety of other methods have been used either as adjuvants – including hot wax, electric massage, electric sound waves, musical EA and vibration – or as alternative point stimulants – including magnetic beads, intradermal needles and saline injection.

## TIMING OF THE INTERVENTION

Length of the induction period   AA does not deliver immediate analgesia; an induction period is required to develop its full effect. Twenty to thirty minutes is the most frequently used time period for a wide variety of operations, although less than 20 minutes has been advocated, mostly for more superficial procedures such as tonsillectomy or tooth extraction. Several of these studies use strong stimulation at Ren-24 and Du-26. The shortest reported times have been 1–5 minutes for endoscopy. By contrast, 40 minutes' induction has been recorded for hysterectomy and 60 minutes for a biceps reconstruction.

Continuing stimulation through the operation   For shorter operations, stimulation should be given continuously throughout the operation; interruptions of more than a few minutes may diminish the analgesic effect. In longer operations, this must be balanced against the tolerance that may arise, for which intermittent stimulation is recommended.

AA for postoperative analgesia   If AA is used entirely for its postoperative effects it nevertheless seems to be most efficacious when administered preoperatively. Even AA delivered after the induction of anaesthesia may not be helpful. This parallels Dundee's findings on use of the point P-6 for the relief of postoperative nausea.

## ELECTRICAL PARAMETERS

Frequency – general principles   Use a low frequency – i.e. 1.5–6 Hz – on peripheral/distal points, and a high frequency on local points: for example, 10 Hz – hernia, 40–80 Hz – thyroid, 100 Hz – cervical discectomy, appendectomy, hysterectomy and 1000 Hz – tonsillectomy.

Start at LF, then build up. The target end-point may be a particular HF range, for example 20–40 Hz, 200–500 Hz, or even 6 kHz (!), or an individual patient threshold (or both) – anything from slight muscle tremor to maximum tolerance or tears/salivation. Kitai pointed out that starting too strongly may aggravate the pain, and suggested the same frequency as the pulse rate, around 1.5 Hz.

Use lower frequencies for children (e.g. 10–15 Hz) than for adults (e.g. 15–20 Hz).

Change the frequency to avoid habituation.

Box 9.13.1 gives examples of different frequencies appropriate for different operations.

Voltage/intensity   As with frequency, voltage has usually been set low at the start and then increased until some kind of tolerance threshold is reached; again, this may mean a comfortable sensation, a heavy, distending one, or something distinctly unpleasant. Maximum voltages of 90 V and 120 V have been reported.

---

**BOX 9.13.1**

**Examples of different frequencies used in different operations**

**Low: 2–8 Hz**

Brain, posterior cranial fossa, anterior cranium, incision for cranial tumour, dental extraction, endoscopy, laparotomy (and various others).

**Medium: 10–30 Hz**

Biceps reconstruction, various abdominal, dental.

**High: 40+ Hz**

Dental, frontal glioma, thyroid with atrial fibrillation (3–5 kHz auricular!), various.

**Variable – wide range**

5–100 Hz – larynx
2.5–20 Hz distal plus 1000 Hz local – tonsillectomy
27–4000 Hz (local) – thyroid
2–100 Hz – cervical discectomy

---

Current   Reported values for currents used in AA break down into two main groups: one at < 1–3 mA and one at 8–12 mA, although Wang suggested the split was 0.4–0.8 mA versus 2.5–3.5 mA and was a matter of preference amongst workers.

Waveform   Some have employed a continuous wave and some a biphasic one, or non-charge-balanced stimulus with polarity reversed every 10 minutes, which may help to avoid adaptation as well as tissue damage.

# Points

## TYPE OF POINT: LOCAL, DISTAL OR AURICULAR

Auricular points have frequently been used or recommended for AA, often without body points. Although most formulae have included proximal and distal points, face and nose microsystems have also been used, as well as ear points. For cranial and facial operations, auricular points may be treated as local.

## TRADITIONAL CHINESE MEDICINE VERSUS NEUROLOGICAL MODELS FOR POINT SELECTION

Although point selection in China in the heyday of AA was determined by clinical experience, operative area and TCM principles, some groups found AA to be most effective in the same and the neighbouring dermatomes. Hence the standard Chinese approach became a combination of TCM, neurology and empirical knowledge. In the West there has been more emphasis on neurology, but still largely within the context of classical acupuncture points. BL-32, for example, which is commonly used in gynaecological operations, is related segmentally to the uterus.

## SPECIFICITY OF POINTS

The analgesic effects of acupuncture may depend largely on physiological reactions not specific to the particular points chosen, and it has been suggested that non-specific sites could provoke generalised anaesthesia. However, Chinese trials have demonstrated differences in success rates between alternative points selected for EAA. This sort of finding prompted the Chinese to develop standard formulae appropriate to specific operative sites.

## IPSILATERAL, CONTRALATERAL OR BILATERAL APPLICATION

If points are chosen on the basis of a common innervation with the operative site, the ipsilateral treatment should produce the major effect – a result demonstrated in comparisons of ipsi- and bilateral auricular points. If the operation crosses the midline, however, bilateral points are chosen, although contralateral procedures have also been used successfully.

## NUMBER OF POINTS

Most formulae involve three or four points (plus or minus the paraincisional sites) but anything from one to 12 or more has been recorded.

## SPECIFIC POINTS WITH GENERAL USE ACROSS DIFFERENT OPERATIONS/SITES

The late eminent Japanese researcher Takeshige Chifuyu expressed the extreme view that only three effective points exist for surgical AA: LI-4, ST-36 and SJ-18. The first two of these are far and away the most frequently employed across a whole range of types of operations, but SJ-18 has hardly been cited at all in the literature. Similarly, Jayasuriya declared LI-4, ST-43 and ST-44 to be most effective, although ST-43 is otherwise anonymous in the literature and ST-44 largely restricted to dental/upper jaw work.

LI-4 and ST-36 may act better together than separately, and ST-36 is often also paired with SP-6, especially for abdominal operations. Cao Xiadong declared LI-4 to be the most effective *yang* meridian point and SP-4 for *yin* meridians (for manual AA). Of the auricular points, *shenmen* is usually chosen and, according to Bensoussan, it and Lung are best for chest and abdominal surgery. The Adrenal ear point may increase blood pressure and thus guard against the danger of operative hypotension.

Box 9.13.2 lists the points used in different areas.

# ADVANTAGES AND DISADVANTAGES OF AA

## Advantages

### INTRAOPERATIVE

- By avoiding or reducing general or epidural anaesthesia, the chances of serious complications or death are greatly reduced. Acupuncture itself is very safe and minimises physiological interference.
- AA can stabilise vital processes such as heart rate, blood pressure and respiration. It also tends to reduce the stress response to surgery.
- AA may reduce blood loss.
- AA avoids or reduces operational damage to nerves, particularly on the head and neck, the recurrent laryngeal nerve being most frequently cited. In addition, a conscious patient may be helpful in other respects, such as with breathing exercises for cardiopulmonary operations.
- Under conditions where there are few trained anaesthetists, AA can be considered an easy and low-cost option.
- Despite their wakefulness, patients are calm.
- There are many examples of specific advantages for particular operations, such as stabilising intracranial pressure in cranial work, or reducing fluid accumulation in lung operations.

### POSTOPERATIVE

These include:
- Reduced pain, analgesic medication and adverse events.
- More stable cardiopulmonary functions.
- Less immune suppression, reduced infection and faster wound healing.
- Less likelihood of intestinal adhesions.

---

> **BOX 9.13.2**
> **Points used in different areas**
>
> On the CD-ROM ⊙ are lists of the points used in AA studies, with details of the most frequently cited points, other reported points, point prescriptions, and notes on how to choose appropriate combinations:
> For example,
>
> **Dental, jaws, lips, facial**
> - Most frequently cited points: LI-4, ST-44
> - Face/head in general: LI-4, P-6, SJ-5, ST-36
> - Upper jaw: ST-44, LI-4 + select from *SI-18, SJ-17, LI-20, ST-2, ST-5, ST-7, Du-26, taiyang (M-HN-9)*
> - Lower jaw: LI-4, P-6, ST-44 + select from *SJ-17, LI-20, ST-2, ST-3, ST-5, ST-6, ST-7*, ST-36, Ren-24, mental foramen (an opening at each side of the lower jaw, level with the second premolars)
> - Lips: ST-44, P-6, *ST-2*
>
> General comment: LI-4 alone has been used in thousands of tooth extractions, but so too have groups of local points with no distal component. Combination of the two may be optimal.
> Choice of points may vary according to type of tooth as well as upper or lower jaw. Local points are in italics.
>
> **Choosing an appropriate prescription**
>
> 1–2 local points + 1–2 distal points +/– auricular points +/– paraincisional points
> This is a general formula for most applications. Choose points particularly from the frequently cited list and in relation to the site of the operation, e.g. ST-7 for upper jaw, Ren-24 for lower jaw, bearing in mind the particular teeth involved.
> Other point lists on the CD-ROM are:
> - Craniocerebral
> - Eye
> - Throat/neck
> - Thoracic
> - Abdomen
> - Orthopaedic.

---

- Faster extubation and earlier activity immediately after the operation (taking food and drink, moving, cooperating).
- A more rapid recovery at all stages, and faster return to self-caring.

## Disadvantages

- AA is usually incomplete and unreliable, unless combined with drugs.
- Muscle relaxation is inadequate and visceral pain (from traction) is not well controlled.
- AA is generally contraindicated for long operations or those where procedural flexibility is needed.

- AA is more time consuming, especially due to the long induction period. Also, extra personnel are required.
- EA apparatus wires may get in the way.

## WHAT PLACE DOES ACUPUNCTURE ANAESTHESIA HAVE IN SURGERY NOW?

Contemporary commentators, both in China and the West, can find no place for AA as a routine procedure unless supported by medication of some kind. Acupuncture-assisted anaesthesia, however, may provide substantial benefits in reducing overall medication, even sometimes to the extent of replacing opioids entirely in lengthy operations. Given an appropriate medication regimen there is no reason to doubt the effectiveness of the combined approach, but, even in China, practical considerations of extra time and personnel mitigate against its widespread use except in areas such as the head and neck.

The place for AA could be as a specialised procedure for certain high-risk patients (especially those with severe heart or lung problems) for whom a general anaesthetic is contraindicated, and for whom an improved postoperative course would be particularly beneficial. It could also be valuable for operations where it is advantageous for the patient to be conscious, for example to avoid damaging nerves, or when alertness on waking is required.

Recent surgical developments look destined to restrict the role of AA still further, however, as much lighter medications are available and epidural anaesthetics replace general anaesthetics for major surgery. It may well be that the value of acupuncture lies more in pre- and postoperative treatment to promote recovery, rather than as an analgesic on the day itself.

## SUMMARY

Some key points in this chapter are:

- The surgical application of acupuncture and associated electrical devices has declined to marginal importance, even in China
- Despite undoubted advantages in postoperative recovery, and with the potential to reduce anaesthetic drug requirements, the drawbacks have been seen to outweigh the advantages
- There may still be scope for the use of AA where it is important that the patient remains conscious during an operation or where potentially reduced blood flow in minor surgery may be an advantage.

**9.13** Summary of relevant studies in the electronic clinical studies database (number of studies)

| Condition | MAA | EAA | Other | Condition | MAA | EAA | Other |
|---|---|---|---|---|---|---|---|
| **AA – Orofacial** | | | | Appendix | 1 | 24 | 2 |
| Nose and sinus | 0 | 13 | 1 | Other gastrointestinal tract surgery | 0 | 3 | 2 |
| Face and jaw | 1 | 17 | 7 | Abdominal (general/other) | 3 | 41 | 15 |
| Dental | 15 | 57 | 72 | Gastroscopy | 3 | 12 | 1 |
| Other oral-related surgery | 0 | 5 | 1 | Colonoscopy | 1 | 5 | 2 |
| **AA – Head (other)** | | | | Cystoscopy | 0 | 3 | 1 |
| Brain surgery | 0 | 61 | 11 | Urinary tract | 1 | 16 | 10 |
| Eye surgery | 0 | 31 | 18 | Prostate | 0 | 6 | 3 |
| *Other eye-related procedures* | 0 | 1 | 0 | Other male genitourinary surgery | 0 | 3 | 4 |
| Ear surgery | 1 | 3 | 0 | Herniorrhaphy | 5 | 28 | 4 |
| **AA – Neck and throat** | | | | OBSTETRIC AND GYNAECOLOGICAL | | | |
| Thyroid | 3 | 94 | 19 | Caesarean section | 7 | 30 | 12 |
| Larynx and oesophagus | 0 | 21 | 3 | Hysterectomy | 0 | 31 | 7 |
| Tonsillectomy | 5 | 17 | 1 | Tuboligation | 0 | 22 | 2 |
| Other (neck/throat) | 0 | 10 | 6 | Other obstetric and gynaecological surgery | 4 | 47 | 20 |
| Spinal surgery (cervical) | 0 | 13 | 1 | **AA – limbs and general points** | | | |
| **Thorax and abdomen** | | | | Limb surgery (orthopaedic and vascular) | 3 | 22 | 12 |
| THORACIC | | | | General orthopaedic surgery | 0 | 8 | 4 |
| Heart | 0 | 60 | 5 | AA studies illustrating general points | 3 | 22 | 30 |
| Lung | 6 | 9 | 14 | Mixed or unspecified locations | 0 | 30 | 17 |
| Breast (cancer, other) | 2 | 11 | 4 | Burn and injury management | 0 | 1 | 0 |
| Thoracic (general) | 1 | 20 | 8 | Cosmetic and plastic surgery | 0 | 8 | 2 |
| Spinal surgery (thoracic or lumbar) | 0 | 8 | 0 | Other skin and soft tissue surgery | 3 | 3 | 1 |
| Other spinal procedures | 0 | 0 | 2 | Miscellaneous procedures | 0 | 1 | 2 |
| ABDOMINAL | | | | **AA – animal** | | | |
| Gall bladder | 1 | 25 | 9 | Veterinary studies | 0 | 23 | 4 |
| Liver | 0 | 0 | 1 | | | | |
| Spleen | 0 | 4 | 1 | | | | |
| Stomach | 2 | 50 | 21 | | | | |

## RECOMMENDED READING

*An early, informative but critical view:*
Murphy TM, Bonica JJ Acupuncture analgesia and anesthesia. Archives of Surgery. 1977; 112: 896–902

*A useful two-part overview:*
Wang BX [Advances of clinical researches in acupuncture anesthesia in China]. Chinese Journal of Acupuncture and Moxibustion. 1988; 1(1): 79–86
Wang BX [Advances in clinical researches on acupuncture anesthesia in China]. Chinese Journal of Acupuncture and Moxibustion 1988; 1(2): 48–53

*A review by one of the major proponents of AA:*
Cao XD Scientific bases of acupuncture analgesia. Acupuncture and Electro-therapeutics Research. 2002; 27(1): 1–14

*A standard work on veterinary AA:*
Klide AM 1992 Use of acupuncture for the control of chronic pain and for surgical analgesia. In: Short CE, Van Poznak A (eds) Animal Pain. Churchill Livingstone, New York (1st edn), 249–57

*For those who read German, the following are excellent:*

*Special journal issue, with contributions from various Western groups included in AA:*
Der Anaesthesist. 1976 May; 25(5)

*A comprehensive textbook on AA:*
Van Nghi N, Van Dong M, Lanza U 1978 Akupunktur-Analgesie. Medizinisch Literarische Verlagsgesellschaft, Uelzen, Germany

*An excellent summary of one particular approach to AA:*
Herget HF [Analgesia by vibration and stimulation at reactive points in the skin]. Physikalische Medizin und Rehabilitation. 1978; 19(2): 71–9

# 9.14 POSTOPERATIVE PAIN

*David F Mayor and Michael W Flowerdew*

> Topics covered here include the different interventions for postoperative pain, treating postoperative pain in specific areas, and the points and parameters used for treating postoperative pain.

Pain following surgery is common. It may be deep visceral or superficial incisional pain, and can be very distressing, compounding the stress and anxiety inherent in surgery.

Pain, or fear of pain, can cause complications such as impaired cardiovascular, respiratory, bowel or urinary function and may impact on immune function, possibly mediating tumour-promoting effects. Reduced mobility increases risks of thromboembolism and muscle wastage. Adequate analgesia, therefore, improves patient outcome.

Using acupuncture for postoperative pain predated and contributed to the development of 'acupuncture anaesthesia' in China and the renaissance of interest in acupuncture in America during the 1970s. Indeed, by 1997 the NIH Consensus Development Conference Panel concluded that there is good evidence for the effectiveness of acupuncture in this field.

TENS, EA, MA and acupressure have all been used to help control postoperative pain. The accompanying decrease in narcotic analgesic usage benefits patients by alleviating possible side-effects – respiratory and immune depression, sedation, orthostatic hypotension, urine retention and nausea, all of which are more likely in debilitated or elderly patients. They are also useful for postoperative functional problems, such as nausea and vomiting (PONV), ileus, urinary retention and hiccup.

Potential postoperative benefits of AA and related intraoperative treatments may include fewer respiratory complications. Acupuncture prior to surgery may also have important postoperative benefits, reducing analgesic intake and chronic postoperative pain. In principle, the combination of pre- and intraoperative acupuncture with postoperative treatment could be correspondingly beneficial; there are many reports of AA during surgery leading to extended periods of reduced postoperative pain. However, the detail remains to be verified in controlled studies.

## DIFFERENT INTERVENTIONS: GENERAL COMMENTS

### MA

There have been many publications on the treatment of postoperative pain using classical MA, in different settings as well as when pain is long term. One particular application is for headache or backache following epidural regional anaesthesia. Various forms of acupuncture have also been used for rehabilitation of trauma patients, for *wei* syndrome (muscle weakness) following surgery and for scar and adhesion pain. However, as an adjunct, acupuncture has been used most successfully in dentistry and relatively superficial operations such as thyroidectomy. Significant changes in pain control tend to occur soon after treatment onset, but may disappear within 30 minutes of needle removal, although subjective changes in pain threshold can last for several hours. Blood pressure and heart rate stability are maintained using AA, with implications for post-trauma shock management.

Other areas where MA has been used include scapulohumeral pain following heart surgery, rectal surgery and abdominal surgery. In an important, robustly designed double-blind RCT, BL-18–BL-24 were used bilaterally for upper and BL-20–BL-26 for lower abdominal surgery. Postoperative analgesia was maintained with epidural and intravenous morphine. Incisional pain, at rest and during coughing, and deep visceral pain were recorded during recovery and for 4 days after surgery using a verbal rating scale. Plasma concentrations of cortisol and catecholamines were monitored. Preoperative acupuncture, with the needles retained throughout surgery, significantly reduced both postoperative pain, analgesic requirement and opioid-related side-effects, as well as the stress-induced overactivity in the sympathoadrenal system that accompanies surgery. The relaxing effects of MA for postoperative pain have been recorded in other studies although, as with many conventional methods for acute postoperative pain, MA is not always successful or may be no better than placebo.

## Auricular and other microsystems

Auricular acupuncture, with semipermanent microneedles, MA, EA or pTENS has been used for pain following a wide range of surgical procedures.

Results with auricular EA are mixed. In one study it performed better than standard care; in others it gave similar results at real and sham points following menisectomy, and did not appear to benefit postoperative pain following cholecystectomy .

Scalp needling has been used for orthopaedic postoperative pain.

The ECIWO ('embryo containing the information of the whole organism') system of 'holographic' points has been used to control pain and shoulder dysfunction associated with nerve damage during thyroidectomy, and was found to be very effective after abdominal surgery in one controlled trial.

## EA

There is a larger literature on the use of EA for control of postoperative pain than that on other forms of acupoint stimulation, with EA demonstrated as superior to conventional treatment in a number of studies. Like MA and TEAS, EA reduces postoperative stress. It may also improve muscular dysfunction due to immobilisation.

## TENS

TENS has been more rigorously investigated for postoperative pain than MA and EA, although the published data are very mixed, both in outcome and quality. TENS may well be an acceptable alternative or adjunct to conventional treatment for acute postsurgical incision pain, but evidence is less clear for serial rib fractures or post-Caesarean pain. A stringent review from the mid 1990s found that, of 19 RCTs of TENS for postoperative pain, only two judged the treatment to be superior to placebo; in contrast, of the 19 excluded non-randomised studies with pain outcomes, 17 judged TENS as having a positive effect. A more recent review identified 21 placebo-controlled RCTs of TENS or ALTENS, involving 1350 patients. For all trials, the mean reduction in analgesic consumption after TENS/ALTENS was 26.5% better than placebo, provided that stimulation was administered in the wound area, with a strong, subnoxious intensity and at an 'adequate' frequency.

TENS has been used to help control pain with varying success following a wide range of operations, including orthopaedic surgery and arthroplasty, spinal surgery, cardiac surgery, hernia repair, appendectomy, cholecystectomy, thoracotomy, obstetric and gynaecological procedures and haemorrhoidectomy, as well as paediatric surgery. Postoperative TENS, TEAS or silver spike point therapy (SSP) may also reduce anxiety and stress more than some medication, thereby reducing discomfort and the need for medication, as well as enhancing early mobility and allowing patients to carry out potentially painful rehabilitation exercises effectively.

As an alternative to EA and TENS when treatment is best applied continuously over several days, wire electrodes have been implanted temporarily, either parallel to the surgical incision or to stimulate specific nerve branches.

## pTENS

Pain was significantly reduced by auricular pTENS immediately after wound care and dressing changes in patients with burns.

## EMS

Electrical muscle stimulation (EMS), a variant of TENS, is a simple and effective method for improving muscle protein synthesis and muscle mass (in the quadriceps femoris muscle) in immobilised patients following surgery or stroke.

## CES

CES was found 'highly effective', compared with control treatment, in one controlled study of postoperative pain following gynaecological interventions, stabilising cardiorespiratory parameters and increasing 'vivacity'. Use of CES during or after thyroid and gastric cancer surgery also decreased the need for narcotic medication and associated side-effects.

## MRT

Following cancer surgery, MRT was found to reduce haemorrhage and atony, enhancing healing without stimulating tumour processes.

## LILT

LILT has been used both before and after surgery to prevent complications, reduce pain, oedema and eventual scar formation and speed recovery time.

## Magnetic fields

Magnets have been applied locally after plastic and spinal surgery, reducing pain and oedema and speeding healing.

## Acupoint injection

Successful pain control has been reported after injecting various substances into acupuncture points, including simple glucose solution and placental suspension. Acupoint injection with homeopathically diluted sodium hydroxide has been used for prolonged postoperative (muscle) weakness.

# POSTOPERATIVE PAIN IN SPECIFIC AREAS

## Dental pain

Because of its limited, predictable course, considerable interest has been shown in using acupuncture for pain control following dental surgery, particularly the extraction of wisdom teeth. In a typical double-blind RCT, patients undergoing third molar extraction were randomised to receive MA or placebo. A statistically significant difference in mean pain-free interval following extraction was found between acupuncture patients (181 minutes) and sham acupuncture controls (71 minutes). Systematic review of 16 similar studies concluded that acupuncture was probably effective for pain after dental surgery and that research should concentrate on refining techniques. MA also reduces orofacial swelling. A possible adverse reaction to MA delivered before or during surgery is increased incidence of 'dry socket'.

EA has been used for pain after mandibular wisdom tooth extraction. In one report of LF EA applied bilaterally at LI-4 and on the affected side at ST-6 and ST-7, in conjunction with 2% xylocaine, pain was reduced only if the teeth were difficult to extract. EA initiated before the local anaesthetic injection was slightly more effective than after extraction. For chronic trigeminal paraesthesia following dental intervention, EA is best initiated within 2 months.

There are few studies on TENS for dental postoperative pain. In one, results were better when TENS was applied postoperatively, rather than before surgery.

Athermal PEMF and small permanent magnets have been used for pain reduction after dental or periodontal surgery.

Locally applied 100 Hz vibration and ultrasound are other possible treatments.

## Other head and neck pain

Both acupuncture and TENS have been used following cataract surgery.

EA has been given after surgery for brain injury, and CES during early rehabilitation following surgery on intracranial arteries. CES has also been used following surgery for thyroid cancer.

A complex programme of interventions, including high-voltage electrical stimulation, MENS, LILT, TENS, moist heat, ultrasound, ice, mobilisation and physical therapy, has been used for rehabilitation following arthroscopic surgery for temporomandibular joint (TMJ) syndrome.

Considering their historical background, it is not surprising that both MA and EA have been used for post-tonsillectomy pain, as have TENS and pTENS.

Auricular EA has been used for pain following cervical laminoplasty.

## Thoracic pain

Pain, severely compromised breathing and respiratory complications following thoracotomy can be particularly distressing. Persistent long-term pain is not uncommon and can be moderately disabling.

EA has been used for postoperative pain in thoracic surgery, reducing pain and improving chest expansion and mobility.

TENS, as well as electrical stimulation via implanted wire electrodes, has been used following radical mastectomy. LILT may help with postmastectomy complications, including lymphoedema, as well as pain.

Most controlled studies on TENS for postoperative thoracic pain do indicate its usefulness for pain control, decreased use of analgesics and rehabilitation. However, TENS is unlikely to be helpful for severe post-thoracotomy pain and may not alter the incidence of pulmonary complications. Benefits are less clear when TENS is used for pain following coronary artery bypass graft surgery. Short-term benefits may be minimal. However, TENS may help neurogenic pain arising months after the operation.

MA has been used for scapulohumeral pain following heart surgery.

LF SSP stimulation may facilitate breathing exercises following thoracotomy.

LA has been used for post-thoracotomy pain.

## Abdominal and inguinal pain

Auricular EA (both HF and at 10 Hz) was not found helpful for postoperative abdominal pain. However, 8–10 Hz EA at body points did result in substantial pain relief, beneficial liver function changes and earlier mobilisation following cholecystectomy.

TENS may be beneficial for postoperative abdominal pain, with the usual benefits of lower narcotic intake, although sham TENS was also effective in some reports. TENS applied before and during cholecystectomy decreased both peri- and postoperative analgesic requirements, although with variable results in terms of lung function and pain itself. Electrodes positioned paraincisionally, or bilaterally at BL-19 (TEAS), gave similar results in one study.

TEAS (7–14 Hz at local points and ST-36, together with auricular pTENS if necessary) has been used for pain and stress following gastrectomy.

CES has been used following surgery for gastric cancer. TCET has reduced analgesic requirement after various types of abdominal surgery.

A single treatment of LILT (6–8 minutes) given immediately after surgery reduced pain following elective cholecystectomy in one RCT.

## Obstetric, gynaecological, urogenital and anorectal pain

Both EA and TENS have been used for pain relief following Caesarean section and uncomplicated gynaecological surgery. They may be combined with low-dose narcotic analgesia. Other benefits include improved central nervous system function, haemodynamic stabilisation and blood coagulation.

Following hysterectomy, EA started immediately after wound closure can reduce pethidine requirement for up to 6 hours after surgery, thus decreasing nausea and drowsiness compared with no-treatment controls. However, in a later and larger study, no significant differences were found in any measure, possibly because high doses of pethidine masked the benefits of EA, or because EA was started only after the induction of anaesthesia.

EA has been used after rectal, renal and other uronephrological surgery, and to assist recovery following transurethral prostate resection.

TENS after Caesarean section lessens requirements for analgesic medication, benefiting both mother and baby, if breast feeding. In this situation, TENS may reduce movement-related cutaneous incisional pain, but not the deeper visceral pain caused by uterine contraction (narcotics are also less effective against the latter). TENS may be less effective for those patients who have used narcotics or abused alcohol prior to surgery, or who received an epidural rather than general anaesthesia.

Local TENS is helpful after colorectal surgery. Motor level TEAS (2/100 Hz DD) unilaterally at LU-7 and LI-4 can also reduce pain and morphine use, and may be more acceptable to some patients than local treatment. TENS may be useful following prostate/penile surgery, but less so after nephrectomy.

CES has been used for pain following various types of gynaecological surgery.

LA has been used after anal and uronephrological surgery, although with less positive results than EA. LILT may reduce complications following episiotomy.

## Pain in back and limbs

Following surgery for lumbar disc prolapse, MA with moxibustion and physical therapy gave better results than electrotherapy. Preemptive MA has been used following knee arthroscopy. Using mainly proximal points, oedema responded rapidly to postoperative MA for hand, wrist and leg surgery.

EA has been used for lumbar surgery and following hip replacement, with excellent analgesia in 75% of patients, absence of postoperative complications, reduced conventional analgesic intake and early comfortable mobilisation.

Rehabilitation following surgery can be painful. Auricular EA prior to exercises (6–8 Hz for 30 minutes at *shenmen* and a point corresponding to the operated area) may be helpful, with the needles retained and occasionally twisted thereafter. Thus auricular EA has improved joint movement and pain after meniscectomy, although not in all studies.

Reduction of pain with TENS enables patients to carry out rehabilitation exercises more comfortably, contributing to early mobilisation. Most TENS studies on postoperative pain following back or limb surgery, although uncontrolled, have reported a significant decrease in analgesic requirements and possibly faster rehabilitation. Results may be better for cervical than for lumbar laminectomy. Although TENS has been used effectively for pain following cancer surgery, it was ineffective in one study after spinal surgery for primary or secondary neoplasm, perhaps because of patient anxiety (CES was still helpful).

TENS used after hip replacement surgery may reduce pethidine requirements, and in several controlled studies was effective for pain following knee surgery. However, after major lower limb amputation, although LF TENS promoted more rapid healing, both active and sham TENS were helpful for pain. Following foot surgery, TENS combined with hypothermia may reduce pain, medication and oedema.

MENS stimulation has been combined with stretching exercises following laminectomy, and may reduce pain after anterior cruciate ligament reconstruction. EMS, used for muscle strengthening after cruciate ligament repair or meniscectomy, can benefit healing.

LILT has been used for swelling and inflammation following hand surgery.

## Postoperative pain in children

MA has been used in children undergoing tonsillectomy. Needling carried out *during* halothane anaesthesia effectively relieved postoperative pain.

EA has been used following paediatric abdominal, thoracic, urological and orthopaedic operations. Less invasive pTENS and SSP have also been used, for pain following thoracic and abdominal surgery, with beneficial effects on cardiorespiratory parameters.

**Comparisons and combinations** Following surgery for lumbar disc prolapse, MA was superior to electrotherapy (both were combined with exercise). Although both MA and EA were superior to electrotherapy (using similar current parameters) for pain following laminectomy, EA was more effective if pain was associated with motor losses, whereas electrotherapy was helpful for motor loss without pain. In their review of acupuncture-based interventions for postoperative pain, Leong and Chernow concluded that EA produced most of the statistically significant changes found. MA was indeed less effective than TENS in one controlled trial. However, TENS may become less effective with extended use. Furthermore, although onset of pain relief may be more rapid with TENS, it may not be as sustained as with EA.

Combining EAA with postoperative TENS, EA/TENS with CES, MA/EA with magnetic field treatment and EA with stellate ganglion block may all be beneficial for postoperative pain.

TENS has been combined with hypothermia for pain and oedema following foot surgery. Both cryotherapy and TENS may be helpful following thoracotomy.

**Points used for postoperative and other post-traumatic pain** Points used in EA vary widely but most commonly are on meridians passing through the affected area, both local and distal, together with points selected on the basis of their TCM functions. Some of the general points used for EAA may be appropriate.

Auricular points are not always helpful, particularly after surgery on internal organs. However, CES may be beneficial. Trigger points and paraspinal points have also been used.

Some acupoints may be inaccessible, covered by bandages or plaster, but it may be possible to treat above and below the affected region using MA, EA or TENS, or to use auricular or paraspinal treatment.

Box 9.14.1 lists some points that may be useful, according to Klide and Gaynor.

Local/distal stimulation is necessary for dental postoperative pain, as for AA. It is insufficient to use LI-4 alone for EA or magnetic stimulation.

Phil Rogers recommends P-6, LI-4 and LI-11 for postoperative healing following thoracic surgery, and ST-36 and SP-6 for abdominal surgery, in addition to general immunostimulant points.

**Dental pain**

- LU-7–LI-4, with MA at local and distal meridian specific points

**Sternotomy**

- EA at either end or either side of incision, with ST-36–SP-6 and P-6–LI-4

**Laparotomy (including Caesarean section)**

- As for sternotomy, but without P-6–LI-4

**Upper limb pain**

- Shoulder: SI-9–SI-11, SJ-14–LI-15
- Humerus: SI-3–SI-9, SJ-5–SJ-14
- Elbow: SI-3–SI-8, SJ-3–SJ-14, LI-4–LI-15
- Radius/ulna: SI-3–SI-9, P-3–P-6, LI-4–LI-15
- Carpal: SI-3–SI-8, P-6–P-8, SJ-3–SJ-14, LU-7–LI-4

**Lower limb pain**

- Hip: BL-40–BL-54, GB-29–GB-30
- Femur: BL-40–BL-54, GB-30–GB-34
- Tibia/fibula: BL-40–BL-60, GB-34–GB-39, ST-35–ST-41, SP-6–SP-9
- Tarsal: BL-40–BL-62, ST-41–ST-44, SP-3–SP-6 (additional points can be used with MA, such as BL-11 following orthopaedic surgery)

Following Caesarean section, EA at GB-34, ST-36, SP-4, SP-6, auricular points and also paraincisional needling have been tried.

After hysterectomy, EA has been used at BL-32, ST-36, SP-6, Du-2 and Du-4, and other points familiar from EAA hysterectomy studies, such as GB-26.

For posthaemorrhoidectomy pain, TEAS was successful at LU-7 and LI-4, unilaterally, rather as in Kaada's protocol. It would be useful if this simple method could be adopted for other postoperative pain.

With CTENS, the standard approach is to use sterile, disposable electrodes parallel to and approximately 1–2.5 cm either side of the surgical incision (or painful area), using 'adequate stimulation'. Electrodes can also be applied proximally/distally, or with one electrode locally and one over the appropriate dermatomal nerve root, over acupoints segmentally related to the area of pain if possible. Four electrodes may be applied parallel to the incision, connected in a 'criss-cross' arrangement, or so that current flows across the wound (Fig. 9.14.1).

There is little evidence that any one configuration is best. In a TENS/TEAS study of pain following cholecystectomy, no difference was found if electrodes were positioned paraspinally or at distal acupoints. For pain after total abdominal hysterectomy or myomectomy under standardised general anaesthesia, little difference was found between 9–12 mA (non-noxious) 2/100 Hz DD paraincisionally or at ST-36; both reduced narcotic requirements and both were superior to sham and non-acupoint shoulder stimulation.

For placement involving joints, more complicated arrangements may be preferable. For knee surgery, placement of electrodes over the medial and collateral ligaments has been advocated. Contralateral EA or TENS is another possibility.

EMS pads should be placed over motor points, where least current is required to stimulate the muscle. If this is not possible, electrodes may be positioned proximally; distal placement will require highest levels of current.

Pekka Pöntinen recommends preemptive LILT applied directly to the operation site and nearby trigger points, if feasible. LA has been used at ST-36 following hysterectomy.

**When to use what – parameters for postoperative and other post-traumatic pain** LF (0.6 or 3 Hz) and HF (60–350 Hz) EA have been used following dental work. Both LF (1–3 Hz) and medium frequency (20–22 Hz) EA were effective in paediatric postoperative pain; curiously, LF EA was more effective in younger and HF EA in older children.

For hysterectomy, a combination of local HF and distal LF is not uncommon, although 2/100 Hz or 10/100 Hz DD is also used. A gradually increasing frequency pattern has been employed, starting at 5 Hz and increasing to 50 Hz. An unusual alternative for spinal surgery is to use 80 Hz and then 5 Hz in each session, alternating every 30 minutes.

Because of cumulative effects, more than one session of EA is needed to treat postoperative pain effectively. As with TENS, whether to treat before as well as after general anaesthesia should be carefully considered.

Both CTENS and LF TENS (not necessarily at high intensity) have been recommended for postoperative pain. Sensory level stimulation is probably best following musculoskeletal trauma or incisional pain; HF TENS at just below patients' pain threshold has also been recommended.

TENS for pain following major gynaecological procedures, using 2 Hz, 100 Hz or 2/100 Hz DD, decreased morphine requirements in one RCT, especially with 2/100Hz DD. All three 'active' treatments reduced analgesia requirements, with accompanying decrease of side-effects. Electrodes were positioned in the dermatome corresponding to the surgical incision. In another rigorous study on pain following low-abdominal surgery, 2 Hz TEAS at LI-4 was alternated with 100 Hz TENS via paraincisional electrodes every 6 seconds. Results were better with high-intensity than low-intensity stimulation, resulting in lower demand for analgesics.

In an unpublished informal review, Michael Flowerdew found that most studies on pain following thoracic, back or limb surgery used paraincisional HF TENS at comfortable or strong intensity. The authors of another review concluded that, if administered with a strong, subnoxious intensity at

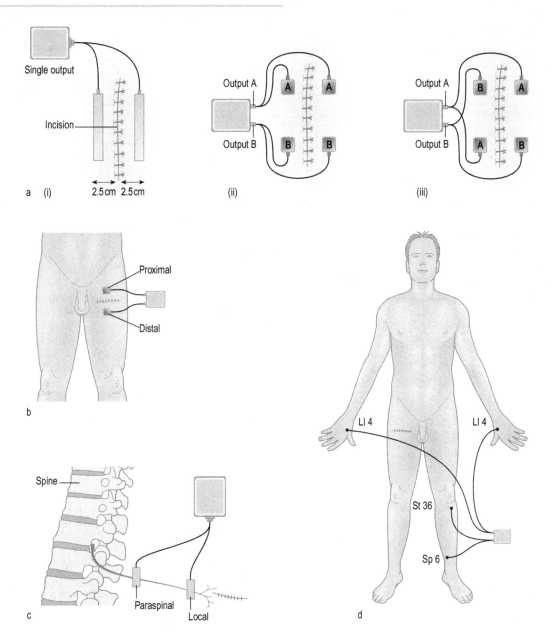

**Figure 9.14.1** Possible electrode locations for postoperative pain. (a) Paraincisional: (i) single output; (ii) two outputs, parallel configuration; (iii) two outputs, criss-cross configuration. (b) Proximal – distal. (c) Nerve root – local. (d) Acupoints. Note possible use of segmental, non-segmental or even contralateral locations.

an 'adequate' frequency in the wound area (~85 Hz for CTENS, or possibly ~2 Hz for ALTENS), TENS can significantly reduce analgesic consumption. However, David Mayor does not recommend ALTENS in immediate proximity to a recent incision and treatment should be comfortable, not painful. In one study, LF TENS following limb surgery

appeared to give better results than HF TENS; however, the former was applied for 1–6 hours, but the latter only for 15 minutes, in each session! Deirdre Walsh suggests that electrodes should be positioned as soon as practicable after surgery and stimulation should begin within 2 hours at 2–100 Hz and high intensity

(9–12 mA), without causing discomfort. However, Russian researchers consider that treatment should begin just as the patient begins to recover from anaesthesia. Treatment prior to surgery is another option.

Following surgery, electrodes can be left in place with continuous TENS stimulation for 48–72 hours; a period of 7 days or longer has been reported, but this may result in habituation. Stimulation may be intermittent (30 minutes every 2 hours, for example). Treatment duration will depend on patient response and surgical procedure and varies widely from study to study.

For the prevention of quadriceps muscle atrophy following major knee surgery, intermittent HF TENS/EMS has been used (200 Hz, 5–6 seconds on/5 seconds off, 1 hour daily, for 5 days each week). Trains of stimuli should be applied briefly initially; treatment duration and repetition rate can be increased as patient confidence increases.

Both red and near-infrared LILT have been used preoperatively by Pekka Pöntinen's group to prevent postoperative complications. 2–4 $J/cm^2$ are used locally, together with 1–2 J/TrP.

## SUMMARY

Some key points in this chapter include:

- Peripheral stimulation, whether MA, EA, TENS/TEAS/EMS or LILT/LA, with early active mobilisation ensures faster recovery by maintaining peripheral input to the central nervous system
- The order of treatment may be important, with stimulation perhaps best initiated when the patient is conscious
- For additional pain relief, tramadol seems to be the opioid of choice, as it does not interfere with immune function and is free from gastrointestinal side-effects
- Epidural and localised anaesthesia are also considered more effective than some conventional methods of pain relief, but can contribute to immobilisation; require expert administration and are much less tolerated than a non-invasive method such as TENS
- In general, postoperative pain treatment is best carried out by a multidisciplinary team rather than a solo practitioner.

**9.14** Summary of relevant studies in the electronic clinical studies database (number of studies)

| Condition | EA | Other | Condition | EA | Other |
|---|---|---|---|---|---|
| **Postoperative pain (obstetric and gynaecological)** | | | Abdomen | | |
| Obstetrics | | | General abdominal surgery | 14 | 29 |
| Caesarian section | 2 | 10 | Upper abdomen (gall bladder) | 6 | 13 |
| Gynaecology | | | Upper abdomen (stomach) | 1 | 3 |
| Hysterectomy | 5 | 6 | Upper abdomen (pancreas) | 0 | 1 |
| Myomectomy | 0 | 2 | Lower abdomen | 0 | 2 |
| Mixed/other gynaecological surgery | 1 | 12 | Herniorrhaphy | 1 | 4 |
| Mixed obstetric and gynaecological | 1 | 0 | Pelvic and proctological | 2 | 6 |
| **Postoperative pain by region** | | | Urinary tract | 1 | 1 |
| Head | | | Male genital | 0 | 4 |
| The eye | 0 | 2 | Orthopaedic | | |
| The mouth | 14 | 11 | Spine | 4 | 12 |
| Throat/neck | 1 | 2 | Extremities | 7 | 21 |
| Thorax | | | Mixed orthopaedic surgery | 0 | 1 |
| Heart | 1 | 10 | Other/mixed surgery | 9 | 26 |
| Lung | 4 | 13 | **Other postoperative factors** | | |
| Breast | 2 | 4 | Burns | 1 | 2 |
| Other/unspecified thoracic surgery | 1 | 8 | Postsurgical tissue repair and oedema | 0 | 9 |
| | | | Muscle condition after surgery | 1 | 2 |
| | | | Other aspects of postoperative recovery | 3 | 5 |

# RECOMMENDED READING

*A useful meta-analysis of TENS:*

Bjordal JM, Johnson MI, Ljunggreen AE Transcutaneous electrical nerve stimulation (TENS) can reduce analgesic consumption. A meta-analysis with assessment of optimal treatment parameters for postoperative pain. European Journal of Pain 2003; 7(2): 181–8

*A selection of interesting studies using very different methods:*

Kotani N, Hashimoto H, Sato Y, Sessler DI, Yoshioka H, Kitayama M, Yasuda T, Matsuki A Preoperative intradermal acupuncture reduces postoperative pain, nausea and vomiting, analgesic requirement, and sympathoadrenal responses. Anesthesiology 2001 Aug; 95(2): 349–56

Leong RJ, Chernow B The effects of acupuncture on operative pain and the hormonal responses to stress. International Anesthesiology Clinics 1988; 26(2): 213–7

Lewis SM, Clelland JA, Knowles CJ, Jackson JR, Dimick AR Effects of auricular acupuncture-like TENS stimulation in pain levels following wound care in patients with burns. Journal of Burn Care and Rehabilitation 1990 July–Aug; 11(4): 322–9

Wang BG, Tang J, White PF, Naruse R, Sloninsky A, Kariger R, Gold J, Wender RH Effect of the intensity of transcutaneous acupoint electrical stimulation on the postoperative analgesic requirement. Anesthesia and Analgesia. 1997 Aug; 85(2): 406–13

# 9.15 ADDICTION

*Ann Brownbill, with additions by David F Mayor and a contribution by Rodney S Robinson*

Topics covered in this chapter include the Western background and TCM theories of dependency, with a review of the acupuncture studies on withdrawing from alcohol, nicotine and drugs, and a look at the possible future role of acupuncture in practice and research.

A number of specifically defined terms will be used throughout the chapter. These are:

*Addiction* – a condition of being dependent on some substance, activity or thought process

*Dependency* – feelings of an inability to cope without the substance/behaviour:

(a) *psychological dependence*, which may involve feelings of tension and anxiety during periods without the drug or a drive to take a substance or act out a behaviour to produce pleasure or avoid discomfort

(b) *physical dependence*, where withdrawal symptoms are experienced when deprived of the drug

The psychological component is an integral part of dependency, whereas physical dependence may or may not be present.

*Tolerance* – a state where there is a reduced response to the effects of a drug caused by its previous administration; hence, in order to induce the effects the drug had previously, larger quantities need to be taken

*Withdrawal* – signs and symptoms, both physical and psychological, which occur and last for a limited time when the amount of a drug is reduced or is stopped altogether

## THE WESTERN BACKGROUND

Theories abound as to why people initially become dependent upon a certain activity or substance, including the 'addictive personality', availability, psychological pain (loss, response to past or present abuse), social influence and curiosity, to give but a few examples. The causes are often varied and complex.

Dependence on a substance may or may not imply physical dependence. It is possible that no physical symptoms occur but that, psychologically, removal of the substance causes intense anxiety or other unpleasant psychological disturbances, which may in turn cause physical side-effects.

However, it may be worth considering whether the physical withdrawal symptoms from a drug are really distinguishable from psychological craving. In some studies, the focus is on physical withdrawal, with little recognition that the accompanying psychological cravings may have very deep roots. Evidence suggests, however, that any treatment programme that tries to assist the 'recreational' drug-dependent person to stop taking drugs or change certain behaviour must involve comprehensive psychological support.

Drugs that tend to be misused appear to share the property of being positive reinforcers: they cause positive experiences such as anxiety reduction, associated with release of dopamine (DA) in the brain. The DA pathways involved are often considered part of a physiological 'reward system'. Some drug misusers may be naturally deficient in DA, reinforcing drug-seeking behaviour. Therefore, DA precursors, such as the amino acid tyrosine, may be helpful in combination with other treatments for drug withdrawal. Other studies suggest a link between alcoholism and low serotonin levels.

## CURRENT PRACTICE IN THE UK

In the UK, detoxification treatment of drug/alcohol dependency is often based either in National Health Service or private psychiatric units, or in specialised clinics. In some cases, 'street drugs' are substituted by a pharmacologically prepared prescription; methadone, for example, is administered in place of heroin. The rationale is that the use of methadone will stop the use of street heroin, as well as keeping clients in contact with statutory services in order to maintain their supply.

Many drug dependency units offer complementary/alternative health treatments, including acupuncture, as an adjunct to more orthodox treatments. The acupuncture offered may be auricular (the National Acupuncture Detoxification Association (NADA) protocol), or may combine auricular with body acupuncture, with or without the use of Chinese herbs. One major problem with these treatment programmes is the retention of clients. Initial withdrawal is one thing; recovery and rehabilitation are very different. As Ellinor Mitchell rather controversially puts it, 'addiction is a relapsing disease'.

For nicotine dependency, much of the treatment available is in the form of self-help, such as over-the-counter nicotine patches. However, since 1998 the UK government has implemented smoking cessation support programmes.

## SOME COMPLEMENTARY/ ALTERNATIVE TREATMENTS

Acupuncture is possibly the most widely used complementary treatment to support those who are substance dependent. Others include nutritional programmes, homeopathy and the use of herbs. Hypnosis, biofeedback, shiatsu, yoga, meditation and other relaxation techniques are also used.

Where studies of these various therapies have been carried out in relation to substance misuse, efficacy has not been consistently demonstrated.

## Dependency and traditional Chinese medicine (TCM)

When examining the role of acupuncture in dependency, it is important to understand its process in terms of TCM. Steve Given has written a clear account of the effects various drugs have on the body and mind, according to TCM. He notes that all misused drugs affect the *shen* (Mind or consciousness) of the user, initially causing an abnormal euphoria, and with continued use, unpleasant *shen* disturbances such as insomnia and restlessness. This would equate with, in TCM terms, an excess condition of the Heart, which may lead to Heart Fire. Likely associated symptoms are agitation and mental restlessness, palpitations, feelings of heat and insomnia. Once the person is dependent on the drug, there follows a cycle of withdrawal followed by self-medication. Administration of the drug leads to Heart Fire, whereas withdrawal equates to Liver *qi* stagnation characterised by depression, melancholy or feeling 'wound up', with a sensation of bloating in the hypochondrium, poor appetite and nausea/vomiting.

Chronic abuse can lead to Heart *qi* deficiency characterised by tiredness, sweating, palpitations and shortness of breath. In chronic abuse, because of regular excessive sweating, possible diarrhoea due to Spleen *qi* deficiency (caused by Liver–Spleen disharmony and malnutrition), and the Heat generated by damage to the Heart and Liver, Kidney *yin* may become deficient, resulting in such symptoms as night sweats, thirst, constipation, dizziness, poor memory and sore, aching back and bones. Given states that this is more prevalent amongst those abusing opiates. First, opiates appear to cause more Liver–Spleen and Stomach disharmonies, resulting in body fluid loss from diarrhoea and vomiting. Secondly, they also appear to cause more *shaoyang* disharmonies (chills and fever). As Kidney *yin* is the foundation of *yin* for the Heart and Liver, both these organs become *yin* depleted, and as Liver *yin* is depleted so Liver *yang* is free to rise, causing anxiety, irritability, headaches and night sweats.

As Kidney *yin* and *yang* have the same origin, a deficiency in one will cause deficiency in the other. Kidney *yang* deficiency may cause a sore, cold lower back, weakness and oedema of the legs, loose stools, sexual problems and a poor appetite. It may also lead to breathing problems as the Kidneys fail to grasp the Lung *qi*. Difficulties with breathing are likely to be exacerbated by Heat and Phlegm in the Lungs, caused either by smoking tobacco, or by drugs.

## ADDICTION AND ACUPUNCTURE

The interest in the use of acupuncture in the field of addiction largely stems from a serendipitous discovery by Drs Wen and Cheung at the Kwong Wah Hospital in Hong Kong in November 1972. They found that auricular electroacupuncture (EA) being used for analgesia during surgery on an addict deprived of his supplies helped to relieve symptoms of acute withdrawal.

Some of the first research on acupuncture and addiction was carried out at the Lincoln Hospital in New York. Initially, EA as opposed to manual acupuncture (MA) was the choice of treatment, with different points selected for different addictions. Gradually there was a shift to what is now known as the NADA protocol, using MA bilaterally at a standard selection of points (*shenmen*, Lung, Kidney, Liver, Sympathetic), whatever the drug of addiction. Lincoln researchers claimed that gentle MA resulted in a more prolonged effect and more consistent outcomes than strong EA. Group treatment was found to enhance the acupuncture effect, with less symptom relief and poorer retention in the programme if fewer than six people were treated at once. Based on this five point auricular protocol, the National Acupuncture Detoxification Association (NADA) was founded in 1985, its function being to provide training and assure specific clinical and ethical standards in withdrawal treatment programmes worldwide.

In terms of Chinese medicine, acupuncture helps to release blockages of energy so that it flows more smoothly, thus aiding the process of detoxification; Western medicine would possibly view this as encouraging homeostasis of the nervous system. Clinically, in the field of dependency, acupuncture appears to relieve withdrawal symptoms, prevent craving and help the client to relax.

## ALCOHOL

Alcohol is a nervous system depressant. Initially, the release of inhibitory neurotransmitters at synapses in the brain becomes depressed and the level of serotonin (5HT) increases, so that the person may feel more sociable. However, if alcohol intake continues, the excitatory synapses also become depressed and 5HT decreases, leading to drowsiness and impairment of both motor and sensory function. People are generally considered to be alcohol dependent if they exhibit tolerance and withdrawal symptoms, and spend large amounts of time obtaining or using alcohol to the detriment of other activities.

Acute withdrawal symptoms may occur within 4–12 hours of reducing or stopping chronic alcohol intake and may include agitation and shaking, nausea and vomiting, sweating, tachycardia and hypertension, insomnia, headaches and transient hallucinations (both auditory and visual). Epileptic seizures are not uncommon.

## MA

MA has been used for alcohol withdrawal since the early 1970s, though with contradictory results. Auricular MA has been used in conjunction with herbal treatment, for example, both for acute alcohol withdrawal and for alcohol-related liver disease. Authors often also emphasise that acupuncture has to be integrated with counselling and social support. Whereas many Western MA studies on alcohol withdrawal use a standard auricular protocol, other ear points include *zuidian*, or Occiput and Subcortex for severe cases.

## EA

There are similar numbers of EA and MA studies. Most EA studies on alcohol-related problems are uncontrolled. Lewenberg, for example, studied 50 clients receiving auricular EA and the antidepressant maprotiline to assist with alcohol withdrawal, and found that no client showed or complained of acute symptoms in withdrawal. Overall, 79% of the clients had improved (abstaining or reduced drinking) at 2–3 months and 64% at 6 months. The maprotiline and acupuncture may have 'acted synergistically'.

Milanov and Toteva studied 25 outpatients with alcohol withdrawal, using EA for tremor. The points HE-7, SI-4, P-6, SJ-5, GB-8, GB-14, LI-4, LI-11, *taiyang* (M-HN-9) and *yintang* (M-HN-3) were treated in varying combinations with 20–60 Hz, 1.5–2.0 mA for 30 minutes (apart from P-6, which received, for unexplained reasons, 1–20 Hz for 5 minutes only) on a daily basis for 15 days. Tremor amplitude, but not frequency, was reduced, although with previous episodes of alcohol withdrawal tremor had mostly resolved only with resumed drinking. Other withdrawal symptoms, such as sweating, elevated blood pressure and heart rate, also improved.

A further study by Toteva and Milanov 3 years later looked at 118 clients; 50 clients received MA or EA (EA if alcohol had been abused for over 10 years) compared with the control group of 68 clients treated with medication and intravenous vitamins. The points used were the same as those mentioned in the study above. In the acupuncture treatment group there was a significantly smaller drop-out rate and a higher rate of voluntary entry into the poststudy psychotherapy group. Depressive symptoms and the desire to start drinking again were less than in the control group.

Rampes et al divided 59 clients withdrawing from alcohol into three groups, all receiving standard treatment. In addition, group 1 received stimulation at auricular points *shenmen*, Sympathetic and Lung 1. Group 2 were treated at auricular points Knee 2, Internal Secretion and Elbow. EA was applied to bilateral Lung 1 in group 1 and Internal Secretion in group 2. Group 3 received standard treatment only. The authors concluded that treating specific auricular addiction points was not advantageous but that EA may be a useful adjunct in the treatment of alcohol dependence.

Bahn and Küblböck report that 5-minute 130–160 Hz EA treatments at bilateral auricular Occiput and Subcortex points, repeated four times at intervals of 2 minutes and allowing the patient to rest for a further 5 minutes thereafter, gives 'excellent' results in withdrawal. Ten treatments are given, initially daily. The same points (with MA or LA) can be used for a hangover.

In addition to MA and EA, pTENS, CES, LA and other acupuncture methods have been used for alcohol withdrawal.

# NICOTINE

In 1997 in the UK, one in five deaths were attributable to smoking. In addition to heart and lung disorders, smoking is associated with depression, anxiety and schizophrenia, male impotence, and substance abuse and hyperactivity in the children of mothers that smoke. Although the prevalence of smoking has declined since its health risks have been advertised, there is an increase in smoking amongst younger people, especially women.

Acute withdrawal symptoms from nicotine may include irritability and craving, restlessness and difficulty in concentrating, anxiety, insomnia and increased appetite.

## MA

Acupuncture for nicotine withdrawal has been carried out in France since the 1950s, with more French RCTs on this application of acupuncture than any other. Nevertheless, controlled studies of acupuncture for smoking cessation are still in the minority.

Requena and colleagues treated 1138 patients using the Gall Bladder nose point as the main point, with additional points in subsequent treatments. Patients were reviewed after 3 months and categorised as excellent (total abstinence or less than five cigarettes daily for 3 months), good (reduction by half or more of cigarettes smoked previously) and failure. After 1 week 82% were abstaining, with 75% still desiring nicotine after the first treatment. At 3 months 61.2% fell into the excellent category, 9.7% into good and 29.1% had failed.

LaMontagne et al compared three highly motivated groups of clients; 25 received acupuncture aimed at smoking withdrawal (auricular Point Zero and Lung), 25 received acupuncture aimed at enhancing relaxation (HE-4, SI-3, BL-60, KI-3, SJ-10, ST-36, ST-45, Ren-7, Ren-17 and 'Ear 24', and 25 were self-monitoring. Acupuncture treatments were given for 20 minutes, once a week for 2 weeks. After 14 days the combined adjusted mean smoking rate of the two acupuncture groups was significantly lower than the self-monitoring group, but there was no significant difference between the two acupuncture groups. At 1, 3 and 6 months there was no significant difference between all three groups, indicating a lack of specific effectiveness for acupuncture.

Similar results have been reported by other groups, although positive long-term outcomes have been reported in uncontrolled studies. Many different acupoints have been used, such as ST-9 and BL-10 bilaterally, or auricular *shenmen* and Lung, sometimes combined with Du-20, Du-26 or *yintang* (M-HN-3).

Press needles or other needle-embedding methods have frequently been used, as well as acupoint injection and pressure using ear seeds.

## EA

Martino's programme for helping people to cease smoking includes stimulation of both auricular and body points, as well as information, herbs and psychological support. The auricular points used are *shenmen*, Kidney, Point Zero, Lung 1 or Lung 2 and Hunger, and the body points are LI-4 and *tim mee* (*tianmei*, 'sweet taste', located close to LU-7, but slightly more towards the dorsal aspect of the wrist, or midway between LU-7 and LI-5). Points are treated on alternate sides at each visit, and 10 Hz electrical stimulation is applied to *shenmen*, *tim mee*, LI-4 and one of the Lung points for 40–45 minutes. Ear press needles or silver pellets are then retained on the auricular points between treatments. Clients receive two treatments the first week, 2 days apart, then two other appointments 1 week apart.

He et al used a combination of ear acupuncture, ear acupressure and body EA administered to smokers twice a week for 3 weeks. The test group received acupuncture to points believed to have an effect on smoking cessation, including EA at LU-6 and LU-7. The control group received acupuncture to points believed to be without effect on smoking cessation. EA was applied first, for 20 minutes at 3 Hz. By the end of the treatment, both groups reported a drop in consumption of cigarettes, and noted that the taste of cigarettes had become less pleasant (more so in the test group), and hence the desire to smoke had diminished. Thirty-one per cent of the test group stopped smoking compared with none in the control group, and serum levels of cotinine and thiocyanate were reduced significantly in the former. Eight months later, both groups had increased their smoking, although this was more evident in the control group. After 5 years there was little further change beyond that noted at 8 months. This seems to be the first study in which the taste of cigarettes was investigated quantitatively, although it has been reported that cigarettes tasted bad after treatment in several studies, whether of EA, TEAS or LA, as well as following use of ear seeds.

In many of the studies using auricular stimulation, Lung or *shenmen*, or both, is needled. Other points used include Sympathetic, Subcortex, Allergy, Antiaggression, Addiction, Mouth and Point Zero – a mixture of TCM and Nogier points. The auricular points receive either electrical stimulation or press needles applied after treatment.

Body points such as LI-4 and Du-20 have been used in several studies. Auricular points are often stimulated bilaterally. In one report by Heidary, for example, using bilaterally linked ear points but unilaterally linked body points, 62% of patients stopped after one session, 14% after two, and 11% after three (only 13% did not stop). No follow-up was mentioned. Others have used a simpler approach: 2–4 Hz EA at the bilateral ear Lung points for 15–20 minutes at a comfortable intensity, followed by placement of ear seeds or semipermanent needles. The author of one such study considered the semipermanent needle to be of psychological value only.

Other studies indicate less favourable outcomes with EA. Martin et al used 1 Hz square waves at LI-4 and auricular Tongue for 20 minutes for one session only. Auricular press needles were inserted into Lung and Hunger points 1 week prior to the EA session and remained in for the ensuing 2 weeks. The authors concluded that acupuncture may help 5–15% of the population to stop smoking for at least 6 months but that EA does not increase the chance of stopping, nor prolong the period for which smoking ceases. Instead they propose that there is a large psychological component attached to the use of acupuncture in smoking cessation.

In general, the number of treatment sessions and the intervals between them varies considerably, from twice daily, over 3 days, to twice weekly, over 6 weeks, to two treatments with 3–4 days in between. Results are more favourable with several rather than a single session. Many authors have emphasised the importance of motivation, that changes in the taste of smoking can be a key to good results, and that the aim must be total abstinence rather than becoming an 'occasional' smoker.

In addition to MA and EA, pTENS, CES, TEAS and LA have been used for nicotine withdrawal.

## Nicotine: reviews and conclusions

A number of reviews now exist of the considerable amount of research carried out on acupuncture and smoking cessation. The benchmark Cochrane review, for example, in line with earlier reports and analyses, considers that no evidence is available that the specific effectiveness of acupuncture for this problem is any greater than that of placebo (sham acupuncture), although in the first 6 weeks following treatment it is probably superior to doing nothing. Other reviewers consider that acupuncture may be as effective as other interventions in the initial stages of nicotine withdrawal, or as effective as nicotine replacement therapy. Failure to demonstrate effectiveness does not mean, however, that the intervention is ineffective. Indeed, in one comprehensive review of 64 studies, involving some 15 000 smokers, the overall analysis indicated that, at the end of treatment, 75.05% abstained, with the highest recurrence rate between 6 months and 1 year.

Trials and reviews of acupuncture for smoking cessation have usually not considered users' degree of motivation or the severity of their habit in coming to their conclusions, whether treatment was carried out in groups or individually, or the possibly different effects of MA and EA. With motivation such an important factor, the bias associated with different methods of recruitment may even affect results more than the treatment itself. However, the more rigorous the review or the trial, the less likely it is to reach a positive conclusion. Nevertheless, one rigorous French meta-analysis concluded that, after all, acupuncture is significantly superior to minimal, sham or no intervention both at less than 6 weeks follow-up and at 6 or 12 months.

Despite the disagreements, clinics where acupuncture is offered as part of a package to assist smoking cessation do appear to have their place. A holistic approach involving diet and exercise, family and workplace support may well improve outcome.

# DRUGS

The majority of acupuncture studies designed to help in the withdrawal from drugs focus on heroin, methadone and cocaine. Heroin and methadone are both opiates, and rapid dependence and physiological tolerance may develop with either. They both have sedative effects, causing sleepiness, respiratory depression, diminished appetite and constipation, as well as the effects desired by the user of euphoria or analgesia, or both. Typical withdrawal symptoms are generally severe and flu-like, with restlessness, nausea and vomiting, and a strong desire for the drug.

Cocaine is a powerful stimulant and produces strong dependency. Its effects are euphoria, increased energy and feelings of greater confidence, but high doses may cause paranoid psychosis. Physical effects include increases in blood pressure, heart and respiratory rates, in some cases status epilepticus or even death. Withdrawal from chronic use causes intense craving, depression, muscle spasms and lethargy, amongst other symptoms.

## MA

Margolin and Avants are two of the leading researchers in this field. In an early single-blind, randomised study they used three auricular points (Lung, *shenmen* and Sympathetic) and one body point (LI-4) for methadone-maintained cocaine-dependent patients. The control group received sham acupuncture within 2–3 mm of the active sites. Both groups were treated five times a week for 6 weeks. Subject retention was good and cocaine use decreased in both groups. The only significant difference between the two groups was a decrease in craving in the test group.

In a later trial, 82 subjects dependent on cocaine were divided into those receiving NADA auricular acupuncture, those receiving sham auricular acupuncture and those receiving non-acupuncture relaxation techniques. More cocaine negative urine samples were found within the NADA acupuncture group. The authors therefore concluded that acupuncture in the treatment of cocaine addiction showed promise. However, a follow-up study, this time dividing 620 cocaine-dependent adults into similar groups, found that, although there was an overall reduction in cocaine use, there was no difference in reduction between the three groups. This time the authors concluded that acupuncture was no more effective than the other treatments for cocaine addiction.

A smaller study examined the effects of acupuncture on the psychological and physiological changes occurring during cocaine withdrawal. The test group was treated at the auricular NADA points and the control group at five points on the auricular helix. Each group was required to watch a 5-minute videotape of the preparation and use of cocaine and crack in order to stimulating craving, before and after receiving acupuncture treatment. No significant differences were found.

In order to encourage retention of inpatients in treatment, Holder et al proposed the use of three auricular points – the Limbic System, the Chinese Brain point and the French Zero point (Fulcrum). When these were combined with auricular *shenmen*, Sympathetic and Kidney for at least 10 days of treatment, numbers completing the dependency treatment programme rose.

The study by Otto et al of 36 cocaine users receiving auricular acupuncture found no difference between the treatment and control groups, whereas one by Lipton et al on 150 subjects dependent on cocaine and crack found that the treatment group showed more favourable urine tests when compared with the placebo acupuncture control group. However, both groups in the latter study reported a significant decrease in the use of cocaine.

Washburn et al studied 100 heroin-dependent patients, randomly and blindly assigned to a 21-day detoxification programme where they would receive either auricular acupuncture treatment (Sympathetic, *shenmen*, Kidney, Lung) or sham auricular acupuncture. Attrition rates were high overall, although higher in the control group. In both the test and sham groups it was found that those who had entered the study with a heavier habit (i.e. injecting at least three times daily), terminated their treatment earlier as they found no relief from the acupuncture. It was also noted that those in the test group were more likely to continue their treatment beyond the 21 days. This study concentrated more on the efficacy of acupuncture as a treatment modality than success in detoxification, and the authors concluded that they had no evidence that those who completed the programme detoxified.

On the other hand, addition of the NADA protocol to the usual care programmes was found to accelerate the process of becoming 'clean' in one mixed substance abuse controlled study in which frequent urine testing was undertaken.

Montazeri et al have used MA at body points to alleviate the severe withdrawal reaction induced by rapid opiate detoxification with naloxone (an approach used earlier with EA by Wen, as well as Kroening and Oleson). Bardellini describes use of the NADA protocol (but with needles retained for some 9 hours) in a comatose patient with combined opioid and benzodiazepine treatment who appeared to have withdrawal symptoms following attempted suicide. Even though the patient was not conscious initially, the protocol was helpful, even dramatically so.

Part of the success of treatment may well be dependent on motivation, particularly if the alternative is a jail sentence, as it is in some US states. Furthermore, those dependent on cocaine and other stimulants can become very agitated during withdrawal. Acupuncture helps to calm patients so that they may be sufficiently relaxed and attentive for long enough to partake in psychotherapy.

In contrast, some researchers have found that cocaine-dependent clients responded less well to acupuncture than those dependent on opioids. Similarly, 51% of users in one small study who identified methamphetamines as their drug of choice responded more poorly to MA than the study group as a whole.

# EA

Most EA studies for drug withdrawal (particularly cocaine) are still uncontrolled. In one such study, 66 heroin-dependent clients in a 28-day detoxification programme underwent a 10-day acupuncture and electrostimulation detoxification course within the 28-day period, once withdrawal symptoms were being experienced. Auxiliary points determined by TCM diagnosis were used in addition to the NADA points, SP-6 and the Jérôme point (located on the tail of the helix, just above the lobule of the ear). Electrodes were connected to SP-6 and Jérôme bilaterally, and patients adjusted the voltage of a portable electrical stimulator after instruction. Each treatment was for 30 minutes. Results indicated that over two-thirds of patients found withdrawal symptoms (chosen by the patient) relieved and craving reduced. The author concludes that complete detoxification is often unrealistic, particularly in younger, possibly less motivated patients, whereas reduction is more achievable. At interview, many clients felt that medication was more convenient for easing symptoms than acupuncture; some found it hard to lie still for 30 minutes and others noted that needling was very painful.

A study by Severson et al used Wen and Cheung's method of EA detoxification, beginning once withdrawal symptoms had started. Treatments were given on demand to bilateral auricular Lung (square wave or modified square wave current at 125 Hz, voltage adjusted by the patient). Other points were used if necessary, such as HE-5, HE-6 or HE-7 for anxiety or ST-36 for abdominal cramps. Within 1 week, five had successfully detoxified, but within 1 month three had resumed use of heroin, and within 4 months only one client was still heroin free.

This study emphasises the importance of controlling physical symptoms and the speed at which detoxification may be achieved. Complete detoxification within a short space of time appears as an impressive outcome. However, although physical withdrawal is an important part of the detoxification process, other equally important changes may not be achieved quickly, and the study does acknowledge that there is a need for psychological care beyond that which is possible in such a short time.

Many of the EA studies reporting good results were conducted by Wen Hsiang-lai, the majority being for opium and heroin and based on a lengthy treatment of three and a half to four and a half hours. This involves 30 minutes of electrostimulation, usually at 125 Hz, 4–5 V to auricular Lung.

He reports that symptoms gradually improve within 15 minutes, and usually almost disappear after 30 minutes. In some studies, injections of naloxone are also administered. Wen notes that with this rapid detoxification, on the first or second day after the treatment, clients reported feeling more alert, had no craving, and had better sleeping patterns, better appetites and normal bowel movements. He writes that it is the combination of electrical stimulation with naloxone that clears the receptor site(s) of the consumed narcotic. In a study by Wen and Cheung of 40 patients receiving electroacupuncture to auricular Lung bilaterally, treatment was between 30 and 45 minutes and was stopped when clients felt fully satisfied (i.e. felt as if they had had the full dose of drug). Subsequent reviews of this study have highlighted confusion as to the duration of time that the 39 clients who were discharged remained drug free after being successfully detoxified.

The addictive potential of many pain-relieving drugs is a matter of concern. Dependence may become a complicating factor in chronic pain, and may itself contribute to a worsening of pain. Somewhat surprisingly, given Wen's original finding that EA can relieve symptoms of acute withdrawal in addicts undergoing surgery, there appears to have been little further research on EA analgesia during or after operations in withdrawing clients deprived of their supplies, for whom the alternative is potentially risky high doses of opiates. Kroening and Oleson combined EA (to bilateral auricular *shenmen* and Lung) and low doses of naloxone, administered to 14 chronic pain patients addicted to opiates. Patients were changed from their opiate medication to methadone at the start of the study. The electroacupuncture parameters were 1–3 Hz alternating with 600–1000 Hz (DD), at less than 200 µA for 2–6 hours. After 45 minutes of electrical stimulation, periodic injections of naloxone commenced. Twelve successfully detoxed in 2–7 days and continued on a total pain management programme (which included TENS, acupuncture and biofeedback). When followed up after 6 and 15 months, none of the 12 had returned to using opiate medication.

There appear to be few studies using electroacupuncture in cocaine withdrawal alone. One study on the use of EA for cocaine users is presented as an anecdotal series of case histories reporting various degrees of success. Treatment combined auricular EA, a small dose of the antidepressant maprotiline, counselling and, in some patients, additional self-administered TENS.

As for benzodiazepines, there is little formal research on the role of acupuncture, despite its potential benefits for the conditions for which benzodiazepines are often prescribed in the first place. Marcus writes that withdrawal may take between 5 days and 2 months, and can include symptoms such as restlessness, tremor, palpitations, insomnia, headache, photophobia, hyperaesthesia and a decreased perception of movement, amongst others. He notes that EA may be useful in helping to shorten and ease symptoms in the withdrawal process. He suggests a combination of a slowly reducing dose of diazepam with EA administered every few days or weekly, presumably at the settings he mentions at the beginning of his chapter (100–125 Hz biphasic, to auricular Stomach, *shenmen* and Lung, plus body points for specific symptoms, for 20–30 minutes). Unlike narcotic addiction, with benzodiazepine dependency inpatient treatment is not necessary.

There are many studies on possible noninvasive alternative treatments such as pTENS, CES and TEAS.

Case study 9.15.1 describes the use of electrotherapy for drug withdrawal

**Points used for alcohol, nicotine and drug withdrawal**
Treatment protocols vary widely, although auricular points are commonly used for both MA and EA. The most popular points in Western studies appear to be the NADA points (Lung, *shenmen*, Sympathetic, Kidney and Liver). Stomach,

---

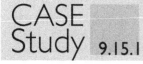
# CASE Study 9.15.1

### Electrotherapy for drug withdrawal
**Rodney S Robinson**

Drug dependence is now a major concern throughout society. There is increasing anecdotal evidence that, used appropriately, electrostimulation (ES) can be a useful treatment in the management of symptoms associated with withdrawal from a range of addictive drugs. However, the effectiveness of ES in treating withdrawal syndrome has not been tested in a robust manner and remains controversial. Nearly all of the studies reported in the literature have employed non-randomised, unblinded designs. A number of studies have linked auricular acupuncture to increased production of endogenous opiate peptides such as β-endorphin and enkephalins; this is thought by some researchers to be the mechanism of the treatment's purported effects on opiate withdrawal.

Traditional opioid detoxification methods include methadone reduction programmes, narcotic antagonists for relapse prevention, and the use of various medications to ameliorate the symptoms of withdrawal. Most acupuncture treatment protocols for addiction and withdrawal have focused on the use of auricular therapy, with points treated either using needles alone or with attachment to electrostimulation devices.

Laser light has been used as a substitute for needle insertion by medical acupuncturists for well over 10 years. Red light produced by a 660 nm light emitting diode (LED) has been used at the CIC – Drug Services centre in Liverpool for treating auricular acupuncture points, with favourable reports from clients suffering acute opiate withdrawal syndrome. The technique has the advantage of being non-tactile. Each auricular point is treated for about 1 minute. A further development is the use of a cluster head probe (a circular array of 51 ultrabright LEDs), which can cover the whole of the auricle and should improve the effect. Initial results look very promising, with favourable reports from clients and observed effects such as rapid relaxation, regulation of respiratory rate and rhythm, and dramatic improvement of aches and pains.

Apparent advantages were discovered in combining auricular and body point stimulation for any form of drug dependence (Fig. 9.15.1). Auricular therapy appears to give more immediate relief, which is further enhanced by a 30-minute session of ES applied mainly through body points. Extended treatments are often applied using tiny magnetic spheres (ion granules) taped directly over a chosen auricular point. This method works by applying constant pressure to the point; the ongoing stimulation can be important in the treatment of craving.

If the client is already showing the first signs of withdrawal syndrome it is important to carry out an auricular treatment immediately. Results should be apparent within minutes of starting the auricular treatment. It will be noticed that some points for certain individuals will produce more dramatic results. This indicates that these points are highly electrically active at that moment in time (the biophysical profile will change according to the physiological state and should be considered a dynamic system). Auricular ES can be given using 10 Hz, or treatment frequency can be chosen according to the Nogier frequency rates for the auricle.

The full auricular treatment takes a few minutes depending on the method of stimulation applied (ES or laser light (Fig. 9.15.2)). If ES is the chosen method of treatment, an auricular probe electrode is held against each point in turn for 30 seconds to one minute. The tip of the probe is moistened with a tiny smear of water-based gel to reduce skin resistance. If no electrical measurement device is used, the treatment probe can be moved gently over the skin, examining one small section of the auricle at a time, checking for sensitivity to the current. Any points can be located this way, with the most sensitive points being treated for the required time. This method is particularly useful for comparing the sensitivity of the Stomach and Lung points, which are indicated for craving (Fig. 9.15.3). An ion granule (acu-dot) should be applied to the most sensitive point.

### Case history – cocaine withdrawal

Peter X attended CIC – Drug Services for the first time having stopped taking cocaine for the previous 3 days. This followed a 4-year consistent and heavy daily habit. The anger and frustration at not being able to give up the drug had been the cause of a suicide attempt the previous

## CASE Study 9.15.1 Continued

week by cutting the wrists and attempted drowning. When he was seen at the centre, Peter presented with anxiety, depression and great craving for the drug. He was lethargic and sleeping a lot.

Peter was given an auricular treatment using an ES treatment (EST) probe for pulsed current treatment over the stress points, each point being stimulated for 30 seconds to 1 minute. Following auricular treatment, Peter appeared much more relaxed and reported feeling general improvement in his symptoms, particularly in levels of anxiety and craving. The auricular Lung point was stimulated, as it was found to have a raised voltage (+60 mV), with increased sensitivity to pressure and electrostimulation. This is always tested, and sensitivity (or voltage reading) compared against that of the of the auricular Stomach point, which is also

effective against craving. An acu-dot was placed in situ to give ongoing acupressure to the point and so alleviate craving.

EST was immediately set up after the auricular treatment, timed for 30 minutes. Points used for stimulation were as follows:

- bilateral Auricular *shenmen*, using auricular clips
- bilateral hand-to-hand, using cylindrical electrodes
- bilateral ST-36, using square TENS electrode pads
- bilateral SP-6, using ankle clamps (see Fig. 9.15.1)

The frequency setting was 80 Hz + 1.1 Hz.

The important aspect of the treatment protocol for cocaine withdrawal is correct choice of frequency. Pulsed frequency stimulation for cocaine withdrawal should be in the 80–200 Hz frequency window. By stimulating production of serotonin, frequencies in this range help to combat depression and lethargy. A delta frequency of 1.1 Hz was mixed with the serotonin-stimulating frequency of 80 Hz.

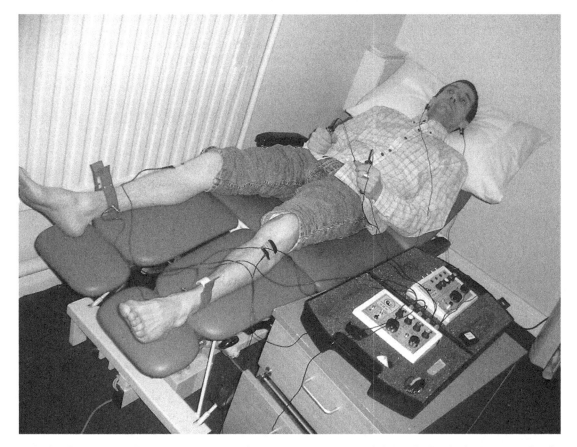

**Figure 9.15.1** Comprehensive Equinox treatment, showing how stimulation can be applied via ear clips, handheld cylinders, gelled surface pads and ankle clamp electrodes. The device used is the AAA-401.

### CASE Study 9.15.1 Continued

Activating these two separate biochemical mechanisms enhances the effectiveness of treatment. Also, 80 Hz by itself can produce some unwanted side-effects of dizziness, headache and nausea. These are minimised by the combined-frequency approach.

Peter showed good commitment to the treatment programme and attended daily to begin with, as advised. On day six of his withdrawal, Peter started to feel his anxiety lifting, although he was still sleepy all the time and very depressed. The SP-6 point was exchanged for SP-2, an acupuncture point effective against depression. The frequency setting was kept at 80 Hz + 1.1 Hz. After 2 more days of treatment, all symptoms were considerably improved. He reported feeling less depressed, anxious and paranoid. His sleep pattern and appetite were back to normal. The treatment stimulation was changed to an alpha 10 Hz frequency for general maintenance and relaxation.

At this stage it is important to explain to the client that there will still be days of anxiety and craving. These symptoms do not simply disappear, and some days will seem particularly difficult to cope with. Also, as stress-coping mechanisms may be several weeks getting back to normal functioning, little everyday stresses will tend to promote an emotional overreaction. I call this the 'storm in a teacup syndrome', but this stage passes quite quickly if EST is continued to help restore equilibrium to the nervous system. Panic attacks are now not uncommon, but if these occur they can be very effectively treated using 2.5 Hz. Continuation of EST is important in order to minimise any panic or stress symptoms. Alcohol is not advised during this period.

Peter felt able to cope with the aid of EST and his attitude remained positive throughout. From day 17, he reported feeling consistently well and looked healthy. Daily treatment was maintained at his own request. On the odd day when he felt a bit low, an 80 Hz frequency was used, which worked very well to lift his spirits. If he had a poor night's sleep, a delta 2.5 Hz frequency was used. His sleep pattern was very good and EST was continued to maintain it. After about 20 days drug free, Peter started to reduce the number of EST sessions gradually, as advised. He started back at full-time work 3 weeks after stopping his cocaine and continued to attend the centre on a weekly basis. We explained that we would continue to work with him for as long as necessary, offering treatment, counselling and support as part of our relapse prevention commitment to our clients.

(This case history, together with some supporting text, has been extracted from the author's comprehensive and informative article, which can be found in full in the CD-ROM ⊙ resource.)

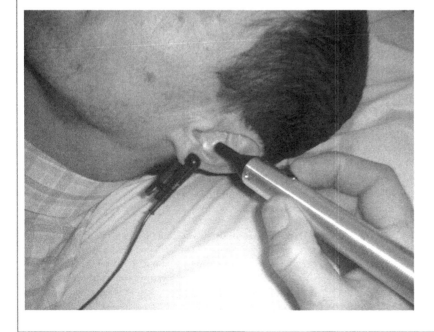

**Figure 9.15.2** Treating ear points: irradiation of the lower concha with the AAA LED attachment. Also visible, ear clip (Body Clock Health Care) at the Jérôme/Sleep point.

CASE Study 9.15.1 **Continued**

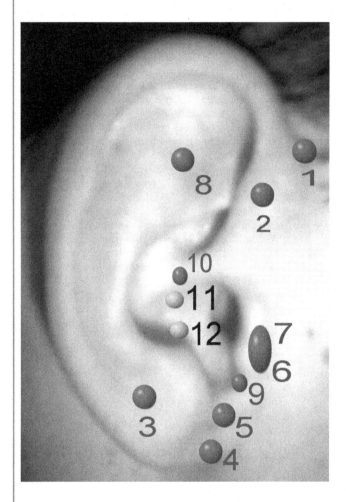

**Figure 9.15.3** Auricular points commonly used in drug dependence at CIC – Drug Services.

Key:
1. Psychosomatic point
2. Weather point
3. Jérôme/sleep point
4. Master cerebral point
5. Antiaggression point
6/7. Outer surface of auricular tragus (6 equivalent to ST-36, 7 to LI-4)
8. *shenmen*
9. ACTH point
10. Point zero
11. Stomach
12. Lung.

Adrenals and Nogier's Antianxiety point are also mentioned. Some researchers will combine these points with a selection of body points, specifically chosen to treat individual symptoms. In China, body points (such as LI-4 and ST-36) are preferred to ear points. LI-4 and P-6 were used in two TEAS (HANS) studies. Ulett and Nichols have recommended using LI-4 alone. Other authors have suggested ST-36 with auricular *shenmen*, the Antiaggression point and Lung (all bilateral, with either EA or LA), or a point 5 mm lateral to the upper end of the nasolabial groove, or LU-7, LI-4 and LI-5 instead of *tim mee* (LA).

It is worthwhile noting that, although some authorities insert needles horizontally under the skin, so that the cartilage is not penetrated, in the NADA protocol needles do penetrate cartilage, to a depth of 1–2 mm. An important question that remains to be addressed is whether results are different with auricular EA if needle (or other electrode) connections are arranged so that current flows from ear to ear, through the head, or simply from one point to another in the same ear.

**Parameters used for alcohol, nicotine and drug withdrawal**
Frequency settings appear to be anything from 5 Hz to 125 Hz, with some researchers using 2/100 Hz DD (Han's collaborators in China), or even modulated frequencies just in the 7–14 Hz range. Han has suggested that, whereas 100 Hz may be appropriate for opiate withdrawal, it is not so useful for treatment of cocaine addiction. Patterson too

recommended ~100 Hz for opiate detox, while the results of prior studies collated by Kroening and Oleson show that poorest results for opiate detox were obtained with 7 Hz stimulation. A number of authors have suggested that 10 Hz may stimulate β-endorphin release, and be appropriate for nicotine withdrawal. Most treatments lasted between 30 and 40 minutes at various intervals, commonly over 1 to 2 weeks. Extra medication was administered in some studies.

With CES, parameters vary considerably depending on which device is used. Some treatments are lengthy – constant stimulation day and night for 7–10 days. Other authors have used shorter treatments of 20 minutes twice daily.

### Caution

Some drugs (including amphetamines and cocaine) can predispose to epileptic-type activity in the brain, particularly during withdrawal. In this situation, patients should be monitored carefully when treated with EA. Seizures can also occur when withdrawing from alcohol (or suffering from alcoholic delirium tremens), and have on occasion been associated with EA.

Because the vagus nerve is stimulated by auricular EA, prolonged and continuous treatment can, occasionally, result in uncomfortable gastric distension. Wen also describes headache, dizziness and even nausea, vomiting and paralytic ileus resulting from overlong bilateral auricular EA.

## CONCLUSION

The misuse of addictive drugs, either self-prescribed or provided through various health care facilities, continues despite a wealth of information available to the public on the deleterious effects of these substances. For acupuncture treatment to infiltrate significantly into a health care system dominated by Western medicine, scientifically conducted, randomised, controlled and blind trials will be necessary to increase knowledge and identify new areas of enquiry. The data collected will also assist in the rational distribution of resources to maximise therapeutic potential.

However, treatments such as acupuncture do not lend themselves to being studied in this way and it is often argued that this reductionist method restricts our view of their potential. There are many subjectively described benefits to alternative therapeutics that we do not yet have the scientific tools to measure. Methods for critically analysing patient narratives would be a useful adjunct to the scientific work so far undertaken.

Many of the studies examined here have been hampered by a high drop-out rate amongst subjects, and difficulties in long-term follow-up. Also, authors have not always stated explicitly whether a study involved manual or electroacupuncture, the exact points treated, the stimulation applied, the duration of treatment, and the precise criteria by which the subjective measure of 'success' is identified. The use of sham acupuncture as a control may also be criticised.

As Reuveny and others have concluded, there are still really no clear indications on whether electrical stimulation adds anything to MA treatment. In part this is because many of the reviews of acupuncture for addiction have not clearly separated out the MA and EA research, but it is also due to a poverty of comparative studies and basic research.

When looking at the many and complex reasons why a person may start to misuse drugs, it is naive to believe that acupuncture alone will help them to detoxify completely and remain free of chemical dependency. To paraphrase Mitchell, the use of acupuncture is a useful adjunct in treating drug addiction, as it allows change rather than forcing it, whilst it nourishes and supports the body and the emotions. The therapist's role is not to take responsibility and 'fix it' for the client. A myriad of social and psychological issues are also likely to need addressing if there is to be lasting success in complete detoxification and rehabilitation.

It is clear that much interesting work has already been achieved and a great deal of data collected regarding the use of acupuncture in the treatment of drug dependence and the management of withdrawal symptoms. The role of acupuncture in rehabilitation and relapse prevention is less clear, however, and may require quite different strategies. It has sometimes been argued, for example, that the value of auricular acupuncture in dependence is not that it helps withdrawal, but that it makes the patient more likely to access other services. For the future, more research, both quantitative *and* qualitative, needs to be carried out in order to identify clearly the place of acupuncture within the overall treatment programme for this group of people.

## SUMMARY

Some key points in this chapter are:

- It is important to distinguish between physical and psychological dependence in deciding treatment strategies
- Many protocols use auricular acupuncture at a standard selection of points
- It is still unclear whether there are advantages to using EA rather than MA
- Most systematic reviews show that acupuncture has not been effective for smoking cessation, although several French trials show good results
- Acupuncture treatment is best used within a wider programme that deals with not only the consequences but also the causes of addiction.

### Additional material in the CD-ROM resource

In the electronic version of this chapter, considerable additional material is presented on addiction in general, treatment using other acupuncture modalities and CES, and details of many specific studies.

**9.15** Summary of relevant studies in the electronic clinical studies database (number of studies)

| Condition | EA | Other |
|---|---|---|
| **Addiction and withdrawal** | | |
| Alcohol | 13 | 37 |
| Nicotine | 36 | 69 |
| Opiates | 35 | 27 |
| Cocaine | 1 | 16 |
| Other drugs | 0 | 2 |
| Mixed/unspecified studies | 11 | 21 |

## RECOMMENDED READING

*An excellent textbook, with contributions by Michael Smith, Wen Hsiang-lai and others:*
Lowinson JH, Ruiz P, Millman RB, with Langrod JG 1997 (eds) Substance Abuse. A comprehensive textbook. Williams and Wilkins, Philadelphia (3rd edn)

*The pioneering report on EA for drug withdrawal:*
Wen HL, Cheung SYC Treatment of drug addiction by acupuncture and electrical stimulation. Asian Journal of Medicine. 1973 April; 9(4): 138–41 [reprinted in American Journal of Acupuncture. 1973 April–June; 1(2): 71–5]

*A good non-technical review:*
Mitchell ER 1995 Fighting Drug Abuse with Acupuncture: The treatment that works. Pacific View Press, Berkeley, CA

*A very useful overview:*
Culliton PD, Kiresuk TJ Overview of substance abuse acupuncture treatment research; Discussion of substance abuse treatment. Journal of Alternative and Complementary Medicine. 1996 Spring; 2(1): 149–60, 161–5

*A small study with some good practical suggestions:*
Choy DSJ, Lutzker L, Meltzer L Effective treatment for smoking cessation. American Journal of Medicine. 1983 Dec; 75(6): 1033–6

*An excellent piece of research on the role of electrostimulation in withdrawal:*
Reuveny G 1999 Acupuncture research: heroin addiction and detoxification. MSc dissertation. Northern College of Acupuncture, York, UK

# 9.16 APPETITE REGULATION AND WEIGHT CONTROL

Topics covered in this chapter are weight gain, weight loss, anorexia and bulimia.

## CRAVING AND CULTURE

Substance abuse and eating disorders, particularly those involving excessive eating, are closely connected. Both can be seen as forms of addiction. There are differences, however, between appetite, hunger and craving. The first is more psychological/emotional, the second more physiological. With the third, a healthy appetite tips over into the pathological, a compulsive want (not need) of food.

## WEIGHT GAIN AND ACUPUNCTURE

Weight gain occurs more commonly in women than men, and tends to increase with age and a slower metabolism. An increase of 20% above the expected weight for gender, age and height can be regarded as abnormal. Being overweight adversely affects health and can shorten lifespan, predisposing to cancer and cardiovascular conditions. It also contributes to infertility in women. Food restriction (within limits) may improve health and increase longevity. Weight loss increases the likelihood of becoming pregnant in obese infertile women. A large number of different Western medical interventions have been attempted for obesity, many of which are of questionable benefit.

TCM syndromes involving obesity may include Spleen and Stomach *qi* deficiency, Liver *yang* excess with Liver *qi* stagnation, and Kidney *qi* or *yin* deficiency. Manual acupuncture (MA), electroacupuncture (EA), probe TENS (pTENS), auricular transcutaneous electrical acupoint stimulation (TEAS) and laser acupuncture (LA) have frequently been used for obesity. Yet, despite the many studies published, and the existence of plausible mechanisms to explain how acupuncture might take effect, randomised controlled trials (RCTs) of MA for obesity have not all had positive outcomes, and in general the evidence is poor that acupuncture is clinically effective for weight loss. In some cases, it was clearly less useful than control treatments.

However, obesity is multifactorial, and acupuncture may influence some contributory factors more than others. In particular, it appears to have more effect on hunger and craving than on weight loss per se. Some authors have concluded that, although there may be short-term benefits from acupuncture, lasting weight reduction depends on being able to establish satisfactory eating patterns and active or aerobic exercise schedules initially, and then sustaining such dietary/lifestyle changes.

Seed (pellet) pressure has been used in a number of studies. In several of these, repeated pressing on ear points (or on seeds in fatty body areas) before meals was an important part of the protocol. Pressure over needles implanted in body points is another approach. Simple body point acupressure has also been emphasised in addition to auricular stimulation. Such disciplined 'reminders' of the aims of treatment could well act to condition patients to modify their behaviour and reduce their food intake, whatever the other effects of acupoint stimulation. For some, it may also distract from cravings.

Magnetic press needles have been used in a similar manner, as well as stimulating an implanted staple with a weak magnet. MA, cupping and magnetic stimulation have been combined. Auricular acupressure without seeds or pellets is another, even simpler approach.

## WEIGHT LOSS, ANOREXIA AND BULIMIA

Weight loss can be associated with many conditions, from iatrogenic nausea and vomiting to cancer. In anorexia and bulimia nervosa, the cause is more psychological than physical, with a distorted self-image and intense fear of fatness, and yet a preoccupation with food (and sometimes exercise).

In anorexia, weight loss due to dieting is often associated with self-induced vomiting and laxative abuse, and may lead to amenorrhoea. Those with chronic anorexia are at risk of osteopenia (reduced bone synthesis) and osteoporosis (loss of bone mass).

In bulimia, which may occur independently from anorexia, satiety mechanisms are deficient and the fear of fatness is in direct conflict with an uncontrollable and intense hunger. It involves an obsessional preoccupation with the adverse consequences of eating, with frequent episodes of ritualistic bingeing (especially on carbohydrates), usually terminated by vomiting. Apart from the psychological suffering involved, it can entail complications such as fluid and electrolyte imbalances (largely the result of purging and laxative abuse).

Ryodoraku has been used for anorexia. Other forms of EA have been explored as well for a possible role in anorexia and bulimia. EA has also been used for stress induced by fasting.

**Points used** According to traditional acupuncture theory, points on the Stomach and Spleen meridians should have specific effects on stomach function. Thus ST-34 EA has been found to inhibit gastric acid secretion and SP-4 EA to decrease gastric peristalsis in cases of obesity. In another EA protocol, targeted specifically at excessive appetite, SP-4 has been alternated with ST-21, with intradermal needling and acupressure at the points between consultations.

Given the possible links between bulimia and nausea in terms of 5HT$_3$ involvement, it would be logical to investigate the effects of P-6 EA on the condition, particularly when P-6 would be indicated from a TCM perspective. The 'AcuOne,' a device specifically for P-6 stimulation prior to meals, is marketed in the UK for appetite control.

Points such as BL-20, ST-36, ST-40, SP-6, abdominal points on the Stomach or Spleen meridians or the Conception Vessel (or other abdominal points local to fatty deposits) and additional points such as SJ-6, LIV-3, LI-4 and ST-37 have also been used.

As for auricular points, both the Stomach and Hunger points have been used. The latter has also been suggested for food craving during tobacco withdrawal. Other points used include Mouth, Spleen, *shenmen*, *sanjiao* and points for other parts of the upper digestive tract, together with further points selected according to the TCM syndrome. Use of auricular points and body points together may have some synergistic benefits.

**Parameters used** Low-frequency (LF) stimulation has been used for craving (at low intensity) and obesity (at high intensity). Strong dense-disperse (DD) stimulation is another possibility. Stimulation at 2 Hz, 100 Hz or 2/100 Hz DD was at all settings found equally effective in preventing weight loss during acute heroin withdrawal.

Short-term therapy (four to five sessions) may be less effective than sustained treatment (cycles of 12 sessions).

## POSSIBLE MECHANISMS

Physiologically, within the hypothalamus there is a feedback loop between the 'feeding centre' (the lateral hypothalamus), and the 'satiety centre' (the ventromedial hypothalamus). Stimulation of the former increases appetite, and of the latter decreases it. The mediobasal arcuate nucleus is also implicated in regulation of food intake.

EA may affect both lateral hypothalamus and gastroelectric activity, leading to appetite suppression. However, EA (at body points) may also counter some physiological effects of gastric distension, so presumably *increasing* appetite There are many contradictions evident in results of further studies on this point; however, it is unclear whether these are due to differences in initial state (obese or not), the acupoints stimulated, or other factors.

Craving and dopaminergic reward pathways are involved in many forms of addiction. Central dopamine (DA) and endogenous opioids are implicated in normal feeding behaviour, and so also in some eating disorders. Serotonin (5HT) is also involved, particularly in those with carbohydrate cravings (carbohydrate and alcohol craving may involve similar serotonergic pathways).

Peripherally, increased 5HT may reduce appetite. Thus both L-tryptophan and 5-hydroxytryptophan (5HTP), the immediate precursor to 5HT, have been used as short-term appetite suppressants. The obsessional nature of some anorexia may involve 5HT$_{2A}$ receptors. Bulimic behaviour, on the other hand, may involve vasopressin and 5HT$_3$ receptors.

Sympathoadrenal hypofunction, with raised aldosterone and saline blood levels, may be responsible for the oedema involved in some simple obesity that is responsive to acupuncture. Vagal hyperfunction, if implicated, would indicate a role for auricular stimulation.

## SUMMARY

Some key points in this chapter are:

- Acupuncture is only a part of the treatment for appetite regulation and weight control
- Motivation, dietary change and active (aerobic) exercise are also key factors
- Without these, treatment is likely to have only a short-term effect
- Treatment is best kept simple, using a few tried and tested points.

Additional material in the CD-ROM resource

There is further information on the topics presented in this short chapter in the CD-ROM resource.

**9.16** Summary of relevant studies in the electronic clinical studies database (number of studies)

| Condition | EA | Other |
|---|---|---|
| **Weight reduction** | | |
| Appetite regulation and weight control | 18 | 30 |
| Lipolysis | 0 | 1 |

# RECOMMENDED READING

*A useful general book, with many practical suggestions:*
Kirschenbaum DS, Johnson WG, Stalonas PM Jr 1987 Treating Childhood and Adolescent Obesity. Pergamon Press, Oxford

*Examples of acupuncture-based popular books on weight loss:*
Blate M, Watson GC 1985 How to Lose Weight Easily: The acugenic method. Arkana, London

Sun XQ 1988 How to Reduce your Weight? A therapeutic method of acupuncture. Shandong Science and Technology Press, Jinan
Warren FZ, Berland T 1978 Lose Weight the Acupuncture Way. Cornerstone Library, New York

*A challenging article on the subject:*
Pöntinen PJ [Acupuncture in obesity, a therapy based upon science?]. Akupunktur. 1995; 23(4): 240–4

# PART THREE
## TECHNOLOGY AND PRACTICE

## INTRODUCTION

Following the account of electroacupuncture (EA) research that forms Part 2 of this book, the next chapters focus on the technology involved and its application in clinical practice.

**Chapter 10** offers an overview of the different families of electrotherapeutic and other equipment that may be of interest to those wishing to expand their repertoire beyond the traditional tools of needles, moxa and cups. Many interesting and some extraordinary avenues have been explored in this very creative field. The chapter ends with a brief discussion on the need for technology in acupuncture.

**Chapter 11** briefly outlines factors to consider when deciding what equipment might be appropriate for your own practice, followed by an account of pertinent design, safety, legal and marketing issues. The second half of the chapter comprises an annotated listing of some commonly used devices, with suggestions on those that may be useful in a general acupuncture practice.

**Chapter 12** covers the practical aspects of basic electroacupuncture and other non-traditional acupuncture methods. The focus is on electrostimulation, although laser acupuncture (LA) and magnets are also briefly described. In the second half of the chapter, the necessary precautions and contraindications are considered. In many ways this is the most important chapter in the book for those who wish to apply the methods described.

**Chapter 13** on the integration of EA in clinical practice, is again in two sections. In the first, intention and an awareness of treatment levels (neurophysiological and TCM, informational and energetic) are emphasised. Illustrations are then given of various possible simple strategies, treatment duration and non-response are discussed, and examples given of how different modalities can be combined.

**Chapter 14** the final chapter in the book, draws together various themes, some obvious, some more subterranean, that have been woven into the fabric of the work. Some of these are enumerated, and the tapestry examined as a whole. The chapter ends with a look to what the future may hold for the rapidly changing field of non-traditional acupuncture.

# Ten

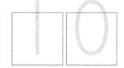

## The technology of acupuncture

### With contributions by Ken Andrews, J Gordon Gadsby and Jacqueline Young

Maintaining a balance between inner awareness and the technology we use to extend this into the outer world in action is a precarious business. In complementary as well as conventional medicine, methods fostering inner rhythm and harmony have too often been supplanted by alien rhythm and discordance. However, some modern inventions definitely have a place in acupuncture practice.

Here the main categories of such equipment are described in brief, touching on their theoretical rationale and major uses. They fall roughly into two classes – those where something is definitely being 'done to' the patient, and those where the emphasis is rather on eliciting some reaction from them in more of a two-way interaction. Among the former are conventional stimulators (EA, TENS/TEAS, pTENS and their variants), vibration, sound and ultrasound, and among the latter integrated measurement and treatment systems (e.g. ryodoraku and its derivatives, EAV), treatments using the body's own signals rather than external stimulation, and polarity agents.

## ELECTRICAL STIMULATION

Acupuncture methods can be subdivided according to whether there is awareness of *deqi* and/or the stimulation itself, and how strongly the latter is perceived. In electroacupuncture (EA), transcutaneous electrical nerve or acupoint stimulation (TENS or TEAS) and handheld probe TENS (pTENS), stimulation is usually strongly perceived.

### EA and TENS/TEAS

EA and TENS machines are very similar, the main difference being that currents for EA are not so strong. Further, EA machines must provide a charge-balanced output, whereas this has not always been thought necessary for TENS. For EA, biphasic charge-balanced square waves are more commonly used today than spike or sawtooth waveforms (see Fig 3.5 on page 30).

## Handheld probes (pTENS)

A common variant of TENS, sometimes known as pTENS (for point or punctate TENS) is the handheld device that applies current to points on the skin surface through a small blunt probe, combining the precision of needling with non-invasive stimulation. Some have different probe tips, and others an array of 'pulse-pins'. Many are small enough to fit in a pocket, but some, connected to a larger unit, are suitable only for clinical use.

## Variants on TENS

Variants on TENS include the Codetron (developed by Bruce Pomeranz's group in Canada in the 1980s), where electrodes are energised in random order, and the Japanese Trimix 303H, which offers a more soothing stimulation through a repeating regular sequence of electrode activation. TSE (transcutaneous spinal electroanalgesia), developed by the British medical acupuncturist Alexander Macdonald, uses electrodes directly over the spine to obtain the effects of implanted spinal column stimulation but non-invasively. There are many other devices that deliver current transcutaneously.

## Piezoelectric stimulators – the art of shock

Piezoelectric stimulators produce brief electrical high-voltage discharges in response to a mechanical shock to a crystal (see Fig. 3.14 on page 35). Generally around 5–10 impulses per point are recommended. These devices are cheap and do not require batteries, but have a limited life. They are employed in some Japanese and German acupuncture systems, and are useful for insect and snakebites.

## Direct current (DC) devices – working at the sensory level

Direct current is generally contraindicated for extended periods of EA. However, stimulation via both needles and handheld probes for only a few seconds is very much part of ryodoraku, one of the most influential of EA systems. A different approach is high-voltage pulsed galvanic (HVPG), a TENS modality using surface pads and very narrow pulses, mostly for non-healing wounds and oedema. HVPG has also been applied to acupoints.

A number of prominent French acupuncturists, including Roger de la Fuye and Paul Nogier, recommended monophasic stimulation. Conventional pulsed galvanic stimulation (using moistened sponge electrodes, wider pulses and lower amplitudes), though unfashionable, still has acupuncture proponents in Europe. Another approach is action potential simulation therapy (APS), in which nerve action potentials are simulated through application of monophasic stimulation.

One particular application of DC or monophasic stimulation is iontophoresis (ion transfer) using surface electrodes. One view is that this occurs via acupoints, where electrical skin resistance is low. In China dampened herbal packs are sometimes employed as surface electrodes, particularly for elderly patients who may not benefit from strong needle EA.

## Microcurrent stimulation – subthreshold systems

The methods described above all use milliampère (mA) currents strong enough to produce a sensation, and so activate afferent nerves. Microcurrent stimulation uses microampère (μA) currents (< 1 mA), may not even result in sensation and produces its effects without involving action potentials in the nerves.

There are few good clinical studies on microcurrent. Its proponents often suggest that it is of the same order as the body's own electrical signals, and invoke the Arndt–Schulz law as a rationale for its use. As Motoyama found, strong stimuli produce a generalised autonomic reaction, but subthreshold pulses a meridian-specific response.

The indications for microcurrent are similar to those of other forms of electrotherapy. However, because it does not trigger nerve discharges, its effects on pain are possibly secondary to changes in microcirculation and resulting reductions in inflammation.

Most microcurrent devices provide some form of monophasic output with much longer pulse durations than TENS or EA. There are protocols for tissue repair, oedema, muscle strengthening and lymph drainage. Handheld probes (or surface pads) can be used to 'sandwich' a problem area, for instance, either side of a muscle or at its origin and insertion. Probes can also be placed sequentially around an area, in circle or spiral patterns (Fig. 10.1). Moist probes can even be used through thin clothing. Microcurrent probes have also been designed for intraoral, nasal and aural application, for a temporary facelift, and for roller application.

Microcurrent originated as an offshoot of ryodoraku, but has grown up in the American physical therapy (PT) and chiropractic communities, so much of the literature emphasises working with muscle rather than meridian flow and acupoints. However, microcurrent (although not called that) was very much part of Paul Nogier's system of auriculotherapy.

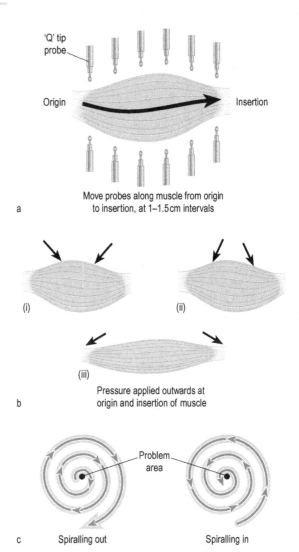

**Figure 10.1** Microcurrent probe applications. (Adapted with permission from Greenlee, Greenlee and Wing 1999.) (a) 'Parallel' technique. (b) 'Series' techniques: (i) to relax muscle; (ii) to strengthen muscle; (iii) Golgi tendon technique (muscle stretched). (c) Circling or 'swirling the dragon', with probes applied around problem area.

There are claims that microcurrent is as effective as acupuncture, with more rapid benefits and carry-over effects lasting longer than those of TENS or EA.

Microcurrent variants include the MicroACE device, a simple method for patients to use at home that appears to have tissue-healing effects in addition to providing pain relief. Better known is the AlphaStim, developed by neurobiologist Daniel Kirsch, with its semirandomised waveform (Fig. 10.2a). The AlphaStim can also be used for CES (see next section), and combines well with other treatment modalities. The Liss pain suppression device and Thomas Wing's Accu-O-Matic are other microcurrent/CES stimulators (Fig. 10.2b, c).

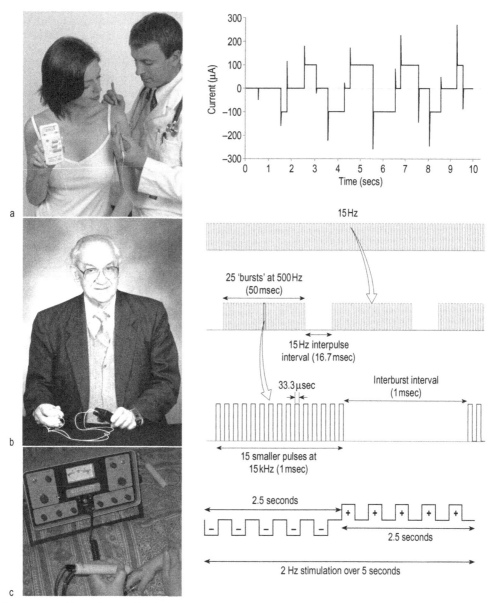

**Figure 10.2** Microcurrent and its application. (a) AlphaStim, with probe electrodes. (b) Saul Liss, holding Liss Cranial Stimulator and sponge electrodes. (c) Accu-O-Matic, with Q-tip electrode. Note different waveforms and methods of application for each device. (a) Reproduced with permission from Electromedical Products International, Inc.; (b) photograph courtesy of Saul Liss, Medi Consultants, Inc.; (c) photograph courtesy of Julian Scott; waveform reproduced with permission from Greenlee, Greenlee & Wing 1999. Patent on Tsunami Wave granted 1984 to Thomas W Wing, DC, ND, LAc.)

## Cranial electrotherapy stimulation (CES)

One form of microcurrent treatment that is a useful addition to any acupuncture practice is cranial electrotherapy stimulation. CES, closely allied to auricular acupuncture, is well documented as a relaxing treatment with potentially beneficial effects in the treatment of depression, anxiety,

insomnia and drug withdrawal. Most forms of CES use earlobe clip electrodes, or mastoid pads. The most researched and sophisticated form of CES is SPES (subperception electrical stimulation). Sadly, this is not currently commercially available.

In a very different variant of CES, 'low-energy emission therapy' (LEET), a lollipop-like emitter is placed in the mouth and energised with athermal radio frequency sine waves modulated at LF. The resulting sleep-inducing effect has been shown in double-blind studies to be attributable to the electrical stimulation rather than oral satisfaction.

## Electrolipolysis

Electrolipolysis, or electrically induced dissolving of fat, was discovered by chance in France when a Vietnamese doctor, Dang vu Nguyen, noted atrophy of fatty tissue during EA treatment. Controlled lipolysis is possible with long needles within the fatty layer under the skin, or using surface electrodes. Results may be good for *peau d'orange*, and better around hips and thighs than on abdomen or arms. A related application is the use of DC microcurrents to treat tumours. The resultant reductions in tumour size are significant, and synergistic with concurrent localised chemotherapy. Both electrolipolysis and tumour treatment should be undertaken only by those properly trained and qualified to do so.

## Electrodes

EA is usually applied through ordinary acupuncture needles. Thinner needles present greater electrical resistance; more current will be needed to achieve adequate stimulation. Needles that are insulated except at the tip ensure that *deqi* is elicited from muscular, not skin, afferents.

Surface electrodes come in various forms (Fig. 10.3). Larger ones, which require less precise point location, also require less current for effective stimulation, so that batteries last longer. Some authors, however, prefer using smaller electrodes (c. 1 cm² in area) on precisely located acupoints. Strips of silicon rubber or wet cotton lint are convenient for nail (*jing*) points. Various types of intraoral electrodes are also available (Fig. 10.4). Moistened 'Q-tip' or felt-tipped

probes (Fig. 10.2), commonly supplied with microcurrent stimulators, enable shorter treatments than surface electrodes.

Surface electrodes, however, remain the mainstay of most electrotherapy practice. Carbonised silicon rubber ones do not have a long life, and may need to be replaced every 6 months or so. Self-adhesive or pregelled electrodes for single-patient use are simpler and more practical to use nowadays, particularly at home. Some types last for 20–30 treatments, or even longer. Low-cost disposables are convenient for clinic use. Self-adhesive electrodes, however, may draw more power from an electrical stimulator than ordinary rubber ones used with a gel.

An alternative to flat surface electrodes is Japanese 'silver spike point' (SSP) electrodes. These combine attributes of both needles and surface pads, being non-invasive but shaped so that pressure and charge are concentrated at a point (Fig. 10.5). They may be more effective than TENS pads, but less so than needles, and are not readily available outside Japan.

For treating ear points, EA or pTENS is usual. However, since it is not practical to give long treatments using a handheld probe, auricular clips are available (Fig. 10.6), although these are not suited to commonly used points such as Lung and Stomach. An alternative approach has been to fill the concha with a mouldable conductive electrode on the principle that current will flow preferentially through the same points of low electrical resistance that are indicated for treatment.

Roller electrodes can be useful sometimes, and come in a variety of shapes and sizes. Voll used a roller with LF monophasic current at comfortable intensity for energy stagnation in, for example, the local treatment of trigeminal neuralgia. Rollers have also been used in some electrical measurement systems.

Electrical and even magnetic versions of the traditional seven-star or plum blossom hammer are available.

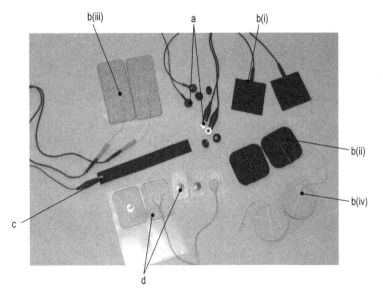

**Figure 10.3** A selection of surface electrodes. (a) Small electrodes. (b) Large electrodes: (i) flat carbonised silicon rubber electrodes, with hole for lead pin; (ii) self-adhesive silicon rubber electrodes; (iii, iv) standard self-adhesive electrodes. (c) Conductive rubber strip used for *jing* Well point stimulation. (d) Large and small electrodes with press stud connectors. (Photograph by Riccardo Cuminetti.)

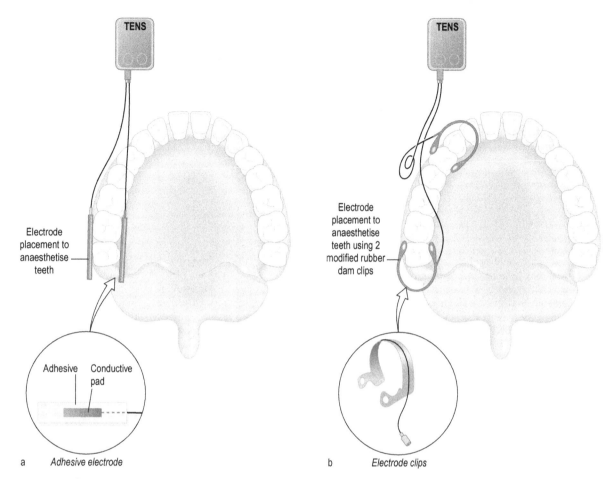

**Figure 10.4** Different intraoral electrode placements. (a) Conductive adhesive strip electrodes. (b) Modified rubber dam clips positioned for working on two teeth in one session. (Courtesy of J Gordon Gadsby and Michael W Flowerdew.)

**Figure 10.5** Close-up of the small electrodes shown in Figure 10.3. (a) Button electrodes, (i) with and (ii) without central magnet. (b) Silver spike point (SSP). (c) Chinese version of SSP, rubberised. (Photograph by Riccardo Cuminetti.)

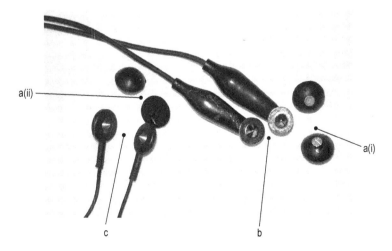

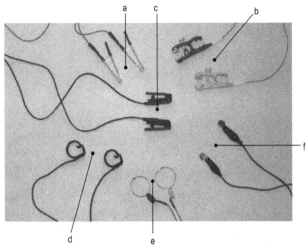

**Figure 10.6** Various ear clip electrodes. (a) AlphaStim (old version). (b) SPES. (c) Body Clock. (d) Healthpoint. (e) Sprung hoops, supplied with some Chinese devices. (Courtesy of Scarboroughs Ltd.) (f) Magnets (note how simply lead clips are held in contact). (Photograph by Riccardo Cuminetti.)

In summary, the only real difference between EA and TEAS is that one employs needles and the other surface electrodes. This restricts EA to clinical use by trained practitioners, whereas TENS/TEAS may be used both in the clinic by minimally trained staff and by patients in everyday life. This may give TENS/TEAS the advantage as it can be available at any time and for longer periods of treatment. It may also be more comfortable.

Handheld probes (pTENS) may be even more convenient in a busy clinic, for patient use, or when travelling. Both sensory and motor level stimulation are possible. However, one limitation they have is that treatment cannot be longer than a minute or so (it may become too uncomfortable), nor can several points be treated at once.

## HEAT AND COLD

Traditionally, 'acupuncture and moxibustion' are considered together as a single form of therapy, *zhenjiu* (*zhen* = acupuncture, *jiu* = moxibustion), acupuncture being particularly useful for acute conditions and moxibustion more appropriate for chronic ones. However, some practitioners (and patients) find the moxa smoke annoying, and may even develop allergic reactions to it, or other respiratory complications. As a result many alternatives have been explored, including brief diathermy currents passed through the acupuncture needles, halogen lamps, even hair dryers and fans, sometimes used in conjunction with herbal applications.

A useful ancillary device for warming larger areas, and an alternative to the moxa box, is the TDP far-infrared lamp. This provides a more deeply penetrating heat than that from standard heat lamps and is easily combined with MA or EA. What differentiates TDP from ordinary heat is the radiation spectrum given out, which is claimed to coincide with the 'biospectrum' of the human body. Far infrared may affect immune function, circulation, sleep and growth. It has been used for fungal skin conditions in children and to enhance lactation in breast-feeding mothers.

This principle of *bioresonance* – applying frequencies that match those of various physiological processes – is used in other, stronger 'multifrequency lamps', claimed to benefit prostatitis, thyroid problems, multiple sclerosis (MS), bronchitis and asthma, and even spinal cord injury.

Unlike heat, cold is rarely used in TCM, and may well be contraindicated in chronic painful disorders. There are a number of acupoint cooling devices, however, and interesting research has been carried out on the effects of cooling needles (for instance, on salivary cortisol concentrations).

## NON-THERMAL RADIATION METHODS

### Microwaves and millimetre waves (extremely high frequency)

Extremely high frequency (EHF) millimetre waves appear to have important clinical applications. Their use in acupuncture, first proposed in 1970, has been most researched in the Ukraine. As with far infrared, their effect seems to depend on resonance with characteristic GHz 'eigenfrequencies' of the human organism. Hence the alternative name for this type of treatment: 'microwave resonance therapy' (MRT).

EHF is generated either at fixed but tunable frequencies or in the form of a random or 'noise' output. Specific frequencies are tuned to resonance in response to the patient's awareness of subjective changes in sensation (the 'sensor reaction'), or using techniques like EAV, muscle testing or even dowsing. However, some practitioners prefer the less specific noise outputs, or devices that scan through a range of possible frequencies (Fig.10.7).

Mikhail Teppone, one of the chief proponents of EHF treatment in the West, advocates that it be used according to TCM principles. Shorter treatment durations may be tonifying (warming), and longer ones reducing (cooling). Saul Liss, in contrast, considers EHF to be primarily reinforcing. Indeed, Liss, together with Norman Shealy, has

**Figure 10.7** Extremely high frequency (EHF) stimulation.
(a) SHeLI TENS. Note use of ordinary TENS electrodes, despite output with a GHz component. (b) Artsakh-03, showing applicator heads on supporting arms. ((a) Courtesy of the Shealy Institute; (b) reproduced with permission from AcuVision Ltd.)

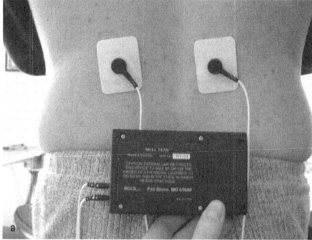

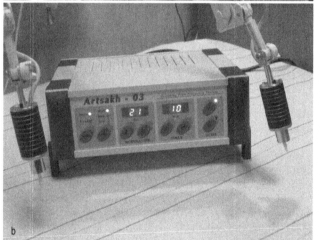

developed an American version of EHF, the 'SheLi TENS', with a noise-like signal similar in some ways to that produced by the 1919 Electreat device that inspired Shealy's pioneering work on TENS in the 1960s. He believes that EHF may be superior to both TENS and microcurrent.

Another noise-like signal is produced by the MRT® Bioenergizer, a handheld device developed by Bob Beck, another American, which produces an 'impulse wave' from a spark discharge.

## Low-intensity lasers and polarised light

The mechanisms of laser acupuncture (LA) can be considered the same as for laser stimulation in general (low-intensity light therapy, LILT). The effects of laser seem very similar to those of the much cheaper ultrasound modality, if possibly more rapid. Whether LA is more effective than other forms of intense monochromatic light or infrared

is still controversial, although there does currently appear to be more research support for LILT than for non-laser light treatment using light-emitting diodes (LEDs), for example.

Proponents of the less expensive and more robust LED devices argue that it is *colour* and intensity, not *coherence*, that is important. Rather than intensity, it may even be the information carried by the light that is significant.

In China, light is often passed through a hollow needle for deeper irradiation, or used in conjunction with ordinary needling. Much Russian research, in contrast, has been devoted to exploring LA as an alternative to MA.

The cheapest lasers are the equivalent of lecture pointers. The more expensive units used by physiotherapists often come with an acupoint locator or electrical stimulation facility, or the option for linking to ultrasound or interferential machines. Surface electrodes have been designed that incorporate LEDs within them, and LILT is also sometimes combined with pulsed or static magnetic field stimulation.

Polarised light is appropriate for superficial conditions, such as non-healing ulcers, skin conditions and joint pain when this is not deep.

An increasingly common method is irradiation of the blood with laser or ultraviolet, either within the body or extracorporeally.

# LOW-INTENSITY ELECTROMAGNETIC FIELDS

## Variable fields – EEG entrainment methods

Of the many different electromagnetic stimulators available, some explicitly combine electric and magnetic fields, whereas others depend primarily on magnetic field effects. The Swiss MitoSan device, for example, emits an unusually wide range of frequencies, from ELF up to a few GHz (in pulses at up to ~220 Hz). The ultraweak signals it produces are applied locally, or over the adrenals or on the feet or neck for a more systemic effect. A version is being developed that provides the body with frequencies measured as 'deficient' in its electromagnetic field.

A similar approach has also been used in a British device, the Empulse, a small pendant that can be individually programmed for a particular patient with up to 16 different electromagnetic frequencies in the EEG range. These may be selected according to the patient's symptom picture, or using a method such as AK (applied kinesiology). Originally frequencies were selected after an analysis of the output from an innovative form of piezoelectric EEG detector. They were then programmed into the device to boost EEG power where it was deemed 'deficient'. Treatment response was apparently better when a fixed frequency at approximately the heart rate was included, along with the individually programmed ones. One version of the Empulse, the Aegis, provides a 28-day standard programme of changing frequencies.

The principle of applying low-power EEG frequencies in treatment has also been used with the 'Vegasom' device by Peter Mandel in what he calls 'brainwave induction therapy',
although here the 'missing' frequencies are determined according to his own idiosyncratic interpretation of Kirlian photography or measurements at auricular or back acupoints. Signals are fed back to patients as standard programmes of electrical stimuli to points on the forearm.

## Static fields

There is a long history of using magnetism as a means of treatment in China and elsewhere. Permanent magnets, which are inexpensive and readily available, are frequently used in conjunction with acupuncture, often on acupoints to prolong the effect of a clinical treatment and on *ashi* points for pain. Some types can double as surface electrodes, and be positioned over press-needles in ear or body points. Small magnetic spheres have been used instead of press-needles; larger magnets can be used in combination to treat the whole body.

Nerve conduction is enhanced by magnetic fields. Thus magnets have been used to amplify and stabilise dowsing responses, the O-ring test and Vegatesting (see below, page 300), all of which involve subtle motor activity on the part of the operator. On the other hand, magnets used by a patient may suppress their symptoms, reduce vulnerability to external perturbation, and so block or bias subsequent electrical acupoint measurements.

# VIBRATION, SOUND AND ULTRASOUND

Although classified as massage equipment in the US, one interesting device is the so-called *Qi Gong* machine (QGM), or '*qigong* energy simulator'(Fig.10.8). To be effective, this does not have to be in close contact with the skin, as it is based on low-frequency sound rather than vibration (it even works through thin clothing). Developed by Lu Yanfang of the Chinese National Institute of Electro-Acoustics, it emits both infrasound and a magnetic field, semirandomly at around 8–14 Hz, and is claimed to simulate at least part of the energy emitted from the hands of healers.

Patients often find the QGM surprisingly relaxing, if not 'hypnotic', and it has some interesting effects on the EEG.

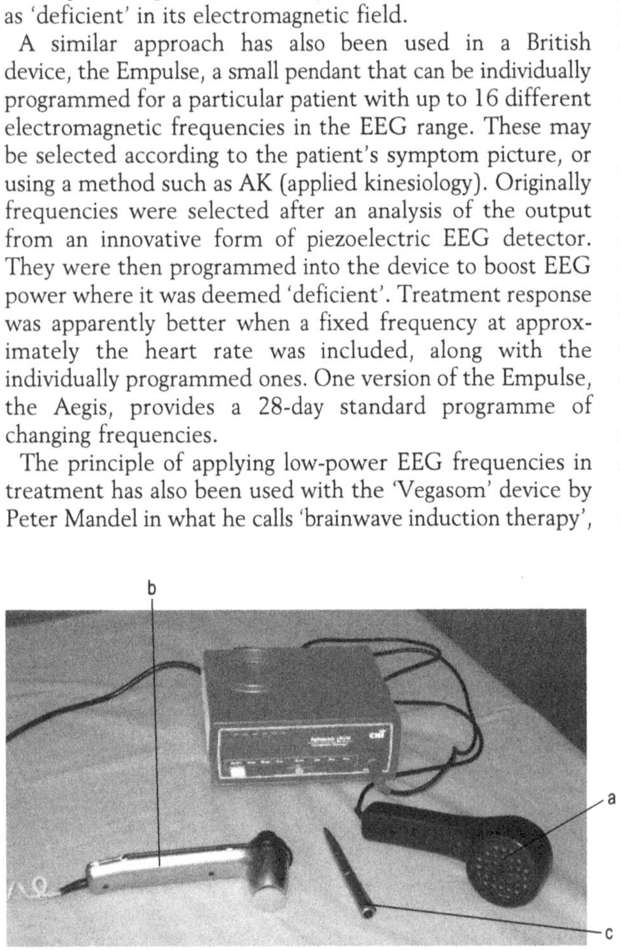

**Figure 10.8** Applying vibration. (a) Infrasound *Qi Gong* machine. (b) Audio frequency Novasonic. (c) Pen style vibrator, suitable for more precise acupoint stimulation. Note relative sizes. (Photograph by Riccardo Cuminetti.)

It is claimed to be beneficial for a wide spectrum of conditions. The QGM is generally applied at midline points, although use at KI-1 can be invigorating.

Audio frequency vibration (at 150–600 Hz) was already used at acupoints in the 1940s by Jean Leplus, an associate of George Soulié de Morant. Leplus considered that lower frequencies were more sedating, and higher ones more tonifying, with a neutral effect at around 300 Hz. Pulse changes were used to guide frequency selection. Other sonic devices for use at acupoints have also been devised, such as Jean Lamy's 'phonophar' in the 1960s.

To prevent tolerance to repetitive stimulation and for relaxation, music translated into electrical signals has been applied to both auricular and body points. In 'sonoelectric acupuncture anaesthesia', inserted needles have even been submitted directly to the loudspeaker vibrations from broadcast radio, with claims that results were better than with conventional AA, and that the method also relieved the decidedly unpleasant sensations of traction on internal organs during abdominal surgery.

A well-known device in Britain is the 'Novafon' or 'nova-sonic' device ('orthosonic' in the USA). This produces vibration at around 200–8500 Hz. The frequency can be tuned to the most effective setting. Like the QGM, the Novafon can be applied through thin clothing. It is used mainly for musculoskeletal problems.

More popular with many acupuncturists has been 'tama-do', a more aesthetic and intuitive approach devised by Frenchman Fabien Maman, using simple tuning forks and traditional ideas of correspondence between notes and acupoints. The 'acutone' system is a variant of this.

Ultrasound offers more precise and repeatable 'doses' of stimulation. Before LILT became widely accepted, ultrasound devices with soundheads small enough for use on auricular and body acupoints were quite popular. Ultrasound is still an important modality to consider, together with phonophoresis (sonophoresis) – the introduction of substances into the tissues using acoustic or ultrasonic frequencies.

## OTHER FORMS OF STIMULATION

Cupping has been combined with LILT, ultraviolet light, electrical heating and various forms of magnetic stimulation. More widely used than these hybrids is acupoint injection, which is sometimes known as 'mesotherapy' or even 'aquapuncture'. Simple saline, vitamins, herbal preparations, drugs have all been injected. Procaine has been advocated for both trigger point (TrP) injection and Huneke's neural therapy. The resulting prolonged local irritation may be more important than the substance used.

Nevertheless, acupoint injection of homeopathic remedies is widely practised, with claims that their combination is more potent than when they are used separately. Less invasively, remedies can also be rubbed into the skin at acupoints, or – in pill form – affixed to the points. Acupuncture needles have been dipped into (hopefully sterile)

homeopathic remedies in 'homeosinatry', and the vaccaria seeds sometimes taped to ear points soaked in herbal solutions before use. There are also herbal 'magnetic plasters', magnetism being claimed to open the skin pores and so enhance uptake.

## ACUPOINT DETECTION AND MEASUREMENT

Many simple devices for measuring electrical skin resistance are available, often combined with a means of stimulating acupoints in a handheld probe. Despite the often-equivocal results of experimental studies on point detection, their continued use would seem to indicate that they definitely have a part to play in acupuncture practice.

## ELECTRICAL AND OTHER IMAGING METHODS

Kirlian photography, although its results are erratic, still fascinates and appears to have a market. Also available are Peter Mandel's variant, 'energy emission analysis', and the Armenian Acuvision device, which can be used as a method of ion therapy as well as imaging.

Thermography and allied methods are quite cumbersome and have never really proved popular with acupuncturists. Simple handheld infrared thermometers, however, can usefully demonstrate bilateral temperature differentials to patients, as well as the marked changes that can occur with acupuncture treatment.

## INTEGRATED SYSTEMS

Various combination systems that offer both treatment and measurement facilities, and some means of interpreting the latter, are now available. They are very attractive to both practitioners and patients, particularly if computerised. Provided a system is not given some magical authority but is used only as a tool, tested against other methods and with its limitations always in mind, then it may certainly be useful as part of the framework for therapeutic decision making.

The various systems can be divided into those using small probe-type electrodes, like ryodoraku and EAV, and those using larger pad-type electrodes, like the SEG, DFM or AMI.

### Ryodoraku and its derivatives

Of the various integrated measurement and treatment systems that use a handheld probe, ryodoraku is the easiest to master. The origins and fundamentals of the measurement side of this integrated system are outlined in Chapter 5, and its practical aspects in Chapter 12. The 'neurometer' used is very simple (Fig. 10.9), producing DC at 6, 12 or 21 V for

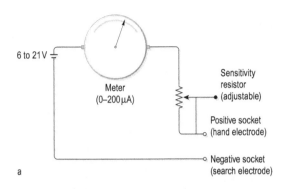

a

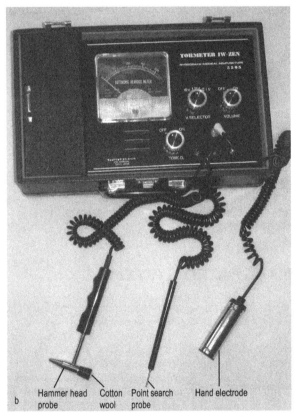

b    Hammer head    Cotton    Point search    Hand electrode
     probe          wool      probe

**Figure 10.9** TORmeter, as used in ryodoraku, with simplified circuit diagram. (Photograph by Riccardo Cuminetti.)

both measurement and stimulation. Current levels are read from a meter. A dry or moistened probe is used.

When gauging the overall state of the patient, measurements are taken at the 'representative measuring point' (RMP) for each meridian. These are identical to the source (*yuan*) points in most cases. Measurements are recorded on a special chart, and those that are higher or lower than an average range are considered significant. Using this chart, it is claimed that a skilled operator may be able to pinpoint a patient's symptoms even before taking a history, and that

ryodoraku can reveal pathology even before it is clinically detectable.

Manual needling, ion granules and 7-second stimulation of points via needles or with the surface probe are used as treatment modalities. For 'total functional adjustment', treatment can be given on traditional lines. For local treatment, the point with the highest reading is stimulated. Readings tend to normalise provided stimulation is directed to the imbalanced ryodoraku. Some practitioners go further, stating that stimulation anywhere will tend to balance readings.

Thomas Wing's 'Accu-O-Matic' (now the 'MENS®-O-Matic'), using Q-tip probes, was developed in 1973 as a gentler alternative to the relatively strong DC stimulation of ryodoraku (see Fig. 10.2c). In addition to microcurrent treatment (and needle stimulation), measurements are possible with minimal probe pressure, and permit rapid ongoing evaluation of treatment. Wing focused on *jing* Well point readings for overall energy assessment, rather than the *yuan* points of traditional ryodoraku.

## Motoyama's AMI

The methods developed by Motoyama Hiroshi for use with his 'apparatus for measuring the function of the meridians and the corresponding internal organs' (AMI) are quite different from those of ryodoraku and EAV. Small (7 × 7 mm) self-adhesive silver–silver chloride (Ag/AgCl) electrodes are positioned on the *jing* Well points. After some minutes, when their electrical balance with the skin has stabilised, they are touched lightly, each in turn, with an electrode probe to allow a brief DC pulse to flow between the *jing* point and two return electrodes, one on each forearm. The resultant readings are automatically recorded and analysed.

The whole process can be carried out in about 10 minutes, is simple, and does not require lengthy training and practice to master. It also has the advantage that pressure and humidity artifacts are minimised, if not eliminated, and there is no feedback loop that might lead the practitioner to influence the measurement process.

In line with other measurement systems, high readings in what Motoyama terms the 'before polarisation' (BP) current (see Fig. 5.12 on page 58) tend to indicate an excited state, and low readings a tendency to chronic disease. He interprets BP as a measure of meridian function. Differences between averaged hand and foot readings are also considered (relatively higher hand readings, for instance, may be associated with a feverish head, emotional excitement and cold feet, and lower hand readings with introversion and a tendency to depression). Complex patterns in BP readings may be easier to interpret if just the highest and lowest AMI readings are considered. Motoyama has found intriguing differences in those with different psychic abilities, and has even shown how BP can be affected by the proximity of others.

# CASE Study 10.1

## The AMI in a patient with lung deficiency
**Jacqueline Young**

### Introduction

The AMI is a high-speed diagnostic electroacupuncture device devised by Dr Hiroshi Motoyama (Fig. 10.10). It measures the electrical conductivity, capacitance and polarisation of the skin tissues and fluids and evaluates the functioning of the acupuncture meridians and their corresponding internal organs.

The AMI measurement yields information on overall vitality, functioning of the nervous system, functioning of the immune system and spinal alignment. In my clinical practice I have found it invaluable for the following:

- *General health screening of 'well' clients and populations.* On an individual level it can clearly identify health strengths and weaknesses. On a wider level it can provide useful epidemiological data for sample populations or clinical groups, for example the classification of different categories of asthma patients according to TCM theory.
- *Accurate evaluation of individual patient's health problems.* The AMI measures can pinpoint the root cause of chronic conditions. It is especially useful in the case of people with multiple, unexplained symptoms that have not responded to orthodox medical investigation and treatment.
- *Evaluation of treatment protocols.* The AMI can be used to monitor and evaluate precisely the effects of ongoing treatment and therapy.
- *Preventive medicine.* The AMI can highlight imbalance in meridian function *prior to* the appearance of obvious symptoms. For example, a person may show elevated immune function and abnormal Lung and Large Intestine measures and then go on to show the first signs of a cold some days later. Early detection by the AMI enables prompt preventive action to be taken.
- *As a 'biofeedback' tool and motivational enhancer for the patient.* Patients find it a useful way of monitoring their own progress. For example, a patient with poor Lung function may be asked to practise simple breathing exercises and can then see the effects of the exercises reflected in subsequent Lung measures.

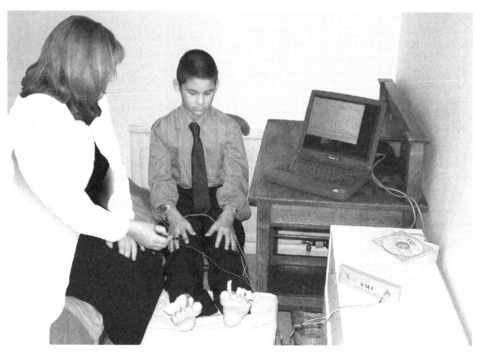

**Figure 10.10** Jacqueline and Michael Young with the AMI device in an informal setting. Note electrodes affixed to *jing/sei* points, only lightly touched with handheld probe, use of two return electrodes, one on each forearm, electrodes on Diaphragm (*kakuyu*) and Stomach branch (*hachiyu*) points, and separation of toes. (Courtesy of Riccardo Cuminetti.)

*(Continued)*

## CASE Study 10.1 Continued

### Clinical practice

I evaluate all new patients with the AMI alongside other standard forms of Oriental medical diagnosis, including pulse diagnosis, tongue analysis, palpation, observation and questioning. Following measurement, the AMI results are explained to the patient and linked in with other diagnostic signs and the patient's current signs and symptoms. The results are used to identify key health targets and to determine treatment strategy. Particular emphasis is placed on the most deficient (*xu* (Chinese)/*kyo* (Japanese)) meridian(s) and on any *yin/yang* (*in/yo*) pair showing marked imbalance. Attention is also paid to overall measures of vitality, nervous system function and immune function. The most excessive meridian(s) is/are also noted. All those showing function within the normal range are identified as the patient's health 'strengths'.

Emphasising evaluation and treatment of the most deficient meridian is a cornerstone of Japanese acupuncture treatment. Although the most excessive (*shi/jitsu*) meridian may be the one most closely linked to any current acute symptoms, the most deficient meridian and corresponding organ is seen as the underlying root cause and the most important one to treat and rebalance.

Treatment may include acupuncture or acupressure based on the acupuncture point recommendations that are part of the AMI printout. These points are based on a series of acupuncture effects tests carried out by Motoyama in the 1980s that looked at the most effective use of front *mu* (*mo*), back *shu* (*yu*), and *yuan* (*gen*) Source points in treating the most deficient meridians. Treatment may also include yoga-based meridian exercises devised by Motoyama and other relevant complementary therapies on the basis of AMI results. On follow-up visits the patient is remeasured with the AMI to evaluate progress

### Case history

#### Presenting symptoms and medical history

James, a 54-year-old male office worker, had suffered from headaches, tiredness and digestive disturbance (bloating and indigestion) for over 10 years. His GP had carried out a range of blood and digestive function tests but all had shown normal. Various medications had been tried but had made no significant difference. There was no previous medical history, apart from a brief recent urinary infection treated with antibiotics, and parents and siblings were all healthy. However, James felt his symptoms were having a very harmful effect on both his working and family life as he constantly felt lethargic, irritable and 'worn out'.

#### AMI test results

Overall measures showed that core vitality (BP = 1717), immune function (IQ = 2720) and nervous system function

(after polarisation, AP = 26.1) were all comfortably within the normal range for the month of measurement (March). However, AMI measures for the individual meridians and corresponding internal organs showed clear imbalance in two meridian pairs: the Lung and Large Intestine meridians and Kidney/Bladder meridians. Of these, the Lung meridian was the most deficient and the Bladder meridian was the most excessive. All other meridians were within the normal range.

### Diagnosis

The normal overall measures were of great importance since they ruled out the possibility that James's fatigue was due to: a lack of core vitality in the body, a nervous system imbalance, or an immune deficiency. The individual measures suggested that the root cause of James's symptoms was Lung deficiency while the Large Intestine and Kidney/Bladder imbalance were linked to his more recent symptoms of bladder infection and increased abdominal bloating following antibiotic treatment. The elevated Bladder reading suggested that some bacteria or bladder inflammation might still be present while the Large Intestine deficiency was likely to be related to imbalance in intestinal flora following antibiotic treatment.

The diagnosis of Lung deficiency was corroborated by tongue and pulse diagnosis since the tongue was pale and flabby with a thin, white coating and the pulse weak and thready, especially in the Lung and Kidney positions.

James was initially surprised by the Lung deficiency diagnosis since he had no obvious lung symptoms or any history of respiratory problems. However further questioning revealed that both his parents had been heavy smokers at home and as a child he had avoided breathing deeply as he hated inhaling the smoke. He had also been exposed to passive smoking in previous jobs and his current job involved sitting in a small, enclosed environment with no opening windows or fresh air. He remained indoors most of the time, both day and night, since his office was attached to his home, and took very little exercise. Examination revealed very poor breathing habits and with mostly shallow breaths. His peak flow measurement was also low at 400 units.

### Treatment

Treatment focused on strengthening James's Lung function and improving his breathing habits. James was taught how to breathe diaphragmatically and advised to practise daily. He agreed to step outside every hour or so at work to take some deep breaths in fresh air and to take a 30-minute walk every evening after work. He was given a respiratory trainer (the Power Breathe™) to improve his respiratory function and taught how to use acupressure on the acupoint Ren-17 to give the lungs a further boost.

## CASE Study 10.1 Continued

He was advised to have a repeat urine test to ensure no infection remained and when this proved negative was recommended cranberry powder to reduce irritation of the bladder. He was also recommended a probiotic supplement to replenish bowel bacteria, a multivitamin and mineral supplement and a zinc supplement to aid tissue repair.

### Outcome

At follow-up 6 weeks later, James reported substantial improvements. He had practised the breathing exercises regularly, taken 'breathing breaks' at work, used the acupressure point and was enjoying his nightly walk. He had much more energy and his headaches had almost disappeared. He also felt more 'mentally alert' at work. His digestion was now almost normal and he experienced indigestion only if he ate certain foods or too quickly. He liked the cranberry juice and had no further urinary symptoms.

The new AMI measure showed substantial improvement in Lung function, with Lung meridian values almost in the normal range. Peak flow had also improved to 550 units. The Bladder, Kidney and Large Intestine measures were all now normal, as were the other individual meridian measures.

### Summary

The AMI measurement clearly identified the root underlying cause of James's symptoms as Lung deficiency linked to poor breathing habits. This meant that simple behavioural changes combined with acupressure and brief supplementation enabled almost total remission of long-standing symptoms to be achieved.

Aside from BP readings, Motoyama further considers the average 'integrated charge' (IQ) as an indicator of general homeostatic metabolic and immune ability, and average 'after polarisation' current as reflecting the state of the autonomic nervous system. AP and BP, the autonomic and meridian systems, appear to maintain a 'dynamic antagonistic functional balance'. Methods such as ryodoraku and EAV all measure AP, not BP.

When it comes to treatment based on AMI measurements, the aim is to increase BP for those meridians where it is low, or for *yin* meridians whose BP is lower than that of the corresponding *yang* meridians, to reduce it where high, and to reduce left–right imbalances. The computerised system analyses the various measures taken, and comes up with a simple selection of *yuan* (gen), *mu* (bo) and back-*shu* (yu) points. It can even allow for seasonal (monthly) changes in readings.

Some of Motoyama's conclusions include:

- Treating the most deficient meridian (often the treatment of choice in Japanese acupuncture) will result in the greatest changes in all meridians, and so the greatest improvement for the patient, with no ill effects at all.
- In particular, stimulation of the *yuan* or back-*shu* point of this meridian results in an overall *qi* increase in all meridians.
- Clinical effectiveness of treating the most excessive meridian (more the emphasis in much Chinese acupuncture) is generally slight.
- In particular, stimulation of the *yuan* point on this meridian results in an overall *qi* decrease in all meridians.
- Stimulation of the *mu* point of the most deficient meridian generates greater *qi* increases in

- meridians in the upper half of the body than in the lower half.
- Conversely, stimulation of the *yuan* point of this meridian produces greater *qi* increase in the lower half of the body.

Another device developed by Motoyama is the 'Chakra instrument', which is sensitive to electrical fields around the body at up to 100 kHz. Readings from particular chakras to some extent correlate with AMI measurements from corresponding meridians.

Case study 10.1 looks at the AMI in a patient with Lung deficiency.

## EAV – Electroacupuncture according to Voll

The original EAV device developed by Voll was built around a conductance meter reading from 0 to 100, the 'norm' being 50 (the full scale represented a reading of around 2 V). Brass electrodes were used, moistened with water, to take readings from acupoints or larger areas. Measurement of 'buccal currents' (DC currents in the mouth) was also possible. These may occur owing to the presence of different metals in the oral cavity, and can clearly affect other bioelectric processes within the body.

EAV, like ryodoraku, has been an immensely influential system, with an impact even in China To recapitulate the fundamentals of EAV, described elsewhere in this book, three basic principles of the measurement side of EAV are: (1) conductance measurement at the acupoint, particularly the indicator drop (ID), reflects physiological function, (2) acupoints, both new and traditional, may have direct relationships to specific anatomical entities (parts of organs), and (3) remedies introduced into the electrical circuit during testing will, if correctly chosen, normalise readings.

Voll found that electrical stimulation of an imbalanced point could normalise its reading more reliably and accurately than with traditional needling, and developed a comprehensive LF therapy system for this using a handheld probe connected to the EAV device. Frequencies could be applied singly, on the basis that each organ might have its own LF resonance, or as a 'wave swing', sweeping through the whole range over about 3 minutes, the assumption being that the body would then select the frequencies necessary to establish balance.

Voll took measurements at the *jing* Well points, reunion points (such as SP-6 and a 'Hypophysis' point for meridians meeting on the head), what he called 'central measurement points', 'control measurement points' (CMPs) to check for stability of remedy testing, and so on. A cynic might argue that, given more than 1100 possible points to measure, statistically some 'problems' are bound to show up, but simplified versions of EAV using only 120 basic points also give useful results.

Case study 10.2 describes a blinded EAV screening test in a patient with various health problems.

In addition to specific point measurements, an initial overall assessment is made using a four-quadrant system, with cylindrical electrodes for the hands and footplates for the feet (Fig. 10.13 on p. 229). High readings indicate sympathicotonia (excess), and low ones vagotonia (deficiency). If readings are low, the patient might require 'charging' through the hand electrodes with alternating LF currents before going on to take individual point measurements. Quadrants should be balanced, so far as possible, prior to point measurement.

Treatment is then first directed at the meridian with the most imbalanced measurements (especially the ID), indicating the most stressed organ. Points can be 'charged' or 'discharged' using different types of current (Fig. 10.14 on p. 230). Measurements are then taken again.

Voll adopted the notion of latent or actual foci of infection that might have a general effect on health and 'block' effective treatment. He also made many complex connections between meridians and specific tonsils, odontons, vertebrae and so on, although these have really only been verified within the context of EAV practice. He also integrated aspects of traditional acupuncture energetics such as the 'mother–son' or 'husband–wife' laws in his work.

Remedy testing is another fascinating aspect of EAV. If a remedy is placed in circuit with the patient and the EAV device, or held in one hand by the patient while being tested, EAV measurements change. An appropriate remedy will normalise an anomalous reading to '50' on the meter, and an appropriate combination of remedies may be found to balance several abnormal readings. On this basis, a 'remedy well' is usually included in the circuit between the handheld return electrode and the instrument itself (see Fig. 10.13c). Ampoules of different remedies (including homeopathic nosodes) and potential allergens or toxic substances are used to show both aetiological factors and what treatment may be required.

The principle that remedies in closed containers are able to affect the patient's state has a long history. Voll attempted to explain it in biophysical terms: he considered that each illness might have its own frequency, affecting not just the diseased organ but other parts of the body too. Remedies, with their own frequencies, would have the ability to interfere with these illness signals and so reduce their negative effects. The remedy test is thus a method of determining *resonance*. On the assumption that transmission of such remedy signals is possible, one colleague of Voll's, Franz Morell, devised a 'test transmitter–receiver' that also amplified remedy signals slightly to make remedy testing easier.

Some researchers investigating EAV have concluded that its measurements have external validity, yet Voll himself stated that further clinical studies and laboratory tests are necessary to verify results, and tended to *precede* detailed EAV measurements with a careful anamnesis, other clinical tests and measurement of overall energy balance.

An allied method is Omura's 'bidigital O-ring test' (BDORT), developed on the basis of experience with applied kinesiology (AK) and skin conductivity testing. Some have shifted their allegiance to the O-ring test from the more complex EAV. Others have evolved their own mix of the O-ring test or AK, auriculomedicine and EAV remedy testing.

Further approaches include Nogier's auriculocardiac reflex (ACR) and AK. To the outsider the variety of these methods is bewildering and even possibly laughable. In the context of clinical practice, however, the situation may be very different; the 'left-brain' style of EAV and 'right-brain' dowsing methods may both have their place.

## Croon's electroneural diagnosis and therapy

Although Richard Croon undertook early work on point measurement, his methods were only really elaborated into a complete system by his son, Rolf Croon, and other collaborators. Impedance measurements (in ohms and nanofarads) can be taken at over 200 points (including acupoints), using a 9 kHz 0.05 mA signal. Readings that differ most significantly from the mean are given most weight, in addition to left–right differences at symmetrical points and global differences between left and right sides of the body. Treatment, with 0.5–2.0 mA exponential pulses of 400–1000 Hz, is claimed to have a regenerating and revitalising effect particularly in chronic conditions. Stimulation automatically stops once readings normalise, and can often be stabilised with repeated treatments (although often as many as 20–40 frequent 15-minute may be required for this).

## The Vegatest – EAV modified by way of BFD

Practitioners who initially adopted Voll's methods with enthusiasm eventually sought to adapt and simplify them. Schmidt, in Germany, used EAV for 10 years before

# CASE Study 10.2

### Blinded EAV screening test
**J K Andrews**

The objective of this test was to establish the efficacy of taking electrodermal screening (EAV) readings from a patient as a way of determining the clinical profile of a consenting volunteer, without the EAV practitioner being aware of the volunteer's medical history, and to assess whether a correlation exists between EAV findings and the volunteer's conventional medical history.

The test would look not only at the patient's overall health profile from EAV readings but also possible underlying causes not found in or thought relevant from the patient's medical history and symptoms through conventional examination or diagnosis. The volunteer had a known verifiable pathology unknown to the tester.

### Conventional medical history of the volunteer

The volunteer was asked by the adjudicator to complete a questionnaire to detail his or her known medical history. Results were as follows:

Patient is a non-smoker and drinks alcohol occasionally in moderation.

### Major health concerns

- Angina pectoris – confirmed by electrocardiogram and cardiac angiogram.
- Hypercholesterolaemia – confirmed by serum blood analysis.
- Arthritic bone structure changes in the lumbar area – confirmed by X-ray.
- Allergy to Septrin (co-trimoxazole).
- Intermittent ischaemia of right foot.

### Minor health concerns

- Occasional respiratory tract infections.
- Occasional lethargy.
- Occasional bleeding gums.
- Occasional sore throats.

### Medical interventions

- Tonsillectomy following reoccurring episodes of tonsillitis.
- Whiplash injury following road traffic accident.
- Childhood illnesses including measles and chickenpox.

- Vaccinations as per the directions of the British National Formulary.
- Reaction experienced following Hepatitis vaccination.

### Current medication

- Zocor (simvastatin) 10 mg and $1/2$ aspirin (acetylsalicylic acid) per night.

### Parents' health

- Mother – pernicious anaemia and diabetes mellitus.
- Father (deceased) – history of ischaemic heart disease.

### Test protocol

Readings were taken from Voll points in the patient's finger and toe areas, including control measurement points (CMPs), using a computerised acupuncture system (Fig. 10.11).

### EAV graph readings/interpretations (Fig. 10.12)

Readings of 50 to 60 mV = a healthy parameter.
Readings *above* 60 mV = start of inflammatory processes leading to total inflammation.
Readings *below* 50 mV = start of degenerative processes leading to total degeneration.
Readings that are all 'black' are functioning areas.
Readings that are black with 'white' tops are priority degenerative readings/underfunctioning areas.

### Initial observations from the EAV graph readings

Hypertension, circulatory problems, lymphatic congestion especially in the head area, hypercholesterolemia, all excretory processes and cellular respiration were underfunctioning.

### EAV test results

Of the 40 CMPs:
- The most degenerative initial reading was left-side Liver.
- The most inflammatory initial readings were Cellular Metabolism and Heart, both right-sided.

Further in-depth readings taken along the meridians revealed the following areas as primary causes in generating the 40 CMP readings:

The *worst priority reading* was the Liver's central venous system, followed by peritoneal lymph vessels of Liver region, and the bile ducts (interlobular).

*Immune function:* leukocyte underfunction was indicated in the upper body (head area), followed by lower body leukocytes.

Erythrocyte and platelet underfunction was indicated.
Macrophage activity was also indicated.

*(Continued)*

CASE Study 10.2 **Continued**

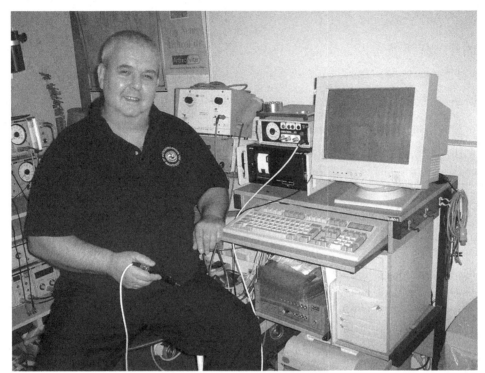

**Figure 10.11** Ken Andrews with some of his treatment room facilities. Behind his right shoulder, two updated MORA II units. Below these, MORA Colour and Indumed instruments. Behind his left shoulder, interferential equipment, with ultrasound below this. To the left of the monitor are the AcuPro II EAV device (with remedy well on top of it) and an ECG unit, with a SEG on the shelf below them. Onscreen can be seen the EAV points of the hand. (Courtesy of Ken Andrews.)

*Allergy vessel left:* readings indicated responses caused by heavy metals, inhalants, dental inhalants, phenolics, antibiotics/hormones, toxins, foods and insects.

*Left lymph vessel:* readings indicated underfunction in jaw and teeth, tubal tonsil, paranasal sinuses, ear, eye and deep cervical lymph nodes. The priority jaw/dental indicated were left lateral lower jaw followed by left lateral upper jaw.

Dental amalgams gave the following mV readings:

Left upper 2nd – 196;  Right upper 5th – 208
　　　　5th – 151;
　　　　6th – 190
Left lower 6th – 17;  Right lower no
　　　　7th 100　　　　amalgam fillings.

*Endocrine* points suggested the following areas as underfunctioning: pituitary, thyroid, parathyroid, thymus; cervical sympathetic ganglia (autonomic); internal secretions of head and body of pancreas; lymph vessels.

*Left circulation* areas of underfunction indicated with summation measurement points (SMPs) for lymph vessels, autonomic coronary plexus, cisterna chyli, and thoracic duct.

*Pancreas* areas of underfunction indicated were as follows: carbohydrates metabolism; lipase metabolism; pancreatic duct; uric acid metabolism; protein metabolism; peritoneal lymph vessels of pancreas region.

*Excretory* systems are all underfunctioning.

**Observations/diagnosis utilising further EAV readings**

(Key to confirmation by patient after completing the EAV testing: confirmed ✓; not confirmed ✗)

Heart/blood pressure problems from a foreign toxin within the body (deceased father had heart problems)　✓
Heavy metal problem　✗
Elimination problems – all systems are showing underfunction　✗
Predisposition to diabetes – (mother has diabetes mellitus)　✓

## CASE Study 10.2 Continued

| | |
|---|---|
| Dental and temporomandibular joint (TMJ) problems | ✗ |
| Tonsil problems – recurring sore throats | ✓ |
| Predisposition to rheumatism/arthritis | ✓ |
| Cervical problems – known whiplash injury | ✓ |
| Tiredness/lethargy – cellular respiration problems from acidity | ✓ |
| Digestive problems – not assimilating foods | ✗ |
| Anaemia | ✓ |
| Hypercholesterolaemia | ✓ |
| Muscular stiffness and joint problems – arthritis | ✓ |
| Allergic reactions to antibiotics | ✓ |
| Anterior pituitary under function | ✗ |
| Bacterial problems in oral cavity — gum related, with possible cavitation – lower left 7th area | ✗ |
| Lymphatic congestion | ✗ |
| Possible iatrogenic damage | ✓ |
| Tendency for haemorrhoids | ✓ |
| Liver underfunctioning | ✓ |
| Parasite problem indicated | ✗ |
| Overall, patient's systems are open to illness/infections | ✓ |

### Follow-up dental examination

A dental examination was arranged 1 week after taking the EAV readings. The dentist was not notified of the EAV testing results/readings prior to his dental examination. He reported:

- Limitation in bilateral jaw movement – left TMJ not functioning properly
- Wear pattern on teeth indicates that patient is clenching and grinding his teeth, causing greater mercury release from his dental fillings
- Larger temporalis and masseter muscles
- Reduced jaw opening, not quite 48 mm
- On opening, jaw deviates to left – TMJ problem
- Six odontons missing
- Overall poor dental hygiene, with decay
- The older fillings, especially on left side, appear poor – lower 7th tooth either dead or dying.

### Panoral (all-round) and digital X-rays, and also odonton examination via camera

The lower seventh tooth has curves in root – tooth has questionable vitality – holes in bone structure either side of tooth.

The 6th and 7th teeth on the left and right lower jaw are drifting and tilting anteriorly.

The upper left 7th has a large amalgam mercury filling with two pins. It is also close to the sinus and has a hole in the bone structure.

### Microscope findings on examination of plaque/saliva sample

- High spirochete activity.
- High leukocyte activity.
- Amoebic parasites detected.
- Probable candida present.
- Very active biological anaerobic bacteria present.

The oral cavity has been bacterially compromised. The initial observation from examination by the dentist is that this could cause increased heart/circulatory and kidney problems.

### Treatment regimen/advice

The patient was advised to see a biological dentist for dental hygiene treatment, amalgam removal, TMJ correction and dental treatment combined with cranial corrections.

Complex homeopathic drainage remedies were given to the patient, along with advice about nutritional support and dietary changes.

### Postscript (more than 3 years later)

To my knowledge, this patient still has not had any dental work done, not even basic cleaning with a dentist/hygienist. Nor has he had his fillings replaced or removed. This presents a problem. The fillings are tantamount to a roadblock in his body and in his meridians, since each tooth has a direct relationship to the organ systems and meridian energy flow. Even though he saw the bacteria and amoeba on the microscope monitor screen, he refuses to believe that this could be a primary cause of his health problems.

### Acknowledgement

With thanks to Bernard Garrett, BSc, MPhil, RMN, SRN, DipAc, Primary Care Cert (Homeopathy), who acted as impartial adjudicator for this test.

*(Continued)*

CASE Study 10.2 **Continued**

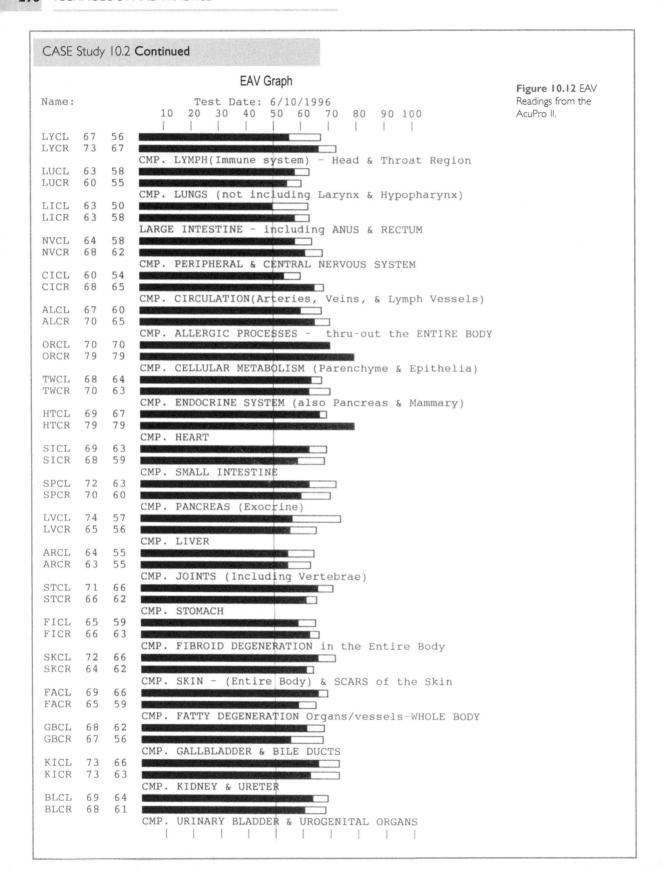

**Figure 10.12** EAV Readings from the AcuPro II.

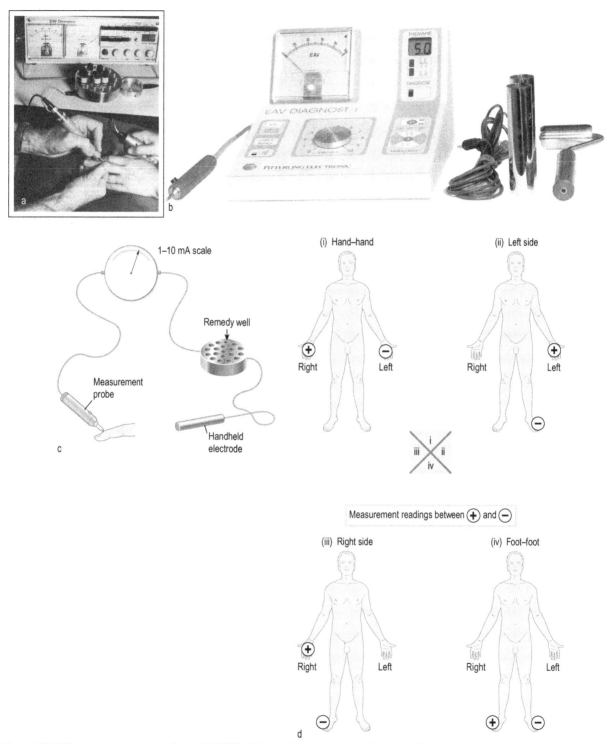

**Figure 10.13** Electroacupuncture according to Voll (EAV). (a) Remedy testing using the Dermatron. (Reproduced with permission from Kenyon 1985.) (b) Diagnost-1, a currently available EAV machine without stimulation facility. (Reproduced with permission from Pitterling Electronic GmbH, Munich.) (c) Schematic of treatment set-up. (Adapted with permission from Kenyon 1985.) (d) Diagram of quadrant measurements, using hand and foot electrodes. (Adapted with permission from Werner & Voll 1979.)

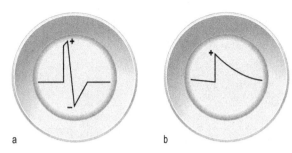

**Figure 10.14** Electroacupuncture according to Voll (EAV). (a) High-intensity biphasic LF current used to 'charge' points in EAV. (b) Very-low-intensity positive sawtooth current used to 'discharge' points in EAV. (Adapted with permission from Werner & Voll 1979.)

transferring to his own system of 'bioelectronic function diagnosis' (BFD) developed with another doctor called, confusingly, Vill. They emphasised that measurements refer to *bioenergetic* functional imbalances, not organ function as Voll believed.

The device they used worked with silver rather than brass electrodes, alternating rather than direct current, a higher current than EAV, and with measurements centring on a meter 'norm' of 40 (rather than Voll's 50). Thus measurements using these different systems are not interchangeable. The BFD measurement technique too is very different from that of EAV, and supposedly gives reproducible results. The ID, so fundamental to EAV, is not considered, although it was Schmidt who first described it in 1952. Again, although Voll had considered measurement mandatory at more than 180 acupoints, in BFD this number was reduced to 54, including the *jing* Well points, with four additional points for overall measurement (hand, foot, under the thigh and under the upper arm). The number of measurement ampoules needed was also reduced.

Schmidt believed that the most significant readings were those that appeared both when the patient's energy was deficient and when it had been recharged (so that, if healthy, all points should then balance). Thus readings were taken before and after the use of LF stimulation in order to recharge the system and highlight these hidden imbalances.

In 1978, on the basis of both EAV and BFD, Helmut Schimmel proposed a new system, the 'vegetative reflex test', now more commonly known as the Vegatest, to simplify BFD still further. The basic device necessary is far less elaborate than those of EAV and BFD, and correspondingly less expensive. As such, it is the simplest and so the most widely used of these 'bioenergetic regulation techniques' (BER), as they are often known.

Schimmel's method is far less invasive than Voll's, at least in terms of physical pressure on the acupoint. However, like EAV, it depends on the use of a handheld probe (silver, as in BFD) and takes considerable practice to master. The acupoint itself is not of primary importance and, rather than measuring a number of points on each meridian, one point is selected for measurement throughout the session. This may be the first point of either left or right Allergy, *sanjiao* (Triple Burner) or Connective tissue degeneration meridians/vessels (see Fig. 5.11 on page 57) (the handheld return is held in the patient's dominant hand). Only about 100 remedies are required for Vegatesting, far fewer than in EAV.

In Schimmel's method the different organs are represented in homeopathic form in closed ampoules in a variant of Voll's remedy test. Thus the fourth decimal potency (D4) of Liver (Hepar) is used in circuit with the patient and the Vegatest device to determine whether there is some abnormal response at the point selected that would indicate a Liver function problem, and so on. Schimmel also developed a set of homeopathic 'meridian complexes' for testing the energetic status of the 12 main acupuncture meridians, as well as some of the eight extra meridians. Other ampoules can be used to amplify readings, check such elusive factors as premalignancy, 'biological age', 'geopathic stress' due to so-called earth radiations or 'psychogenic stress', as well as the usual toxins, foods, nutritional factors and so on. Filter ampoules serve to determine the most severely stressed organ or whether a condition is inflammatory or degenerative.

Another difference from EAV and BFD is that the body is first 'stressed' using a piezoelectric stimulator. Readings are then taken while the body is still reacting to this (over about 15 minutes) and are considered more useful than if the body is in a state of relative balance in the first place. The first priority is to obtain a stable reproducible reading (the so-called 'disorder control'), using a toxic substance guaranteed to disorder the most balanced reading. However, one informal study of three experienced testers found that they could differentiate between the toxic sample (paraquat) and water with only 70% accuracy, so even at this stage clearly Vegatesting is not an infallible procedure.

Thus, as Schimmel himself is fully aware, the Vegatest is not an objective method. Rather, as others have put it, it is a 'perception enhancement device' that at the same time involves more than simple intuition, or 'an effective means of clarifying one's intuition of a patient'. As such, on the one hand some believe it is similar to such methods as AK or radionics, even if dressed up in somewhat more impressive gear. Ampoules have an effect because of a mental 'resonance' of ideas. On the other hand, it is possible to consider this resonance in terms of radiation (as Voll, Morell and others have done).

Thus Vegatesting has been regarded by some practitioners as a form of 'electronic dowsing', useful for monitoring patient progress but not to be relied upon for medical diagnosis. As with dowsing, Vegatest results do seem to depend on factors such as the patient's mental attitude, geopathic stress in the test place, and the practitioner's state of health, level of training or unique sensitivity (more 'right brain' intuitive than 'left brain' critical). To reduce the effects of these factors, Schimmel devised a special 'absorber' ampoule that is supposed to screen out 'interference signals' from both tester and the immediate environment, making the procedure less tiring for the tester and enabling more reproducible results.

Whatever one may think of this, and despite its short-comings, Vegatesting may be a useful adjunctive *back-up* method within a given therapeutic context and relationship. On the basis of the readings obtained, using a sophisticated analysis in terms of 'causal chains', it is possible to fine tune the determination of appropriate treatment. However, used carelessly, the Vegatest may become just a medium for the expression of unconscious fantasies or fixed ideas. There is a tendency to look for (and find) patterns that that may perhaps have relevance within the therapeutic encounter, but are unlikely to have any objective reality outside it.

In the 1980s, Cyril Smith and colleagues in Britain began to investigate electromagnetic signals that affected electrically sensitive patients in the same way as particular homeopathic remedies or allergens. They found, as Morell had done earlier, that higher homeopathic potencies corresponded to higher frequencies. Smith also discovered that the signals could be transferred to water via simple coils, so that the water took on some of the characteristics of the original remedy/allergen. Julian Kenyon, one of the most experienced British practitioners in this area, claims that electronically patterned water works just as well as the real remedy for sensitive patients.

Jacques Benveniste's group in France has taken this a stage further, demonstrating that such data can be transmitted and stored in digital form. Then, in the 1990s, Gerhard Braun and Martin Lehman of Vega Grieshaber devised a system of 'individual frequency storage' (IFS) that enabled recording signals directly from ampoules on to electronic chips within a specially shielded chamber. Using this technology, Vega Grieshaber have gone on to develop advanced versions of the Vegatest, such as the Vegatest Expert, which permits stimulation using LF modulation of remedy signals through a roller or probe, and the VegaSelect, which stores the patient's own signals in magnetic memory. Using a pulsed magnetic field as a carrier, they are then transmitted back to the patient for therapeutic purposes. Alternatively, therapeutic signals can be stored on cards, which are worn by the patient.

## Schimmel's Segmentalelectrogram (SEG) – before and after

Voll's measurement of overall function using large hand and foot electrodes (see Fig. 10.13) was echoed in other German developments. Helmut Schimmel, for example, created the 'Segmentalelectrogram' to give a more rapid, objective and broad overview of energetic processes in the body than is given by EAV and other derivative small-electrode systems. In the original 'long programme' version, 10 silvered 6 cm diameter electrodes are positioned on the body on the fore-head, chest, abdomen, pelvis and (as with BFD) the posterior thighs (Fig. 10.15a). Measurements are taken between each pair of points in turn. After an initial measurement, as with the Vegatest, the pair is 'stressed' using a 13 Hz 'non-thera-peutic' frequency, while the readings continue.

The SEG results are interpreted in terms of energy reserve or 'positive regulatory capacity', inflammation (increased activity) or reduced energy flow/rigidity in organs of the corresponding body 'quadrant'. Rigidity may result from malignancy, toxicity or geopathic stress. Depression may show up as a complete lack of regulatory control, with low energy in all quadrants. Regulatory capacity is considerably reduced in patients on steroids, for example. Causal chain analysis is possible, as with the Vegatest. However, as Tiller suggests, SEG measurements may in fact have only local significance.

A further development is the DFM, or 'diagnostic system for functional medicine'. This successor to the earlier SEG uses a simpler electrode array (since adopted in later versions of the SEG itself), with measurements between forehead, palms and soles (so that only shoes and socks need be removed) (Fig. 10.15b). The authors of the one book so far published on the DFM emphasise that it should not be regarded as a diagnostic machine, but rather as 'a source of ideas which give valuable indications about regulatory behaviour and energy condition'.

## Computerised systems – the new generations

There are a number of computerised and other acupuncture treatment and measurement systems in China, but these are little known in the West, where most are based on EAV. The first to design such a computerised system was an American, James (Jim) Hoyt Clark, in 1979. He explicitly states that what he calls 'computerised electrodermal screening' (CEDS) cannot be used to diagnose and treat disease, but rather measures and treats energetic imbalances. It has sometimes been described as a form of 'stress testing'.

The testing is done using Voll's original 100-point scale, with a 5 V 30 µA DC signal through brass electrodes. Focal problems are addressed first, followed by treatment of imbalanced meridians in order of their importance. Clark places less emphasis on the ID than Voll, looking also at the lowest and highest readings and the rise rate of the measurement. Including treatment, the average screening protocol takes around an hour, and Clark claims that two properly trained testers ('technicians') should obtain very similar screening results.

Jim Clark's original LISTEN system (the 'Life Information System Ten'), like the latest Vegatest Expert, contained 'samples' of thousands of different remedies and other substances in software form. These were encoded in binary form as so-called 'capsules' taken to represent the substance, a concept that Clark and his coworkers held from the begin-ning, even before the results of Smith and Benveniste were known. If this electronic form tests as an appropriate remedy for a particular patient, treatment can be given by potentising water with a reproducible signal based on the remedy code. Alternatively, personalised capsules can be electronically loaded into a pocket-sized unit for home use by the patient, or into a clinical treatment unit. The remedy information in the capsule acts on the body via a modulated electromagnetic carrier wave (as with the MitoSan device), or TENS-type stimulation. Unlike homeopathically potentised

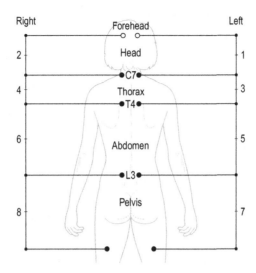

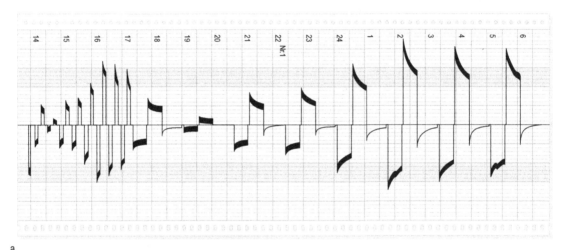

a

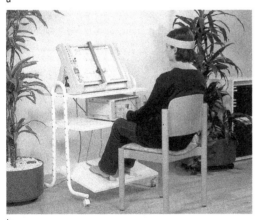

b

**Figure 10.15** Whole body measurement systems. (a) Segmentalelectrogram (SEG) 'long programme' electrode locations (all dorsal, except for those on forehead), with sample of a grossly imbalanced printout. (b) Diagnostic System for Functional Medicine (DFM), showing simpler handheld and foot plate electrodes, with printout in action. ((a) Adapted with permission from Schimmel & Grieshaber 1982; (b) courtesy of Noma (Complex Homoeopathy) Ltd.)

remedies, digital capsules are not affected by X-rays, heat or light. Acupuncture meridians too have their particular frequency patterns.

Jim Clark lost the rights to use the name LISTEN, which, together with the name BEST, is now applied to another computerised system based on different technology. This has been called 'hololinguistic'. As far as I can understand, this means that no signal is generated and *intention* is the key operating principle. The ohmmeter and 'virtual library' software program become essentially a pendulum and word list... purely subjective and non-reproducible. Thus hololinguistic methods represent a melding of acupuncture and radionics. Clark's main CEDS device is now called the ORION.

Bill Nelson's 'Eclosion' is the best-known hololinguistic computerised measurement system, incorporating elements of EEG, FFT (fast Fourier transform) and ECG as well as EAV, with electrodes at forehead, wrists and one finger. Actual samples of the substances tested are contained within the device. Now superseded by the 'EnergyScan' or 'Quantum Xeroid' device, Nelson's theories on how it and its successor work are very difficult to follow. A key principle is that the machine should analyse all the data, leaving the practitioner free to concentrate on the therapeutic relationship with the patient. However, the result of analysing the measurement data is a vast range of readouts that appear quite meaningless to the uninitiated. Nelson goes out of his way to spell out the historical relationship between his method and radionics. Thus it is questionable whether this approach really offers any advance in terms of objectivity on other methods where the tester uses a handheld probe.

All in all, given the sometimes dubious theories invoked and the inconsistencies in basic measurement methodology and results, expensive computerised integrated systems should be approached with caution. There is also a risk that greater reliance on such technology can distract, rather than assist, the practitioner.

## Down to earth – the Equinox system

### By J GORDON GADSBY

A group of British scientists and clinicians interested in electroacupuncture and biophysical measurements of the acupuncture system formed the Society of Biophysical Medicine (SBM) in the 1980s. In contrast to the complexities of EAV, they developed a clear and systematic approach to diagnosis and treatment that eventually became known as the Equinox system.

The SBM approach integrates methods of investigation and treatment at three distinct levels: basic, meridian system and symptom Together, these form a complete stand-alone system of electroacupuncture. The first level of investigation is the assessment of electrical resistance from the hands and feet, using a standard multimeter. This technique is fast and easy, giving an overall assessment of the patient's energy levels. Readings can be differentiated into normal, inflammatory, degenerative and indeterminate.

Meridian activity may then be evaluated by a variety of methods or their combination, including *jing* Well point measurements of voltage and its changes (in a manner somewhat similar to EAV measurements of conductance and 'indicator drops'), Kirlian photography, auricular organ point voltage measurements, linking symptoms to the meridians in association with the basic resistance readings, and conventional history taking and diagnosis.

Treatment is aimed at the three levels (the basic resistance imbalance, the meridian system level and the symptom level) with a variety of electrostimulation techniques that use dedicated high-quality biphasic charge-balanced electroacupuncture units.

Assessment of the basic electrical resistance is the cornerstone of biophysical measurement and electrical diagnosis. The multimeter is used with cylinder electrodes to measure the electrical resistance in kilohms between the hands, between the feet, and between the left and right sides of the body. Correction of any basic imbalance found is an important part of the treatment programme. Many conditions will improve using this treatment alone. Correction of imbalances is made possible by passing selected current frequencies through the electrodes, either hand to hand or foot to foot (see Fig. 9.15.1 on page 270). Inflammatory conditions are treated with 2 Hz low-frequency electrostimulation (EST), degenerative conditions with high frequency (80 Hz), and indeterminate ones with a stabilising 10 Hz frequency.

Correction of meridian imbalances uses electrostimulation of tonification and sedation points with needle or surface electrodes, or of the *jing* Well points with wet lint or electroconductive rubber strip electrodes. EST may be used to stimulate, sedate or stabilise depending on the frequency used. This is determined by the meridian measurements in association with the basic electrical resistance readings, taking into account too whether the condition is acute or chronic. The use of neuroelectric (or needleless) acupuncture (NEAP) and surface electrodes has become the norm for most SBM practitioners, and the use of needles is no longer considered necessary. NEAP stimulation of ear organ/meridian points is usually with a point stimulator.

Treatment of pain and restricted range of movement is a first priority, using probe electrostimulation of ear points, together with organ, local and anti-inflammatory points. Treatment of the basic imbalance and the meridian system is then carried out until all three levels have been treated and balanced.

The SBM integrated approach is relatively simple, adaptable and does not exclude a more complex approach to point and meridian measurement and assessment. The NEAP technique means that patients with chronic conditions can also treat themselves at home under the direction of a suitably qualified practitioner. NEAP appears to be just as effective as needling with electrostimulation, but is non-invasive and almost devoid of side-effects.

(Note: NEAP corresponds to TEAS and pTENS in this section.)

## ACMOS from France

Another simplified version is René Naccachian's ACMOS method, based on measuring potentials at hand and foot points. As usual, higher values indicate excess energy (inflammation) of the associated organ, and low a deficiency. Treatment is via a basic handheld probe offering facilities for tonification and sedation.

## Back to the USSR – automated biofeedback

A rather different form of integrated instrument is the Skenar (Scenar) or Kosmed device developed as part of the Russian space programme for maintenance of astronauts' health when away from Earth. The device is handheld (the size of a TV remote control) with inbuilt concentric metal electrodes. Signal characteristics are in part decided by the user, but also vary automatically in response to impedance measurements from the body during treatment, so that the stimulus keeps changing and habituation is not a problem. Treatment location is primarily local to the problem area, with the operator searching for particular dynamic changes in impedance (signalled by an audible signal, as well as different sensations of 'stick' as the device is moved about). Larger zones rather than acupoints are usually targeted.

## MORA – THE NEW WORLD OF MORELL AND RASCHE

All the treatment methods described so far involve external stimulation to the patient. 'MORA' therapy (from the names *M*orell and *Ra*sche), in contrast, uses the *body's own* signals, building on Morell's and Voll's insight that disease is 'a state in which pathological oscillations exist'. This is the first principle of MORA.

The second MORA principle is 'inverse switching'. The totality of the patient's oscillations ($A$) can theoretically be subdivided into 'harmonic oscillations' ($H$), those of a healthy body, which are supposedly ordered and coherent, and 'disharmonic' ones ($D$), which are irregular and unbalanced. A 'separator' filter for $H$ and $D$ enables them to be modified and returned to the body independently. If $D$ is then 'inverted' ($D_i$) before being fed back, the initial disharmonic signal is in some sense cancelled out or reduced (Fig. 10.16). $A_i$ (the total body signal inverted) tends to be used for *yang* (e.g. inflammatory) conditions, $H$ for depleted patients, $H + D_i$ for *yin* (e.g. chronic degenerative) conditions, and so forth.

Initially a 2–3-minute MORA 'basic therapy' is carried out using hand (or foot) electrodes. The body's own signal A is passed to an input electrode in the left hand. Within the MORA device it is amplified and frequency filtered in various ways and then transferred intermittently to an output electrode in the other hand (the input and output are linked optically, not via an electrical conductor).

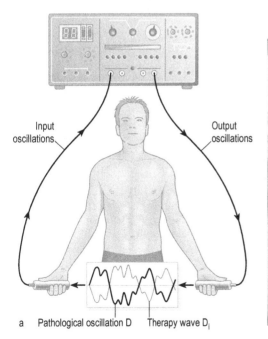

Input oscillations  Output oscillations

a   Pathological oscillation D   Therapy wave D_i

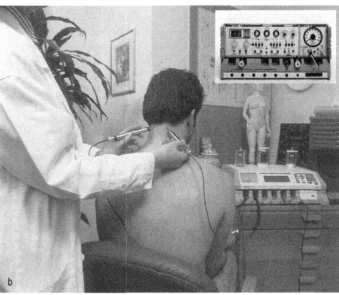

b

**Figure 10.16** MORA®. (a) The MORA principle of inversion, showing cancellation of pathological oscillation *D* and inverted therapy wave, the result being elimination of the pathological oscillation. (b) Twin probe application using MORA-Super⁺. (Inset shows MORA® III.) (Courtesy of Med-Tronik GmbH)

Basic therapy is intended to have an overall balancing effect and to make subsequent more specific treatment simpler, perhaps even unnecessary.

MORA therapy can also be applied using large-area or roller electrodes, and via a handheld probe to acupoints, scars, *ashi* points and so forth. It is even possible to use signals from the patient's own bodily secretions. Remedies, serially diluted allergens, even procaine (as injected in neural therapy) can also be individualised using the patient's own oscillations (and the oscillations of allergens or addictive drugs inverted and passed to the patient). However, patient signals are not stored in the MORA device.

Treatment is directed to those points with the greatest remaining pathological values, or those most clearly connected with the disease in question. Since there is congruence between the body's oscillations and those applied, only very short treatments are necessary. Input and output probes can be used on the same meridian or its contralateral partner, or on different meridians. The point giving the highest reading can be used as input, and that with the lowest measurement or ID, or both, for the output probe. There is little local sensation from treatment, and there are no known side-effects.

Various other devices can be linked to the basic MORA unit, such as the MORA 'rotation tester', which is used to test for the presence of geopathic or electromagnetic stress in a patient that may possibly block the effects of treatments such as MORA therapy itself, as well as acupuncture.

There is also the 'Indumed' magnetic therapy device, developed by Wolfgang Ludwig. The output signal, using various waveforms of very low intensity (0.25 G) and very brief pulses, was originally described as 'an almost natural field' more in harmony with the energy of the body than stronger magnetic treatments. Frequency can be varied over a large frequency range, up to around 10 MHz (the so-called 'waveswing'). Two frequencies can be applied simultaneously.

The magnetic field is applied via special non-self-inductive heads for a deeply penetrating homogeneous effect. However, the uniqueness of Indumed is that the treatment heads are impregnated with trace elements found naturally in the earth's crust, the magnetic field acting as a carrier for their frequencies within the patient's body. The purpose of this multifrequency stimulus is thus to normalise the whole of the human biospectrum, which is potentially disturbed or depleted by man-made electromagnetic smog and other environmental disturbances (particularly in the urban environment). On the basis of Cyril Smith's research, *brief* exposures to such multiple frequencies are claimed to excite harmonic (health-promoting) resonances of the body, but not harmful ones, which take longer to build to coherence. Indumed sessions last around 15–30 minutes (or less, if coupled with MORA therapy).

Ludwig also developed smaller units for home and clinic use, employing the same trace elements as the Indumed and with magnetic frequencies related to those naturally occurring in Schumann waves. Current MORA instruments no longer make use of the Indumed technology. Instead, static magnetic fields are used as 'carriers' for the patient's own oscillations.

Finally there is the MORA colour instrument. A number of 'colour acupuncture' systems have been developed. The MORA version was one of the first, translating colour signals into LF electrical beat frequencies that are supposed to have the same therapeutic effect as light, but with deeper penetrative power, especially when delivered via the Indumed. The principle is similar to that of Indumed: to replace colours that are depleted in the human biospectrum. There is also a facility for combining colour and sound therapy through the same outputs.

MORA technology has developed considerably over the years. Now MORA colour and magnetic stimulation are included in the main unit. And, as with Vega, digital storage is used for homeopathic remedy information.

Other approaches to colour include those of Nogier, with colour correspondences for different zones of the ear, and Manaka, who applied not just coloured light but also coloured inks to acupoints. Colour acupuncture treatments have also been designed with reference to tonification or sedation of the different meridians, or to the chakras. Mandel, in his system of 'colorpuncture', has elaborated an even more esoteric ('esogetic') and idiosyncratic scheme of 'zones' to which coloured light can be applied. He also uses colour and sound together, although this approach is by no means unique to him.

## Bioresonance therapy – an alternative to MORA

In 1987, a rival to MORA appeared, called the BICOM, with many more treatment programmes preinstalled, and a profusion of different applicators. The MORA principles were renamed as those of 'bioresonance therapy'. There were also more fundamental changes: for example, magnetism was now employed as a 'transport medium' rather than for any therapeutic effect it might have. The new BICOM permitted not only amplification but also attenuation of signals. In addition to the 'waveswing', 'wobbling' of a narrow frequency band around a central frequency was used to emphasise effective therapy signals.

Another approach is 'multiresonance therapy', which is designed to restore bioresonance signals missing from our twenty-first-century environment. Examples are the use of different elements to emit radiation compatible with that of the human body when excited by heat (as in the Chinese TDP device), the use of various frequencies of the electromagnetic field to counter both global geomagnetic and local Schumann wave depletion (Indumed), and the use of colour (as in MORA colour therapy).

The Multicom device applies different frequencies of colour, sound and even the energies of different metals and precious stones, by means of a low-intensity laser acting as a carrier and applied to acupoints. Different frequencies and colours can also be individually applied, or automatically through whole ranges using a magnetic field as carrier, in the form of physical vibration, or through surface electrodes for longer treatments. Modulation from an external music source is also possible, and the Multicom even incorporates a small pyramid. Such multiple possibilities are reminiscent of Georges Lakhovsky's multiwave oscillator from the 1920s, which was intended to re-establish health through 'the harmony of multiple radiations', and also of radionics where there is a strong tradition of using sound, colour, magnetism and gemstones as transducers for more subtle energies.

While Voll and others in Europe considered that remedies and their target organs might have particular resonant frequencies, in America Royal Rife and later Hulda Clark believed that different organisms might also have specific frequency characteristics. Clark developed her own measurement device, the 'syncrometer™', a kind of blend of EAV and radionics intended to detect the resonances of different pathogens (viruses, parasites, etc). Rife had determined in the 1920s that irradiating viruses and bacteria at particular audio-modulated radio frequencies could kill them. In the late 1980s Clark first used radio frequency signals and then a simple 'zapper' that supposedly kills pathogens indiscriminately over a wide frequency range if used correctly.

A related method was developed in the late 1980s by Bob Beck, using electrical stimulation at different frequencies applied via footplate electrodes. Later, on the basis of in vitro experiments on HIV using microcurrent and a resulting US patent for electrically treating blood outside the body to inactivate pathogens, he proposed a different approach. This involved treating blood circulating *within* the body by stimulating a point on each ankle (~KI-3) or foot (~KI-2) over prominent arteries for some 2 hours daily at around 4 Hz. This was to be combined with application of a 1 T (10 000 G) magnetic pulse generator over the lymph glands, and ingestion of colloidal silver. My own experiences with Bob Beck's and Hulda Clark's methods have been inconclusive.

# BIOCIRCUITRY AND THE POLARITIES OF THE BODY

The body has polarities of left and right, back and front, and head and foot, sometimes described in terms of *yin* and *yang* It would make intuitive sense, then, to try to balance such polarities by somehow connecting them together. In the 1920s, Leon Eeman (1888–1958) devised a 'circuit' that would do just that (Fig. 10.17). In this 'relaxation circuit' people tended to feel relaxed, whereas in a 'tension circuit' they might feel tense or restless. In the relaxation circuit, blood pressure was likely to drop if it was high, but

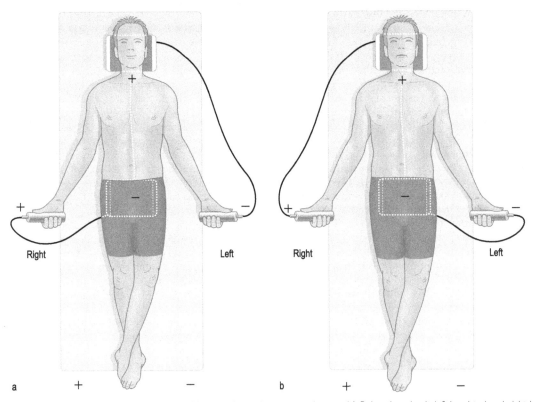

Right        Left        Right        Left

a     +     −     b     +     −

**Figure 10.17** Eeman's circuits, using cylindrical handheld electrodes and copper mesh mats. (a) Relaxation circuit, left hand to head, right hand to pelvis. (b) Tension circuit, right hand to head, left hand to pelvis (this would be a relaxation circuit for someone with reversed polarity).

rise if low. Some of these findings were confirmed in a small RCT in 1991.

Consistent use of the relaxation circuit (20–30 minutes, daily to start with) is beneficial for insomnia, fatigue and illness, and for many conditions that are also considered amenable to acupuncture. As with acupuncture, some patients might experience temporary aggravation of their condition. Eeman noted that with the relaxation circuit even intractable wounds healed more effectively, while the bleeding of an acute injury would be staunched, restarting if the circuit was interrupted. Eeman eventually developed what he called 'cooperative healing', linking two or more people together with more complex circuits. Japanese acupuncturists have used a related form of 'connection therapy', connecting acupoints in a patient with the corresponding points in a healthy person.

Eeman, like Morell, believed some form of energy, 'the X force', travelled through his circuits. This was not electricity, as circuits made of silk were just as effective as his original ones of copper wire, if not more so. This X force could span gaps in the circuit of a few centimetres. From 1927 onwards, Eeman investigated the effects of different drugs and other substances (in solution), in circuit with patients. Like Morell and his German colleagues, he found that they acted more rapidly than when taken orally.

## POLARITY AGENTS

Magnets, with their opposite poles, are the archetypal polarity agents. A number of Japanese acupuncture systems use magnets on the master and coupled points of the eight extra meridians, or *qi jing mai* (N pole towards the skin on one, S pole downwards on the other). In Korean *su jok* hand acupuncture, N and S pole magnets are placed in a specific order along the meridian to tonify or sedate it. For a pain problem, magnets of opposite polarities can be positioned locally and distally along the same meridian.

Metals also have their differences. Gold and silver needles, for example, are employed in some Western methods of acupuncture. Similarly, copper and zinc have a place in some Japanese systems, the former being considered tonifying, the latter sedating. Other metals, such as steel or titanium are sometimes thought to have an intermediate or 'balancing' effect. Gold and silver contacts rather than needles have also been used in the West, and small copper and zinc discs (*kikai*) on the master and coupled points of the eight extra meridians in the Japanese *toyohari* system (in *toyohari*, needles made of other metals are used as well). There are also small 'acumed' patches that combine magnetism with the effects of copper and zinc.

Metal in contact with living tissue produces an electrical potential. Different metals result in different potentials according to a well-established hierarchy. Thus if needles of different metals are inserted at different acupoints, there will be a slight potential difference between them, and a small current may flow from one to the other. As with magnets, gold and silver needles positioned at AcPs along

the same meridian can thus be used to tonify or sedate, depending on the order of the needles (some practitioners connect the two needles together).

The best-known protagonist of polarity agents was Manaka Yoshio. Rather than using simple connections between different parts of the body like Eeman, or highly technical equipment like Morell, his well known 'ion-pumping cords' consist of a conductive lead with needle clips at each end and a rectifying diode in the middle. If there are differences in electrical potential between the two needles, a small current will flow between them. However, the diode permits this microcurrent to flow preferentially in one direction only.

Manaka first devised this system to 'pump' positive ions from injured (burned) tissue to contralateral healthy tissue. With Tany Michio, he found that pain was reduced and healing enhanced if the diode was one way round, but that only the pain decreased if it was oriented the opposite way (Fig. 10.18). On the basis of this simple discovery, he went on to erect an elaborate system involving the eight extra meridians and other meridian points, their use being confirmed by abdominal and other subtle palpatory methods of diagnosis.

With ion cords, needles are only superficially inserted, and may even be taped to the skin without penetrating it. Thus, what Manaka called the 'X-signal system' appears to operate via non-neurological, superficial stimulation, as opposed to the strong stimulation of EA. Intriguingly, there are reports that Manaka's ion cords still work when used with plastic-handled (non-conductive) needles. Thus the diode cords and the other polarity agents that Manaka used may not be acting electrically at all.

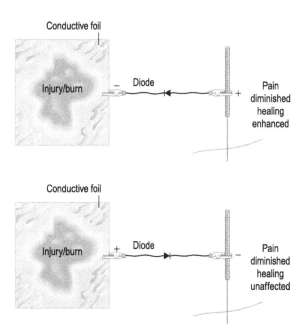

**Figure 10.18** Ion pumping cords. An early application – wound healing.

Indeed, his 'X-signal' may be the same as Eeman's 'X force'. One practitioner, Joseph Odom, has in fact combined ion cords with Eeman's circuits, using diode cords in circuits that include different substances (herbs or vitamins) in solution, and claiming better and more rapid results with this '*qi* and microcurrent' combination than with needles alone. Unlike Morell, he has not found amplification important for lasting benefits. He also uses much deeper needling than Manaka, and still obtains good results.

Willem Khoe, in the 1970s, used ion cords in conjunction with EAV measurement, connecting the 'positive' end to a needle in the point with the lower reading. In the case of pain, he attached the 'negative' end to a needle in the *ashi* point, and the other end to LI-4 or ST-36. Unlike Manaka, he found that reversing the polarity could sometimes exacerbate pain.

## SOME VERY SUBTLE APPROACHES

In the Japanese *toyohari* tradition, some treatments are given without needles penetrating the skin or even contacting the body. Another subtle energy system has been promoted by Korean industrialist Kim Chi Kyung, who developed it to treat his wife after a severe stroke. Known as Genesen, its 'acutouch pointers' make use of the effects of magnetism, far infrared and negative ions to 'accelerate the life forces around us'. However, the probes are very sharp, and both this and the lengthy treatments recommended make it rather impractical for most people.

At the subtle end of the acupuncture technology spectrum, what is being manipulated and measured sometimes appears to be idea, and sometimes energy, like *qi* itself. Conventional medicine may consider some of acupuncture's effects 'psychosomatic' but, as Felix Mann has said, 'the success of acupuncture lies somewhere between the mental and physical aspects'. The presence of mind (or the interaction between two minds) is a necessary part of the process.

## CONCLUDING THOUGHTS: IS TECHNOLOGY ULTIMATELY REDUNDANT?

Non-traditional methods of acupoint stimulation are very diverse. Broadly, they can be separated into those whose main effect is mediated through neurological mechanisms (afferent nerve activation) and those where this may not be so. The former give a relatively strong sensation, whereas the latter are subtler. As Manaka wrote, methods using strong physical stimulation can achieve desired results quickly, but may easily overshoot optimal levels of stimulation, whereas polarity agents nudge the body back to adjust slowly to the desired condition, with less chance of adverse reactions. Microcurrent, depending on the mode used, may offer a middle way.

Despite their diversity, both strong and subtle approaches have often been justified as attempts to replicate signalling parameters used within the body, the former with pulses shaped like those of neuronal action potentials, or with naturally occurring frequencies, and the latter in terms of microcurrent levels or with the body's own signals. The gentler methods may also give a more differentiated effect depending on the parameters used. In particular, there is a persistent view that polarity in some way plays a role in the more subtle approaches when the whole person of the practitioner is involved in determining how the treatment is to be applied and in monitoring resulting changes.

The aim of treatment is of course to help patients regain their own homeodynamic balance in life and dispense with external gadgetry, rather than becoming dependent on it. However, in many instances of severe illness, there may be long-term dependence on some of the stronger forms of nerve stimulation.

With measurement rather than just simple point detection, there are again a number of currently used methods that, apart from the AMI, all involve the practitioner in a feedback loop with the patient and some kind of meter. Thus they appear to be aids that amplify and bring to awareness what in a sense we may already know. Some experienced testers experience such signals directly within their own bodies and do not actually need the apparatus any longer. This is not to say that the equipment is unnecessary. It may very well be needed to focus and train inner awareness, may become necessary again after a period of lack of practice, and may have other subsidiary functions in the 'trialogue' of patient, practitioner and intermediary technology. Nevertheless, like the treatment device, the measurement system may become redundant in time.

---

## SUMMARY

Some key points in this chapter are:

- A distinction is made between methods such as EA and TENS, in which stimulation is usually strongly perceived, and microcurrent systems, including CES, where stimulation may even be subliminal
- Because microcurrent does not trigger nerve discharges, its effects on pain are possibly secondary to changes in microcirculation and resulting reductions in inflammation
- EA systems can also be divided between those in which something is done to the patient and those in which there is more of a two-way interaction

- Many advanced systems involve treatment based on electrical readings at body points. The practitioner is closely involved in the feedback loops that result. Expensive computerised integrated systems should be approached with caution
- Bioresonance systems, applying signals that match those of various physiological processes, may well become more important in future.

## Additional material in the CD-Rom resource

The full version of this chapter in the electronic research resource contains further details on the devices mentioned here, together with information on treatment protocols for some of them. Other equipment is also introduced.

## RECOMMENDED READING

*Heavyweight TENS textbook:*
Mannheimer JS, Lampe GN 1984 Clinical Transcutaneous Electrical nerve Stimulation. FA Davis, Philadelphia, PA

*A useful account of microcurrent from an acupuncture perspective:*
Starwynn D 2002 Microcurrent Electro-Acupuncture: Bio-electric principles, evaluation and treatment. Desert Heart Press, Phoenix, AZ

*A good introduction to ryodoraku:*
Hyodo M 1975 Ryodoraku Treatment: An objective approach to acupuncture. Japan Ryodoraku, Autonomic Nerve System Society, Osaka

*A comprehensive report by Motoyama:*
Motoyama H 1997 Measurements of Ki Energy Diagnoses and Treatments: treatment principles of Oriental medicine from an electrophysiological viewpoint. Human Science Press, Tokyo

*A basic introduction to Voll's work:*
Werner F, Voll R 1979 Electro-acupuncture Primer. Medizinisch Literarische Verlagsgesellschaft, Uelzen, Germany

*A very readable biography of Voll (in German):*
Rondé G 1998 Dr Reinhold Voll 1909–1989, Arzt, Forscher, Lehrer: Elektroakupunktur nach Voll – ein ganzheitliches Diagnose- und Therapiesystem. Medizinisch Literarische Verlagsgesellschaft, Uelzen, Germany

*The basic MORA textbook:*
Morell F 1990 The MORA Concept: Patients' own and coloured light oscillations. Theory and practice. Karl F Haug, Heidelberg

*The corresponding book on the BICOM device:*
Brügemann H 1993 Bioresonance and Multiresonance Therapy (BRT): New, forward-looking forms of therapy with ultrafine body energies and environmental signals. Documentation on theory and practice. Haug International, Bruxelles

*The master's book on polarity methods:*
Manaka Y, Itaya K, Birch S 1995 Chasing the Dragon's Tail: The theory and practice of acupuncture in the work of Yoshio Manaka. Paradigm Publications, Brookline, MA

*A fascinating account of Eeman's research:*
Eeman LE 1947 Co-operative Healing: The curative properties of human radiations. Frederick Muller, London

*Sources for figures:*
Greenlee C, with Greenlee DL and Wing TW 1999 Basic Microcurrent Therapy Acupoint and Body Work Manual. Earthen Vessel, Kelseyville, CA
Kenyon JN 1985 Modern Techniques of Acupuncture. A critical Review of European Developments in Electro-acupuncture III. A Scientific Guide to Bioelectronic Regulatory Techniques and Complex Homoeopathy. Thorsons, Wellingborough, UK

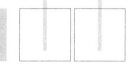

# Tools of the trade

This chapter is intended to help you decide what equipment you may want to use in your own clinic. It should be read in conjunction with Chapter 10, which offers an overview of the equipment available.

## YOU AND YOUR PRACTICE

There are many questions to consider before you invest in a device:

- Are you an expert or a beginner?
- Are you rich or are you poor?
- Are you adventurous and exploratory, or conservative and cautious?
- Do you have the time and inclination to attend courses and learn demanding and complex new skills, or do you just want an adjunctive tool as a backup to use occasionally and which you can handle after an afternoon's tinkering?
- Are you trained in an acupuncture tradition where strong stimulation is the norm, or are you happier with subtler methods?
- Do you feel comfortable around electricity and needles, or do you like the idea of stimulating the body to do its own thing with less-invasive modalities such as light and magnetism?
- Are you satisfied with your current ways of diagnosis, or do you believe more can be learned from the body by other means?

Take your time, ask questions and remember that very little is 'proven' in electrotherapy. As Richard Kovacs wrote in 1949, 'There is danger in too much and too complicated apparatus for therapy, just as there is danger of too much apparatus for diagnostic purposes when one's five senses and clinical experience, unaided, should be adequate to solve many problems.'

## WHAT TO LOOK FOR IN A DEVICE

There is no point in purchasing new equipment unless it is genuinely going to increase your versatility and effectiveness in the clinic. Suggestions of unique benefits over and above those of similar devices should be supported by *independent* research. Even the most ardent gadget lover will rarely need more than a few different machines.

The factors mentioned here are applicable primarily to TENS and EA, but some may be appropriate for other types of equipment too.

### Type

Once you know which modality interests you (EA, LA, microcurrent, etc.), you need to consider your working style. Would you prefer a handheld device for brief stimulation of a number of different points in quick succession (in which case you are very much part of the procedure), or do you prefer to set up a treatment such as TENS that can run by itself for a certain time, leaving you free to focus on other things? Or would you consider investing in a multifunctional machine so you are free to choose how you work as your experience develops?

### Size

A large clinic unit may look hopelessly out of place and intimidating in a homely traditionalist treatment room. A lightweight, portable and compact unit may be more easily tidied away, and be more practical for a multiclinic practice or home use by patients.

### Design

Equipment should be sturdy, conveniently shaped and presentable, with controls clearly and simply laid out. Exotic design features, fancy push-buttons and lights do not relieve pain. For smaller items, a belt or pocket clip might be useful.

## Controls

Controls need to be of a convenient size and shape, easily adjustable and accessible, yet protected from accidental knocking or disturbance (this is especially important with TENS). They should not be too stiff, small or poorly marked. In particular, although this may sound ridiculous, amplitude controls should be marked so that they are not likely to be turned up instead of off at the wrong moment. They should also provide finely graded and precise changes, preferably linear, with no sudden or unpredictable increments.

## Amplitude

Is the amplitude sufficient for your requirements? Is it still strong if all outputs are active at once? Do quoted current figures refer to peak or average levels – even if the former is high, if the latter is low it may not be very useful (see Ch. 3, page 30). Many EA devices are built with such a large safety margin that they are not strong enough for use with surface electrodes (for TENS, currents of up to 80 mA into a 500 Ω load, or 60 mA into 1 kΩ, should be available). If you wish to use surface stimulation, output parameters should enable a deeper sense of *deqi* from skin pads or probe but preferably without eliciting uncomfortable skin sensation (you can check for this on yourself, at LI-4 for example). Most stimulators have a 'constant current' output (see Ch. 3, page 37), and should be 'voltage limited', with a maximum current density of around 4 mA/cm² to avoid such discomfort. For constant voltage output, if this is > 40 V, current should be limited to 1 mA. Some authorities suggest maximum output should not exceed 16 V. A microcurrent stimulator should provide a minimum of at most 20 μA.

## Amplitude range switch

Some machines can be very strong. A clearly marked amplitude range switch, to reduce output volume when using needles rather than pads, could be a useful safeguard. For EA, output of 20 mA into 1 kΩ is generally ample.

## Waveform

A variety of waveforms may be useful, but you are unlikely to find this except in the more expensive machines. Nowadays, for EA and TENS more and more provide symmetrical biphasic charge-balanced square-wave output (see Ch. 3, page 32). In some cheaper devices there may be spikes that are uncomfortable if amplitude is too high.

## Charge balance and asymmetry – the polarity switch

If manufacturers claim a device is charge balanced, you need to check whether this is so over the whole output

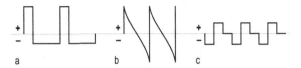

**Figure 11.1** Stimulation feels uneven. Three situations in which charge-balanced stimulation may not feel symmetrical to the patient. (a) Greater amplitude in phases of one polarity. (b) More rapid rise time in phases of one polarity. (c) Negative polarity phases lead.

range you are likely to use therapeutically. If a device is *not* charge-balanced and is being used for EA, you will need to keep treatments short (less than 3 minutes, in some instances) to avoid electrolysis of the needles. If longer treatment is required, polarity will have to be reversed (maybe more than once) during a session. Some machines have a switch so you can do this without having to unclip the leads to swap them over. Such a switch may also be useful even with some devices that are charge balanced, and when you are using surface pads. As shown in Figure 11.1, the sensation may be stronger if the amplitude of one pulse is greater than that of the return pulse, or if it is always the negative phase of a biphasic pulse that leads. If the patient is to experience roughly the same sensation at both electrodes, these will need to be switched over. Being able to select polarity can be an important asset in microcurrent treatment.

## Pulse duration

Some devices will automatically alter pulse duration with frequency or amplitude changes so that the amount of charge transferred is much the same whatever the setting. Most do not, and it is useful in any case to be able to control pulse duration independently, so that different diameters of nerve fibre can be selectively stimulated. A good range would be 50–250 μs. Longer pulse durations are the rule when using microcurrent.

## Frequency

A wide frequency range is useful, perhaps with some preset frequencies you are likely to use. Output frequency should be both stable and accurate; numbers round frequency dials are often not precise, particularly at low frequencies. A useful range would be 2–200 Hz. If you wish to use EA for investigational rather than clinical purposes, frequency and other output parameters should be properly calibrated. In one study of three 'representative' EA devices available in the US, for example, at least two measured parameters were not within 25% of the manufacturer's claimed values. In another study of six commercially available devices, frequency was accurate to less than 1% in only two, with errors of 15–50% in the others!

## Modulation and patterns of stimulation

An EA or TENS machine should be able to produce both continuous and interrupted patterns of stimulation. For EA, dense-disperse (DD, alternating two different frequencies) is essential. For TENS, different sorts of modulation are often provided: amplitude, pulse duration or frequency modulation (the latter a gentler form of DD). Some devices provide various options.

Modulation can produce a pleasant massage-like effect, and is also important as a means of dishabituation. To reduce habituation, some devices introduce random elements ('noise'), 'jitter', or even musical elements into the stimulus, or add a second frequency out of step with the main treatment frequency.

Some simple machines offer only a few parameter combinations. Even the more complex devices may offer only preset programmes. Consider whether these really suit your needs. On the other hand, without presets you may be left floundering in a sea of uncertain options.

## Battery or mains?

Any mains-powered device should incorporate some form of safety override control. Battery rather than mains operated is perhaps best for EA devices. Some machines come with a non-removable rechargeable battery, for which a specific mains adaptor is supplied. Others may use readily available rechargeables, or may work properly only with non-rechargeables. It is useful to know how often a battery needs changing, how long it takes to charge, whether a device has a reliable low-battery indicator, and whether treatment can be given while an internal battery is being charged. Generally speaking, the more parameters that can be adjusted and the wider the range of adjustment, the greedier the device will be for power.

## Outputs

How complicated are your treatments? Do you want two, three or four outputs? Are output channels isolated, and with independent amplitude controls, or might there be 'cross-talk' between electrodes from different outputs, or unpredictable changes on one channel when changing the parameters of another? Do you want to be able to use different frequencies as well as amplitudes on different outputs at the same time (as in interferential, or for optimising local/distal treatment effects)?

## Plugs and sockets

Plugs should not be loose when inserted in the output sockets, nor so tight as to be a struggle to get in or out. With changes in US and European legislation on stimulator design, the simple 3.5 mm diameter jack plug has now almost disappeared in favour of supposedly safer variants. Some of these may not be as sturdy. Sockets of 2.5 mm diameter are still sometimes used; adaptors for converting 3.5 mm jacks for these (or 2.5 mm jacks to 3.5 mm sockets) can be found in electronics stores.

If you intend to use a TENS/EA device for obstetric use, a patient handheld 'booster' switch and appropriate socket should really be available. A few electrostimulators also come with a socket for a handheld LED probe.

## Leads

Leads should neither be too short, nor so long as to tangle in use or in storage. Around 120–140 cm is generally adequate. They should also not be so heavy and rigid as to pull on needle clips; some thin modern ones are stronger than they look. Colour-coded leads can be an advantage.

## Clips and connectors

Needle clips should not be too chunky. Various miniature or lightweight ones are available (Fig. 11.2b). High Street stores can provide lead 'splitters', which are useful for treating several points of similar sensitivity at the same time, provided the stimulus from the one output is strong enough and standard jack plugs are used (Fig. 11.2a). Some companies provide splitters suited to the socket design they use. For disposable surface electrodes, most provide standard connectors (with 12 mm long, 2 mm diameter connector pins). Crocodile clips that fit on to these can be found in radio supply catalogues, although they are quite heavy (Fig. 11.2a).

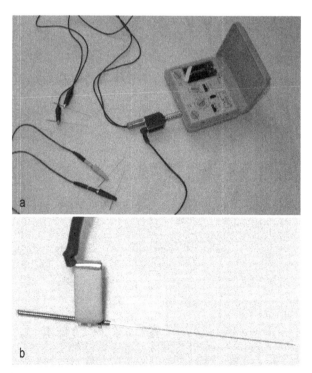

**Figure 11.2** (a) V-TENS device, with lead 'splitter', standard 'crocodile' clips (above) and more cumbersome clips for converting TENS leads to EA use (below). (b) One design of lightweight clip. (Photographs by Riccardo Cuminetti.)

## Point detector/stimulators

If a point probe is provided separately from the main unit, it is much easier to switch from detection to treatment mode if the switch is on the probe itself. Test it in detection mode for accuracy and definition of response; many are not very reliable. The best will use a biphasic microcurrent for detection, and will have a spring-loaded probe. Make sure the probe tip is not too sharp.

## Extras

A timer can be useful, especially for home use. Check whether the treatment duration offered fits with your preferred way of working, and whether the device switches off completely when treatment ends.

A 'ramp' function may make stimulation more acceptable to some patients and is standard in many microcurrent devices. With this, the amplitude of trains of pulses increases gradually, rather than abruptly.

Being able to treat different points with different stimuli simultaneously (e.g. CTENS locally, ALTENS at related trigger points) is becoming more common with more sophisticated electronics. Once a device is processor driven rather than just a matter of hardware, much more becomes possible, from PC links to biofeedback interaction with the patient, to treatment recording, and so on.

Do make sure your device comes with all the right accessories (mains adaptor, matching plugs and sockets, no 'hidden extras').

## Gels

Any electrode gels supplied should be non-allergenic, non-staining and preferably chloride free.

## Instructions

Is the manual illustrated, clear and comprehensive? Is there a helpline? If a training course is offered, try to speak to someone who has already attended to find out how useful or necessary it may be, and whether it offers good value for money. Such courses may not be independent of marketing pressures. You need to know whether they properly qualify you to use the equipment, and whether your practitioner insurance covers this use. Remember too that advice from sales personnel on safe and effective operation may not always be reliable.

## Warranty and service

How long is the warranty? What does it cover? Does it include defects in material or workmanship, shipping damage (if reported within a defined period), labour and parts (perhaps for different periods)? It is unlikely to cover leads, damage from misuse or neglect, and is probably invalidated if the unit is opened by anyone unauthorised.

Carefully check the terms of the manufacturer's liability in case of adverse events. It may also be sensible to find out how long the company has been in business.

Is there a reliable and rapid maintenance service? (Maybe find out from someone who has used it!) How expensive is this? Is regular service a requirement for continued use of the device? Is a loan machine available while yours is repaired or serviced? If service by the manufacturer or supplier is not an option, will they provide the necessary details for someone else to do the job? What is the expected lifetime of the device? Can you find out how many have been manufactured, and what the repair rate is?

## Trial, or tribulation

Some companies offer a 'try before you buy' option, which can be helpful. During such a trial period, you can assess a device for its usefulness and effectiveness. If you work in a hospital or other medical setting, you may be required to have someone who understands electromedical equipment assess it for safety and compliance with standards. This may not be so easy if you work outside such institutions, but would be sensible nevertheless.

## Price and purchase

In the UK, if a patient with chronic pain is purchasing a device, they can sign a form (giving their practitioner's address) that states this. Under group 14 of schedule 5 to the VAT Act 1983, this will generally mean they are not liable for VAT (value added tax) on the purchase. Of course, practitioners who purchases such a device solely to treat their own chronic pain will not be liable for VAT either.

Some acupuncture suppliers will give 10% reduction to *bona fide* students of acupuncture. Mail order companies in the UK generally offer a 30-day money back guarantee in addition to statutory rights (a handling fee is usually deducted).

Be very cautious with secondhand equipment, particularly if you see adverts for several practitioners trying to get rid of the same device. If the price is high but you are convinced that this is what you really want, consider a leasing agreement, but consult your financial advisor first.

Be a little wary of special offers. Sometimes warranty terms are not so good with these, and sometimes old stock is being sold off to make way for more up-to-date equipment.

Shop around. The differences between some European and British prices, for instance, can be quite astounding. Beware, however, of importing untried cheap equipment from the Far East. Apart from the legal problems that may be involved, some copies of established lines, even with similar names, may not perform as well as the originals.

## Safety

A number of safety features may be incorporated. In some machines, it is impossible to activate electrodes if any output amplitude is not at zero first. In others, output may revert to zero if parameters (other than amplitude) are changed during treatment, or if the device malfunctions. Some indication may also be given if there is a poor connection or a broken lead. There should also be one simple control that a patient can use to switch the device off if for some reason you need to leave them unattended for a short while.

## Standards

There may be local state legislation you need to know about (or, in Europe, legislation for your country that is slightly different from the overall European rulings). In Europe it is now illegal to sell devices without a CE mark, numbered, to indicate the manufacturer. You may need to consider this when disposing of older equipment. Further information on standards and legislation may be found in Appendix 2.

If you purchase a device that requires a mains adaptor, do make sure this is suitable for medical use, and has been passed for use with the device.

# LISTINGS

The following listings offer an introductory overview of some of the equipment available. A much fuller list, together with technical information on the different devices, is included in the CD-ROM ⊙ resource version of this chapter. Entries on older devices and curiosities can also be found there.

(Much of this information was obtained from manufacturers' websites, product literature and advertisements, so should be read with discrimination. Prices and output parameters, where given, may not be current. Although inclusion should not be interpreted as recommendation, I have indicated some personal favourites of my own. For details of suppliers and other sources of information, see Appendix 1.)

## Electrical stimulation

### EA, OR EA WITH TENS

AAA-301 (Harmony) (the AAA-401 is shown in Fig. 9.15.1 on page 270) This is a three-channel stimulator with nicely coloured control knobs and matching crocodile clip sleeves (the sleeves could be tighter). Has a zero-output safety feature, with LED indicator if all outputs are not at zero when device is switched on, battery level indicator and timer. Is a successor to the Equinox meridian devices (developed in association with the Society for Biophysical Medicine and others). With very comfortable pulses, it is suitable for both EA and TENS.

Acus (Cefar) This is a processor-driven purpose built EA device, with four outputs and nine preset programmes. Each pair of channels can output a different programme.

Display indicates battery level, as well as current setting and programme for each channel; 30-minute timer for all programmes (timer can be deactivated). Powered by an internal rechargeable NiMh battery. Light microhook needle clips.

Agistim Duo (Sédatélec) This is a top class machine, beautifully engineered. There are two pairs of independent outputs (i.e. four in all), each pair with its separate signal generator, a charge-balanced asymmetrical pulse (but no electrode reversal switch), suitable for needles or pads, and an adjustable timer. Very clear LCD display for time elapsed, total time and treatment parameters. Various safety features include a zero-only start, and rezeroing if any parameters other than amplitude are altered during treatment. A number of disadvantages include the large 'footprint' (when using on a small couch), the need to switch it off even if using the timer, and that it is mains powered (the manufacturers advise against use during a thunderstorm!). The frequency scan can feel a little abrupt if you set it to run repeatedly from 1–100 Hz (better might have been for it to increase and decrease alternately). Although the clips are very attractive to look at, I found them a little fiddly when attaching to needles difficult to access. In one unit tested, there was considerable cross-talk between outputs. Make sure you get the appropriate mains adaptor for your country.

AM System B and AM3D Acupunctoscopes (AcuMedic) These are similar to the Ito IC-4107 and AWQ-104B in conception, although pricey and a little limited in some ways compared to the Ito device. The AM3D incorporates a digital frequency meter. Both have robust, fairly sensitive controls, and with output strong enough for TENS as well as EA, polarity reversal and amplitude (TENS/EA) switches. Supplied with three slightly heavy leads and medium-sized crocodile clips (lighter clips available). The point location/treatment probe is basic, and its amplitude control is poorly labelled.

AS Super 4 Needle stimulator (Schwa-Medico) This has four independent outputs (no point locator), with two separate generators, so that HF and LF can be used simultaneously (e.g. for local HF, distal LF stimulation). The internal 9 V battery is rechargeable in a handy 4 hours. Patented short-circuit facility. Good informative manual. Disadvantages are that the minicrocodile clips supplied can be awkward, springing off needles without warning, and the unnecessary complication of a separate box into which the electrode leads are plugged.

AWQ-104B (Plenty Source) This is a cheap and cheerful four-channel unit, with point location/treatment probe, but may be a little confusing for the beginner (the manual though is quite clear and detailed, with good instructions on point location). Although now made in Hong Kong, test before purchase, as with all low-cost Chinese devices!

Electro-Stimulator 4-C, 6-C and 8-C (Pantheon Research) These have four, six or eight independent channels, respectively. They are US made, with inbuilt clip, lead and battery tester. Auricular 'microclips' are included; an extra facial probe (interchangeable Q-tip or rounded steel probe), is available. Two-year warranty is standard (excluding clips).

ES-160 (Ito) This six-output eight-programme device is impressive, a lot easier to use than the completely push-button 'Trio' series, although without an option for simultaneous use of different programmes through different outputs, as with the Trio or Cefar's products. Otherwise it has a good range of facilities, although parameters are surprisingly limited in some respects. Has a battery level indicator, and 0–60 min timer adjustable once stimulation has started (thankfully the electronic bleep that sounds when treatment is completed can be disabled). Frequency and pulse duration can also be adjusted during treatment. Various safety features include zero-start, output cut-off if output increases abruptly, and emergency stop button. I found the long leads tended to tangle, particularly with the rather angular (and heavy) crocodile clips used. The leads were also difficult to separate to stimulate points far apart. Usefully incorporates ryodoraku – readings can be stored in memory.

G-6805/2 (SMIF, Shanghai) This is a Chinese classic, used in hundreds of clinical and experimental studies. Available in various models. The usual multioutput design is capable of CW, intermittent and DD output (in some versions fixed at 4/20 Hz), as well as point location. Satisfyingly strong – up to 200 V! (for surface electrodes such as the lead plate ones supplied). However, for needles the output is not completely charge balanced. Sturdily built, with some good extra features. Can be used with batteries (but takes a lot of power) or mains (not recommended). Unfortunately, with some models a very tinny 'Happy Birthday to You' plays when the inbuilt timer switches off! Has some safety functions. Controls are horrendously non-linear, and one test some years ago showed output voltages completely different from those given in the manual. The meter is not really adequate to indicate output frequency, as it claims to. Comes with an interesting selection of electrodes, with useful coloured leads. The manual is quite skimpy for a device with so many knobs and buttons. I do not know whether it is available with a CE mark.

HANS LY257 (Healthronics) 'Han's acupoints and nerve stimulator' (HANS) exists in various models. Designed for use with surface electrodes, the HANS produces quite a kick, but this looks more unpleasant than it feels. Slight overshoot spikes could make this uncomfortable with needles (although in practice none of my patients complained of this). The two outputs can be selected to operate synchronously or alternately, to reduce tolerance (also useful for stimulating muscles and their antagonists). Has an automatic 30-minute timer, after which the low-battery indicator LED will flash as a reminder to switch off the device and conserve power. The Singapore-manufactured HANS has a much sturdier feel to it than the usual Chinese devices. The little user manual is quite detailed. The press-stud electrode connectors are not quite as simple or flexible as the standard ones. Unfortunately, although an excellent machine, the HANS is not as yet CE marked.

Helio EA-2 (Helio) This is suitable for EA and TENS, with a point detection facility (not the best I've used). It is neat, cheap, but limited (with no frequency indicator, for instance, and the probe cannot be used to stimulate, although the tip can be removed for autoclaving). In the unit I tested, the leads were flimsy and the controls unduly stiff. Warranty covers only 3 months for labour. The manual is clear and simple.

IC-1107 EA device (Ito) This is a neat little three-output device with a good range of useful semipreset frequencies, a high/low-intensity switch, and battery check., but no frills (CW only, no intermittent or DD settings). The output is not charge balanced at high intensity, and even then is too weak for using with surface electrodes. There are optional magnetic button electrodes at two different strengths.

IC-4107 (Ito) (see Fig. 9.3.2 on page 120) This has four outputs (sockets to current US/European standards). It is elegant and impressive, yet small enough to place on a treatment couch (only $200 \times 126 \times 44$ mm, and 363 g). Has good controls and safety features (zero-output start function; virtually no cross-talk between outputs), continuous, intermittent, or DD biphasic charge-balanced output, high/low-intensity and frequency range controls. There is insufficient output for surface electrodes. Has a timer (10, 20 or 60 min) and battery monitor (takes $6 \times 1.5$ V AA batteries). A nice point location/treatment probe is provided, with a well-rounded tip and a switch on the probe itself (but an inordinately long lead!). The manual is a bit computerish, and a slight current surge is occasionally experienced when switching outputs on or off. Comes with colour-coded leads with clip connectors for needles, optional magnetic button electrodes at two different strengths, and is my favourite of the midrange devices. Sadly, the manufacturers have now discontinued production in favour of the ES-160.

Nomapulse 4 (Noma) This has four independent channels. Antisurge protection means there is no output if amplitude is not at zero when switching on, if electrode contact is lost during treatment, or if amplitude increases too rapidly. The single (eight-way) output lead is a recipe for a tangled muddle, the off-the-shelf sleeves for the crocodile clips are annoyingly slippery, and the built in rechargeable battery may take 16 hours to charge (awkward if you're in a hurry!) – disappointing overall.

V-Tens Plus (Body Clock) **(see Fig. 11.2a)** This is a compact and versatile TENS machine, with virtually charge-balanced output, so suitable for EA as well. Leads for surface electrodes or needles are available. The pouch it comes in, as with other Body Clock devices, can be worn on a belt, as can the device itself. An AC/DC mains adaptor is available (CE approved). Produces a slight surge on switching on the first output (so it may be best to connect electrodes after switching on, ensuring amplitude controls are at zero). Pulse duration and frequency can be selected (although the dials are not particularly well calibrated, and are a little small and fiddly). Has a timer (15, 30, or 60 minutes), LED low-battery and frequency indicators. An 'intraoral universal ring electrode' is available from one supplier for use in dental anaesthesia. Size is only $104 \times 89 \times 38$ mm.

WQ-6F (57-6F) electronic acupunctoscope (Donghua, Beijing) This is a modified version of the earlier 57-6D and WQ-10C models (like the G-6805, the 57-6 was used in many clinical and experimental studies). Has a sturdy design, with a handle that doubles as a stand; stable and powerful output, for needles, pads or saline-soaked cotton wool in cup electrodes, is battery or mains powered, with mains adaptor supplied, but no point location function. As with a number of Chinese machines, a small plug-in monitoring loudspeaker is provided, which is useful to familiarise yourself with the different output possibilities. Like the AgiStim Duo and the AS Super 4, it contains two independent signal generators, so that two sets of output sockets can provide different parameters. The seven independent outputs can also be linked in various ways, which can be a bit confusing for beginners, but this is a very good machine once you've got the hang of it. Unfortunately, at the time of writing, this machine has not been CE marked.

## TENS

There are hundreds of different TENS machines available, of which only a few are mentioned here.

804 OB (Body Clock) This is an obstetric TENS, with patient hand switch. It is small, neat, but not charge balanced.

AngioTENS (Nidd Valley) This is a specialised TENS unit developed for treatment of angina in collaboration with the Cardiothoracic Research Centre at Broad Green, Liverpool.

Obstetric Pulsar TENS (Biomedical Life) A patient hand switch converts stimulation from burst mode to boost (continuous mode) during contractions.

Primo (Cefar) This is a neat, well-engineered charge-balanced TENS device. Two independent channels allow simultaneous treatment with two different stimulation profiles (for local/distal points, or different types of pain). A key-lock safety feature ensures amplitude cannot be inadvertently increased (without turning it down first), programmes cannot be changed without first zeroing output, and the unit automatically switches off if left unconnected for 2 minutes. Has an LCD display (shows programme in use, current amplitude on each channel, safety key feature in operation, and low battery), and cleverly designed lead storage, using the case profile and belt clip. Two 1.5 V batteries are used instead of one 9 V battery for longer stimulation time and reduced running costs. For those who select their parameters on the basis of patient preference, the range of presets may feel restrictive compared with those of the V-TENS (for example). Another (dis)advantage is that, although charge balanced, the amplitude of the leading pulse is far greater than that of the return one, so that sensation is much stronger at one electrode than the other (this can be offset to some extent by swapping over leads halfway through treatment).

ReliefBand® (Woodside Biomedical) This is a wristwatch-style TENS, purpose designed for P-6 antiemesis stimulation. It is approved by the FDA as an over-the-counter product for motion sickness, and available from various sources. Available in disposable (48- or 144-hour) and reusable models. Output amplitude may be controlled. Conductive gel is required.

Trio 300 (Ito) This is a pocket-sized device with two *independent* channels. Incorporates TENS, EMS and microcurrent. Supplied with four TENS electrodes and hydrogel pads, and can also be used for EA at a stretch (needle leads an optional extra). A mains adaptor is available, as well as handheld microcurrent probes and vaginal electrode. Extremely versatile, it has space for five user programmes (retained in memory even if the battery fails). It may even be programmed with different programmes for each output (though microcurrent cannot be used with TENS or EMS), or a sequence of different settings (although these cannot then be cycled repeatedly). Safety features include an error message if output is abnormal or circuit is broken, 'zero-start' output and keyboard lock. Includes a digital timer (up to 30 min, with automatic power off) and low-battery warning. In common with many LCD screen devices with only a few buttons (keys) to push, it is hard to get accustomed to a faint screen, and easy to get confused by which key does what. Keys for output intensity are not a good idea – they respond very slowly compared with standard rotary controls (intensity also increases in 1 mA steps – appropriate for TENS, but too gross for EA). It is very good value, if a little fiddly.

## HANDHELD PROBES (pTENS)

Treatment with a small-diameter probe can sometimes be uncomfortable if it just irritates the skin without eliciting (muscle) *deqi*. If for no other reason, it is sensible to try before you buy. Check too for a smooth tip that will not cause minor abrasions and measurement artefacts. When measuring, a sprung probe may give more reliable results.

Acupoint (Plenty Source) This is exactly the same as the Pointer Plus, but comes with a 186-page handbook that could be useful as a guide for self-treatment by patients, and so is more expensive.

Acupoint Avance (Allied Health) This is a British version of the original Acupoint, marketed through the same company, but with very different output parameters (a much lower current, for one thing). Polarity reversal is possible. Has a visual display, but the controls are somewhat fiddly. After the Pointer Plus, I found this disappointing, but it may perhaps be suitable for home use by patients.

AM Neurostimulator (AcuMedic) This is one of the best devices I have found for point location, but a bit awkward in some ways (the handheld probe is not self-contained, but linked to a unit for the controls and batteries). Different polarities or higher frequencies can be used. With its strong output, it is claimed to be useful for deep trigger point work. Surface electrodes can be connected in place of the probe. Version 'M' includes a meter, and so is suited for ryodoraku, in place of the dearer Japanese TORmeter.

MibiTech Tao (MibiTech) This is a beautifully designed point locator/stimulator with silver-plated probe tip. A pressure-sensitive switch activates the pen at approximately 15–20 g. A desk holder includes an optional recharger. A planned version includes a Bluetooth™ PC link. It applies 50–300 µA pulses to the acupoints for about 40 seconds, claimed to trigger the body's own healing system. A long-term goal is to develop a method for adapting stimulus frequency to the patient's skin characteristics.

NeuroTrac 3A™ (Verity Medical) This is a two-channel digital TENS and pTENS (incorporates acupoint detector). There are 12 preprogrammed TENS modes (including burst, modulation and conventional TENS) and two preprogrammed pTENS modes, and facilities to set up customised conventional TENS and pTENS programmes. The LCD displays parameters, programme mode and time (countdown).

Pain Master (Skylark) This provides a combination of either electrical or vibratory stimulation (or both) with static magnetic field, applied via carbonised rubber electrodes in a handheld unit (not to be confused with the Painmaster). It is suitable for patient use, although the handle may be a little cumbersome for those with arthritis. Frequency of electrical stimulation is adjustable.

Pointer Plus (Plenty Source) (see Fig. 9.11.4 on page 229) This provides a strong but comfortable stimulus (stronger than the Stimplus, for example, but has no timer and is a little more expensive). It is identical to the Acupoint but comes only with a single sheet of instructions and no manual.

Has useful interchangeable (screw-in) sprung probe tips. A good rugged device for clinical use, with simple sensitivity and intensity controls, but requires fairly frequent battery changes. Includes a cylindrical return electrode for practitioners who do not like to receive treatment at the same time as their patients, and in some countries an optional probe accessory that converts the device into a dual-point stimulator. Chan Gunn uses it in contact with needles for trigger point stimulation.

PuTENS (Schwa-Medico) This is a 'punctiform TENS' developed by Alf Heydenreich, and used in many of his impressive studies on pain and headache. It comes with a fine sprung probe and a wonderful roller long enough to treat your own back. Gives a powerful – and effective – kick!

Stimplus (see Fig. 12.3 on page 329) This is an elegant little point locator/stimulator, with an earphone for the practitioner so you can use it on ear points without driving the patient crazy. Has a timer (30 or 60 seconds, or continuous), and six intensity levels, but even at maximum is considerably weaker than the Pointer Plus (so when treating a patient with dry skin, you may well need to use some form of moisturiser to get an effective stimulation). Amplitude is regulated by a rather tedious push-button control, and a somewhat annoying safety feature is that when switched off the amplitude reverts to the lowest setting. But patients like it.

## Other equipment

### PIEZOELECTRIC STIMULATORS

Akupunkt-Impulser PM-2002, or Piezo-Impulser PM-2002 (Vega) This has an adjustable impulse strength.

Pain Gone (Unique International) According to the manufacturers, the device lifetime is 100 000 discharges or 2–3 years, whichever is the sooner.

Piezo-DX (via most acupuncture distributors) Has a lifetime of 100 000 discharges.

### DIRECT CURRENT (DC) DEVICES – WORKING AT THE SENSORY LEVEL

Micro-Z™ (Prizm Medical) This is a pulsed DC neuromuscular stimulator, used with Electro-Mesh™, Silver-Thera™, and Stim-Support™ garment electrodes (gloves, sleeves, socks or lumbar supportive back brace). These can be worn in bed for easy night-time use (no gel required), are washable and durable (estimated life 90 days). It is used for diabetic neuropathy, carpal tunnel syndrome and other chronic pain problems.

### MICROCURRENT STIMULATION – SUBTHRESHOLD SYSTEMS

AlphaStim 100 (Electromedical Products International) (see Fig. 10.2 on page 283) This is probably the most commercially successful CES/microcurrent device. It is provided with earlobe clips, probes and electrode pads. If the latter need replacing, this should be with high-conductivity silver/silver chloride ones, not standard TENS pads. Has an LCD display and timer.

Liss bipolar cranial and body stimulator model SBL202-M (Pain Suppression Labs) (see Fig. 10.2 on page 283) This is very easy to use (only one control). It is battery powered, and uses old-fashioned moistened sponge electrodes that can be positioned over body acupoints, or over the temples for CES (less convenient than earclip electrodes). My own very limited use of the device with 11 patients left me unconvinced of its benefits, but it is a favourite of Norman Shealy's.

MENS®-i SUPER C (Earthen Vessel) This has two independent channels (each with main and auxiliary outputs for simultaneous use of probes and pads). Frequency, current, polarity (+, −, biphasic) and waveslope are adjustable independently for each channel, with 11 preset protocols in addition, and 'search threshold' (sensitivity) control (so that only points with conductance over a certain threshold are detected). Has a timer, with optional alarm (seconds and minutes ranges), analogue meter, and low-battery LED indicators for each channel (once on, output does not degrade for a further 16 hours of treatment). A variety of electrodes and probe tips include patented retractable 6 × Q-tip interferential probes that permit 'combing' of contoured areas.
  'MENS®' was intended to stand for 'minimal electrical non-invasive stimulation,' but more commonly now is taken as 'microcurrent electrical neuro/nerve stimulation.'

MicroACE Programme™(formerly ACE – Arthritis Care Electrostimulator) (MSL) This is one of the first devices to use preset dosages instead of treating at levels dependent on patient tolerance. It is very simple for patients to use at home, although it is easy to switch on inadvertently.

## CES – CRANIAL ELECTROTHERAPY STIMULATION
Please note that, in the US, CES devices are sold only to licensed health care professionals.

AlphaStim SCS (Electromedical Products International) This is a slimmed-down (CES only) version of the AlphaStim 100 (listed under Microcurrent devices above).

Nustar II, Nustar Custom, Wavestar (Nustar) Nustar devices, based on research by the late Michael Hercules, use a four-electrode headband rather than earclips.

Oasis (Comptronic) This is a stereo CES. It may be synchronised with Comptronic's light/sound stimulators.

SPES® Rx750 (SPES Technology) This was developed by scientists rather than clinicians, and is probably the most

researched of the lesser-known electrotherapy treatment modalities. Used for chronic intractable pain, anxiety and depression, and abstinence symptoms in drug withdrawal. Despite a fundamentally simple design, it is awkward to use (it is so sensitive that ensuring proper contact with the needle-clip ear electrodes can be quite fiddly, for example). It is temporarily unavailable.

## INFRARED AND MICROWAVE
Handheld infrared lamps for home use, like Skylark's 'Infrarex' (ST-302) are still a popular item, although standard infrared is considered a rather outdated modality by some. On the other hand, 'far infrared' is quite a current buzzword.

Firard III™ TDP lamp (via most acupuncture distributors) This is a basic far-infrared unit. The ceramic emitter in version III contains 33 minerals (version I had only eight), is more powerful and larger than earlier versions (250 W, 16.25 cm diameter). Has a 1500 hours ceramic plate life (spares are available, and easy to replace). It is classified as an infrared lamp in the US. Purchasable for home use without prescription. A small low-temperature portable version is available (11.25 cm diameter, charge time 2 minutes).

## MILLIMETRE WAVES (EXTREMELY HIGH FREQUENCY, EHF)
Artsakh (AcuVision) (see Fig. 10.7b on page 287) This is an EHF stimulator with fixed frequency (60.0 and 118.0 GHz, the oxygen absorption frequencies) or noise-like output, modulated randomly or according to a 1–99–1 Hz waveswing. Output is via a plastic waveguide. It was developed at the Institute of Radiophysics and Electronics in Armenia, and is named after the former capital of the country. One version includes pulse and respiration rate sensors, for monitoring the effects of treatment.

MRT Bioenergizer (Becktron) This is a handheld EHF device for local pain, inflammation or lymphatic congestion.

Porog-3NN (ICPI NSA RF) This is a microwave resonance therapy apparatus, used in many clinical trials, giving a low-power white noise output. It is supplied with an auriculotherapy attachment.

## LIGHT THERAPY: LOW-INTENSITY LASERS, LED, POLARISED LIGHT AND COLOUR DEVICES
Numerous companies produce lasers suitable for LA, classed as IIa devices unless otherwise stated. The most up-to-date information on this field can be found at Laser World (www.laser.nu). This should be browsed before deciding whether to purchase laser or LED equipment, for instance. Although many companies still supply low (1–10 mW) output devices, a more recent trend has been towards more powerful lasers (30–200 mW), not least because treatment time is then reduced. For the same reason, multisource diode arrays continue to be popular, for treating

open wounds, for instance (dosage can also be more accurately calculated than with manual 'scanning'). Portable rechargeable units are useful for sports injury work. Many other forms of light therapy equipment are listed in the CD-ROM ⊚ resource version of this chapter.

If tempted to buy a cheap lecture-style laser pointer, remember than if the light source is recessed within it, away from the tip, the power may be insufficient for treating all but the most superficial points in sensitive patients.

## LOW-INTENSITY ELECTROMAGNETIC FIELDS

### Variable fields – EEG entrainment methods

Many small PEMF devices have come and gone over the years. Most owe a considerable debt to the pioneering work of Wolfgang Ludwig in Germany, but his are the only ones to use coil cores 'doped' with particular combinations of trace elements.

#### Medicur (Snowden Healthcare)

This is a magnetic field therapy unit for home use. Effective through clothing, it is very easy to use (for just $3 \times 10$ minutes daily). The iron core is treated with 64 trace elements (similar trace elements are included in skin gels that can be used with the device). The basic version delivers 7.8 Hz, with a 2.5 kHz modulated carrier, producing a subharmonic frequency of 3.9 Hz and 'balanced' harmonic frequencies up to 1.25 GHz. A more sophisticated model delivers 3 Hz (for insomnia and stress), 7.8 Hz and 20 Hz (for stimulation and chronic pain), together with 'solar frequencies' and 2 kHz (claimed to stimulate endorphin production). The field penetrates 30 cm, and the device is safe to use near the head. Some of my patients have found this useful ('it's a comfort knowing you've got it'), but others not. Unusually, it has a 10-year guarantee.

### Whole-body and local exposure devices

There are many of these, and even proposals for a simple coil applicator that could be used with any TENS or EA stimulator (I do not believe this ever made it past the ideas stage).

#### MagPulser™ (Quantum Techniks)

This is a neatly designed handheld pulsed magnetic field therapy acupoint stimulator. As with other magnetic field devices, it can be used through clothing. Has been used for a number of acute and chronic pain conditions.

#### MitoSan (Vitatec)

This is an interesting but unnecessarily expensive variant of PEMF, using flexible 'biotrodes'. Two different signals may be applied simultaneously in some models. Has a facility for applying external (e.g. homeopathic) signals, or analogue colour frequencies. There is no measurement capability (some form of energy-testing procedure is required such as ACR, AK or EAV to determine optimum parameters, although a 'colour pass' enables a complete spectrum sweep for those that do not use such methods).

## VIBRATION, SOUND AND ULTRASOUND

There are numerous vibratory therapeutic devices, in part because vibration overlaps with massage. Leaving aside the larger chairs and beds that vibrate, oscillate, roll and heave, or play music into your chakras, there are many smaller machines that can be used in acupuncture practice.

#### QGM PE501 (various suppliers)

(see Fig 10.8 on page 288) This is the most recent ('chaotic') version of the *Qi Gong* machine (QGM), and clearly a machine for clinic use (although patients can use it unattended). Earlier versions (without the words 'chaos therapy' on the front panel) are available at lower prices. As a 'mechanical massage device', it is covered by most US medical insurance companies. It combines well with many other treatment modalities.

#### Novasonic (Novafon)

(see Fig 10.8 on page 288) This is an audio frequency vibration device. Unlike the QGM, which is chunky enough to place on or next to a patient without having to hold it, the Novafon requires active involvement, either by patient or practitioner, and is not experienced as relaxing in the same way. The short mains lead can also be a drawback. However, its low price means it is quite suitable for home treatment, and the smaller size of the two treatment heads can also be an advantage for focused stimulation. A deluxe version comes with an extension handle.

## INTEGRATED SYSTEMS

### Ryodoraku and its derivatives
#### AAA-401 (Harmony)

This is a four-channel version of the AAA-301. It incorporates ryodoraku facilities.

#### I-W Zen Automatic Nerve Regulator (various distributors)

(see Fig. 10.9 on page 290) The 'TOR-meter' is a nicely chunky ryodoraku neurometer, also useful for auricular treatment. It is simple to use, but needs a little perseverance to develop proficiency.

### Motoyama's AMI
#### AMI (IARP)

(see Fig. 10.10 on page 291) A new version of this 'apparatus for meridian identification' is now available, after several years' delay. BP resolution is increased eightfold over earlier models. It is compact, portable and reasonably priced.

### EAV – electroacupuncture according to Voll

There is a large range of devices suitable for EAV. As one 1988 survey pointed out, measurement parameters used are not all identical, and not all in accordance with Voll's original requirements. This should be borne in mind when considering purchase.

#### Cutatest IA (Reckeweg)

This is for EAV and BFD, with the facility for remedy and dental testing. Has an additional 10–100 Hz surface probe treatment facility, and linked 'Akutest' PC software with data on AcP location, indications and recommended remedies; repertory can be individualised.

## Dermatron ST (Pitterling)
This is a standard EAV machine from Voll's favoured manufacturers, now with automatic skin moistness adaptation and optimum pressure indicator.

## EAV Diagnost-1 (Pitterling)
(see Fig. 10.13b on page 299) This is a new model of the original Voll machine, a scaled-down version of the Dermatron ST.

## EAV Porty (Medizinische Bedarfsartikel)
This is an attractively designed EAV machine, with digital readout (rather than analogue meter with ID, though an analogue dial can be provided), optional buccal current and quadrant measurement facility, PC link, and a built-in remedy well/ honeycomb. Skin potential measurement is a future option.

## Mini-Expert-DT (Imedis)
This is a Russian EAV device (EAV diagnostics, remedy testing and treatment), with optional Expert–Voll software and buccal current facility. Preset and customisable programmes are available for specific addictions, or for diseases due to specific pathogens.

### Other integrated systems
## Acutron Mentor (Microcurrent Research)
This is very versatile, with 19 preset programmes for different aspects of electrotherapy (microcurrent, interferential, Russian stimulation, diadynamic, 'electric moxing', etc.), four independent channels, for probes or pads, and an internal 12 V rechargeable battery. It is also capable of EAV, ryodoraku and Akabane-style measurements. Has a PC link (one of the earlier machines with this facility). It is good value if you want to have an all-in-one device, but not cheap, and quite chunky too (31 × 26 × 19.5 cm W × H × D, 6 kg).

## MORA, BRT AND MORE
As with EAV, this is a complex area, and should not be entered unless you are willing to devote considerable time and funds to exploring it properly. Only a few items are listed here.

## Inversion (Bio-Medscan)
This is a very slimmed-down version of MORA, incorporating the same amplification and inversion technology, and the facility to 'copy' remedies. It may be used with roller electrode or magnetic probe (optional extras).

## MORA Century (Med-Tronik)
This is a recent version of the MORA with even more capabilities than the MORA-Super. Modular, with EAV and quadrant measurements, magnetic and current stimulation,

PC and printer connectivity, as well as the usual MORA facilities.

## MORA-Super (Med-Tronik)
(see Fig. 10.16 on page 304) This is a MORA device offering EAV, BFD and Vegatesting facilities.

# SOME CONCLUSIONS AND RECOMMENDATIONS

There is clearly a huge and fascinating variety of equipment that can be used in acupuncture practice. For basic electroacupuncture, you will not need more than a point locator/stimulator and a clinical treatment unit with three or four outputs. It is also useful to have TENS units available for lending to patients.

For patients who wish to purchase a locator/stimulator, I usually suggest the Stimplus or Medisana as a good buy (although you may need to prepare better and individualised instruction sheets for them). In the clinic, I prefer the Pointer Plus (Acupoint). It gives a stronger output, though is less sensitive for point location.

For a multioutput clinic unit, there are many possibilities. These include the Ito EA units, although the IC-1107 has only three outputs, and the amplitude is not really strong enough for surface electrodes (the same goes for the IC-4107). The AcuMedic Acupunctoscopes are more powerful, but also expensive. If money is not a problem, the Cefar Acus 4 or Sédatélec Agistim Duo are both very nice machines. The relatively new AAA series has many features that have been designed with EA, TENS, ryodoraku and even LA in mind.

Two (or even three!) V-Tens units would be a lot cheaper, give extra outputs, and more treatment possibilities. Using two smaller units can also result in less lead tangles than a bigger device with more outputs.

For home use, the Cefar Primo may be suitable for lending to patients, whereas the V-Tens may be too complicated for some, despite offering greater versatility. Many other cheaper TENS machines would also suit.

For obstetric use, the 804 OB is quite adequate as a TENS machine. However, it is not suitable for use with needles, and if you want to have the option of using EA during childbirth, none of the equipment currently available offers all the necessary facilities.

**Note**
These recommendations are based on my knowledge of products available primarily in the UK when this book went to print. Equipment may cease to be available, or may be marketed or used legally only in certain countries, specifications may change without notice, and new and better devices may be developed. Always look around before you buy.

# SUMMARY

This chapter has outlined factors that may influence how decide what type of equipment to purchase, what design features to consider, as well as safety, legal and marketing issues of which you should be aware. The listings are subdivided according to the types of device described in Chapter 10: EA, TENS, pTENS, piezoelectric, microcurrent, CES, etc. The chapter then concludes with suggestions on a few basic devices that may be useful in a general acupuncture practice.

## Additional material in the CD-ROM resource

In the electronic version of this chapter, additional material can be found on all the families of equipment mentioned here, and on others under the headings:

- Variants on TENS
- Ionisation devices
- Microcurrent stimulation – patches and membranes
- Electrolipolysis
- Electrodes, gels and leads
- Electrical heating methods
- Cold
- Static magnetic fields
- Thermography
- Automated pulse diagnosis
- The Vegatest
- Dental measurement
- The segmentalelectrogram, DFM and related systems
- Integrated computerised systems
- Kosmed/Skenar
- Multiresonance therapy
- Polarity agents

# RECOMMENDED READING

*Most textbooks on EA and TENS include section on equipment. Examples include:*

Myklebust BM, Robinson AJ 1989 Instrumentation. In: Snyder-Mackler L, Robinson AJ (eds) Clinical Electrophysiology: Electrotherapy and electrophysiologic testing. Williams and Wilkins, Baltimore, MD, 21–58

Zhang ZF, Zhuang D, Jiang XP 1994 Fundament and Clinical Practice of Electroacupuncture. Beijing Science and Technology Press, Beijing

*Books by Mannheimer and Lampe (see Ch. 10), Schoen (Ch. 6) and Walsh (Ch.4) are other examples.*

*An important overview of different devices:*

Kenyon JN 1983/1985 Modern Techniques of Acupuncture. A critical review of European developments in electro-acupuncture (3 vols). Thorsons, Wellingborough, UK

*Useful articles:*

Lytle CD, Thomas BM, Gordon EA, Krauthamer V Electro-stimulators for acupuncture: safety issues. Journal of Alternative and Complementary Medicine. 2000 Feb; 6(1): 37–44

Niemtzow RC, Clydesdale D, Cho ZH, Oleson T, Son YD, Johnstone PAS Are frequency outputs of commercial electro-acupuncture stimulators accurate? Medical Acupuncture. 2002. 14(1): 41–4

*A review of LILT:*

Mayor DF Light, light ... and more light: on LEDs, lasers and lunacy. Traditional Acupuncture Society Newsletter. 1995 Aug; (54): 6–7

# Practicalities and precautions:
the basic do's and don'ts

This chapter covers practical aspects of basic electroacupuncture (EA) and non-traditional methods of acupuncture treatment and point detection for clinical use, together with suggestions on the home use of transcutaneous electrical stimulation of nerves or at acupoints (TENS or TEAS). The focus is on electrostimulation, although laser acupuncture (LA) and magnets are also briefly described. In the second half of the chapter, which assumes familiarity with the basic clinical skills of acupuncture, the necessary precautions and contraindications are considered.

All electrical equipment brings with it special responsibilities. If in any doubt about procedures the reader should refer to the instruction manuals provided with their equipment, or to their suppliers or manufacturers.

## ELECTROSTIMULATION: CLINICAL PROCEDURES FOR EA AND TENS

### The patient and preparation for treatment

Many people are apprehensive when receiving electrical treatment for the first time. It may be advisable to use more traditional methods of manual acupuncture (MA) before offering them EA. They may, of course, be coming to you specifically for EA or, if needle phobic, for TENS or other non-invasive forms of stimulation, but you may still need to put them at their ease.

You should explain the treatment and the procedures involved in a simple, business-like manner, outlining the advantages, possible side-effects and what the patient will experience during treatment. This is not only reassuring, but is a prerequisite of *informed consent*. In particular, emphasise that the current administered should never be more than can be comfortably tolerated, and that the patient is always to let you know if this is not the case. You might also describe what the patient is likely to feel: tingling, a gentle electric fluttering, or muscle movements that may at first be disconcerting. For those who do not easily tolerate strong MA, it may be helpful to clarify that EA may well be more comfortable.

As with any acupuncture consultation, the patient and the condition must be properly assessed following your usual methods, and treatment designed accordingly. Using EA does not change your responsibility for this, although it may provide additional and important information. You should carefully enquire whether the patient has ever lost consciousness for any reason, or received other forms of electrotherapy or any strong electric shocks You will also need to find out if the person has any form of indwelling pacemaker or other prosthetic device (e.g. a metal hip joint), and consider the contraindications to electrical stimulation detailed below.

For the treatment itself, the patient should be in a well-supported position that can be maintained comfortably without movement for up to 20 to 30 minutes. If using low-frequency (LF) stimulation at points likely to activate a specific muscle, it should be comfortably relaxed, not in a position of maximum flexion or extension. However, some authors recommend that the most painful or electroconductive *ashi* points be sought and treated with the patient in a position that elicits *most* discomfort. If treating denervated muscle, you should provide physical resistance to resulting muscular contractions.

Once you have decided where treatment is to be applied, this area should be inspected for any peculiarities of skin or underlying tissue. Vigorous EA may aggravate existing tissue damage (e.g. recently healed tissue, scars or open wounds) or nerve compression in the area. The presence of severe skin lesions or infection may be a contraindication to treatment, and if bruising is present it is best to ask the patient about it before proceeding.

It may also be important to assess the electrical resistance of the skin or tissue. If this is low (where there are cuts or abrasions, for instance), attempting electrical measurement will be futile, and treatment intensity will have to be carefully moderated. In contrast, if there is some sensory nerve damage, so that sensitivity is reduced, treatment may need to be stronger to be effective. However, since this can increase the risk of skin damage, especially with TENS used for repeated home treatment, it may be better to apply stimulation somewhere else altogether. Muscle atrophy or fibrosis, oedema, fat or scar tissue may all reduce current flow and the effectiveness of stimulation. Some electrotherapists recommend briefly warming an area to reduce skin resistance before using TENS.

If using self-adhesive reusable surface electrodes, it may be as well to wash the skin and remove any dry flaky bits, since this will not permit optimal TENS stimulation, and may shorten the life of electrodes. Skin should also be free of grease or cosmetics. Moistening skin increases its electroconductivity, whereas swabbing with alcohol may dehydrate it.

One advantage of EA over TENS is that points in hairy areas can be stimulated, although some electrodes have particularly thick gel layers, suited to use where body hair grows more densely. If there is still too much hair to permit proper electrode adhesion, it can be close clipped, but only in accordance with patients' wishes!

## The apparatus, its storage and troubleshooting

*No piece of equipment should ever be used without reading the instructions first!* Even simple devices may have nonstandard features for which an understanding of EA in general terms may not prepare you. More complex equipment may necessitate attending training courses. In particular, before using a device in clinic you need to check whether amplitude controls are linear and indicated frequencies are accurate.

Equipment also has to be properly looked after if it is going to function as designed. When not in use, it should be stored carefully in a dry, dust-free place, away from volatile strong chemicals or direct sunlight. For laser equipment, there may be legal requirements on storage that have to be observed. Any removable batteries should be taken out if you are not using a device for an extended period. Avoid dropping, banging or vibrating equipment, or exposing it to excessive moisture or extremes of temperature. If water has got into it, it must be serviced before reuse.

Long electrode leads need to be stored so they do not get tangled. They can be slung over hooks or a rack or secured to a 'washing line' (if unsecured, they tend to slide together). An alternative with a portable stimulator is to wrap them round it, although if they are kept plugged in this may lead to damage of the sockets if it is inadvertently dropped. Repeatedly coiling leads too tightly, however, may shorten their lives.

The two most common problems with electrical stimulators are batteries and leads. If reliability and a steady output are critical (as when stimulating peri- or postoperatively), it is best to use disposable batteries. For many applications, though, rechargeable ones suffice. Batteries tend to last less long when using stronger stimulation, higher frequencies or greater pulse durations. Thus it is as well to keep a supply handy, as well as some spare leads.

The output from the socket can be tested using a multimeter and leads you know to be intact, or a small loudspeaker plugged directly into the unit (see Ch. 11, page 317). If there is no 'low-battery' indicator on your stimulator, you can also check the battery with a meter. However, even if this indicates it is producing the right voltage, there is unfortunately no guarantee that it can still provide enough current to drive the device. If you are having problems, check that the battery is connected correctly – sometimes cleaning a battery's terminals will improve performance.

If using standard rechargeable batteries, they need to be carefully managed for a full working life; one tip is to discharge them across a 100 $\Omega$ resistor before charging them again, as otherwise the residual charge they hold prevents subsequent full recharging. Once charged, they are best stored in a cool place. Remember, though, that they do not stay charged forever, and in general their charge lifetime is less than that of many 'longlife' alkaline batteries.

Leads should never be disconnected from either treatment unit or electrode by pulling on the lead itself. They tend to break near or in the connectors at either end, which may not be easy to spot visually if the outer insulating sheath is still intact. If the output socket tests normal, and there is no output through the lead, then use another lead. When reordering, ensure the jack plug on the lead is the right diameter and design for the sockets in your unit, and specify what type of electrode the lead is to be used for; standards and designs have changed rapidly in recent years.

If leads and battery show no problems, and there is still no output from the stimulator, then you will have to go through a troubleshooting process specific to your device. This may (should!) be outlined in its accompanying manual. It is best not to attempt to dig around inside it in the hope that you can repair it yourself, but to take advice from your supplier.

Other faults than just reduced output may develop, particularly with equipment that is poorly engineered in the first place. Indicator lamps or controls that function only sporadically can be particularly frustrating. If you suspect that equipment is defective in some way, it is important to label it clearly with a description of the problem, and remove it from where other practitioners might inadvertently use it. Depending on where you work, you may need to file a report of any adverse incident arising from the defect, but in any case a record should be kept and a copy sent to the product supplier or manufacturer. Repairs made should be documented in the device manual, which should be easily accessible at all times.

Mains-powered devices in particular require regular (generally annual) testing and maintenance by qualified personnel, as do laser devices. They must be used only with appropriate power supply units that have been passed for medical use. If using a directly mains-powered unit for EA it is best to have prior knowledge of the manufacturer and experience with their products.

## Setting up the treatment

Position the treatment unit on a stable support close to the patient, so there is no risk of disturbing any electrode leads or the unit itself during use. If the patient moves about during treatment, it is sensible to check that leads are still properly attached and needles or pads are not pulled out of place.

For current to flow, each of the two leads from a treatment unit output socket has to be attached to the patient by means of an electrode, whether you are using only one output or all of them. It is generally best to use the same form of electrode for both leads from the same output socket, whether these are needles or surface pads, unless you specifically want stronger stimulation at one of the two points stimulated. If, for example, you only want to stimulate one point with EA, the return could be a handheld cylindrical electrode: with its surface area much larger than that of the needle, the patient will feel much less sensation than at the point treated. It is important to ensure that electrodes do not come into contact with each other (short circuit), and that each lead is attached to only one electrode. Dry cotton wool balls can be placed between auricular needles that might otherwise touch.

With a device having a limited number of output sockets, it is possible to use a 'lead splitter' (see Fig. 11.2a on page 313) so that more points are treatable (or larger areas not flat enough for a single large electrode), although it then becomes more difficult to adjust output intensity to achieve equivalent stimulation at all the points stimulated.

Arrange leads loosely so their weight does not pull unduly on any needles, especially those not deeply inserted – in ear points, for instance. It may be necessary to secure these, or other electrodes that are not self-adhesive, with some form of tape, over either the electrode itself or the leads (Fig. 9.15.1 on page 270, Fig. 12.1). Micropore™ or other hypoallergenic tape can be used, although some electrodes come with proprietary, specially shaped fixers. For auricular needles, one creative solution is to use a hairgrip to hold the leads. This has been found to be effective even in active childbirth.

There are various forms of clips for attaching leads to needles (see Ch. 11 for some example), and different diameters of connector pin or press-stud for different surface electrodes. With most surface electrodes, no metal connector surfaces should be left exposed to accidental contact. With needles, clips should be attached to the handles as close as possible to the skin to minimise lead pull. Some suggest attaching the clip to the needle shaft in case of poor electrical contact between shaft and handle, but this could potentially be problematic in terms of cross-infection. If you want to stimulate more than about four points simultaneously, it is sensible to colour-code your leads or connectors/plugs if this has not already been done by the manufacturer, so that you know which output to adjust if stimulation at a particular point is insufficient or too strong.

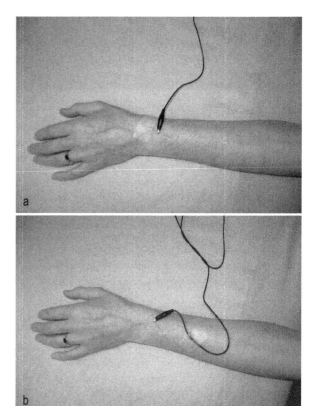

**Figure 12.1** Securing leads. Note how tape can be applied (a) over a bent over needle handle, or (b) over the lead. (Photographs by Riccardo Cuminetti.)

Some of the pros and cons of self-adhesive pregelled and non-gelled electrodes have been discussed in Chapter 10 (page 284). If gelling up your own electrodes, do ensure the whole electrode is covered to avoid skin irritation, using reflected room light. As silicon rubber electrodes age, they may become less flexible and electroconductive, so should be replaced if this occurs. Self-adhesive electrodes may themselves last for 6–8 weeks of daily use, or even longer if the skin is well prepared and they are stored carefully. They may require damping evenly with a few drops of tap water if they are too sticky at first (and can be revived by the same means if they become a little dry). Some patients may find a moisturising skin cream applied after TENS to be helpful.

Needles for EA are little different from those used traditionally. The handle and needle shaft have to be electrically conductive (not silicon or parylene coated or plastic covered, for instance). To take the weight of clip and lead, it may be sensible to use thicker needles (30–32 gauge/0.25–0.30 mm diameter, or even 28 gauge/0.35 mm diameter); this is especially important if there is any suspicion that the stimulator output is not charge balanced (see Ch. 3, page 30).

If this is the case, EA should not be applied for longer than an hour at the very most, and needles discarded after use. Thicker needles also have lower resistance, so less power will be needed from your stimulator to achieve the same effect, and with less discomfort.

Most practitioners in the West now use disposable needles. However, where this is not the case, it is important to remember that needles should not be reused if they have already had current passed through them for lengthy periods, particularly if you are using LF and the needles are subjected to repeated stresses with resultant muscle movement. Unless you have a specific reason to do so, and understand the consequences, the same current should not be passed through two needles of different metals (e.g. silver and gold plated from the same output).

Whether you decide to use needles or surface electrodes, they must be compatible with your stimulator. It is not appropriate to use needles with most TENS machines if they are not charge balanced, or produce too strong a current, or pads with EA machines that may produce only smaller currents suitable for needles.

## The treatment: beginning

Once the patient is comfortable, electrodes are in place, leads properly connected and the stimulator has been checked:

1. *Always check that output amplitude controls are at zero before switching on!* Some devices are designed so that this happens automatically, others so that, if they are not, no output is allowed until they are rezeroed. Some devices may give a brief surge through output sockets when switched on, even if amplitude is supposedly zero. If you find this is the case, it may be best to connect the second electrode of each pair to its lead only *after* switching on the unit or individual output (but before turning up the amplitude), to avoid startling the patient.
2. Select the *frequency*, frequencies or frequency range you wish to use, whether low-frequency (LF), high-frequency (HF) or dense-disperse mode (DD), for example.
3. If there is a *pulse duration* control, adjust this to a convenient initial setting (50 μs for HF, 200 μs for LF, for instance).
4. Switch on the stimulator.
5. For LF, high-intensity stimulation (conventional EA, CEA, or acupuncture-like TENS, ALTENS), gradually increase the *amplitude* setting/s to a level that is 'strong but comfortable'. Remember that not all amplitude controls give a smooth linear increase as you turn them up, and that once a patient can feel stimulation, it may take very little further current for this to feel quite strong. Muscles (and needles, if used) may well twitch visibly if motor points are stimulated – this should not be painful. With HF, low-intensity stimulation (TENS-like EA, TLEA, or conventional TENS, CTENS), strong stimulation may result in muscle spasm rather than twitch, and is to be avoided.

You might want to consider the order in which you turn up the amplitude of different outputs, in terms of where you have positioned electrodes (rostral to caudal, for instance, or vice versa).

Optimally, using identical electrodes, treatment sensation should be the same at both, and, if treating pain, should also reach the problem area. In practice, the patient may well draw your attention to different sensations at the points treated, even when these are symmetrical and stimulated from the same output socket. This may have no bearing on outcome, but if it is the case, you may want to consider the following factors:

(a) How did you locate the points? Using a point detection device, or according to traditional methods?
(b) If you are treating with TENS, was the skin resistance similar at the two points; if with needles, were there similar sensations of *deqi*?
(c) Differences in sensation can also result if stimulation is not charge balanced.
(d) Differences in sensation may depend on the order of phases in a biphasic train (positive preceding negative, or vice versa), even when the output is charge balanced.

It is as well to check which lead gives the stronger sensation before you treat. It may then be necessary to relocate electrodes, or swap leads over, if either the patient or you are not happy with these differences. Some units have a switch to reverse polarities without physically having to disconnect and reconnect pads or needles.

It is important to remember that, according to conventional neurophysiology, sensation is necessary for TENS and EA to be effective, and that in some cases optimal results will require more stimulation ipsilateral to a problem, whereas in others bilateral stimulation may be preferable. Remember too that some points (e.g. on the face) may be particularly sensitive, and that needles from the same output should therefore be paired in regions of comparable expected sensitivity.

6. Within the range you have selected as appropriate, you may now wish to adjust frequency for maximum comfort. It may also be possible to increase pulse duration to give a stronger stimulation that *feels* deeper or more extensive, without becoming uncomfortable, although generally it is best to use the minimum pulse duration that the patient finds effective.
7. If the device has a *timer*, now that you have adjusted the output would be a logical time to set it.

## The treatment: middle

If it is necessary to make *adjustments* during treatment, whether to compensate for different sensations at treated points, to change output parameters in any major way, or to replace the battery, always turn the intensity control gently to zero before doing so. This is not necessary if you are just turning up the amplitude or changing frequency slightly to compensate for the habituation that tends to occur with continuous (especially HF) stimulation.

Always monitor the patient during treatment, and if you leave the room ensure that the person knows about and has easy access to some kind of 'panic button' to summon you. Depending on your style of practice, you may wish to give control of treatment amplitude to the patient, but if you do, ensure it is at a suitable level, adequate but not overly strong, and ensure the patient understands why this is necessary.

Some patients may not be satisfied unless they get the strongest zapping they can stand. But remember: 'wants' don't equal 'needs', and 'more' is not necessarily 'better'! Overtreatment may lead to undesirable, if temporary, consequences. It may be best to delay introducing strong stimulation until the patient is familiar with the procedure. Intensity can then be increased from session to session. Some patients, by contrast, can become more sensitive as treatment progresses, and may no longer be able to tolerate the strong stimulation they could to start with.

EA is not a form of torture. If the patient reports any unpleasant sensation, the amplitude of the associated output should be turned down. If there is no immediate relief, turn it off entirely, and once the patient is comfortable again then turn it up again carefully. If the patient still experiences discomfort, check electrodes for poor contact, too much pressure, or needle position. Remove leads and reapply the electrode(s) or shift the needle until discomfort lessens (but never insert or remove needles while current is flowing through them). If different stimulation parameters do not help, electrical stimulation should be abandoned for the session: either the patient has become sensitised to treatment for some reason, or a fault may have developed with your equipment.

Many reports on Chinese acupuncture, as well as Western electrotherapy, emphasise the importance of concurrent active movement exercises during treatment for musculoskeletal conditions. Passive movement and massage may also be helpful.

## The treatment: end

As a rule of thumb, 30 minutes of treatment is usually sufficient with EA or TENS/TEAS, although some authorities recommend that stimulation should end when the patient no longer experiences reduction in a pain that is being treated. When concluding a session:

1. Turn amplitude controls slowly to *zero,* perhaps considering the order in which you turned them up in the first place.
2. *Switch off* the stimulator. With some devices this can induce a current surge along the output leads. If this is the case, it may be best to disconnect one electrode of each pair from its lead *before* switching off the unit or individual output (but after turning down the amplitude). Some inbuilt timers can cause a surge on switching off as well. If this is so, it is best to use some form of external reminder to circumvent this.

3. *Disconnect* leads from all electrodes and tidy away the stimulator unit and leads, making sure you don't pull on leads that may now be underneath the patient.
4. *Remove* all surface electrodes and needles, taking particular care if the skin is clearly delicate. If you use surface electrodes on more than one patient and these cannot be autoclaved (e.g. some magnetic ones), you need to consider how to ensure there is no risk of their contamination with blood when you are using both these and needles in the same treatment.
5. Needles should be dealt with according to your usual practice. In the West, most needles are for single use only, but if needles are to be reused then carefully *examine and cleanse* them before autoclaving, to ensure that any possible electrolytic changes will not adversely affect subsequent treatments.

   Dry wipe silicon rubber electrodes to remove gel, tape adhesive or skin debris, which may reduce future electrical conductivity (do not use alcohol or detergent on rubber). *Store* safely if they are to be autoclaved, and store self-adhesive electrodes according to their accompanying instructions, remembering that they are for single-person use only. Some (but not all) electrodes may store best in a 'fridge. If a patient perspires a great deal, self-adhesive electrodes may need to be left to dry out for a while before storage.
6. *Remove* any tape or gel *residue* from patient's skin, and examine for any *reactions* (e.g. hyperaemia).
7. Allow the patient to rest for a few moments; patients are more likely to feel a little dizzy on getting up than after MA.
8. Explain what might be expected from this particular treatment, if there is anything the patient should do between treatments, and when to come again. If treating for a pain problem, you may wish to reassure that any aggravation of pain is likely to be temporary, but also warn that a lessening of pain does not necessarily mean the problem has suddenly and entirely vanished.
9. Later on, if necessary, wash silicon rubber electrodes using mild soap and warm water, rinse and pat dry. Autoclave or dispose of electrodes, as appropriate. You may wish to cleanse needle clips from time to time, although it is generally not possible to autoclave them. Clean other forms of electrode, such as CES (cranial electrotherapy stimulation) ear clips, according to suppliers' instructions. Brass electrodes in particular become discoloured easily and should be washed in soap and water.

## Home treatment

Home use of TENS or microcurrent modalities may be appropriate for anyone with a chronic condition who requires more than one palliative treatment per month, or whose pathology is progressive. Sadly, although TENS, for instance, is increasingly available and offered to patients via pain clinics or other channels, people are often given insufficient instruction on how to use it. Patients, and possibly their families, need to be educated in the proper use of TENS, precautions to be observed and limitations of the treatment. Written instructions should be given and, if lending or renting out a device, you may even wish to draw up a contract for patients so that all parties are clear who is responsible for the unit in case of damage, equipment failure or adverse treatment response.

If recommending a device for home use, always go through a trial treatment with the patient. Done properly, this may well take a full hour. It may even be necessary to spend more than one session with the patient to determine the most effective electrode locations. If a patient is already finding acupuncture beneficial, it can be helpful to combine TENS/TEAS with acupuncture in at least one session.

You will need to:

1. Determine the type of pain involved (nociceptive or neurogenic, for example), whether in principle TENS is appropriate and what parameters are most likely to be beneficial (see Subchs 9.10, 9.11). Different parameters may be needed for each new pain treated.
2. Ensure pain is not aggravated by use of the device.
3. Familiarise your patient with the device and the sensations it produces.
4. Assess if the treatment may give pain relief.
5. Check for any immediate skin reaction.
6. Instruct the patient in use and care of equipment, especially the electrodes (and their storage, if reusable).
7. Encourage the patient to compare the effects of different frequencies and waveforms (continuous, intermittent, modulated), giving each a careful trial. Although some patients quickly find what is best for them, others may need systematic guidance with this.
8. Also suggest the patient may alter positioning of electrodes 'within reasonable limits'.
9. Ensure the patient knows how to contact you immediately if there are any problems.
10. Review home treatment at sessions, or, if you are not seeing the patient regularly, every month, at least initially, then at 6 months and a year. It is important not to treat without being able to evaluate change. There are now various validated outcome measures available that are simple to use and analyse, for instance, the MYMOP (measure yourself medical outcome profile), visual analogue scale (VAS) and numerical rating scale (NRS) for particular problems such as pain.

It is obviously important to record all pertinent treatment settings, as well as the device used. Such records can be useful when reviewing individual cases, as well as for clinical research. Sometimes changing just one parameter can make all the difference between success and failure, so such changes need to be carried out carefully, in accordance with a protocol that feels comfortable to both you and the patient.

# SOME OTHER USEFUL TREATMENT PROCEDURES

## The 'electric hand'

The combination of massage and electrical stimulation is a time-honoured technique (Fig. 12.2). One lead from a stimulator output socket is attached to you, and one to the patient. This can be via two handheld (cylindrical) electrodes, or two surface pads. The circuit is completed when the practitioner touches or massages the patient with a free hand. It is even possible to use two outputs: affix one pad from each output to each of your own forearms, and the other two to the patient near to an area that would benefit from massage. Low-intensity stimulation can then be applied to an area, rather than just specific points.

Gordon Gadsby suggests using around 2.5 or 10 Hz to discharge a local trigger point (TrP), *ashi* or even auricular point, or a small area, using your dominant thumb or first two fingers, treating each point for 30–60 seconds with soft massage technique, for a total not exceeding 3–4 minutes. With more of your hand in contact, larger areas of spasm or pain can be massaged. Adjust intensity to your own tolerance and use before, or preferably after, a main treatment. Gadsby has found this useful for neck, hip or acute back pain, for sports injuries, and over areas of neurological pain (e.g. postherpetic or trigeminal neuralgia, diabetic or other neuropathy).

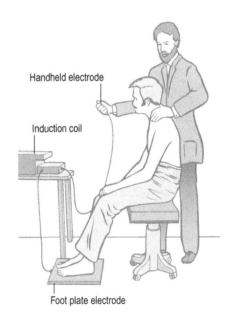

Handheld electrode

Induction coil

Foot plate electrode

**Figure 12.2** The 'electric hand': a method widely used in the late 1800s, with therapist and patient connected via the massaging hand and an induction coil. (After Oschman 2000.)

## Trigger point massage

If you prefer to keep your hands free, you can affix all the pads to TrPs on the patient (flexible self-adhesive ones in preference to the harder silicon rubber variety, and not electrodes with a central press-stud connector). Pressure can then be applied to the points through the electrodes. Application of pressure to the pad may increase electrical sensation to the patient if the stimulator produces a 'constant voltage' rather than 'constant current' output.

## Using a handheld treatment probe (pTENS)

Electroacupressure with handheld probes can be very effective, a technique that was possibly originated by chiropractors. This can be at *ashi* points or TrPs, as well as ear points. Using a point stimulator with a rounded tip (such as the 'Pointer Plus') on one point, the circuit is completed by your thumb massaging at another point. Stimulation can be pulsed (on/off) steadily, at around 2 seconds on, 1 second off. Again, you will feel this through your own thumb (don't forget to warn the patient it may be uncomfortable!). This technique will work best if the two points are not more than about 20 cm apart. It can also be used with piezoelectric stimulators.

Rather like a seven-star hammer, smaller-diameter probes can be used with a percussive action on hypertonic muscle, or to crosshatch a painful area to produce hyperaemia, as with *guasha* (these methods have been suggested for a positive polarity probe).

For sensitive patients, some thinner metal probes can be inserted into the end of a moistened Q-tip, which may provide more comfortable stimulation than the bare metal. Probes with moistened Q-tips or felt tips are often employed with microcurrent stimulators (see Fig. 10.2 on page 283). They should be used on only one patient, and not redipped into a container of wetting solution that will be used for another patient. Some microcurrent practitioners still use bare metal probes, just turning down the output intensity if this causes discomfort.

For strong stimulation, the probe tip can be positioned in contact with an inserted needle (Fig. 12.3), rather than directly on the skin (a technique used by Chan Gunn).

## A technique from ryodoraku

Needling, like local injections, may be experienced as painful. Mild electrical stimulation around the site of needling using a handheld probe (or even HF TENS) may reduce such discomfort. This principle has been used in a Japanese design for concentric surface electrodes.

## A technique from EAV

With one electrode in contact with the sole of the foot and another in the patient's hand, it is possible to stimulate one

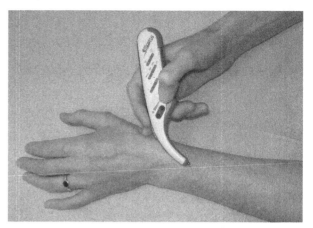

**Figure 12.3** A combination treatment: touching the Stimplus probe tip to a needle (Chan Gunn's technique). (Photograph by Riccardo Cuminetti.)

side of the body, while with electrodes between the feet or hands the lower or upper body as a whole respectively can be treated. Voll's biphasic LF tonification mode (see Fig. 10.14a on page 300) has been used with the unilateral method for oedema, lymphatic swelling and haematoma, and bilaterally (foot to foot) for joint problems, varices, thrombosis and even thrombophlebitis. However, local stimulation (particularly of negative polarity) is often considered as contraindicated in these last two conditions, and this needs to be taken into account.

Gadsby states that LF stimulation with handheld or footplate electrodes is the most effective technique to stimulate β-endorphin (βEP) release, and so is useful both in the clinic and at home for the relief of generalised and local pain, migraine prevention, premenstrual tension, anxiety, stress, depression, drug withdrawal and so on. Which pair of extremities to treat may be determined by simple electrical resistance measurements (see Ch. 10, page 303).

## Checking for the active electrode and charge balance

It is important to find out which lead, if either, from a particular output socket gives the stronger stimulation. You can check on yourself if one electrode is more 'active' than its paired partner, as follows.

With identical electrodes connected to the same output, place one over a motor point (such as LI-4 or LI-11) and the other over a bony prominence. Using around 2 Hz, turn up the amplitude slowly and record the setting when you first sense the flow of current, and then again when you first sense a muscle contraction. Reset to zero, reverse the electrodes, and again record the settings. Compare the settings to determine whether one electrode is more active than the other.

Once you are clear which is the more active lead, you should mark it. However, there is no guarantee that it will remain so if used with a different device, or even with other output sockets in the same one.

In addition to this test, if you have more time you can check for charge balance by connecting two acupuncture needles to the same output and immersing in normal saline solution for 3–4 hours (make sure the needles are not in contact) (see Fig. 3.12 on page 33). If on inspection you can clearly see corrosion or discoloration in one or other of the needles, or bubbles around one of them (possibly around both), this indicates that the output from the device is not charge balanced, and it should not be used for EA except for very short stimulation periods indeed (≤ 10 seconds, according to some sources). However, current amplitude is more important than stimulation duration, or distance between the needles. Net DC currents of more than 10 µA can damage tissue.

A very simple and quick method of checking charge balance is to measure any residual DC between the two leads of a given output using a standard voltage meter set to check DC rather than alternating current (AC).

# THE USE OF HEAT

An alternative to moxa is a TDP far-infrared lamp (see Ch. 10, page 286). This takes about 10 minutes to warm up, and heat is also given out for 5 minutes or more after switching off. The device head is positioned some 30–45 cm from the skin (further for children), nearer than many conventional heat lamps. Moxa essence or other herbal preparations can be applied to the skin before it is heated, and moisturisers afterwards, and inserted needles can be heated using this method.

# THE USE OF LOW-INTENSITY LASER (OR POLARISED LIGHT)

> **Note**
> Low-intensity laser therapy should be used only if you have received adequate hands-on training.

LILT and polarised light (PL) can be used on open wounds, regions of musculoskeletal injury/pain, or specific acupoints. There are both contact and non-contact methods, although it is not yet clear whether non-contact LILT methods are really effective except in the treatment of open wounds, especially if a divergent beam is used.

Probe heads needs to be kept scrupulously clean, and skin must be cleaned before treatment too.

Heavy 'clusters' of LEDs or laser diodes may need some form of support. Protective goggles appropriate for the wavelength of LILT used have to be worn by both patient and practitioner. Treatment should be carried out in a well-lit area.

# Wound healing

LILT can be applied (contact method) at intervals around the wound edge, followed by non-contact application of a cluster (or a single probe for particularly deep or recessed areas). It may be unnecessary to irradiate the whole wound.

## Injury

Accurate location and maximum exposure of the affected area are important. If injury is within a joint the patient may need to move it, 'gapping' the joint, so the beam can penetrate more easily. LILT may be applied even within 48 hours after injury, although the possibility that any bleeding might be aggravated should be borne in mind.

## Acupoints

Margaret Naeser has published a useful protocol for the self-treatment of carpal tunnel syndrome or repetitive strain injury (RSI) using a 'laser pointer', 5 mW 670 nm LILT. She points out that this is only really useful for shallow points (e.g. the *jing* Well points at the ends of the fingers, or some other hand points), although it may be used at any body acupoint in babies or children (5–10 seconds/pt, as opposed to 3 min/pt in adults). On very painful joints, she suggests even up to 6–12 minutes (2–4 J) and combines LA with MA on deeper points. She points out that with a battery-powered device it is best, with long treatments, not to wait for the laser beam to weaken but to replace batteries every 3 hours or so.

# THE USE OF MAGNETS

Permanent magnets are a very simple and useful adjunct to acupuncture. They can be used with or instead of needles, and can even double as surface electrodes. Between sessions, patients can apply magnets themselves directly to *ashi* points or TrPs using some form of hypoallergenic tape intended for long-term use. For larger areas, several magnets (with the same orientation) can be used.

Magnets are best used for no more than 4 days at a time, then if there is some improvement the patient can take a break for 2 days to see if it is maintained without them. If not, they can be reapplied. In the longer term, it is also sensible not to continue using them once symptoms have improved. Small 'ion granules', however, which are unmagnetised despite the name 'magrain' under which they are often marketed, can be left on for a week at a time.

Skin should be clean and dry before applying magnets. If a patient experiences an aggravation that is clearly due to using them, it may be worth leaving them off for a few days and then reapplying either for a shorter time with the same polarity, or with the opposite pole to the skin. For a deeper, perhaps more diffuse pain, the region may be 'sandwiched' between two stronger magnets with opposite poles towards the skin, so that there is a strong field between them. Magnet sandwiches can also be used on ear points if a single magnet appears ineffective. Using acupressure over magnets can enhance their effect.

## THE USE OF VIBRATION AND ULTRASOUND

> **Note**
>
> As with LILT, ultrasound should be used only if you have received adequate hands-on training.

Equipment, particularly for ultrasound, must be properly maintained and regularly calibrated, and an appropriate coupling gel used (sterile if treatment is over broken skin). To avoid tissue damage, only the lowest intensity that produces the desired effect should be used, and the applicator moved constantly throughout treatment (this is important to remember if considering ultrasound stimulation at AcPs or TrPs). *Pulsed* ultrasound also reduces the risk of damage. If any additional pain occurs during ultrasound application, intensity should be reduced so that the pain subsides, or the treatment abandoned. If in doubt, do not use!

Much simpler to use is the '*Qi Gong* machine' (QGM) (see Ch. 10, page 288), which is easy to position adjacent to, under or on appropriate parts of the body. If Velcro is fixed to the back of the transducer head, it will not then slip off the abdomen if a towel or blanket is placed over it.

## ELECTRICAL MEASUREMENT AT ACUPOINTS

Several methods of electrical measurement at AcPs have already been explored in some detail in Chapters 5 and 6, and an account of the associated equipment given in Chapter 10. Those sections include much practical information, and can usefully be read as a background to the following brief account of the techniques involved.

### Point location

When using a handheld probe to search for points of low skin resistance (SR), hold it vertical to the skin and search using constant pressure. Using more pressure or keeping the probe in one position for too long will lead to false positives. As with handheld devices for treatment, you will need to contact both patient and the inbuilt conductive handgrip if there is no return electrode (this may be cylindrical, for the patient to hold (see Fig. 10.9 on page 290), or a bracelet strap for the wrist). Develop the habit of searching at a steady pace without going over the same area repeatedly,

whether you search in lines or spirals – passing over the same area several times will also lead to false positives. Resistance over superficial veins or bony prominences may anyway be low. Although treatment using a handheld probe is rapid, point location in itself takes time.

Skin conditions vary from place to place, so comparing readings in different parts of the body is not particularly meaningful. However, as readings do depend on overall state, if you have time it might be as well to allow the patient to relax for 10 minutes or so before measuring. If there is a handheld return electrode separate from the probe, the person can lightly hold this while resting, so that hand–electrode contact can reach some equilibrium. If the skin is overly moist, you may need to dry it with a paper towel, use lighter pressure, or adjust the sensitivity control on your unit. If the skin is very dry, you can use saline, a dampened Q-tip, a water-based gel or cream, or a conductive oil to facilitate current flow, waiting for it to be absorbed before measuring, since rubbing or wiping too vigorously will affect electrical readings. Otherwise it is not usually necessary to prepare the skin in any way.

Points on the hands, face and ears are generally easier to locate than others. It is best to set the sensitivity level of the detector so that it just gives a reading at certain reference points. If you set it too low, it will pick up very few points; if too high (more current) too many points will appear and, furthermore, the high current used will start to act as a treatment. The usual reference points for setting sensitivity are:

| | |
|---|---|
| in the ear | Point zero (Fulcrum), or sometimes *shenmen* |
| on the body | *yintang* or LI-4 |

If readings remain low whatever you do, sometimes if you strongly stimulate Point zero for 10 seconds this will increase conductivity generally at ear points. However, do not forget that the state of your own skin will affect readings if you are part of the measurement circuit.

Measurement probes should not be used where there is local infection, and if you use a device with an inbuilt conductive handgrip this may need cleansing from time to time, as will the probe tip.

Electrical skin measurement can be used to monitor progress, confirm diagnosis and even give some idea of prognosis, as well as for point location, but it is subject to considerable error. As well as depending on the visual or auditory feedback your device gives you, you may wish to double-check against what the patient feels at different points (more of a tingle, some discomfort even on light pressure – or nothing at all).

Gadsby's method of 'electroacupressure' can be adapted to locate points over peripheral nerves likely to give good results using EA. Using 30–50 Hz at low intensity, probe a potentially useful area with your own finger while increasing the intensity until you find where you experience the most paraesthesia in your fingertip, and the patient also experiences radiating sensations from the point.

# Ryodoraku

Ryodoraku (see Chs 5 and 10) is one of the most accessible and simple to learn of the EA systems that integrate some form of meridian diagnosis with treatment. For those with a knowledge of traditional acupuncture, it is reassuring that most of the main 'representative measuring points' (RMP) coincide with the *yuan* (Source) points. The basic principle is to take measurements at these 24 points using a probe, average them, and then compare individual readings with this average. The most 'reactive electropermeable points' (REPP) are used for local stimulation.

The first step is to calibrate the device (the 'neurometer') (see Fig. 10.9 on page 290). With the 'voltage selector' control at 12 V and the 'volume' control switched on but not turned up, the point probe is placed in contact with the handheld return electrode and the volume increased until a reading of 200 µA is obtained on the meter (this also serves as a battery check). The typical ryodoraku probe (Fig. 10.9) offers two alternatives: a rounded metal end, and a plastic cup into which cotton wool soaked in physiological saline or 30% isopropyl alcohol is inserted; the cotton wool should protrude only 1 mm or so. Most people find the metal probe is simplest to use initially, but after a little practice it is best to use the more comfortable moist probe, with the metal one for more accurate detection or in hairy areas. Nakatani noted that with the moist probe the difference between REPP and other areas is small (only around 20–50 µA on the meter) and suggested that to pinpoint REPP the volume be adjusted to give a reading of ~150 µA; when the point is precisely located, the meter reading may increase considerably. Point location may also be easier with 21 V than 12 V.

Points should be located using a smooth spiral or zigzag movement, with a light uniform pressure, and the probe held vertical to the skin. When low SR (high meter) readings are found, stay on these points for a standard 2–2.5 seconds and record readings as you go along. If taking measurements at points whose location you know, do not press, scrub or touch them repeatedly beforehand, but just apply the probe for the same length of time. Touching the patient during measurement can result in artificially high readings. Readings can also be affected if the patient changes the return electrode from one hand to the other, or pressure on it, by exercise, eating or a bowel movement within 10 minutes prior to measurement, or if points are warmed beforehand.

The same output is used for both measurement and treatment. With a little pressure on the point, the metal probe, and even the moist one, can be used to treat children or sensitive adults, although in general ryodoraku uses needle stimulation, with needles alone or weak EA for reinforcement and stronger EA for reduction. Stimulation is usually for around 7 seconds per point.

# Electroacupuncture according to Voll (EAV)

EAV and its various progeny are more complex and difficult to master than ryodoraku, and EAV is unlikely to give useful results without proper instruction and the investment of considerable time and effort. Repeated practice is the key to success.

Once practical technique is mastered, there are different ways of extracting useful information from the many point measurements involved in a basic EAV test. In addition to control measurement points (CMP) for each meridian, akin to the RMP of ryodoraku, there are several other major measurement points on the meridians that may be useful. To simplify matters, Prince recommends paying particular attention to the point with the 'worst' reading. Having interpreted your measurements, there are many ways to design resultant treatments, depending on your own particular background knowledge, experience and interests. Many practitioners use only the diagnostic side of EAV-based systems, preferring to treat with a mixture of homeopathic, naturopathic or allopathic means.

# SAFETY PRECAUTIONS AND CONTRAINDICATIONS

Some form of risk–benefit analysis is essential when considering any treatment. In the following sections, familiarity with the normal precautions and contraindications for acupuncture is assumed.

## Precautions during treatment

### YOUR OWN CONDITION

If as practitioner your use of equipment entails that you are subjected to stimulation as well as your patients, possibly for extended periods, the contraindications outlined below may apply to you too. This might be relevant, for instance, when you use a handheld treatment probe.

### OTHER DEVICES

Electrical devices may sometimes interact. Hearing aids are best removed. EA and TENS devices, unless you know they are properly shielded, should not be operated less than 3 metres away from shortwave or microwave devices, possibly even mobile phones. The electrode leads may act as aerials, and output may be affected, even so far as causing burn injury at the site of needles.

Although it is unlikely that output levels will be affected, electrostimulators should be used with caution when watching TV close up or using a computer. Interactions with such equipment are more likely to occur with microcurrent devices such as subperception electrical stimulation (SPES), although proximity to household electrical devices like electric blankets during some forms of treatment may indeed negate their effects.

Concurrent ECG or EEG monitoring will usually be affected by EA and TENS.

### ELECTRODES AND THEIR LOCATION

When using strong stimulation, larger-surface electrodes ($\geq 4$ cm$^2$ in area) are more comfortable. If they are as large as 16 cm², nociceptors are not activated. However, with large electrodes it is difficult to stimulate specific muscles or points and for very precise work, as in re-educating single muscles following stroke or in multiple sclerosis patients, needles may sometimes be preferable.

Electrodes should not be located too close together – as this may lead to uncomfortable 'edge effects' – but at least one electrode diameter (or 4 cm) apart. When using needles, some authors suggest that they should not be positioned closer than about half an inch (1.25 cm) apart.

It has also been suggested that it is best not to link *yin* and *yang* meridians with electrodes from the same output, a point selected for reinforcement with one for reduction, or points on both sides of the spine (at least above Du-3), but in most cases there seems to be little justification for these cautions provided stimulation intensity is not set too high.

Electrodes with a central press-stud connector, or the use of stainless steel acupuncture needles, may give problems in those with a nickel allergy.

## ELECTRODE GELS
Adverse skin reactions are the primary reason that otherwise successful TENS treatment is discontinued. Hydrogels, used with most self-adhesive TENS electrodes, tend to be relatively hypoallergenic, and the electrodes themselves may be sufficiently permeable to discourage bacterial growth beneath them.

## MUSCLE SPASM
Never use HF stimulation so intense that muscle goes into spasm. In particular, strong stimulation over trigger or other points in already spastic muscle, as in torticollis for instance, may aggravate the condition, as may EA at TrPs in fibromyalgia.

## ACUPUNCTURE ANALGESIA
If using EA as a method of operative analgesia, it may be sensible to have a backup device available, and certainly spare batteries and leads.

## AURICULAR EA
Treating ear points can have a direct effect on the vagus nerve. To avoid vasovagal effects, the patient is best treated lying down, not seated.

## HOME USE OF TENS
If TENS is used for long periods and is not charge balanced, patients must be warned that skin irritation can occur where the electrodes are applied – if they are kept on during sleep, for instance. Using the same electrode locations repeatedly for months can even lead to lasting skin changes. Patients should vary electrode sites, change electrodes periodically and use different gels from time to time. If skin reactions do occur, reduction of pulse duration may be helpful. Prolonged stimulation for many hours, even with biphasic charge-balanced TENS, may damage muscle.

One problem with overlong or overfrequent treatment is that tolerance can develop to stimulation. A change of electrode sites, as well as stimulation mode (CTENS, burst or modulated), can delay this. Sometimes if the patient takes a break from treatment for a week or two this can re-establish treatment effectiveness.

Patients must be able to understand your instructions. They should be warned not to use TENS or other home treatment units while operating a motor vehicle or other hazardous equipment, and to keep medical devices out of reach of children (when not themselves being treated). Mains-powered equipment should be properly earthed (grounded) and is best not used during a thunderstorm.

# Contraindications to EA or TENS

## ABSOLUTE CONTRAINDICATIONS
- Electrotherapy should be avoided during the first trimester of pregnancy, although some authorities suggest that careful treatment is permissible for hyperemesis, for example, particularly if alternative treatments are potentially harmful to the fetus.
- Stimulation over or close to the uterus is forbidden at any stage of pregnancy prior to labour.
- Electrostimulation should not be administered to a patient in shock or coma, unless its use has been medically advised (e.g. at Du-26).
- Other conditions in which EA and TEAS are not permitted include acute febrile disease (temperature > 38° C), septicaemia, tuberculosis and other local active infection.
- Stimulation should not be applied to the head in children younger than 12 years. It is important to remember that seizure susceptibility may be greater in younger patients.
- EA or TENS should not be used over the carotid sinus in case of hypotensive response, or near the larynx in case of airway restriction, especially at high frequencies (see Fig. 9.11.2 on page 223).
- Electrodes from the same socket should not be positioned over the anterior chest wall in patients with a history of serious or unstable cardiac problems, particularly arrhythmia, and they should be used on upper back points only for short treatments, and not at high intensity.
- Electrostimulation should be used cautiously in cases of apparent but undiagnosed sprain, unless actual fracture has been ruled out.
- Stimulation is contraindicated if a patient uses a demand-type (synchronous) cardiac pacemaker, whether atrial or ventricular.
- Strong stimulation (especially at HF) should be avoided if a patient has high blood pressure.

## RELATIVE CONTRAINDICATIONS
- *Epilepsy:* strong or sustained stimulation should not be used, particularly over the motor cortex at high frequencies. Stimulation at points well away from the head might be possible if undertaken carefully, but in patients with unstable epilepsy even this should be avoided, at least initially. As mentioned above, caution

should be exercised with children. Any sign of rhythmic myoclonic jerks occurring in time with applied stimulation (or at a harmonic of that frequency), particularly in a patient with a personal or family history of epilepsy, should be viewed as a contraindication to continued treatment (mild local muscle twitching in response to EA or TENS occurs commonly, and should not be confused with myoclonus).

- *Cancer (active):* the World Health Organization has recommended that acupuncture should not be used to treat malignant tumours.

Robert Becker wrote in his influential book *The Body Electric* (1985) that 'at this time, I must conclude that high-current electrodes might enhance the growth of any preexisting tumor cells in the electrical path'. Although long-term stimulation could conceivably have an immune suppressive effect, brief non-stressful treatments, as with PEMF, are more likely to slow tumour growth. On the other hand, LF electrostimulation, with its documented effects on circulation, might indeed encourage metastasis. A balanced view on this issue is important.

- *Undiagnosed (undocumented, progressive) pain or swelling:* it should be remembered that stimulation that is not charge balanced might have an adverse effect on oedema, if incorrectly applied.
- *Unstable spine:* whatever the cause, removal of protective spasm could potentially be disastrous.
- *Pregnancy from the fourth month on (except for breech presentation, during labour or for its induction):* strong stimulation on the legs is to be avoided in particular. The safety of electrical stimulation during pregnancy or delivery has not been established.
- *Debilitated patients, those with a deficient (xu) constitution, prone to needle shock or clearly hypotensive:* such patients are best treated with MA initially, and with EA only if lying down.
- *If a patient is hypertensive, has had a cerebrovascular accident (e.g. menangioma or aneurysm) or is liable to transient ischaemic attacks:* monitor carefully when stimulating the head or upper cervical region.

In particular, patients with recent cerebral haemorrhage should be treated cautiously. Strong currents to the head (at > 2 Hz), particularly if not charge balanced, should be avoided. Even subthreshold microcurrent stimulation to the head should be used cautiously.

Patients with spinal cord injury at or above T8 can be liable to 'autonomic dysreflexia', with raised blood pressure in response to stimulation. Such patients should also be monitored during treatment, particularly if already hypertensive.

Generalised vasodilation can occur after a series of EA or TENS treatments, in patients with normal as well as high blood pressure. It may be possible to reduce hypotensive medication in the latter, but this of course should only be done if blood pressure is carefully monitored.

- *In particular, use only low to medium intensity if treating ear points bilaterally:* although CES is both effective

and safe, sudden changes in applied current can lead to dizziness or nausea.

- *If there is some defect in the skull, congenital or otherwise:* avoid placing electrodes nearby. Local EA is similarly contraindicated if there are postoperative scars on the scalp.
- *Exercise caution if stimulating over or near eyes* or other delicate structures.
- *In a patient with a history of cardiac (especially Heart xu) problems:* avoid passing current between both arms. EA is best avoided in cases of arrhythmia or recent heart attack (< 3 months). Ventricular fibrillation can be triggered using a variety of electrode configurations.
- *Electrostimulation is contraindicated in acute venous conditions:* overstrong motor level stimulation could, for instance, dislodge a deep-vein thrombus leading to embolism, and may also disrupt clotting.
- *If a patient has some form of metal implant (e.g. a metal hip joint):* electrodes should be arranged so that the current pathway does not pass through it, or even its vicinity. Any unusual sensations around the implant during treatment should be reported to the practitioner.
- *Needling should not be performed on a severely, or even moderately lymphoedematous limb:* this is due to the risk of cellulitis, and especially applies where the lymph nodes to the limb have been removed during radical mastectomy. Some sources regard all forms of acupuncture as contraindicated after lymph node removal.

## Aggravations, adverse effects and the amount of stimulation

If any intervention consistently aggravates a problem, or is of no benefit within a predetermined number of treatments, it should be modified or terminated.

Feelings of tiredness or sleepiness after acupuncture are not uncommon, particularly early on in treatment. If a patient tends to experience drowsiness or euphoria after treatment (as may occur with 'strong reactors'), use only very-low-intensity stimulation. Advise the patient against operating a motor vehicle or other hazardous equipment in this condition.

In general, do not overstimulate. This may aggravate an inflammatory acute condition, or exhaust a patient already depleted by chronic pain. If aggravations occur, consider reducing intensity or pulse duration. If they persist, you may need to switch to another modality. In particular, if a patient is a strong reactor and treatment is progressing well with MA, it is best not to add electrical stimulation.

Patients with predominantly 'psychogenic' pain or who 'somatise' (express in their bodies what may be primarily psychological problems) may not respond to EA or TENS, and may indeed be worsened by it, no matter what treatment parameters are used. A cumulative pain response with repeated treatment ('hyperstimulation syndrome') may even occur in highly sensitive individuals. This may indicate an underlying neurological, neurochemical or endocrine disorder.

As with traditional acupuncture, EA is contraindicated if the patient is in shock, drunk, unduly hungry, angry, or tired, or has just had a heavy meal. Alcohol, a hot bath or vigorous exercise should also be avoided for 3–4 hours after treatment.

Certain points are forbidden to traditional acupuncture. EA should also be considered as contraindicated at these points.

Stimulation of TrPs if a patient is already experiencing an exaggerated response to a previous treatment (acupuncture or otherwise) is liable to result in hyperstimulation syndrome, as can repeated TrP treatment during acute episodes of chronic myofascial pain disorder. Local electrostimulation is best avoided in these situations, and it might be prudent to revert to gentle traditional needling at other points until the treatment response has dissipated or the acute episode has passed.

If using EA to assist drug withdrawal, ensure there is no concurrent medical condition that would preclude abrupt withdrawal.

## Limitations on the use of EA and TENS

- Those with constant, disabling pain, or who tend to anxiety or severe depression may respond less well to treatment.
- Acupuncture may be more effective against pain in younger patients than in the elderly, or those with long-standing pain.
- Parkinson's disease, which decreases cerebral levels of 5HT, might reduce the effectiveness of EA and related methods.
- Prior surgery, particularly multiple operations for pain, may lead to a less positive outcome, as may previous exposure to a variety of other pain reduction modalities.
- CTENS or TLEA may give insufficient pain relief if it is not possible to cover or even locate the painful area.
- CTENS or TLEA, especially if not charge balanced, may not be suited to peripheral neuropathy with hyperaesthesia or serious sensory loss. Treatment on the affected limb(s), whatever it is for, may not be effective if nerve conduction is impaired.
- CTENS or TLEA is not suited to 'central pain states' from spinal injury, or to 'thalamic syndrome'.
- In general, CEA or ALTENS requires intact muscle afferent nerves to be effective. If there is 'denervation' of muscle (no nerves, motor or trigger points to stimulate), progress will be difficult.
- As with other forms of electrostimulation, discomfort may limit effectiveness when stronger stimulation is required, for instance if muscle is buried deep beneath adipose tissue.
- Visceral pain may not be directly amenable to peripheral electrical stimulation, as it is difficult to elicit paraesthesiae in internal organs.
- In general, local electrical stimulation may aggravate or reproduce acutely painful neurogenic pain, such as postherpetic neuralgia, although electroacupressure here is usually comfortable and effective. Tic douloureux (trigeminal neuralgia) and chronic regional pain disorder (CRPD) are also liable to aggravation, the latter more so if points distal to the damaged area are stimulated.
- If CEA or ALTENS does not help pain, or the effect wears off quickly, there may be a 'block' in the form of focal infection (in teeth/jaw, tonsils or sinus), intestinal dysbiosis or even a tumour.

Of course, like all treatments, EA and TENS do not help everyone, and it is difficult to predict which patients will respond well.

## Drug interactions

Be aware of potential interactions with prescription drugs (especially those affecting neurotransmitters).

The effectiveness of EA or TENS will be reduced in the case of drug addiction, and may be limited (or delayed) by use of drugs such as diazepam, codeine, corticosteroids or narcotics. Thus those currently on high doses of analgesics may respond less well. 'Rebound' pain on withdrawal from benzodiazepines or steroids may also be less amenable to acupuncture. Even those who have used narcotics for more than 2 weeks in the 6 months before treatment may show cross-tolerance effects with TENS.

Amitriptyline may affect sensitivity to TENS. Monoamine oxidase inhibitors (MAOI antidepressants) may affect serotonin levels (and hence the effectiveness of EA) for up to 3 months after use. L-DOPA (for Parkinson's disease) may also deplete 5HT, but sertraline, which inhibits 5HT reuptake and is often given for Parkinson's, may improve response.

Barbiturates may (usefully) raise the convulsion threshold for electrical stimulation, but may also inhibit some EA effects when used in anaesthesia.

Botulinum injection may reduce responsiveness to local stimulation, since nerve endings can be destroyed by the toxin.

It has been suggested that patients receiving gold treatment for rheumatoid arthritis should not receive any form of acupuncture. Those on warfarin or other anticoagulants should be treated with caution, especially if you are strongly stimulating head points. However, there do not appear to be any reports on the safety or otherwise of EA in patients on anticoagulants, although only light acupuncture with minimal insertion of needles has been recommended for use on patients taking warfarin.

Certain drugs may predispose to epileptiform activity in the brain, and electrostimulation should be used with caution when these are being taken.

Caffeine may increase sympathetic activity and, like theophylline, may reduce the effectiveness of HF stimulation, whether EA, TENS or vibration, through its antagonistic effects on adenosine. Drinks or foods containing these stimulants should therefore be avoided for some hours prior to HF (and probably LF) EA or TENS/TEAS treatments.

It is possible that calcium channel blockers such as nifedipine could reduce the clinical effectiveness of LILT and LA.

For further information on drug interactions, see Appendix 3 in the CD-ROM ◎ resource.

## Precautions and contraindications with other forms of treatment

**Note**
Proper training in physical therapy methods should be undertaken before they are used in the context of acupuncture treatment.

### HEAT (INFRARED)
Contraindications to infrared are given in the standard textbooks. The TDP lamp should not be used in cases of high fever or TB, and should not be directed to the head in a patient with hypertension.

Thermal damage to skin or muscle occurs with sustained temperatures of 45°C, but not with short exposures. When using the TDP (for instance), patients who are in any way incapacitated, or who have diminished sensitivity to heat, should not be left unattended.

In all treatments that might induce vasodilatation, if the patient has been lying allow them time before rising, lest they feel faint.

One manufacturer of far-infrared equipment for whole body irradiation recommends that patients with severe adrenal suppression, systemic lupus erythematosus or multiple sclerosis should discuss far-infrared therapy with their doctor prior to use. They consider far-infrared therapy as contraindicated for haemophiliacs, pregnant women and nursing mothers.

A standard contraindication for any form of diathermy includes application over a metallic implant. Diathermy may activate dormant infections, and aggravate infection, inflammation (including arthritic processes) or oedema.

### MILLIMETRE WAVES (EXTREMELY HIGH FREQUENCY, EHF)
Contraindications include acute abdominal pain requiring surgery, pregnancy and menstruation, since treatment may enhance or prolong bleeding.

According to one protocol, irradiation should not exceed 10 min/point (20 minutes per session) if the patient is receiving daily treatment. Ten-day courses should be separated by not less than 3 and preferably 4 weeks.

As with some other forms of electrotherapy, prior surgical intervention may reduce the effectiveness of EHF.

### LOW-INTENSITY LASERS AND POLARISED LIGHT
Many surveys and accounts of LILT focus on its safety aspects. David Baxter lists the following *contraindications*:

- Direct treatment of the eye.
- Irradiation of fetus or pregnant uterus.

- The presence of active neoplasm.
- Haemorrhage (locally).

and the following *cautions*:

- Regions of hypoaesthesia (especially to heat or pain).
- Infection.
- Epiphyseal lines (e.g. the fontanelle) in children.
- Over sympathetic ganglia, the vagus or cardiac region in patients with heart disease.
- Gonads or prostate (the latter commonly treated in China).
- Patients with impaired reflexes.
- Over photosensitive skin.

Some authors have suggested LILT be avoided in cases of venous or arterial disease, or skin damage following radiotherapy. Others have noted temporary adverse effects when irradiating the thyroid area. For some, epilepsy is an absolute contraindication, whereas implanted prostheses or pacemakers are clearly not.

Using a class III laser (for example, 5 or 20 mW, whether red or infrared) at dosages up to 8 J/cm$^2$ is not known to present any cumulative risk, so may be used safely for years, even with children.

### LOW-INTENSITY ELECTROMAGNETIC FIELDS
Magnetic stimulation should not be used if there is bleeding or risk of bleeding, fever, or a low white blood cell count. Their use is also contraindicated in severe acute disease such as cardiac infarction, abdominal pain or dehydration.

In general, the only major risk appears to be that blood pressure may be reduced temporarily. However, it is best to avoid local treatment if there is untreated infection or a metal implant in the treated area, within 48 hours of acute injury and in cases of severe atherosclerosis. Application to the head is contraindicated in epilepsy, and until there is further evidence the list of contraindications should also include pregnancy, presence of a pacemaker, active systemic viral or tubercular infection, myasthenia gravis, malignancy, psychosis and endocrine dysfunction.

#### Static fields
Prolonged exposure to static magnetic fields may result in insulin insufficiency. Roger Coghill, on the basis of official figures on magnetic exposure, calculates that applying a 4000 G magnet for 8 hours daily should be quite safe. However, in epileptic patients, even 10–20 G static fields may elicit epileptiform activity, and he suggests that if larger magnets than those for point application are used then treatment time should be limited to an hour (for 1000 G). Michael Tierra recommends 30 minutes maximum, not more than twice daily, with 3000 G magnets.

It has been suggested that 8–10% of patients undergoing *auricular* magnetic therapy may experience side-effects such as dizziness, palpitations, nausea, temporary dyspnoea, pruritis, insomnia or lassitude. Use of too many magnets or strong magnets should be avoided, particularly in hypertensives, in case blood pressure drops rapidly. When using ion granules on auricular points, if dizziness or hypotension is experienced then treatment should be interrupted for a few days before you try them again.

The use of magnets may alter the effects of some drugs (such as aspirin, cortisone, digoxin and pilocarpine).

Some magnets are nickel plated to prevent corrosion. This may cause problems for nickel-sensitive patients.

Most magnets cannot be autoclaved, but can be disinfected with alcohol.

### Variable fields

In addition to the contraindications mentioned, PEMF should probably be avoided in mycosis and juvenile diabetes. Slowly rotating fields may induce migraine or disturbing psychological states.

## ULTRASOUND AND VIBRATION

Contraindications to ultrasound are covered in standard physiotherapy textbooks. In particular, it has been suggested that ultrasound should not be used on the same day as other electrotherapy treatments such as shortwave diathermy, infrared or X-rays, in case of synergistic effects.

'Infrasound' (the semirandom longitudinal vibrations produced by the QGM) is much simpler and safer to use, the main contraindication being simply to avoid direct contact with very inflamed or infected skin areas, or over the calf if thrombosis is a possibility. The only caution is that if used over the lower abdomen during menstruation it may aggravate heavy bleeding.

## SUMMARY

This chapter covers the basic information required to use EA, TENS/TEAS and other treatment approaches safely in everyday practice. If there is only one chapter you read in this book before you start to use these methods, this should be the one. However, knowledge alone is insufficient. Proper clinical training or supervised apprenticeship is also vitally important.

### Additional material in the CD-ROM resource

In the electronic version of this chapter, additional material can be found on most of the topics mentioned here, including additional techniques and practical tips, with further details on the use of magnets in particular. The reasons behind some of the precautions and contraindications to be observed are also explored in more depth.

## RECOMMENDED READING

*Two non-technical guides on TENS, suitable for patients:*
Gadsby G 2000 An Easy Guide to TENS Pain relief. Body Clock Health Care, London
Tippey KE 2000 TENS: The user's guide to pain relief. A systematic approach. Nidd Valley Medical, Knaresborough, UK (revised edition)

*Two articles that include practical hints for the EAV novice:*
Prince JP How to learn remedy testing in EAV (electroacupuncture according to Voll). American Journal of Acupuncture. 1982 Oct–Dec; 10(4): 347–51
Madill P The uses and limitations of acupuncture point measurement, German electroacupuncture or electroacupuncture according to Voll (EAV): reflections on five years of practice. American Journal of Acupuncture. Jan–March 1984; 12(1): 33–42

*A basic text on safety in acupuncture:*
Zhang XR et al 1999 WHO Guidelines on Basic Training and Safety in Acupuncture. World Health Organization, Geneva

*A selection of thought-provoking articles on possible adverse effects of EA:*
Brattberg G Acupuncture treatment: a traffic hazard? American Journal of Acupuncture. 1986 July–Sept; 14(3): 265–7
Fujiwara H, Taniguchi K, Takeuchi J, Ikezono E The influence of low frequency acupuncture on a demand pacemaker. Chest. 1980 July; 78(1): 96–7
Pöntinen PJ Acupuncture hyperstimulation syndrome. American Journal of Acupuncture. 1979 April–June; 7(2): 161–5
Tillu A, Gupta S Is acupuncture safe in patients with morphine hypersensitivity? Acupuncture in Medicine. 1998 Nov; 16(2): 105–6

# Thirteen

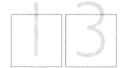

Developing an integrated approach

This chapter explores in general terms how electroacupuncture (EA) and other acupuncture technology can be integrated into clinical practice.

## PHILOSOPHICAL PREAMBLE

### Intention and evolution

Acupuncturists are individuals with different skills, sensitivities, interests and trainings. No one form of acupuncture could possibly suit everyone, and as we develop we each tend to develop our own personal styles. How we work is very much part of our life pattern, contributing to our growth, growing out of who we are. Our tools and our intention, our technique and our understanding, are all part of what we do. We work both with matter and with idea, and with the mysterious dialectic between them. Both are necessary; neither is fundamental.

Our patients are also individuals, coming to us at different stages in their lives, searching for keys that will help shift them through their own particular blocks and difficulties. Their acupuncture treatment grows out of these and, we hope, contributes to their growth in some small way.

In the healing encounter, both acupuncturist and patient play their part. Whatever the beliefs of practitioner or patient, what actually happens may be too rich to define in causal terms. We may have particular models in mind (segmental, trigger point, TCM, Five Element, gross or subtle), we may use particular methods (EA, low-intensity laser therapy (LILT), manual acupuncture (MA), gentle touch), but for all we know change may not occur because of these at all. Whether we consider acupoints do not exist, that treatment is a matter of neurostimulation and traditional methods are just a matter of sticking a needle in a metaphor, or that subtle energetic balance is our goal and anything less is gross

materialism, all we can hope to do is to maintain awareness, 'sensory intent', and act appropriately.

This may sometimes feel more like *wu wei*, actionless action, than a 'doing to', but the importance of intention-to-affect cannot be overemphasised. As Oschman has shown, 'intentions are not trivial'. What Bob Charman has called 'the intention-to-heal mindset' can, for example, result in significant EEG changes in both healer and healed.

EA, therefore, is only part of the clinical picture and there is no one 'right way' of incorporating it into clinical practice, although fundamentals have to be learned and respected. Like any intervention, it is not the 'final answer for all those difficult patients', or something to hide behind when we cannot engage with them. Even EAV practitioners, with all their sophisticated methods (see Ch. 10, page 293), may find in the end that patients who respond are those who 'commit themselves to making consistent and responsible changes'.

### The question of levels

Physical therapists focus on physical bodies, and practitioners of energy medicine on energy bodies. In actual practice, however, we can't 'work' on one level without influencing others. Indeed, in the therapeutic encounter we may be 'working the interfaces', as David Reilly has put it. It is a tantalising exercise to hold both neurophysiology and TCM in mind without reducing one to the other, or emphasising only one and excluding the other. Both may usefully contribute to intention and treatment.

A useful metaphor is that of root (*ben*) and branch (*biao*). For most of us, it is probably more of a challenge to attempt to sort out the *ben* (underlying pattern) and easier to focus on *biao* (in the sense of symptoms), to treat the location of pain rather than attend to what one could call 'constitutional' factors or reflect on the various aspects of the patient's life that may be contributing to it. What is construed as *ben* depends, of course, on what sort of acupuncturists we are, and how we perceive our patients. Medical acupuncturists, physical therapists and those traditionally trained will all have different (and valid) perspectives on this.

Although for the holistic model the Western medical habit of labelling a particular part as 'the problem' and dealing solely with that makes little sense, there is little concrete evidence as yet that treatment that takes *ben* into account is more effective than symptom-based treatment. Personally I believe it is important to feel comfortable with both, and to be flexible: sometimes a patient will require one approach, sometimes the other and sometimes both.

Which level does EA address, however – *ben* or *biao*? And is EA a part of acupuncture, or a modality of electrotherapy? That depends on what is understood by 'EA'. For instance, I was quite surprised, on a visit to Holland in 1997, to find that 'EA' there is generally taken to be EAV, and not a form of peripheral stimulation.

Acupuncture can be used for its more specific analgesic effect (for instance) or as a form of therapy. My own image is of two main levels: a more physical one grounded in the neurophysiology of neural pathways and endorphin release, and a subtler energetic one where the emphasis is on eliciting homeostasis and harmony. The points treated may be the same, but the intention and intervention may be very different. Stronger stimulation (what Becker calls 'high energy transfer') affects the physical level more, whereas gentler treatment (with a 'minimal energy' or 'energy reinforcement' technique) is subtler in effect. With the 'more is better' approach, precision of point location and attuned therapeutic intention become less important, whereas they are prerequisites for successful minimal intervention. On one level, you are definitely 'doing to', and on the other maybe more 'listening to', 'doing with' (or even simply 'being with').

Two levels of treatment or measurement have been a key consideration in several Japanese acupuncture systems. In ryodoraku, Nakatani differentiated between local points reactive in disease and those of the meridian system, although both could be located and treated by electrical means. Manaka differentiated between the advanced and complex nervous system and a more primitive 'X-signal system', which manifests and is manipulated with minute stimuli that clearly cannot affect the nervous system, and so remains unexplainable by current neurophysiology. As he states, 'it is important that we do not confuse the neurological and humoral effects of acupuncture, so thoroughly researched and described in needle analgesia and anesthesia research, with the signal system effects ... We should not think of using acupuncture anaesthesia methods for treatment of general or subtle problems.'

If both systems are activated together, we may not be able to recognise the effects of the low-level stimuli. As Manaka also pointed out, strong treatment may give quick results, but at the risk of 'overdose', whereas short simple stimuli involve much more of an interplay between patient and practitioner as the body is encouraged to adjust towards harmony. When it comes to measurement, Motoyama too very clearly differentiates between autonomic function (as indicated by the AMI device 'AP' readings) and overall meridian or *qi* function (as indicated by AMI 'BP' readings). Misumi Taiji

considers *qi* itself as 'dualistic', as both information and energy, corresponding to the wave–particle duality of quantum physics.

Because my own background is in J R Worsley's Five Element system, which focuses more on homeostasis than symptom, I favour using a traditional and gentle ('information') approach initially with many patients who have chronic problems, and leaving EA and other stronger ('energy') interventions until I judge them appropriate, have consolidated my TCM or Five Element diagnosis or have found that MA is just not enough. However, symptomatic and homeostatic are like the two wheels of a cart, in Manaka's simile.

Some practitioners consider EA as compatible with both Five Element ('meridian style') and TCM approaches. Often – and I am not alone in this – I have no qualms about using strong EA and subtler methods in the same session, whereas those with other biases may believe that electrotherapy-style EA blocks more refined approaches. In acute situations I may use EA alone.

The acupoints I use will also reflect this: local or segmental acupoints (trigger points, motor points or *ashi* points) with stronger stimulation, or meridian points for balancing energy more gently. When the points for the two types of intervention coincide, whether to use EA or not has to be weighed up in the context of the moment. My main superstition is that I tend not to use strong EA on the master and coupled points of the eight extra meridians, if only because of their association with Manaka's methods.

# PRELIMINARY CONSIDERATIONS

The primary goal of treatment is to help patients. Is EA really necessary, or is MA quite sufficient? If EA is indicated, is it the best, most economical method, and safe? Or is it an excuse for the practitioner to focus on technicalities rather than developing a relationship with patients, or a means to cram more into a busy schedule, delegate treatment to assistants and cut costs? Or a grasping at straws when nothing else seems to help? A device can be a powerful placebo for all concerned, but this should not be abused.

Undoubtedly one 'advantage' of EA is that it can reduce contact time with patients. You can park them, wire them up and leave the rest of the treatment to underlings. Repeated needle manipulation is no longer required. If you are using transcutaneous electrical nerve or acupoint stimulation (TENS/TEAS) rather than needles, you can even just mark the points to be used and leave it at that – and your assistants will require only minimal training. When a patient requires more frequent treatment than you can give them, this may be a useful low-cost option for them and for you. It might, however, be yet more cost effective for the patient to rent or buy a home treatment unit for daily or frequent treatment between sessions in the clinic. It may be less effective than acupuncture, but the more frequent use may well compensate for this.

Many people prefer to treat themselves rather than seeing a professional, and a TENS or probe TENS (pTENS) device can be useful for their whole family, provided it is used carefully for diagnosed problems, with the clear understanding that there is more to acupuncture than gadgets, and that sometimes it is essential to consult a health professional. Yet, for those who might feel rejected or discouraged by this emphasis on self-reliance, it can be important to maintain personal contact and continue regular treatments that nourish the patient at a different level.

In many conditions, acupuncture can be a useful alternative to medication, and EA is sometimes particularly welcomed as a means of mobilising the body's endogenous resources. However, just as drugs can be used to suppress unwanted reactions, so too can EA or TENS. They are not panaceas and have to be used sensitively. They may not always provide cures and solutions, but may enable patients to cope more easily with their particular predicaments, or break cycles of pain for long enough that other healthier patterns can be encouraged to take root. However, some patients may have found a better equilibrium in living with pain than they would if their pain were removed, and for some pain there is no satisfactory treatment. It may not be right in such situations to attempt to alleviate pain.

Individuals vary in their response to EA and other non-traditional acupuncture methods, just as to MA. For the 'strong reactor' to acupuncture, vigorous electrostimulation may be unnecessary, and should in any case be used with caution at first. For the 'non-reactor', in contrast, even switching to the strongest EA may make little difference. Felix Mann points out that the most 'difficult diseases' may respond to acupuncture in the former, but not of course in the latter, nor in the 'normal reactor'. It may be in the last group that EA is most appropriate. Women may be less tolerant of strong electrical stimulation than men (at least with TENS) and this too has to be taken into account.

## THE TREATMENT PLAN

When to treat depends on the history of the condition. In general, earlier treatment gives a better response.

EA, laser acupuncture (LA) and other types of 'techno-puncture' have to be part of an overall strategy that addresses different aspects (or levels) of the patient's needs. They may be used as part of acupuncture treatment, or as adjuncts to other approaches (physical therapy, osteopathy or chiropractic, for example). Although in some situations they may be the sole form of treatment, they are best used as part of a comprehensive strategy. In China, even MA is often combined with other interventions, and not necessarily viewed as a stand-alone treatment.

In the acupuncture context, the treatment plan could include several 'patrons': local TrP or *ashi* point stimulation, or auricular points, with accompanying distal points, and constitutional treatment of some sort in more complex cases. This could be based on TCM, Five Elements or the eight extra meridians in traditional terms, on modern methods of ryodoraku- or EAV-style meridian balance, or on correction of 'basic' (quadrant) readings in the SBM system. Whatever system of feedback you use, whether it is taking the traditional pulses, Nogier's ACR, Omura's O-ring test, ryodoraku or EAV (see Ch. 10), it is important to maintain an energetic dialogue with the patient and check how readings change in response to what you do.

In the physical therapy context, it is useful to remember that exercise after treatment may enhance and prolong the effects of acupuncture-like TENS (ALTENS) or conventional, low-frequency high-intensity EA (CEA). Even brief (10-minute) low-frequency stimulation may bring some life into a muscle before other hands-on interventions. Many osteopaths and chiropractors find the combination of EA and manipulation is very effective. Stretching, mobilisation or active exercises have been combined with microcurrent (MENS), either before or after treatment. Exercise accompanying stimulation may, indeed, be vitally important to stimulate neurological pathways, both central and peripheral, for example following stroke, or with a recalcitrant joint problem.

Details of parameter and point selection have been covered elsewhere in this book. However, everyone differs in their response, and you may need to explore different stimulation parameters and unusual point combinations for maximum benefit. In whatever way you do this, a simple sequence of procedures is necessary, to avoid confusion.

You will need to consider what type(s) of stimulation to use. For instance:

- EA.
- TENS/TEAS.
- Handheld probe (pTENS).
- Some form of electromassage.
- Heat.
- Cold.
- Extremely high frequency (EHF).
- LA.
- Magnets.
- Cranial electrotherapy stimulation (CES).
- *Qi Gong machine* (QGM) or ultrasound.
- Other.

You will also need to consider what parameters to use. In the case of electrical stimulation, for instance:

- Low frequency, high intensity – ALTENS (CEA).
- High frequency, low intensity – CTENS (TLEA).
- Intermittent.
- Dense-disperse (DD).
- Microcurrent.
- Other.

And what points to use:

- Local (TrP, *ashi* points, points with low electrical skin resistance).
- Auricular.
- Segmental points (dermatome, myotome, sclerotome) – e.g. paraspinal points, MPs, distal points on related meridians or nerves.
- Points with general effect, such as LIV-3, LI-4, or ST-36.
- Points for 'constitutional' or *ben* treatment, according to principles of TCM, Five Element or other systems.

How many points to use, needle depth, and whether or not to elicit *deqi* prior to EA, may be a matter of personal style as well as theoretical understanding.

## Some brief examples

Do you want to achieve rapid pain relief so that you can then move on to work at a deeper level or with stronger CEA? In that case you might consider initial use of CTENS at local points in conjunction with brief intense stimulation at auricular points, followed by treatment on distal meridian points. Alternatively, if your equipment allows it, you may wish to apply TLEA locally, and CEA simultaneously on distal meridian points or points with general effect.

Many anecdotal accounts state that the combination of auricular and body points may be more effective than use of either alone. Or, perhaps, if relaxation is required, you may find simple needling of ear points to be sufficient, in conjunction with CEA at general effect body points. Or you may wish to position press-needles or 'ion granules' (small metal beads) on ear points for the patient to maintain treatment effect between sessions.

In an acute *shi* case (e.g. musculoskeletal trauma), strong stimulation may be applied immediately. In chronic deficiency (*xu*) conditions, you may want to build stimulation intensity more gently. Alternatively, you may wish to use EA in a phase of acute pain, and MA when the patient is pain free. In this sense, you might aim at matching stimulation and condition.

Of course, the patient may want you to give some attention to a problem area, and you may need to respect this, although without being distracted from designing the treatment that you consider to be appropriate. The same goes for some idiosyncratic attitudes or sensitivities to electrostimulation. Darren Starwynn, for example, has presented a four-step approach when using microcurrent, adapted from Manaka's work. He starts by balancing meridians using the master and coupled points of the eight extra meridians, proceeds to back-*shu* point stimulation, then 'structural balancing' with electromassage, for example, and only then to symptom control treatments.

## THE COURSE OF TREATMENT

How long treatment should continue, and how frequently, can be quite an issue. In China, 10-day courses are the norm, with a break of a few days between courses, and treatment continues as necessary for a number of courses. In the West, the general pattern is to treat relatively frequently at first (once to three times per week, depending on whether the condition is chronic or acute), spacing treatments out over time and abandoning treatment if there is no response within six to eight sessions, but continuing longer if there is some response, then reassessing changes after 10–15 sessions. It is important to remember that response may be delayed for several weeks after a last treatment, so it may be as well to interrupt rather than abandon treatment after a first course of six to eight sessions if there appears to be little change, reassessing after a further few weeks. It has even been suggested that the less vigorous stimulation used in some forms of Western acupuncture may mean longer courses of treatment than are required in China.

After a while, treatment effects will plateau, whatever the intervention. It may then be appropriate to consider home treatments in addition to clinical sessions. Alternatively, you could combine a modality that is partially effective with others, or switch to a different one, especially if its supposed mechanism is completely different from that of the modality already tried. If treatment effects last for a few weeks or months and then taper off, a further course can then be offered.

## TREATMENT RESPONSE AND NON-RESPONSE – WHAT TO DO NEXT

There is a spectrum of response, from swift immediate improvement (suggesting only infrequent treatment is needed), to a slow but sure improvement (treat more frequently?), with aggravation or adverse treatment reactions such as drowsiness or agitation indicating probable overtreatment (use less frequently, for shorter periods or at lower intensity). An initial generalised response after the first session, with improved sleep, more energy and a sense of greater relaxation, may occur with many different acupuncture treatments. However, even though this is prognostically encouraging, it gives little clue as to the effectiveness of the specific intervention used.

Some patients may respond poorly or not at all. Possible reasons for this have already been reviewed in Chapter 12 (page 335) and include:

- Constant disabling or psychogenic pain, central pain, thalamic syndrome, or visceral pain.
- Secondary gain.
- Anxiety or depression.
- Age.
- Other prior treatments.
- Parkinson's disease, malignant tumour.
- Intestinal dysbiosis.
- Focal infection (teeth/jaw, tonsil, sinus) or scar tissue.
- Inappropriate use of CTENS or TLEA.
- Aggravation of conditions through inappropriate use of strong stimulation.

The following is a further checklist for when treatment is not effective:

- Is your diagnosis correct?
- Is acupuncture (and EA in particular) an appropriate treatment?
- Is your selection of acupoints correct and well balanced (in terms of laterality and use of rostral and caudal points)?

- Have you focused too much on local treatment?
- Is your acupuncture technique correct (and EA parameters in particular)?
- Is there appropriate management between treatments?
- Are there other pre-existing conditions that should be taken care of?
- Has the primary cause been resolved?
- Are potential secondary complications being monitored?
- Has the condition progressed beyond its ability to respond to acupuncture?
- Are there genetic or acquired conditions inhibiting response?
- Are there behavioural or environmental factors to consider?

CEA/ALTENS may not be effective if the stress of prolonged or severe pain or illness has led to a condition of 'endorphin depletion'. Furthermore, tolerance can occur with repeated or prolonged use of the same treatment parameters, particularly TLEA or CTENS. Within a treatment, this habituation can be remedied to some extent by turning up the current amplitude when the patient no longer feels it. Some devices have modulation settings where amplitude, frequency or pulse duration is automatically varied, or such variations can be applied manually. It is also worth exploring whether needling or massaging other points during EA could effectively reduce tolerance.

Using a rather different approach, neurotransmitter depletion or blockade, whether due to chronic illness, poor uptake of nutritional precursors, or the action of endogenous antagonists such as cholecystokinin, may be reversed to some extent by preadministering nutritional precursors or cofactors such as D-phenylalanine, vitamin B6 and L-tryptophan or 5-hydroxytryptophan for serotonin, as outlined in Chapter 6.

## COMBINING EA OR TENS WITH OTHER MODALITIES

Traditionally, acupuncture is only one of a whole spectrum of interventions and practices. It does not exist in isolation. Although it may be very effective on its own, in many situations it may best be combined with other modalities.

Knowing the effects of different interventions, such as EA or TENS, heat, LA, magnets, vibration and so on, you may find it effective to combine them. Examples are:

- EA locally with manual reduction using needles at distal meridian points.
- Preheating the area prior to stimulation, or concurrently heating needles used for EA.
- Electric plum blossom needling.
- Using a roller electrode to produce erythema and 'discharge' painful areas.
- Combining EA and LA, or EA and PEMF, especially for wound healing.

- Cupping adjacent to EA needles or TENS pads, to enhance effects on circulation.
- Using different forms of electromassage.
- Applying magnets, press-needles or acupressure on points between sessions.
- Combining EA with homeopathy, in 'homeopuncture' (potentised heroin as an adjunct in treatment for withdrawal, as an extreme example).
- Exercise (stretches), which may be an important aspect of combined treatment for musculoskeletal problems, as may heat and massage, *tuina*, or cryotherapy (cold).
- Drinking more (perhaps even before a treatment), which has been suggested as helpful with microcurrent or PEMF treatment.
- If you are a real techno-head, you may consider combining photic and electrical methods of stimulation.
- Combining EA with nerve block, but preferably in that order.
- Combining EAA with conventional anaesthetic agents, which can be very effective.

Thus there are almost endless possible combinations of peripheral electrostimulation with other modalities. However, sometimes it is good to keep things simple. If you use more than one intervention at a time, it becomes unclear which of these is helpful, and which just self-indulgence.

## SUMMARY

Some key points in this chapter are:

- the importance of intention and an awareness of treatment level (neurophysiological or energetic, for example)
- the need for EA and TENS to be applied sensitively in each individual case
- the variety of possible treatment strategies
- how to decide treatment duration and handle non-response
- how different modalities can be combined.

### Additional material in the CD-ROM resource

The electronic version of this chapter in the CD-ROM resource is only slightly longer than this. As throughout the book, it is fully referenced.

## RECOMMENDED READING

*Thought-provoking material on the practitioner, intention and healing:*

Charman RA 2000 Healing by intention – a research-based overview. In: Charman RA (ed) Complementary Therapies for Physical Therapists. Butterworth-Heinemann, Oxford, 55–77

Reilly D 2001 Some reflections on creating therapeutic consultations. In: Peters D (ed) Understanding the Placebo Effect
in Complementary Medicine: Theory, practice and research.
Churchill Livingstone, Edinburgh, 89–110

Tiller WA, Dibble WE Jr, Kohane MJ 2001 Conscious Acts of
Creation: The emergence of a new physics. Pavior, Walnut
Creek, CA

*An example of how simple measures can enhance treatment:*
Shealy CN Vitamin B6 and other vitamin levels in chronic pain
patients. Clinical Journal of Pain. 1987; 2(3): 203–4

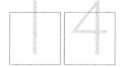

## Conclusion, and the view ahead

Any book is a journey, chapter unfolding after chapter. Starting from basic definitions, looking at history, traversing the cityscape of electrotherapy, and then plunging into the burgeoning jungle of neuroscience with its mysterious inhabits, to emerge, blinking, on to the seemingly endless prairies of clinical studies and experience, descending again into the factory rattle of gadgetry, the suburban classroom of do's and don'ts, we have ended by reflecting on how to integrate this particular journey into our lives, our practice.

But where have we arrived and, if we want to travel further, where next? The intention, of course, is that this book will assist practice, give knowledge, strengthen skills. I hope it will also hone rational scepticism, embolden creativity and allow space for intuitive forays, safely. It has become a cliché that acupuncture is both science and art. This is as true for treatment that uses electrical or other devices as it is for traditional methods. The two are not mutually exclusive. Sometimes I think even machines may have souls, if we do.

The complementarity of *yin* and *yang*, subtle and gross (wave and particle), East and West, meridian and point, information and energy, or energy and neurophysiology, of *ben* and *biao*, are themes that weave their way through this book. Reason, boundary, legislative limitation; insight, openness, innovation – at some times, and in some places, emphasis has shifted more to one side or to the other, but not for ever. From the interplay of black and white come infinite shades of grey.

There are many ways to join in the play of *maya*, many levels of understanding, diverse approaches, different intentions. My belief is that rather than just doing what we have been taught as the norm, as *the* right way, whether our training is biomedical or traditional, we need to be open to exploration, cross-fertilisation and pluralism. Knowing more than one language enriches us. Certainly part of the satisfaction for me in creating this book has been in bearing witness to the sheer ebullient variety and richness of contemporary acupuncture, and its protagonists. A strong message from this book is that there are many roads to healing.

I definitely do not agree with Edzard Ernst's statement that 'One day there will be only one medicine.' Yet, while the currently fashionable emphasis on evidence-based medicine is reductionist and potentially restrictive of practice, possibly even self-defeating (the more precisely we limit our field of vision, the less we can see), as practitioners we all have a need to question what we are taught, and to look at research, at what others have found that may differ from accepted truths, to find our own. I hope that the emphasis on research in this book will encourage this.

One of my agendas in looking at so much research has been to try to find and explore patterns that may not be altogether obvious. Many of the experimental findings, for example, particularly on what I think of as the homeodynamic (regulatory) effects of acupuncture, are very much in keeping with basic biological laws, such as the Arndt–Schulz law, or the law of initial values, or epitomise the workings of the autonomic nervous system. Another evident trend is the development of instrumentation to mimic, not just amplify, what occurs naturally. As with art, we put it 'out there', so we can be aware of it. In a sense, much of the instrumentation of acupuncture is itself another form of art.

Something else that has fascinated, even obsessed, me is frequency. Here traditional and modern methods part company, in some respects, as electroacupuncture and associated methods can be very finely tuned, whereas few people consider frequency when manipulating needles or burning moxa.

Everything is vibration, whether in the string theory of quantum physics, the electrophysiology of the brain, or the bioenergetic theories of Wilhelm Reich. I have looked for patterns in the frequencies of EEG responses, peripheral nerve discharge, resonances between stimulation parameters and their physiological echoes. And of course, with my particular blinkers on, I have found them, or think I have.

So, where next?

As someone who knows, I know how little we know, how the horizon will always be a horizon, if never the same one we thought it was. Knowledge and research are potentially endless. Bearing in mind the difference between strong stimulation, 'doing to', with its physiological consequences (*biao*), and subtle treatment, 'being with', enabling underlying energetic change (*ben*), my vision is of an evolution in the latter that will allow us delicately to tune our electrical (or light, or magnetic, or sound or vibrational) instruments, and so affect, at the same time, the enfolding interaction of our patients and ourselves – in the flow, acknowledging the inherent rhythms and currents of the body, unravelling the blocks. DC as well as AC. Cybernetics with awareness.

Of course it is possible to twiddle a few knobs, stand back and watch as patients shudder in time with monotonously repetitive electrical impulses, programming the release of specific neurochemicals. The assembly line of humans as machines, all given identical treatments. Or we can let the machine dictate what is to be done and go and have a cup of tea. But treatment can be more than this. We only have to find our ways, each of us. And, who knows but at the end, once we have experienced the to and fro of resonance in the patient–practitioner relationship, we may be able to discard the gadgetry and return to simplicity. Although maybe, for some of us, a certain synergism with electronics or machines will always be necessary.

Technology is often only an expression in material form of what we can already do at another level, but we cannot know how it will develop, and science and therapeutic methods with it. Traditional, modern – not good, not bad, only labels. Although there is certainly a danger with technology, as with pharmacology, that it may usurp the rhythms of our own bodies, lead us away from ourselves and entrain discord in our lives. If we let it. Again, we need to hold the balance between gross and subtle, chemistry and current. And also the balance between the established (traditional, conventional) and the new. There is no need to be a Luddite, or a neophiliac, for that matter. Technology does not have all the answers, but nor does tradition.

In terms of another critical issue – neurophysiology and integration with conventional medical practice, or energetic healing, outside the medical establishment – I do not think such rigid separations are realistic, in practice. There will always be an ebb and flow between them. Can we keep our feet in both camps?

With all these issues, we have to be aware, but need not be afraid.

# Appendix

## Resources: information, organisations and suppliers

This Appendix includes information on some relevant internet resources, organisations and suppliers. Inclusion in these listings does not constitute endorsement of products, services or organisations, although those I have found particularly useful are marked with an asterisk (*). The date an address was last contacted or a web address accessed is given in square brackets in some cases.

Suppliers are listed only once. If their products span a number of areas, you may need to search for them under a different heading. The products mentioned are those described in Chapter 11.

The listings in the CD-ROM resource ⊙ version of this appendix are nearly three times as long as those here, with more information provided about individual suppliers as well.

## ACUPUNCTURE

*There are many resources available now for those wanting to explore the world of acupuncture without having to trek to major libraries. These include:*
*Medical Acupuncture Research Foundation (MARF):
    website: www.medicalacupuncture.org/aama_marf/journal
*MARF's associated *Acubriefs* newsletter:
    website: www.acubriefs.com
*The Medical Acupuncture webpage:
    website: http://users.med.auth.gr/~karanik/.

 *Two useful mailing lists are:*

The Acupuncture List [2005]
email: Acupuncture© jiscmail.ac.uk
website: www.jiscmail.ac.uk/mailinglists and [2005]:
*The Professional Acupuncture List (PA-L):
    email: pa-l@yahoogroups.com;
    website: www.yahoogroups.com.

## SOURCES FOR OTHER INFORMATION

Laser World, Swedish Laser Medical Society, Box 1031, 181 21 Lidingö, Sweden;
    tel: (0046) 08 765 0044; fax: (0046) 08 767 27 06;
    email: slms@laser.nu;
    website: www.laser.nu.

*A very useful website on all aspects of laser therapy.*

*Therapeutic Resources Inc., PO Box 12608, Mill Creek, WA 98082-0608 USA [2001];
    tel: (001) 425 745 8505; fax: (001) 425 338 9463;
    email: tri@everett.net, al@sisna.com
    (cestech@tm.net.my for Asia);
    website: www.painsolutions.com/ati14/cesfaq.htm
    [no longer accessible, 2005, May 4].

*Comprehensive information on CES.*

## ORGANISATIONS

### Canada

Planetary Association for Clean Energy (Andrew Michrowski), 100 Bronson Ave no. 1001, Ottawa, Ont K1R 6G8, Canada;
    tel: (001) 613 236 6265; fax: (001) 235 5876;
    email: pacenet@canada.com;
    website: http://pacenet.homestead.com.

*Useful for information on EM environmental issues. See also Essentia below.*

### France

Groupe Lyonnais d'Études Médicales (GLEM), 49 rue Mercière, 69002 Lyon, France [2005];
    tel: (0033) 04 72 41 80 08; fax: (0033) 04 78 37 55 13;
    email: isabelle.glem@wanadoo.fr;
    website: http://isabelle.loras.free.fr or www.glem.org

*Information on auriculotherapy, acupuncture and homoeopathy, based on Paul Nogier's work.*

## Germany

Internationale medizinische Gesellschaft für Elektroakupunktur nach Voll eV, Am Promenadenplatz 1, 72250 Freudenstadt, Germany [2004];

tel: (0049) 7441 918580; fax: (0049) 7441 9185822;
email: IMGfEAV@t-online.de;
website: www.eav.org.

*The major organisation for EAV (electroacupuncture according to Voll).*

## Japan

International Association for Religion and Parapsychology (IARP) and Motoyama Institute for Human Science, 4-11-7 Inogashira, Mitaka-shi, Tokyo 181-0001, Japan [1981];

tel: (0081) 422 48 3535; fax: (0081) 422 48 3548;
email: irp@bekkoame.ne.jp.

*For information on the work of Hiroshi Motoyama and the AMI.*

## United Kingdom

Association of Bioenergetic Practitioners (Chris Dunk, Hon Secretary), Cherry Tree Cottage, Pickford Place, Chapel-en-le-Frith, High Peak, Derbyshire SK23 0EL, UK;

tel: (0044) 1298 813355;
email: getenergetic@aol.com;
www.bioenergy.co.uk.

*Information network for members interested in EAV, EEG neurofeedback, ozone therapy, the Skenar device, and related topics.*

British Biomagnetic Association, 31 St. Marychurch Road, Torquay, Devon TQ1 3JF, UK;

tel: (0044) 1803 293346;
email: grahamgardener@biomagnetics.freeserve.co.uk.

*Courses in the Ito method of using magnets on acupoints (see Ch. 10 in CD-ROM ⊚ resource).*

Society for Biophysical Medicine, Rodney Robinson, CIC – Drug Services, Duncan House, 64–66 Islington, Liverpool L3 8LG, UK [2005];

tel: (0044) 151 207 1133; fax: (0044) 151 207 1146;
email: rodney@biophysicalmedicine.com;
website: www.biophysicalmedicine.com.

*Acupuncture-based electrotherapy courses, with an emphasis on drug withdrawal.*

## United States of America

Electro Therapy Association, 9736 East 55th Place, Tulsa, OK 74153-1189, USA;

tel: (001) 918 663 0297; fax: (001) 918 663 0298;
email: electro@electrotherapy.com;
website: www.electrotherapy.com.

*Auriculotherapy training and seminars.*

International Association for Religion and Parapsychology (IARP), US Branch, and California Institute for Human Science, 701 Garden View Court, Encinitas, CA 92024, USA [2003];

tel: (001) 760 634 1771; fax: (001) 760 634 1772;
email: cihs@adnc.com;
website: www.cihs.edu.

*For information on the work of Hiroshi Motoyama and the AMI.*

Occidental Institute Research Foundation [Walter D Sturm], PO Box 2950, Oroville, WA 98844-0088, USA [2002];

tel: (001) 250 497 6020; fax: (001) 250 497 6030;
email: support@oirf.com;
website: www.oirf.com.

*EAV and MORA information, courses and products.*

# SUPPLIERS

## General acupuncture suppliers

AcuMedic (Man Fong (Benny) Mei), 101–103 Camden High Street, London NW1 7JN, OK [2003];

tel: (0044) 0207 388 5783/6704; fax: 0207 387 5766;
email: info@acumedic.com;
website: www.acumedic.com.

*Mostly 'own brand' devices, but also the Piezo-DX and other equipment. Offers 10% discount to acupuncture students.*

Acuneeds Australia (Dorian Ribush), 622 Camberwell Road, Camberwell, VIC 3124, Australia [2003];

tel: (0061) 3 9889 4100; fax: (0061) 3 9889 1200;
email: acuneeds@acuneeds.com;
website: www.acuneeds.com.

*Ion-pumping cords, Piezo-DX, Pointer Plus and other devices.*

Chinese Medical Center (CMC Tasly Group), Geldersekade 67–73, 1011 EK Amsterdam, Netherlands [2003];

tel: (0031) 20 623 50 60; fax: (0031) 20 623 36 36;
email: info@shenzhou.com;
website: www.shenzhou.com.

*Numerous products, from this centre associated with Shenzhou Open University of TCM. One of the largest catalogues of Chinese devices available in the West.*

Electro-Therapeutic Devices Inc (ETD), 570 Hood Road, Suite 14, Markham, Ont L3R 4G7, Canada [2003];

tel: (001) 905 475 8344 or (001) 416 494 7997;
fax: (001) 905 475 5143;
email: etdinc@on.aibn.com;
website: www.etd-acupuncture.com.

*AWQ-104B, Ito IC-1107, IC-4107, Pointer Plus (and probe accessory), Piezo-DX, TENS and much other equipment.*

*Harmony Medical (Philip Choy), 629 High Road, Leytonstone, London E11 4PA, UK [2005];
tel: (0044) 208 518 7337; fax: (0044) 208 556 5036;
email: sales@harmonymedical.co.uk
website: www.harmonymedical.co.uk.

*AAA line. Distributors for Sédatélec and Ito.*

Health Point Products, Inc., 1804 Plaza Avenue, Suite 21, New Hyde Park, NY 11576, USA;
tel: (001) 516 328 6671; fax (001) 516 328 6926;
email. earthtec@mindspring.com;
website: www.1hpi.com
*Pantheon Research EA stimulators, WQ-6F, Pointer Plus, Piezo-DX, TDP, etc.*

Helio Medical Supplies, 2080 A Walsh Ave, Santa Clara, CA 95050, USA;
tel: (001) 408 748 9585; fax: (001) 408 748 9378.

*Parent company to Oxford Medical, selling the same lines.*

Lhasa Medical (now Lhasa OMS), 539 Accord Station, Accord, MA 02018-0539, USA [2005];
tel: (001) 617 335 6484; fax: (001) 781 335 6296;
website: www.lhasamedical.com.

Noma (Complex Homoeopathy) Ltd (Sylvia Austen), Unit 3, 1–16 Hollybrook Road, Upper Shirley, Southampton, Hants SO1 6RB, UK [2003];
tel: (0044) 2380 770513; fax: (0044) 2380 702459;
email: noma@complementary-medicine.com;
website: www.complementary-medicine.com

*VEGATEST and other hitec devices, as well as conventional acupuncture supplies, TENS and EA (AWQ-104B, Schwa-Medico, as well as some 'own brand').*

OMS (Oriental Medical Supplies) Inc.
(now Lhasa OMS), 1950 Washington St, Braintree, MA 02184, USA [2005];
tel: (001) 781 331 3370; fax: (001) 781 335 5779;
website: www.omsmedical.com.

Oxford Medical Supplies Ltd (Ewan Urquhart), Units 11 and 12 Horcott Industrial Estate, Fairford, Glos GL7 4BX, UK [2003];
tel: 0800 975 8000; fax: 0800 975 8111
(in the UK only);
email: ewan@oxfordmedical.co.uk;
website: www.oxfordmedical.co.uk.

*Helio EA-2 (with SureGrip™ needle clips), Ito ES-160, TENS and Microcurrent TENS, Piezo stimulators, Firard TDP III™ lamp and spares, moxa essence spray for use with TDP.*

*Scarboroughs Ltd (Mrs Evelyn Scarborough), 9 East St, Crewkerne, Somerset TA18 7AB, UK [2003];
tel: (0044) 1460 72072; fax: (0044) 1460 75733;
email: info@scarboroughs.co.uk;
website: www.scarboroughs.co.uk.

*Comprehensive catalogue includes several different lasers and stimulators (including the Pointer Plus, for example). Distributors for Ito and Sédatélec, among others. 10% discount to acupuncture students.*

## EA and related stimulation devices

Acuvision Ltd (Karina Markarian), Birchwood, Pine Walk, Chilworth, Southampton SO16 7HN, UK;
tel: (0044) 2380 760640; fax: (0044) 2380 760629;
email: karina@acuvision.org;
website: www.acuvision.org.

*Artsakh and other devices.*

Allied Health, 89–91 Atholl Road, Pitlochry, Perthshire, PH16 5AB, UK [2004];
tel: (0044) 1796 482100; fax: (0044) 1796 482111;
email: info@allied-health.com;
website: www.allied-health.com.

*Acupoint. Also TENS, Novasonic and other devices.*

Aquadent GmbH (Heinrich Schramm), Brockhagener Str. 40, D-33803 Steinhagen, Germany [2005];
tel: (0049) 5204 5544; fax: (0049) 5204 2432;
email: AquadentGmbH@aol.com;
website: www.aquadent.de.

*The V-TENS and intraoral electrode.*

BioMedical Life Systems Inc., 2448 Cades Way, Box 1360, Vista, California 92085-1360, USA [2002];
tel: (001) 760 727 5600; fax: (001) 760 727 4220;
email: information@bmls.com;
website: www.bmls.com.

*Obstetric Pulsar and other TENS devices.*

*Body Clock Health Care (Marilyn Bash), 108 George Lane, South Woodford, London E18 1AD, UK [2005];
tel: (0044) 208 532 9595; fax: (0044) 208 532 9551;
email: sales@bodyclock.co.uk;
stimplus@bodyclock.co.uk;
website: www.bodyclock.co.uk.

*VTENS and other TENS, Stimplus, various massage units and other home treatment devices. 10% discounts to certain agreed groups.*

CEFAR Medical AB, Ideon Science Park, Scheelevägen 19F, 223 70 Lund, Sweden [2005];
tel: 046-38 40 50; fax: 046-38 40 60;
email: info@cefar.se;
website: www.cefar.se.

*High-quality EA and TENS devices.*

Cerebrex (Edward Courtney), 5 Franklin Rd, Landenberg, PA 19350, USA [2001];
tel/fax: (001) 610 255 0750;
email: cerebrex@cerebrex.com; arcangel@conectiv.net;
website: www.cerebrex.com.

*CES and many other products.*

Comptronic Devices Limited (Dave and Nancy Siever), 9008 - 51 Ave, Edmonton, AB T6E 5X4, Canada [2005];
tel: (001) 780 450 3729; fax: (001) 780 461 9551;
email: info@mindalive.com;
website: www.mindalive.com.

*Oasis stereo CES device.*

Earthen Vessel Productions, 9781 Point Lakeview Rd no. 3, Kelseyville, CA 95451, USA [2005];
tel: (001) 707 279 9621; fax: (001) 707 277 7088;
email: lynnem@mchsi.com;
website: www.earthen.com.

*MENS®-i SUPER and other microcurrent stimulators, developed by Thomas Wing.*

Electromedical Products International, Inc, 2201 Garrett Morris Parkway, Mineral Wells, TX 76067-9484 USA [2005];
tel: (001) 940 328 0788; fax: (001) 940 328 0888;
email: richard@epii.com or dan@epii.com;
website: www.alpha-stim.com.

*The AlphaStim microcurrent/CES device.*

Fysioett AB, Box 828, 191 28 Sollentuna, Sweden;
tel: (0046) 8 92 90 26; fax: (0046) 8 35 73 74;
email: medicfitness@fysioett.se;
website: www.fysioett.se.

*Comprehensive catalogue of electrotherapy equipment, including Schwa-Medico EA stimulators and needles and the PuTENS handheld probe.*

Healthronics Innovations Pte Ltd, 41 Kallang Pudding Road #05-07, Golden Wheel Building, Singapore 349316 [2003];
tel: (0065) 6 8441669; fax: (0065) 6 8441670;
email: info@healthronics.com.sg;
website: www.healthronics.com.sg [no longer accessible 2005 May 4].

*HANS LY257 stimulator.*

Institute of Pathophysiology and Immunology, National Sciences Academy of the Russian Federation [ICPI NSA RF], Sanatori-profilactori, 23 Gagarin Ave, N. Novgorod, 603022, Russia [1999];
tel: (007) 8312 649 965, 657 973; fax: (007) 8312 656 030, 649 863;
email: newmed@unn.runnet.ru.

*MRT apparatus (Porog-3NN) and other innovative equipment.*

Ito Co Ltd, or 3-3-3 Toyotama-Minami, Nerima-ku, Tokyo 176-8605, Japan [2001];
tel: (0081) 03 3994 4619; fax: (0081) 03 3994 1465;
email: Itocoltd@itolator.co.jp;
website: www.itolator.co.jp.

*EA, TENS, etc., a key supplier to Western distributors.*

MED Servi-Systems Canada Ltd, 8 Sweetnam Dr, Stittsville, Ont K2S 1G2, Canada;
tel: (001) 613 836 3004; fax: (001) 613 831 0240;
email: info@medserv.ca;
website: www.acupuncturesupplies.com.

*Sédatélec's outlet in North America. Much else besides.*

Medi-Rep, 1807 N Elm, Suite 313, Denton, TX 76201, USA;
tel: (001) 940 387 2539;
email: jlhester@gte.net;
website: www.medirep.com [no longer accessible 2005 May 4].

*Liss Body Stimulator and other electrotherapy equipment.*

MibiTech Aps, Frederiksborgvej 399, Postbox 30, DK-4000. Roskilde, Denmark [2002];
tel: (0045) 4677 5937; fax: (0045) 4632 1919;
email: info@mibitech.com;
website: www.mibitech.com.

*MibiTech Tao.*

Microcurrent Research, Inc (Paul Davis OMD, President), 3810 East Desert Cove Ave, Phoenix, AZ 85028, USA [2003];
tel: (001) 602 494 5626; fax: (001) 602 953 0544;
email: microcurrent@neta.com;
website: www.microcurrentresearch.com.

*Acutron Mentor.*

MSL Medical, Suite 3L, Cooper House, 2 Michael Road, London SW6 2AD, UK [2003];
tel: (0044) 870 44 25 900; fax: (0044) 20 7 736 3573;
email: info@mslmedical.com;
website: www.mslmedical.com.

*Distributor for the MicroACE Programme™.*

*Nidd Valley Medical Ltd (Craig Smith), Conyngham Hall, Knaresborough, N Yorks HG5 9AY, UK [2005];
tel: (0044) 1423 799113;
fax: (0044) 1423 799115;
email: NVML@aol.com.
website: www.niddvalley.co.uk.

*TENS and TrP stimulators, electrodes. Offers 5 year guarantee on most products, including leads.*
*10% discount to acupuncture students.*

Nustar, 283 Columbine no. 137, Denver, CO 80206, USA [2001];
tel: (001) 303 698 1749;
email: nustarii@juno.com.

*Nustar CES devices.*

Pantheon Research, 626A Venice Blvd, Venice, CA 90291, USA [2002];
tel: (001) 310 822 4965.

*Electro-Stimulator 4-C, 6-C and 8-C. Also red and infrared lasers.*

Prizm Medical Inc, 3400 Corporate Way, Suite I, Duluth, Georgia 30096, USA [2003];
tel: (001) 770 622 0933; fax: (001) 770 662 9392;
email: webmaster@przm-medical.com;
website: www.prizm-medical.com.

*Micro-Z™ and associated garment electrodes.*

RDG Medical, 429 Brighton Road, Croydon, Surrey CR2 6UD, UK [2002];
>tel: (0044) 208 660 4374; fax: (0044) 208 660 9417;
email: admin@rdgmedical.com;
website: www.rdgmedical.com.

*A useful source for electrodes and accessories. Importers of Ito equipment.*

Remington Medical Equipment Ltd, 9-401 Bentley Street, Markham, Ont L3R 9T2, Canada [2003];
>tel: (001) 905 470 7790; fax: (001) 905 470 7787;
email: mail@remingtonmedical.com;
website: www.remingtonmedical.com.

*North American distributor for Cefar, Verity Medical and others.*

*Schwa-Medico Medical Equipment and Supplies, Export Dept, Gehirnstr 4, D-35630 Ehringshausen-Daubhausen, Germany [2003];
>tel: (0049) 64 43 83 33 110;
fax: (0049) 64 43 83 33 766;
email: zentrale@schwa-medico.de;
website: www.schwa-medico.com.

*One of the largest European manufacturers of electromedical products.*

Sédatélec, Chemin des Mûriers, 69540 Irigny, France [2001];
>tel: (0033) 4 72 66 33 22;
fax: (0033) 4 78 50 89 03;
website: www.sedatelec.com.

*Various electrostimulators and lasers, mostly based on Dr Nogier's approach, with a good network of suppliers worldwide.*

Skylark Device and Systems Co, Ltd, 12th Fl 34, Sec 3, Chung Shan N Rd, Taipei, Taiwan, ROC [2001];
>tel: (00886) 2 597 9005; fax: (00886) 2 591 2344;
email: skylark@ms1.hinet.net;
website: www.skylarkdevice.com.

*Taiwan's wholesaler to the electrotherapy industry, including many acupuncture suppliers. A large range of EA, TENS, microcurrent, laser and infrared devices, personal ultrasonic and vibrational stimulators, speciality electrodes (rollers, glove, earclip), and even EAV and pulse diagnostic devices.*

Tower Health/Healthtec/No.1 Health Shop (Jonathan Timms), Tower House, 32 Musters Rd, West Bridgeford, Nottingham NG2 7PL, UK [2003];
>tel: (044) 115 982 6306 (helpline: (044) 115 982 6335);
website: www.no1healthshop.com.

*Pain Gone piezoelectric stimulator, Pain Master.*

Verity Medical Ltd, Uplands Place, Drove Road, Chilbolton, Nr Stockbridge, Hampshire SO20 6AD, UK [2003];
>tel: (0044) 1264 860354; fax: (0044) 1264 860825;
email: sales@veritymedical.co.uk;
website: www.veritymedical.co.uk.

*NeuroTrac 3A™, as well as EMG, TENS and EMS devices, vaginal electrodes and other accessories.*

Woodside Biomedical, 1915 Aston Avenue, Suite 102, Carlsbad, CA 92008, USA [2002];
>tel: (001) 760 804 6900; fax: (001) 760 804 6925;
email: rbinfo@woodsidebiomedical.com;
website: www.ewoodside.com [no longer accessible 2005 May 4].

*ReliefBand® antiemesis products.*

## Accessories

*Cuminetti Cancelli Designs (Riccardo Cuminetti PhD), 43 Daniells, Welwyn Garden City, Herts AL7 1QY, UK [2005];
>tel: (0044) 1707 896578; fax: (0044) 1707 896578;
email: rc603@btopenworld.com.

*Neat ultralight clips for auricular work (as marketed by Helio and Oxford Medical); audio mini-tester for checking output sockets. May also repair stimulators if feasible.*

Henleys Medical Supplies Ltd, Brownfields, Welwyn Garden City, Herts AL7 1AN, UK [2005];
>tel: (0044) 1707 333164;
fax: (0044) 1707 334795;
email: sales@henleysmed.com;
website: www.henleysmed.com.

*A useful source for a variety of electrodes, translucent probe covers suitable for lasers, and other incidental supplies.*

## Other general suppliers

China Healthways Institute (CHI), 100 Avenida Pico, San Clemente, CA 92672, USA [2001];
>tel: (001) 949 361 3976; fax: (001) 949 498 0947;
email: chi@exo.com;
website: www.chinahealthways.com.

*QGM (qigong machine) and other products.*

Essentia Communications (Monique Michrowski), 100 Bronson Ave, no. 1001, Ottawa, Ont K1R 6G8, Canada [2003];
>tel: (001) 613 238 4437; fax: (001) 613 235 5876;
email: essentia@essentia.ca;
website: www.essentia.ca.

*See too Planetary Association for Clean Energy. One of the longest established suppliers of 'alternative' devices.*

Exclusive Products [Philip Braham], PO Box 1000, Indooroopilly Centre, QLD 4068, Australia;
>tel: (0061) 7 3371 6126; fax: (0061) 7 3876 7828;
email: exclusive@peg.apc.org.

*EA, TENS and related equipment.*

Telstar Innovations, Inc, 4734 Topeka Ave, Oakford, PA 19053, USA [2003];
>tel: (001) 215 355 4959; fax: (001) 215 355 2332;
email: info@findhealer.com; telstar@voicenet.com;
telstar@dplus.net; telstarinc@home.com;
websites: www.chinamed.org,
www.findhealer.com/mall/telstar,
www.myholistic.com.

QGM, TDP and other acupuncture-related equipment.
Up to 20% discount to health professionals (distributor
and rental options).

## Light therapy

Lasers suitable for acupuncture application are marketed by
most acupuncture suppliers. A useful list of laser manufacturers can be found at:
www.laser.nu/lllt/manufactures.htm.

## Pulsed electromagnetic field devices

Quantum Techniks Ltd (Rory Orr), Marriot House,
28 Harborough Road, Kingsthorpe, Northampton, NN2 7AZ,
UK [2003];
   tel: (0044)1604 846800; fax: (0044)1604 845381;
   email: enquiries@qtluk.com; rory@qtluk.com;
   website: www.qtluk.com [no longer accessible 2005
   May 4].
   MagPulser™.

Snowden Healthcare (Des Snowden), The Old Surgery,
32 Turney Street, Trent Bridge, Notts NG2 2LG, UK;
   tel: (0044) 115 859 9270, fax: (0044) 115 952 1689;
   email: snowdenhealth@proweb.co.uk.

   Medicur magnetic field therapy units.

Vitatec Medical Systems Ltd, The White House, Church
Lane, Guilsfield, Powys SY21 9NH, UK;
   tel/fax: 01938 556800;
   email: chris.wright@vitatec.com;
   website: www.vitatec.com.

   MitoSan device.

## The Motoyama AMI

International Association for Religion and Parapsychology
(IARP), US Branch, and California Institute for Human
Science (Dr Gaetan Chevalier), 701 Garden View Court,
Encinitas, CA 92024, USA [2003];
   tel: (001) 760 634 1771; fax: (001) 760 634 1772;
   email: lab@cihs.edu;
   website: www.cihs.edu.

   For the latest model of this 'apparatus for meridian
identification', in the UK:
Healthcheck Clinic (Jacqueline Young), 144 Harley Street,
London W1G 7LE, UK;
   tel: (001) 208 449 7771;
   email: healthjackie@aol.com.

## EAV and other integrated systems

Imedis (Centre of Intellectual Medical Systems),
Krasnokazarmennaya st. 14, Moscow 111250, Russia [2005];
   tel: (007) 95 362 73 90, 273 08 39;
   fax: (007) 95 362 73 90;
   email: imedis@mtu-net.ru;
   website: www.imedis.ru

   Group of engineers and doctors who have developed a range
   of computerised Ryodoraku, EAV and related systems.

Medizinische Bedarfsartikel GmbH, Im Grauen berg 24,
D-56414 Wallmerod, Germany [1999];
   tel: 06435 1369 or 06435 961249; fax: 06435 1417;
   website: www.mba-gmbh.de.

   EAV and MORA.

Pitterling Electronic GmbH, Lindwurmstr 117, 80337
München, Germany [2003];
   tel: (0049) 89 74 66 24 0 or (0049) 89 77 80 7273;
   fax: (0049) 89 725 0887;
   email: pec@eavnet.com.

   Dermatron EAV devices and accessories.

Dr Reckeweg (UK) Ltd (Kath Chapman), Dalton
House, 33 Leigh Road, Westhoughton, Bolton, Lancs
BL5 2JE, UK;
   tel: (0044) 1942 811444; fax: (0044) 1942 819821;
   email: reckeweg@complementary-medicine.com;
   website: www.complementary-medicine.com.

   Reasonably priced EAV-style system, with
   intensive weekend training courses, complex
   homoeopathy supplies.

## MORA and bioresonance therapy

Bio-Medscan (Stan Richardson), Back Sload Farm,
Balkram Edge, Wainstalls, Halifax, W Yorks HX2 0UB,
UK;
   tel: (0044) 1422 249399; fax: (0044) 1422 243015;
   email: stan.richardson@messages.co.uk.

   UK agent for MORA. Also markets the lower cost
   Inversion unit.

Med-Tronik GmbH (Erich Rasche), Daimlerstr 2, D-77948
Friesenheim, Germany;
   tel: (0049) 7821 6333 0; fax: (0049) 7821 6333 50;
   email: info@med-tronik.de;
   website: www.med-tronik.de.

   MORA devices and training courses.

# Appendix

## Technology in practice: assessment, legislation and insurance

## INNOVATION AND ASSESSMENT

There are literally hundreds of devices promoted as useful additions to an acupuncture or physical therapy practice. The traditionalists among us may wish to ignore them, satisfied with needles, moxa and our hands, the age-old tools of the trade. However, if our concern is for the welfare of our patients, we need at least to be aware of the potential benefits of some of this new technology, and we need also to be able to assess it in some way before we invest in it.

Innovative technologies are usually introduced against a background of accumulated theory. If a technology does not conform to accepted paradigms, it tends to be rejected. However, medical discoveries often arise from individuals playing with new techniques or instruments to see what happens. Historically this has been especially true in the field of electrotherapy. This has consequences for assessment; instead of relying on preconceived notions, an innovative technology is better judged on its individual merits. A foundation of basic explanatory research studies is often less important than pragmatic comparisons of the new method to existing treatments in terms of benefits, risks and, of course, costs.

### Some factors in assessment

Assessment of new treatments is essential for many reasons. Primary amongst them are considerations of risk and of patient safety, which are often overlooked in the excitement of discovery. Formal assessment procedures can become a nightmare to the uninitiated, and before embarking on such a process it is first necessary to weigh up its pros and cons. Some of the general considerations to be taken into account when assessing new technology are:

- How prevalent is/are the condition(s) to be treated?
- What is the morbidity associated with the condition(s)?
- What is the economic burden imposed by the condition(s)?
- Does current practice already offer several options for treatment?

- What is the aggregate cost of using the new technology?
- What would be the potential of an assessment to improve health outcomes or affect costs associated with the condition?

These are necessary questions even for the smallest of informal studies.

It is also important to distinguish between 'efficacy' and 'effectiveness'. *Efficacy* concerns the benefit likely to be generated under ideal conditions of use. However, actual practice conditions are generally less than perfect. A technology's *effectiveness* is its likelihood of benefit under these conditions. Many efficacious devices may not be very effective in actual practice: patients may find it too difficult to follow protocols, for example.

Clearly, although efficacy and safety may be the basic starting points in evaluating the overall utility of a new technology, financial constraints – the emphasis on economic *efficiency* – may mean that a promising technology is never developed.

### Clinical assessment studies – some ethical considerations

Whether research studies are therapeutic or purely scientific, they have to follow guidelines. Some of these, according to the World Medical Association (WMA), are as follows:

- Biomedical research involving human subjects must conform to generally accepted scientific principles and should be based on adequately performed laboratory and animal experimentation and on a thorough knowledge of the scientific literature.
- Such research should be conducted only by scientifically qualified persons and under the supervision of a clinically competent medical person (who remains responsible for the subjects, even if they give their informed consent).
- Doctors should abstain from engaging in research projects involving human subjects unless they are satisfied that the hazards involved are believed to be predictable.

These guidelines are very much biased towards science-rather than technology-led innovation. If followed to the letter, they would make it difficult to carry out any research based on TCM principles, for instance. They would also place research beyond the reach of any small company trying to launch a new product, let alone any practitioners. Furthermore, 'belief' about the 'hazards of a new treatment' will inevitably be biased by many variables. So, if you wish to explore the potential of any new technology, or even a new application of an accepted one, however benign you may 'believe' it to be, you cannot go it alone, but must be medically supervised and work with those who are scientifically qualified. However sensible and well meaning the intentions behind these guidelines, they could well discourage innovation.

However, according to one authority, there is a loophole:

> In the treatment of the sick person, the doctor must be free to use a new diagnostic and therapeutic measure, if in his or her judgment it offers hope of saving life, reestablishing health or alleviating suffering.

Thus new and untried methods *can* be used, provided medical supervision is available. However, such use has legally to be approved by the Medical Devices Agency (MDA) in this country *before* it is carried out. In addition, according to the MDA, there is a difference between the 'clinical investigation' of a new technology and 'just' research using it. In the former case, selection of the medical overseer involved has to be justified to the MDA. Furthermore, any decisions on statistical analysis and group size have also to be verified by the MDA.

# LEGISLATION – THE 'CE' MARK, MARKETING AND MANUFACTURE

Legislative requirements from both Brussels and Westminster for electrotherapy devices have changed rapidly and significantly over the past few years, placing a huge burden on the smaller manufacturer. Even finding out the details of the various rules and regulations can prove difficult. There has been continuing debate on the meaning of the technical terms employed in legislation and, although things are becoming clearer, the interpretation may still depend on the person to whom you're speaking.

In Britain the MDA, now merged with the Medicines Control Agency to form the Medicines and Healthcare products Regulatory Agency (MHRA), is responsible for overseeing the implementation of legislation and ensuring that products on the UK market are safe. The relevant EU legislation is the 'Medical Devices Directive 93/42/EEC' (MDD), the British rubber stamp for this being the 'Medical Devices Regulations 1994 (SI 1994 No. 3017)', which came into effect on 1 January 1995, with a transition period that ended on 13 June 1998. Independent certification organisations called 'notified bodies', such as the British Standards Institute (BSI), check that medical devices meet the essential requirements of the legislation and thus enable manufacturers to apply the CE marking to their products.

## What is a medical device?

For the purposes of EU legislation, a medical device is defined as:

> Any instrument, apparatus, appliance material or other article, whether used alone or in combination, including the software necessary for its proper application intended by the manufacturer to be used for human beings for the purpose of diagnosis, prevention, monitoring, treatment or alleviation of disease … and which does not achieve its principal intended action in or on the human body by pharmacological, immunological or metabolic means, but which may be assisted in its function by such means.

Furthermore, an *active* medical device is:

> Any medical device operation of which depends on a source of electrical energy or any source of power other than that directly generated by the human body or gravity and which acts by converting this energy.

Thus an acupuncture needle is a medical device, but not an active one, whereas an electroacupuncture stimulator is an active medical device. However, devices that merely enhance the well-being or comfort of subjects without achieving, or claiming, any demonstrable medical improvement in their condition directly related to their use of the device are probably not medical devices within the meaning of the MDD, although devices acting upon a subject's EEG or EMG and thereby affecting a physiological process *do* fall within the scope of the directive.

## CE marking and some consequences

The 'CE' mark now has to appear on virtually all items marketed in Europe. Medical devices with the CE mark must conform to relevant directives like the MDD; devices without the mark cannot be marketed within Europe, nor even, according to some MDA officials, used with patients. However, devices that have not been placed on the market do not come under the jurisdiction of the MDD, which is important for users of non-marked equipment.

The purpose of the CE mark is to indicate conformity to the requirements essential for a device 'to be considered safe and fit for its intended purpose'. It guarantees quality of conformity to *legislation*, not to a particular *standard*. In other words, this is a risk/benefit exercise; part of the 'essential requirements' is to provide evidence on performance, namely that a device does perform *some* useful function, and that 'the performance characteristics of the device are those intended by the manufacturer'. Initially it was proposed that clinical proof of efficacy would be required before a device could obtain the CE mark, although this extremely restrictive requirement was dropped. However, any claims of medical efficacy must be adequately supported with test results and records of relevant experience.

Non-medical electrical devices also have to carry a CE mark. Some electrical stimulators have the mark because they have been marketed as just that, without any specific medical claims being made for them. Immediately medical claims are made, or claims on the medical effects of performance, then these have to be justified with supportive documentation. Clearly, it is in the manufacturers' interests to keep claims as simple and as non-medical as possible. However, electrical and other parameters, including waveform, numbers of outputs and so on, *do* have to be carefully specified within certain limitations. Even with an existing type of device, if any 'new' waveforms or other parameters are produced the risks and benefits may have to be documented.

## Class consciousness

In addition to test results and clinical data, in order to obtain CE marking any electromedical equipment has to pass stringent safety tests, depending what 'class' it is in. Class I devices are generally regarded as low risk (e.g. conductive gels, non-invasive electrodes or adhesive plasters), class IIa and IIb as medium risk, and class III as high risk. Decisions on class are made by the organisation affixing the CE mark, whether this be the manufacturer or a distributor, and it is its responsibility to follow the conformity assessment procedure appropriate for the class concerned.

## Selling, buying and importing

It is now illegal for a manufacturer or distributor to sell any new medical device without a CE mark, or even to lend or give one to somebody who will then use it. Contraventions can lead to fines or even imprisonment. For the practitioner, in contrast, there are no such legal requirements, according to the MDD. Any older device not bearing the CE mark that has been purchased in this country (or elsewhere within the EU), since it has *already* been placed on the market, can still be used and even sold on second-hand. If it has been stripped down and rebuilt ('refurbished'), however, then the refurbisher will have to provide it with a CE mark.

Furthermore, whereas in the past you may have quite legally imported a device without a CE mark from outside the EU for use with your own patients, should you wish to sell it later within the EU you would not be able to, since this would be the first time it is placed on the market. In addition, although you may still quite legally purchase a non-marked device for your own *personal* use while in China and bring ('hand carry') it into the EU yourself, you cannot *send off* for the same device and expect not to have difficulties with Customs and Excise. In this case the Chinese manufacturer or distributor would be considered as placing the device on the market, and would be required to CE mark it.

Instruction manuals accompanying a device are required to include the information to use it safely and to identify the manufacturer, taking account of the training and knowledge of the potential users. This means, of course, that adequate information on cautions and contraindications has to be included. Manuals may also have to bear a CE mark.

## Clinical investigation – or research?

Obtaining the CE mark for a new technology is not cheap. It is also not just a one-off procedure: in many cases, different production batches have to be monitored, and any changes in specification require retests. 'Clinical investigations' of devices may also be required by the MDD, specifically to demonstrate or establish data on performance, and safety or side-effects, unless this can be adequately demonstrated by a review of existing scientific studies. The MDA fee alone for their part in this procedure was £2000 in 1998.

Importantly, new 'clinical investigations are required in the case of devices already authorized to carry the CE marking but where the device is to be used for a new purpose'. In other words, 'devices supplied to a practitioner in order that they might be used outside the conditions of use for which a CE declaration of conformity has been made become devices for clinical investigation and must be regulated as such'. Even a note in the accompanying manual to the effect that clinicians may find the device useful for further conditions than those specified 'might be construed as a performance claim', and so require clinical investigation.

There is, however, a difference between a 'clinical investigation' and 'research'. The latter falls outside the scope of the directive, so that a practitioner may decide to use an approved device for a use unintended by the manufacturer (an 'off-label use'), and if the manufacturer is unaware of this, then this constitutes *research*. This would be the case, for instance, if a practitioner decides to use a *veterinary* device on humans, without informing the manufacturer. On the other hand, if the manufacturer is aware of such use, then research becomes clinical investigation and the MDA has to be informed.

Fortunately, devices to be used in regulated clinical investigation do not require a CE mark for the intended use under investigation. Furthermore, for products that have been established for a number of years, it is likely that a critical review of existing clinical experience rather than a full clinical investigation would suffice.

The situation is different for organisations such as clinics or hospitals. Without having to obtain the CE mark, these can build devices for their own 'in-house' use provided the devices satisfy essential safety requirements. So, if you are a company, or another organisation employing or in some way legally liable for its practitioners, you could provide them with equipment in this way. Unfortunately, this would not stretch to a professional body whose members constitute a separate legal entity from the organisation itself.

## Transition

Until the end of the transition period on 13 June 1998, medical devices did not have to conform with the MDD, but with an 'electromagnetic compatibility directive'

(EMCD) in effect since 1992. This involves knowing the pedigree of every single component in an electronic device, for instance. From 14 June 1998, this was still required, but was no longer sufficient. Medical equipment manufacturers are now able to affix CE mark labels only when supervised by a notified body. However, class I devices may not have to be assessed by a notified body, provided that no medical claim is made for them, and also that they have no 'measuring function' (if a device does not show specific values, or only 'specific values of no direct relevance to patient safety', it is not considered as having a measuring function).

## Comparisons – and costs

In the USA, the 'premarket approval process' is often based on original studies on treatment efficacy, and can be very slow indeed. This process can be slowed up even more if demonstration of 'efficacy' is taken to mean that a device has to be shown to be as good as, or better, than a standard treatment. In the UK there is no legal requirement for comparison with standard treatments, although of course if such claims are made by a manufacturer or distributor they have to be substantiated.

# INSURANCE

The insurance position for those using electroacupuncture devices depends on the extent to which their use falls within what is considered the normal scope of acupuncture. A surprising variety of devices satisfies the scope statements from many US states, and is also considered normal within UK training. As a general rule, however, a practitioner using such a device should have proof of adequate training and obtain a patient's informed consent to meet the insurer's conditions, together with explicit approval for anything that could fall outside the recognised scope. If in doubt, ask your insurers before use.

This, of course, raises the issue of adequate training – which is not generally supplied by manufacturers or distributors of acupuncture equipment. In terms of any but the most run-of-the-mill EA devices, it is not provided by training colleges either, and even then training does not necessarily imply competence, nor does it necessarily provide insurance for the practitioner's subsequent use of the devices.

The issue of using devices that are not yet generally accepted by the profession, or of using accepted devices according to non-standard protocols or in research rather than 'the normal course of events', is another complex one. An obvious example of this would be using a TENS machine with needles. Although this has been accepted practice for years in some quarters, according to the MDA 'if a TENS unit has been CE marked for use only with surface electrodes, according to the manufacturer's intended purpose, then any person using needles or an alternative set of electrodes to provide stimulation would do so under their own responsibility'.

Any claims resulting from damage or injury caused by defects in a device will be passed on by insurers under their product liability cover to the vendor/supplier of that device, whether it is one that has an established history of use or is a novel form of technology. Manufacturers who sell direct, as well as their distributors, will (should!) have their own liability cover for (a) defects of design or production of their equipment, and (b) random failure or premature wear of components and so forth. Their policies should cover claims arising from these, provided the user has followed their guidelines on use. Such guidelines should provide full information on possible misuse of a device, but may not include recommendations on treatment; if they do, a failure to follow the approved protocol will certainly invalidate the cover.

Manuals may include statements on the responsibility of the user to ensure regular maintenance and calibration of equipment according to manufacturer's recommendations. Although it is not a legal requirement for equipment to be regularly serviced, if the manufacturer's instructions are not followed, and an 'incident' occurs that is attributable to this, then this is a 'user issue' and the practitioner's insurers will have to pick up the claim. The party carrying out any maintenance work will need to be qualified to do so, and have its own insurance cover for that purpose. Further, all maintenance or repair work will have to be thoroughly documented.

A new requirement from many insurers is that the insured 'at his own expense shall maintain accurate descriptive records of all professional services and equipment used in procedures'. It is important, therefore, not to mislay instruction manuals for any equipment used, and to ensure you have some record of its electrical characteristics. In addition, treatment records should include details of treatment parameters used: intensity, frequency, waveform, pulse duration, stimulation duration and any other variables under operator control. Because these output characteristics will vary with battery life, it is also necessary to keep a check on this, and to keep a note of when batteries are changed.

It is most important to record any serious malfunctions of equipment. Legally these have to be reported by the device manufacturer to the MDA. Manufacturers also have to report any reasons leading to systematic recall of particular products. It is therefore imperative, and not just sensible, that practitioners in turn inform manufacturers of any serious faults in the devices, as well as any long-term side-effects that may not have been evident in original clinical investigations.

In lending low-cost equipment to patients for home use outside the clinic, it is the practitioner's responsibility to ensure that a device is in safe working order before release, and also that recipients clearly understand the treatment, its indications and risks, and what they need to do to carry it out for best effect. In case a device lent or rented out is lost or damaged, you might wish to ask patients to sign an agreement that they will be responsible for loss or damage, but if you intend to do this on a regular basis it would be advisable to have a solicitor look over the wording first.

## RECOMMENDED READING

*Basic information for practitioners:*

Devices in Practice Working Group 2001 Devices in Practice: A guide for health and social care professionals. Medical Devices Agency, London. Online. Available: www.medical-devices.gov.uk/mda/mdawebsitev2.nsf/webvwSearchResults/65E4753084 1EF41800256AD8003E1970?OPEN [accessed 2005 May 4]

*In-depth coverage of some of the issues involved in using technology within a healing/medical context:*

McNeill BJ, Cravalho EG 1982 (eds) Critical Issues in Medical Technology. Auburn House, Boston, MA

Reiser SJ, Anbar M 1984 (eds) The Machine at the Bedside: Strategies for using technology in patient care. Cambridge University Press, Cambridge

*A useful website for US acupuncture legislation:*

www.acufinder.com/Laws_and_Legislature.asp [accessed 2005 March]

### Disclaimer

The information in this article is intended for guidance and should not be used in place of proper legal or other appropriate advice. In particular, it must be clearly understood that those comments quoted from staff of the MDA cannot be construed as legal advice. Furthermore, the original article on which this appendix is based was prepared in 1998. Some of the information here may therefore now be out of date.

### Additional material in the CD-Rom resource

A longer version of this appendix is included in the CD-ROM resource, containing information relevant to those practising in Australia, New Zealand and the USA.

# Glossary

This glossary covers both specialist biomedical and electrotherapy terminology. A basic knowledge of the former is assumed. Thus 'pituitary' is not included, but 'hypothalamus' is, 'hypertension' is not, but 'ischaemia' is, 'asthma' is not, but 'arrhythmia' is. Some words are included just as reminders. Others may be completely unfamiliar to most readers. The vocabulary of traditional Chinese medicine (TCM) is not covered.

Important terms are usually in *italic* type the first time they are used in the book. An expanded version of the glossary can be found in the CD-ROM ⊙ resource.

**5-hydroxytryptophan (5HTP)** ▓ Serotonin precursor, derived from the amino acid tryptophan

**Acetylcholine (ACh)** ▓ Neurotransmitter at neuromuscular junction

**Acetylcholinesterase (AChE)** ▓ Enzyme that breaks down acetylcholine (ACh)

**Action potential (AP)** ▓ Brief increase in positive potential within a nerve relative to that outside it, when initial stimulus exceeds a certain threshold. Action potentials propagate along the nerve fibre

**Acupoint (AcP)** ▓ Specific points on the body where acupuncture stimulation is applied. Fixed points may be located along meridians, or off meridians (miscellaneous points, new points). *Ashi* points are those that become spontaneously tender with disease or injury. They are not fixed

**Acupuncture** ▓ From the Latin words *acus* and *pungere*, the insertion of needles into the body at specific points, together with the treatment of such points using non-invasive techniques that include electrostimulation and laser

**Acupuncture-balanced analgesia** ▓ Combination of acupuncture analgesia with reduced doses of anaesthetic medication

**Acupuncture-like TENS (ALTENS) or TEAS (ALTEAS)** LF (2–5 Hz), high amplitude (15–50 mA), with long pulse durations. Perceived as relatively strong and may activate muscles (motor level)

**Adenoma** ▓ Benign tumour of the epithelium (tissue lining a surface or cavity)

**Adenosine** ▓ Purine neurotransmitter

**Adenosine triphosphate (ATP)** ▓ Nucleotide involved in energy metabolism. Also classified as a purine neurotransmitter

**Adrenaline (Adr)** ▓ Monoamine neurotransmitter in the ANS, acting more on β-receptors

**Adrenocorticotrophin (ACTH)** ▓ Pituitary peptide that induces cortisol release from the adrenal cortex

**Aerotitis media** ▓ Traumatic inflammation of the middle ear due to rapid descent in altitude. Also known as barotitis

**Afferent** ▓ Afferent nerves carry signals towards the central nervous system from the periphery

**After polarisation current (AP)** ▓ Measured with Motoyama Hiroshi's AMI device. Considered to reflect autonomic nervous system function

**Allergy (or allergy and vascular degeneration) vessel** ▓ One of Reinhold Voll's new vessels, starting at the ulnar nail point of the middle finger

**Allodynia** ▓ Hyperaesthesia to normally innocuous temperature or touch stimuli

**Alpha (α)** ▓ 7–12 Hz frequencies in the EEG

**Alternating current (AC)** ▓ Current that flows one way, then the other, with a sinusoidal waveform

**Amaurosis** ▓ Blindness without obvious lesions

**Amblyopia** ▓ Reduced visual acuity

**Ametropia** ▓ General term for alterations in the shape of the eye

**Ampère** ▓ Unit of electric current

**Amplitude** ▓ Amount, as of current or potential

**Amyotrophic lateral sclerosis (ALS)** ▓ Motor neuron disease with muscle weakness, hypertonia and abnormal tendon reflexes, but usually without sensory loss

**Arcuate nucleus** ▓ Mediobasal nucleus within the hypothalamus, major source of βEP within the brain

**Anaesthesia** ▓ Absence of sensation

**Analgesia** ▓ Absence of pain

**Anaphylaxis** ▓ Toxic shock

**Aneurysm** ▓ Sac formed by dilatation of a blood vessel wall

**Angiotensin II** ▪ Circulatory peptide. Neurotransmitter with vasopressor action

**Anion** ▪ Negative ion

**Ankylosis** ▪ Immobility and consolidation of a joint

**Anode** ▪ Positive electrode

**Anosmia** ▪ Absence of sense of smell

**Anoxia** ▪ Total lack of oxygen

**Anterior horn** ▪ Grey matter, projecting into the white matter towards the front of the spinal cord. The anterior horns are bilateral and associated with motor function

**Antidromic** ▪ Conducting impulses in the opposite direction to normal

**Antinociception** ▪ Reduction of sensitivity to pain

**Anxiolysis** ▪ Reduction in anxiety

**Aphasia** ▪ Impaired spoken or written language

**Apoplexy** ▪ Stroke

**Applied kinesiology (AK)** ▪ Method of muscle testing to assess changes in body function

**Aquapuncture** ▪ An alternative name for acupoint injection

**Arndt–Schulz law** ▪ This states roughly that above a certain threshold a weak stimulus enhances activity, while a strong one inhibits it, and if strong enough can be destructive

**Arrhythmia** ▪ Variation from normal cardiac rhythm

**Arteriopathy** ▪ Arterial disease

**Ascariasis** ▪ Infestation by the large roundworm ascaris lumbricoides

**Ascending** ▪ Used of a pathway or signal that travels towards the brain, or to the higher centres within it

**Asthenopia** ▪ Easily tired eyes, accompanied by eye pain, headache or dimness of vision

**Asymmetrical waveform** ▪ Waveform in which positive and negative phases are not identical

**Atopic** ▪ Atopic dermatitis is chronic, with a hereditary susceptibility to pruritis. Scratching often leads to eczema. Atopic asthma is that due to extrinsic causes, while non-atopic asthma does not appear to be immunologically mediated

**Atypical facial pain** ▪ Diffuse pain in the maxillary or mandibular region, persistent rather than overtly painful or shooting. Onset may be gradual, and the pain may be accompanied by symptoms indicating autonomic dysfunction

**Auriculocardiac reflex (ACR)** ▪ Method of assessing changes in the body in response to auricular stimulation, using the radial pulse. Developed by Paul Nogier

**Autonomic dysreflexia** ▪ Exaggerated response to stimuli following spinal cord lesion at or above T8, with paroxysmal hypertension, bradycardia and other symptoms

**Autonomic nervous system (ANS)** ▪ Nerves controlling the functioning of glands and smooth muscle

**Average** ▪ The average value of a rectangularly pulsed DC is the product of the duty cycle and peak value

**Axonotmesis** ▪ Degeneration of nerve beyond the point of injury

**Azoospermia** ▪ Absence of sperm in the semen

**Baroreceptor** ▪ Internal receptor sensitive to pressure changes

**Basal ganglia (basal nuclei)** ▪ Caudate and other connected nuclei deep within the cerebral hemispheres and upper brainstem

**Beat frequency** ▪ Frequency of resultant waveform when two signals of different frequencies interfere

**Before polarisation (BP) current** ▪ Measured with Motoyama Hiroshi's AMI device. High readings tend to indicate an excited state, low readings a tendency to chronic disease

**Beta (β)** ▪ 12–30 Hz frequencies in the EEG

**Bias** ▪ Patients, practitioners, publishers, cultures can all be biased. A bias in study design may even make a meaningful outcome impossible

**Bidigital O-ring test (BDORT)** ▪ Method of assessing changes in body function developed by Yoshiaki Omura, closely allied to applied kinesiology and dowsing

**Bilateral** ▪ Pertaining to both sides (of the body)

**Biliary** ▪ Pertaining to bile or the gall bladder

**Biologically closed electric circuits** ▪ Pathways for ionic flow within the body, postulated by Björn Nordenström and providing a possible explanation for some meridian phenomena

**Bioplasma** ▪ Streams of subatomic particles, proposed as a model of the energy field of the body by Viktor Inyushin

**Bioresonance** ▪ Treatment applying frequencies that match those of various physiological processes

**Biphasic current** ▪ Current that flows in one direction, then the other

**Blinding** ▪ Procedure used to minimise performance bias in a study. Patients, practitioners and assessors may or may not be blinded

**Block, blockade** ▪ Inhibition of nerve transmission, usually with regional anaesthesia by means of injection of anaesthetics close to the nerve, but also for instance by anodal stimulation or, in theory, by repetitive stimulation of the same or adjacent nerves

**Bradycardia** ▪ Heart rate slower than 60 beats per minute

**Bradykinin** ▪ Peptide neurotransmitter, also classified as a kinin

**Brainstem** ▪ The midbrain, medulla and pons

**Bruxism** ▪ Tooth grinding

**Buccal currents** ▪ DC currents that may occur due to the presence of different metals in the oral cavity

**Buerger's disease** ▪ Thromboangiitis obliterans, an inflammatory disease of the peripheral blood vessels, particularly in the legs, in which the vessels are destroyed, leading to ischaemia and gangrene

**Burst current** Wave trains repeated at short, millisecond intervals

**Calcitonin gene-related peptide (CGRP)** Postsynaptic neuropeptide activating NMDA receptor

**Calculus** Stone

**Capacitance** Ability to store electric charge

**Carotid artery** Ascending artery, divides into external and internal carotid arteries, the former supplying the neck, face and skull, the latter the middle ear, eye and brain

**Catecholamines** Small molecule neurotransmitters, producing more rapid synaptic effects than the larger neuropeptides. Adrenaline, noradrenaline and dopamine are catecholamines

**Cathode** Negative electrode

**Cation** Positive ion

**Cellular immunity** Immunity mediated by T lymphocytes

**Central nervous system (CNS)** The brain and spinal cord

**Central pain** Pain due to damage to pathways within the brain or spinal cord

**Central serous retinopathy** Acute, usually self-limiting detachment of retina in the region of the macula, with farsightedness

**Cerclage** Encircling with a ring or loop, for instance of the cervix if it does not remain sufficiently closed during pregnancy

**Cerebrovascular dementia** Dementia resulting from a series of small strokes, atherosclerosis, or possibly cervical problems, rather than degeneration

**Cervical syndrome** Symptoms of radiating neck pain, paraesthesia and muscle weakness or spasm due to irritation and/or compression of cervical nerve roots

**Cervicogenic** Originating in the neck or its dysfunction

**Charge** Amount of electricity

**Charge balance** If both phases of a current transfer the same amount of charge, the current is charge balanced

**Cheilitis (chilitis)** Inflammation of the lips

**Chloasma** Patchy darkening of the skin, usually on the face and symmetrical

**Cholecystectomy** Removal of the gall bladder

**Cholecystitis** Inflammation and distention of the gall bladder

**Cholecystokinin (CCK)** A gut peptide

**Cholecystolithiasis** Gallstones within the gall bladder

**Cholelithiasis** Gallstones

**Chorea** Ceaseless rapid, complex, jerky and involuntary movements. In Huntingdon's chorea, this is progressive, accompanied by mental deterioration

**Chronic fatigue syndrome** A form of neurasthenia characterised by persistent debilitating fatigue and muscle weakness, sometimes headache and depression. May be associated with prior viral infection

**Chronic obstructive pulmonary disease (COPD)** Emphysema or chronic bronchitis, with chronic typically irreversible airway obstruction resulting in a slowed rate of exhalation

**Chronic pain** Pain that has lasted at least three months, often idiopathic

**Clonus** Rapidly repeating spasms

**Clunial nerve** Nerve innervating the skin of the buttock (clunis), with three divisions (superior, middle and inferior)

**Coherence** A signal is coherent if it consists of waves with identical parameters of frequency and amplitude that are also in phase

**Compartment syndrome** Impaired circulation in a tightly packed and enclosed muscle region, with pain, muscle weakness, sensory loss and eventual necrosis

**Complex regional pain disorder (CRPD)** Pain, affecting one or more extremities, often intense and quite disproportionate to underlying pathology. Type I, formerly called reflex sympathetic dystrophy (RSD), is more likely to be diffuse. Type II tends to have a more clearly somatic origin, and corresponds to causalgia (pain and hyperalgesia, confined to the distribution of an injured peripheral nerve). Not only sensory but also sympathetic nerves can be involved

**Concomitant strabismus** Squint due to faulty insertion of eye muscles

**Conductance** Ability to conduct

**Connective tissue (or fibroid) degeneration vessel** One of Reinhold Voll's new vessels, starting at the medial nail point of the middle toe

**Constant current** A device has a constant current output if current remains unchanged when impedance between patient's body and electrodes is varied

**Constant voltage** A device has a constant voltage output if voltage remains unchanged when impedance between patient's body and electrodes is varied

**Continuous current** Current with constant amplitude, duration and frequency

**Contralateral** Pertaining to the opposite side

**Control** A control group is one receiving a control treatment that is different from that administered to the study group. A controlled trial is one in which there are one or more control groups. Comparison between outcomes in the different groups is used to determine the relative efficacy of the study and control treatments

**Conventional EA (CEA)** LF high-intensity EA, with long pulse durations

**Conventional TENS (CTENS) or TEAS (CTEAS)** HF (50–200 Hz), low–amplitude (10–30 mA) stimulation, with short pulse durations. It is perceived as relatively gentle (sensory level)

**Cor pulmonale** Heart disease with enlargement of the right ventricle

**Crack cocaine** An easily prepared form of cocaine that can be inhaled for a more rapid effect

**Cranial electrotherapy stimulation (CES)** Electrical stimulation using electrodes either on both sides of the head, or frontally and occipitally

**Craniotomy** Any incision or operation on the skull

**Critical fusion frequency (CFF)** Frequency at which neuron frequency following response gives way to more continuous firing

**Crossover study** A crossover study is one in which a different treatment is given to each of two (or more) groups. After a washout period, the groups are reversed, each receiving the treatment the other received before

**Cross-talk** Lack of isolation between different outputs from a stimulator, so that the controls for one may affect the current from another

**Current density** Amount of current applied per unit area, in mA/cm²

**Current modulation** Changes to overall pattern of current rather than its individual pulses

**Current of injury** Current that flows from a skin wound to the surrounding surface

**Cushing's disease** Excessive adrenocortical activity secondary to excessive pituitary corticotrophin

**Cycle** Alternating current consists of a succession of regularly recurring cycles

**Cystalgia** Bladder pain

**Decompensation** In cardiac decompensation, the heart struggles to maintain adequate circulation, with shortness of breath, engorged veins and oedema

**Dehydroepiandrosterone (DHEA)** Androgen corticosteroid, most abundant steroid hormone in human bloodstream (synthesised in both males and females). Precursor of both oestrogen and testosterone

**Delta (δ)** 0.5–3 Hz frequencies in the EEG

**Demyelination** Loss of the neural myelin sheath

**Denervation** Interruption of nerve supply to tissue. May be partial (following neurapraxia) or total (with neurotmesis)

**Dense-disperse (DD)** A current with trains of two different frequencies alternating regularly

**Depressor** Blood pressure reducing

**Deqi** Sensation of numbness (*ma*), heaviness (*zhong*), distension (*zhang*) and possibly soreness (*suan*) experienced by patient when needled

**Dermatome** Skin area innervated by afferent nerve fibres from a single posterior spinal root. Dermatomes are symmetrical

**Dermatosis** Any skin condition

**Descending** Used of a pathway or signal that travels away from the brain, or from the higher centres within it

**Desensitisation** Method of decreasing hypersensitivity reactions by administration of graded doses of allergens

**Detrusor** Smooth pubovesical muscle that pushes down to empty the bladder

**Diathermy** Method of heating body tissues, usually with high frequency (longwave, shortwave, microwave) electromagnetic radiation or electric currents, though also with ultrasound

**Diffuse noxious inhibitory control (DNIC)** Widespread pain suppression following intense stimulation at AcPs or non-AcPs, regardless of distance between area of pain and applied stimulus

**Direct current (DC)** Current that flows continuously in one direction

**Dopamine (DA)** 3-hydroxytyramine, a monoamine neurotransmitter

**Dorsal horn** Grey matter, projecting into the white matter towards the back of the spinal cord. The dorsal horns are bilateral and associated with sensory and pain transmission

**D-phenylalanine (DPA)** Amino acid enkephalinase inhibitor

**Dynorphins (Dyn)** Opioid peptide neurotransmitters that attach preferentially to κ (kappa) receptors. They play an important role in EA in the spinal cord

**Dyskinesia** Disordered movement, as of the biliary system

**Dyspareunia** Difficult or painful intercourse

**Dysphagia** Difficulty in swallowing

**Dysphonia** Vocal impairment

**Dysplasia** Abnormal development of cells

**Dysuria** Difficult or painful urination

**ECIWO** Holographic system of acupuncture using points along the second metacarpal or other long bones of the body, developed by Zhang Yin Qing

**Eclampsia** Convulsions in women during pregnancy or after childbirth

**Ectomy (-ectomy)** Excision or resection

**Edge effect** Changes in intensity of stimulation due to uneven distribution of charge over the surface of an electrode

**Eeman's circuit** A method of linking different parts of the body to induce relaxation and other effects (described in Chapter 10 of the CD-ROM ⊙ resource)

**Effectiveness** The likelihood of benefit from an intervention under normal conditions of practice

**Efferent** Efferent nerves carry signals from the central nervous system towards the periphery

**Efficacy** Benefit likely to be generated by a treatment under ideal conditions of use

**Efficiency** Ratio of useful output of a system to its total input

**Eigenfrequency** Inherent resonance frequency

**Electrical muscle stimulation (EMS)** Similar to TENS, but with the object of eliciting muscle contraction rather than stimulation of sensory nerve fibres

**Electroacupuncture (EA)** (a) *broad sense*: All procedures based on measurements or therapy derived from Chinese acupuncture, using modern electronics; (b) *narrow sense*: Electrical stimulation of acupoints exclusively through needles

**Electroacupuncture according to Voll (EAV)** Influential system developed by Reinhold Voll from the 1950s onwards, involving both measurement and treatment at acupoints, as well as *remedy testing*

**Electroacupuncture analgesia (EAA)** The induction of analgesia using EA

**Electroanaesthesia** A general term for anaesthesia induced electrically, but more usually limited to stimulation applied to the head

**Electrode** Medium through which current is applied to an object

**Electroencephalogram (EEG)** Recording of skin potentials on scalp, the sum of many different electrical events in the cortex

**Electrogastrogram** Record of the electrical activity of the stomach

**Electrolysis** Process that occurs when current is passed through an electrolyte

**Electromyogram (EMG)** Recording of electrical activity (extracellular) in skeletal muscle

**Electrotherapy** The treatment of patients by electrical means

**Embolism** Sudden blocking of an artery by material carried from elsewhere by the blood

**Endomorphin-1** An endorphin

**Endorphins (EP)** Opioid peptide neurotransmitters that attach preferentially to μ (mu) receptors

**Endothelins** A group of vasoconstrictive peptides

**Endpoint measure** What is being measured to determine the outcome of a study. The primary endpoint should be decided in advance

**Energy** The capacity for doing work

**Energy density** How much energy is applied over a given area, measured in joules/cm$^2$

**Enkephalinase** Enzyme that degrades enkephalins (Enk)

**Enkephalins (Enk)** Opioid peptide neurotransmitters that attach preferentially to δ (delta) receptors

**Epinephrine** Adrenaline

**Epiphora** Excessive watering of the eyes

**-ergic** Involving the neurotransmitter whose name precedes the suffix, as in endorphinergic, or dopaminergic

**Evoked potential (EP)** An electrical voltage change, usually measured from the scalp, in response to peripheral stimulation

**Explanatory research** An explanatory clinical trial tests the efficacy of an intervention, in an ideal situation, unlike a *pragmatic study*. Experimental research aims to maximise internal validity (accuracy of results) by assuring rigorous control of all variables other than the intervention

**External auditory meatus** Passage of outer ear leading to tympanic membrane

**Facial nerve** Cranial nerve VII

**Faucitis** Inflammation of the fauces, the passage between mouth and pharynx

**Feeding centre** Lateral hypothalamus

**Fibrillation** Uncoordinated localised muscle contractions, usually small and rapid

**Fibromyalgia syndrome** Condition characterised by a history of widespread pain for at least 3 months, and pain upon palpation of at least 11 of 18 designated 'tender points' over a minimum of three of the four body quadrants. Other typical symptoms include severe daytime fatigue, unrefreshed sleep, irritable bowel, chronic headache, morning stiffness, cognitive or memory impairments, reduced coordination and decreased physical endurance

**Field** An electric or magnetic field is present wherever electrical or magnetic effects are evident

**Frequency** Number of cycles or direction changes per second

**Frequency following response (FFR)** Response of nerve fibre, with each applied stimulation pulse triggering it to fire

**Functional magnetic resonance imaging (fMRI)** Application of nuclear magnetic resonance for obtaining images of soft tissue changes, without the use of a contrast medium

**Galvanic current** Direct current

**Gamma (γ)** ~40 Hz frequencies in the EEG

**Gamma-amino butyric acid (GABA)** An amino acid neurotransmitter

**Ganglion** Group of nerve cells, usually located outside the CNS

**Gapping** Moving a joint to create more of a gap, so that a laser beam may penetrate more easily

**Gastrin** A gut hormone

**Gastroptosis** Downward displacement of the stomach

**Gate control theory of pain** Theory that a 'gate' at the first synapse of the thinner (slow) pain fibres in the dorsal horn of the spinal cord can be closed by stimulation of larger myelinated afferents, preventing transmission of pain signals on to the brain. Devised by Ronald Melzack and Patrick Wall in 1965

**Gauss (G)** Unit of magnetic flux density

**Geopathic stress** Stress on the body due to so-called earth radiations, considered a common factor in many conditions by some practitioners

**Gigahertz (GHz)** 1 GHz = 10$^9$ Hz

**Glossodynia** Tongue pain

**H reflex** ▓ Monosynaptic spinal reflex, usually evoked by submaximal stimulation of tibial nerve or soleus muscle with an electric shock

**H1 and H2 receptors** ▓ Histamine receptors

**Habituation** ▓ Adaptation, a decline in response when stimulation is sustained. Sometimes used interchangeably with *tolerance*

**Haemarthrosis** ▓ Bleeding into a joint

**Haematemesis** ▓ Vomiting blood

**Haematoma** ▓ Blood-filled swelling

**Haematuria** ▓ Blood in the urine

**Haemoptysis** ▓ Coughing up blood

**Hertz** ▓ Unit of frequency. 1 Hz = 1 cycle per second

**Heterosegmental** ▓ Pertaining to another segment

**High-voltage pulsed galvanic (HVPG)** ▓ TENS modality using surface pads and very narrow pulses, mostly for non-healing wounds and oedema

**Hippocampus** ▓ Part of the limbic system in the brain, with memory and learning functions

**Histamine** ▓ Monoamine neurotransmitter

**Homeodynamic** ▓ A dynamic alternative to 'homeostatic'

**Hot plate test** ▓ Pain threshold test, assessing limb withdrawal response to noxious thermal stimulus

**Humoral immunity** ▓ Immunity mediated by antibodies in the blood

**Hyperaesthesia** ▓ Increased, sometimes extreme, sensitivity to stimuli

**Hyperalgesia** ▓ Pain of abnormal severity following noxious stimulation

**Hyperbilirubinaemia** ▓ High levels of plasma bilirubin

**Hyperemesis (gravidarum)** ▓ Severe, excessive vomiting (during pregnancy)

**Hyperopia** ▓ Hypermetropia, farsightedness

**Hyperplasia** ▓ Abnormal increase in normal cells

**Hyperstimulation syndrome** ▓ Cumulative pain response with repeated treatment

**Hypoalgesia** ▓ Reduced pain, as opposed to analgesia (absence of pain)

**Hypocapnia** ▓ Reduced carbon dioxide in the blood

**Hyposmia** ▓ Reduced sense of smell

**Hypothalamus** ▓ Below the thalamus in the brain. Coordinates the ANS and behaviour generally, in particular temperature regulation and the physical expression of emotion

**Hypoxia** ▓ Partial lack of oxygen in blood or tissues

**Hysteroscopy** ▓ Inspection of the inside of the womb using a hysteroscope

**Ictus** ▓ Seizure, sudden attack

**Idiopathic** ▓ Of unknown cause or spontaneous origin

**Ileus** ▓ Obstruction of intestines

**Immunoglobulin** ▓ Glycoprotein antibody. There are five types: IgA, IgD, IgE, IgG, IgM

**Impedance** ▓ Term for resistance when alternating or biphasic current is used

**In phase** ▓ Two signals are in phase if there is no phase difference between them

**Inclusion criteria** ▓ Basis on which patients are included in a trial

**Indicator drop (ID)** ▓ Decrease over time of skin conductance at an acupoint

**Infarct** ▓ Area of necrosis due to local ischaemia

**Infectious mononucleosis** ▓ Glandular fever, usually caused by Epstein-Barr virus

**Infrared (IR)** ▓ Radiated heat, with a lower frequency than visible light

**Infrasound** ▓ Vibration below the frequency of audible sound

**Integrated charge (IQ)** ▓ Measured with Motoyama Hiroshi's AMI device. Taken as an indicator of general homoeostatic metabolic and immune ability

**Interburst interval** ▓ Time between two bursts

**Interference** ▓ The interaction of two or more waves to produce a resultant wave

**Interleukin** ▓ A type of cytokine. Most interleukins are produced by different types of immune cell

**Interpulse interval** ▓ Time between two pulses

**Interrupted current** ▓ Wave trains at intervals of 1 second or more

**Interstitial cystitis (IC)** ▓ Cystitis with inflammatory lesions, leading to urinary urgency, frequency and bladder pain as the bladder fills or empties, symptoms unresolved by antibiotics

**Ion cord** ▓ Electrically conductive lead containing a diode, applied clipped to inserted acupuncture needles so that any current preferentially flows one way between them. Devised by Manaka Yoshio as a polarity agent

**Ion granule** ▓ Small metal sphere used to apply pressure to specific areas of the skin for extended periods

**Ipsilateral** ▓ Situated on the same side

**Ischaemia** ▓ Reduced blood supply, usually due to functional constriction or obstruction

**Joule** ▓ Unit of energy

**Keratitis** ▓ Inflammation of the cornea

**Keratoconjunctivitis sicca** ▓ Dry eye syndrome

**Kilohm (kΩ)** ▓ One thousand ohms

**Kindling** ▓ Spread of neuronal activity in space and time, even after the initial trigger has gone

**Kraurosis** ▓ Drying and shrivelling, particularly of the vulva

**Lacuna** Small cavity

**Lagophthalmus** Incomplete closure of the eyelid

**Laparotomy** Surgical incision through the flank (below the ribs and above the pelvis)

**Laser acupuncture (LA)** Application of laser to acupoints, either transcutaneously or through an inserted needle

**Laser** Light Amplification by the Stimulated Emission of Radiation. Laser light is monochromatic, both spatially and temporally coherent, and collimated

**Latency** Time lag between stimulation and response

**Leiomyoma** Smooth muscle myoma

**Leucine** Essential amino acid

**Leu-enkephalin (LE)** Simple pentapeptide neurotransmitter with amino acid leucine at one end

**Leukocytopenia** Leukopenia, white blood cell count below about 5000/mm³

**Leukoplakia** White patches on the mucous membrane

**Lichen planus** Inflammatory pruritic skin disorder characterised by violet, flat-topped scaly papules, sometimes coalescing to form plaques

**Limbic system** Group of structures such as the septum, hippocampus, caudate nucleus, amygdala and nucleus accumbens, sometimes somewhat erroneously termed 'the emotional brain'

**Lipoprotein** Fat–protein complex in which fats and fatty acids are transported in the blood. High-density lipoprotein (HDL) carries cholesterol to the liver to be excreted as bile. Low-density lipoprotein (LDL) carries cholesterol to extrahepatic tissues

**Lithogenesis** Formation of stones

**Lithotripsy** Fragmentation and washing out of gall- or urinary stones within the body

**Low-intensity laser (or light) therapy (LILT)** Therapeutic application of low output power (< 500 mW) lasers and monochromatic 'superluminous' diodes at athermal levels

**Lymphadenopathy** Disease affecting lymph nodes

**Lymphoedema** Chronic oedema of an extremity as a result of impaired lymphatic circulation. May be bilateral

**Malar** Pertaining to the cheek

**Mammary hyperplasia** Fibrocystic breast disease, mastosis

**Manual acupuncture (MA)** Needling, without adjunctive electrical or other nontraditional stimulation

**Mast cell** Connective tissue cell that forms granules that contain histamine and, in rodents, 5HT. On degranulation, these are released

**Measure yourself medical outcome profile (MYMOP)** A self-rating measure useful in holistic research where more than one outcome is being assessed

**Medulla oblongata** Part of the brainstem, between the *pons varolii* above and the spinal cord below

**Megohm (MΩ)** One million ohms

**Ménière's disease** Disorder of the labyrinth of the inner ear, with symptoms of deafness, tinnitus and vertigo

**Menorrhagia** Menstruation with excessive flow

**Meralgia paraesthetica** Pain and paraesthesiae in the lower two-thirds of the anterolateral thigh, due to nerve compression or injury in the groin

**Meridian complexes** Complex homoeopathic remedies corresponding in symptom picture to the acupuncture meridians, developed by Helmut Schimmel

**Mesolimbic loop** A circuit in the brain postulated by Han Jisheng, involving the periaqueductal grey, nucleus accumbens, habenula and other nuclei

**Meta-analysis** A specific statistical technique of pooling data from several independent studies

**Met-enkephalin (ME)** Simple pentapeptide neurotransmitter with amino acid methionine at one end, central to the mechanism of EA in the spinal cord

**Mho** Unit of conductance

**Microampère** One millionth of an ampère

**Microcurrent** Stimulation with microampère (μA) currents (< 1 mA) that may not result in sensation, and produces its effects without involving action potentials in the nerves

**Microwave resonance therapy (MRT)** Treatment method using EHF millimetre waves, often generated by spark discharges within a resonant cavity

**Micturition** Urination

**Milliampère** One thousandth of an ampère

**Millimetre waves** Extremely high frequency waves, at 30–300 GHz (30–300 × 10⁹ Hz)

**Millitesla** Unit of magnetic flux density. 1 mT = 10 G

**Millivolt** One thousandth of a volt

**Mitogenic** Inducing or causing mitosis, cell division

**Modulation** Change. A signal may be amplitude, frequency or pulse duration modulated

**Monoamine** Compound containing one amino (—NH₂) group

**Monophasic current** Interrupted direct current

**Monopolar** Method of electrode placement in EMG or EMS where one electrode is positioned in the muscle concerned, and the return electrode elsewhere

**MORA** Principle of and device for using the body's own signals as the basis for treatment

**Motilin** A gut hormone

**Motoneuron** Motor neuron, activating muscle fibres via motor end plates

**Motor end plate** Where axon of motor nerve interfaces with striated muscle fibre

**Motor level** Stimulation sufficient to activate motor nerve fibres

**Motor line** ▦ Intramuscular or intermuscular groove, along which stimulation yields muscle twitch, and in some cases possibly correlating with an acupuncture meridian

**Motor point (MP)** ▦ Point on skin where electrical muscle stimulation will result in maximum contraction

**Motor unit** ▦ Motor nerve, its end plates and the muscle fibres that it activates

**Mucositis** ▦ Inflammation of mucous membrane

**Muscarinic receptor** ▦ Receptors for ACh, excitatory (M1) in the cerebral cortex, and inhibitory (M2) in the basal forebrain and brainstem

**Myelopathy** ▦ Spinal cord pathology

**Myoclonic** ▦ Used of shock-like muscular contractions, sometimes occurring synchronously in different areas

**Myoelectrical** ▦ Pertaining to the electrical properties of muscle

**Myofascial pain syndrome** ▦ Musculoskeletal pain without an obvious cause, usually associated with muscle shortening and the formation of trigger points, with nerve entrapment and neuropathic (sensory, motor or autonomic) manifestations

**Myogelosis** ▦ Area of hardening in a muscle

**Myogenic** ▦ Originating in muscle or its dysfunction

**Myoma** ▦ Benign muscle tumour

**Myotome** ▦ Group of muscles innervated from a single spinal segment

**Naevus** ▦ Congenital skin lesion, usually pigmented

**Naloxone** ▦ The major opioid antagonist used experimentally

**Nanometre** ▦ Unit of length. 1 nm = $10^{-9}$ m

**Narcolepsy** ▦ Irresistible drowsiness occurring several times daily

**Natural killer (NK) cell** ▦ A type of immune cell

**Necrosis** ▦ Cell or tissue death

**Neural therapy** ▦ A method of treatment using local anaesthetic injections, discovered by the brothers Ferdinand and Walter Huneke in the 1920s

**Neurapraxia** ▦ Conduction block in injured nerve that recovers relatively quickly (sometimes spelled 'neuropraxia')

**Neurasthenia** ▦ A group of symptoms resulting from some functional nervous system disorder, usually due to prolonged and excessive expenditure of energy. It is marked by a tendency to fatigue, lack of energy, back pain, memory loss, insomnia, constipation and loss of appetite

**Neurinoma** ▦ Neoplasm of a nerve's myelin sheath

**Neuritis** ▦ Nerve inflammation, with pain, tenderness, anaesthesia and paraesthesiae, as well as paralysis and muscle wasting

**Neurodermatitis** ▦ Eczematous skin disorder, possibly psychogenic. More strictly, a lichenoid eruption limited to the axillary and pubic areas and associated with a nervous disorder

**Neuroelectric acupuncture** ▦ Transcutaneous electrical acupoint stimulation (TEAS) or probe TENS (pTENS), the application of electrical stimulation to acupoints via surface electrodes. Also used as a variant of acupuncture-like TENS (ALTENS)

**Neurofibromatosis** ▦ Condition characterised by changes in the nervous system, muscles, bones and skin, including multiple soft tumours distributed all over the body

**Neurogenic bladder** ▦ Any bladder condition caused by central or peripheral nervous system lesion

**Neurogenic pain** ▦ Pain arising from damage to neurons, although sustained by CNS changes

**Neuroleptanalgesia** ▦ Analgesia using an opioid analgesic together with a neuroleptic agent such as droperidol. The result is a state of quiescence as well as absence of pain

**Neuroleptic** ▦ Drug producing a state of apathy and reducing emotional response

**Neurometer** ▦ Device for measuring and adjusting sympathetic nerve excitation

**Neuromodulation** ▦ Electrical stimulation of central or peripheral nerves, usually for relief of pain

**Neuromodulator** ▦ Chemical that modulates synaptic transmission, although not a neurotransmitter itself

**Neuropathy** ▦ Functional disturbance or pathological change in peripheral nervous system

**Neuropeptides** ▦ Single chains of amino acids, forming the largest neurochemical family

**Neurosis** ▦ Mental disorder in which the ability to distinguish reality from fantasy is unimpaired

**Neurotmesis** ▦ Complete severance of a nerve

**Neurotransmitter** ▦ Substance released from presynaptic boutons of one neuron, crossing synaptic cleft to affect target cell

**Nicotinic receptors** ▦ Receptors for ACh in brainstem and spinal cord motoneurons

**Nitric oxide (NO)** ▦ Gaseous neurotransmitter. Not to be confused with nitrous oxide ($N_2O$)

**Nociception** ▦ Ability to feel pain

**Nociceptive pain** ▦ Pain arising from activation of nociceptors

**Nociceptor** ▦ Pain receptor

**Nogier frequency rates** ▦ Stimulation frequencies for use in different regions of the ear

**Noradrenaline (NA)** ▦ Monoamine neurotransmitter in the ANS, acting more on α receptors

**Norepinephrine** ▦ Noradrenaline

**Noxious level** ▦ Stimulation sufficient to activate nociceptive C fibres

**Numerical rating scale** ▦ Method of rating a response such as pain, using numbers, usually 0–10 or 0–100, with 0 representing 'no pain' and 10 or 100 'the worst pain imaginable'

**Nystagmus** ▦ Involuntary movements of the eye

**Ohm (Ω)** Unit of electrical resistance

**Oligospermia** Low sperm count

**Orchitis** Inflammation of the testes

**Orphanin (nociceptin)** Peptide neurotransmitter with opposite effects in different regions of the CNS

**Oscillopsia** Apparent movement of objects

**Osteochondritis** In Russian studies, this may refer to spondylitis rather than inflammation of both bone and cartilage, its standard meaning in the West

**Osteochondrosis** In Russian studies, this may refer to spondylosis rather than juvenile kyphosis

**Osteopenia** Reduced bone synthesis

**Otalgia** Ear pain

**-otomy** Surgical incision

**Outcome** Result (of a study)

**Overflow incontinence** Leakage of small amounts of urine after the bladder has contracted to its limit

**Pad** Type of surface electrode, used either with a conductive gel, or self-adhesive

**Pain** An unpleasant sensory and emotional experience associated with actual or potential tissue damage, or described in terms of such damage

**Pain threshold (PT)** Lowest level of input at which pain is expressed, frequently assessed in experimental research on EA

**Palpebritis** Blepharitis, inflammation of the eyelids

**Pancreatic polypeptide** A hormone and neurotransmitter, secreted in the pancreatic islets and elsewhere

**Paraesthesia (plural, paraesthesiae)** Abnormal tactile sensation, such as burning or prickling, often occurring without external stimulus

**Paralytic strabismus** Strabismus usually due to lesions of the nerve supplying the affected extraocular muscles

**Paraplegia** Paralysis of the lower trunk and limbs

**Paraspinal (paravertebral)** Beside the spine (vertebrae)

**Parasympathetic nervous system** Craniosacral division of the ANS, more active in periods of rest and tranquillity

**Paresis** Partial paralysis

**Peak amplitude** Measure between greatest value and zero of a DC or monophasic waveform

**Peak-to-peak amplitude** Measure between greatest positive and negative values of a biphasic waveform

**Peptides** Compounds containing amino acids. The constituent parts of proteins. There are many families of peptides (opioid, pituitary, circulatory, gut and so on)

**Percutaneous electrical nerve stimulation (PENS)** Much the same as electroacupuncture, if not at traditional points

**Percutaneous** Of electrodes, used to stimulate intramuscularly, beneath the skin

**Period** Duration of a cycle

**Permanent magnet** Magnetic material producing a constant magnetic field

**Peyronie's disease** Autoimmune condition, in which inelastic plaque is formed that does not expand with erection and therefore causes curvature of the penis and pain

**Phase** That part of a cycle in which current is flowing in one direction only

**Phase duration** Duration of a phase

**Pheochromocytoma** A rare form of adrenal tumour

**Phlebitis** Inflammation of a vein

**Phonophoresis (sonophoresis)** Introduction of substances into body using acoustic or ultrasonic frequencies

**Phrenic nerve** Mixed nerve, controlling the diaphragm

**Piezolelectric effect** Contraction or expansion of a crystal in response to an applied electric field, and the converse phenomenon: production of an electrical pulse when pressure (stress) is applied to a piezoelectric crystal

**Pilomotor** Pertaining to the muscles that cause erection of the hair

**Piriformis syndrome** Symptoms that mimic those of discogenic sciatica spasm, but are due to contracture or injury of the pyriformis muscle and compression of the sciatic nerve

**Plantar fasciitis** A painful inflammation of the fascia between the heel and metatarsal heads

**Platelet aggregation** Part of the process leading to formation of a blood clot

**Polarity agent** Various bipolar agents, such as magnets or ion cords, that appear to act in some way to balance the body's energy

**Polarity** Electric charges of positive and negative polarity may have opposite effects. Opposite poles attract, like poles repel

**Pollinosis** Hay fever

**Polyneuropathy** Simultaneous neuropathy of several peripheral nerves

**Postpolio syndrome** A condition, similar to fibromyalgia or chronic fatigue syndrome, that may ensue even years after the initial viral infection and seeming recovery

**Potential** The electric potential at a point in a field is the potential energy per unit charge of a positively charged particle placed at that point

**Potential difference** The difference in potential energy between two points in a field

**Potential energy** The capacity to expend energy

**Power** Rate at which work can be done

**Pragmatic study** Study of treatment *effectiveness*, under normal clinical conditions involving many variables, as opposed to *explanatory research*. Pragmatic research aims to maximise external validity (generalisability)

**Presbycusis** Progressive, bilateral hearing loss with age

**Pressor** Blood pressure increasing

**Probe** Handheld device for treatment or measurement, generally at points on the surface of the body

**Probe, point or punctate TENS (pTENS)** Electrical treatment using a small diameter handheld probe at points on the surface of the body, often acupoints

**Proctitis** Inflammation of the rectum

**Projection zone** (of an organ) Cutaneous region segmentally related to the organ

**Proprioception** Awareness of the body

**Prostaglandins** A family of potent mediators of many physiological processes, mostly synthesised from arachidonic acid

**Proton** Particle with charge equal and opposite to that of an electron, but with much greater mass

**Pruritis** Itching, an unpleasant sensation in which C fibres are activated

**Pseudobulbar paralysis** Spastic weakness of muscles innervated by cranial nerves

**Psychosis** Mental disorder in which the ability to distinguish reality from fantasy is impaired

**Pulse** Brief flow of current. Sometimes an interrupted current is said to be pulsed

**Pulse duration** Total time for a complete pulse

**Pulse repetition rate (PRR)** The correct term for frequency when applied to pulses

**Pyelonephritis** Inflammation of the kidney and renal pelvis due to bacterial infection

**Q-tip probe** A type of handheld probe used with some microcurrent devices

**Quadrant measurements** Electrical measurements, generally between hands, feet, and hands and feet, used to assess the overall state of the patient

**Radiation** The transmission of energy through a medium as waves or particles

**Radiculitis** Inflammation of a spinal nerve root

**Radionics** A method of assessment and treatment, sometimes in the absence of the patient, utilising specially designed instruments based on unconventional electrical or electronic circuitry

**Randomisation** Assignment of patients to groups according to a defined method which ensures that distribution of any characteristics between the groups varies only by chance. Used to reduce error and bias in clinical trials

**Raynaud's phenomenon** Intermittent bilateral ischaemia of the extremities, and sometimes ears or nose, often accompanied by paraesthesiae and pain

**Reflex incontinence** Subtype of urge incontinence, in which voiding occurs periodically without advance warning

**Regulatory effect** A treatment has a regulatory effect if it reduces overfunctioning or increases underfunctioning of some aspect(s) of an organism, but has little influence on an organism already in equilibrium

**Remedy testing** Procedure used in EAV and some other systems, whereby appropriate remedies are selected in accordance with the interpretation of electrical acupoint measurements

**Resection** Partial excision

**Resistance (R)** Opposite of conductance. Used in relation to direct or monophasic currents, not if alternating or biphasic

**Resonance mode** Major operating rhythm, often characteristic of a particular brain region

**Resonant frequency** Frequency at which an object or circuit vibrates or oscillates occurs naturally. If an external signal is applied at this frequency, resonance occurs

**Retinitis pigmentosa** Retinal disorder, often hereditary, with retinal atrophy, clumping of retinal pigment and contracted field of vision

**Rhizopathy** Nerve root disorder (radiculopathy)

**Rigor** Muscle rigidity

**Rise time** Time taken for a pulse to reach maximum amplitude

**Rostral** Towards the oral and nasal region, as opposed to *caudal*, inferior

**Rotator cuff** Muscles and tendons around the capsule of the shoulder joint

**Ryodoraku** Integrated acupoint measurement and treatment system developed by Nakatani Yoshio in the 1950s

**Sample size** Number of patients required in a study to ensure it has adequate statistical power, with an outcome that is unlikely to be due to statistical error

**Satiety centre** Ventromedial hypothalamus

**Schizoaffective disorder** Condition in which symptoms of schizophrenia may be associated with mania or depression

**Schumann resonance** Standing wave resonance occurring in the cavity between the earth's surface and the ionosphere

**Scleroderma** Chronic hardening and thickening of the skin, occurring as a systemic connective tissue disorder as well as locally in some conditions

**Sclerotome** Areas of bone innervated from a single spinal segment

**Segment** A spinal segment consists of the dermatome, myotome and sclerotome innervated by a particular pair of spinal nerves, together with the viscerotome innervated by sympathetic nerves from the same level of the spinal cord

**Semiconductor** Substance whose conductivity is intermediate between that of a conductor and an insulator

**Sensor reaction or response** Sensations experienced in response to EHF stimulation, used as a guide to frequency selection in microwave resonance therapy (MRT)

**Sensory level** Stimulation sufficient to activate sensory nerve fibres

**Sensory neuron** Nerve transmitting signals from sensory receptors

**Sequela (plural, sequelae)** After-effect

**Serotonin (5HT)** 5-hydroxytryptamine, a monoamine neurotransmitter

**Shin splints** Strain of the flexor digitorum longus muscle, with pain along the shin

**Shock** Circulatory collapse, with inadequate perfusion of vital organs

**Shoulder–hand syndrome** A form of complex regional pain disorder (CRPD)

**Siccus** Dry

**Silver spike point (SSP)** These electrodes combine attributes of both needles and surface pads, being noninvasive but shaped so that pressure and charge are concentrated at a point

**Singlet oxygen** Oxygen in the form of single O atoms rather than the usual $O_2$ molecule

**Sjögren's syndrome** Symptom complex of dry eyes (keratoconjunctivitis sicca), xerostomia and a connective tissue disorder, of unknown aetiology

**Somatostatin** A neurotransmitter and hormone secreted by the pancreatic islets and hypothalamus that inhibits release of insulin, glucagon, growth hormone and other hormones

**Somnambulism** Sleep walking

**Sonopuncture** Application of ultrasound to acupoints

**Spike** Waveform with short rise and decay times

**Spinal cord stimulation (SCS)** Electrical stimulation of the spinal cord, usually for chronic pain, sometimes called dorsal column stimulation (DCS)

**Spirography** Registration of respiratory movements

**Splitter** Plug containing two sockets, so that one output can supply more than two electrodes

**Spondylarthrosis** Disorder of the joints of the spine

**Spondylitis** Vertebral inflammation

**Spondylosis** Used here in the sense of degenerative spinal change due to osteoarthritis. May refer to reduced movement of the intervertebral joints

**Status asthmaticus** Severe episode of asthma, responding insufficiently to standard treatment, possibly requiring hospitalisation

**Status epilepticus** Continuous series of seizures for more than five minutes without return to consciousness. Life-threatening

**Stenosis** Abnormal narrowing of a duct or canal

**Stomatitis** Inflammation of the oral mucosa

**Stomatodynia** Mouth pain

**Strangury** Slow, painful urination due to spasm

**Stress incontinence** Involuntary passage of urine when intra-abdominal pressure is raised

**Stridor** High pitched breathing sound

**Strong reactor** Felix Mann's term for someone who is likely to respond strongly to acupuncture

**Subarachnoid haemorrhage** Bleed beneath the delicate middle membrane covering the brain

**Subluxation** Partial dislocation

**Submaximal** Of stimulation that is less than the greatest normally possible for the tissue being stimulated

**Subperception electrical stimulation (SPES)** A form of CES

**Substance P (SP)** A gut peptide

**Substantia nigra** Region of the brainstem containing relatively large amounts of dopamine and iron. Loss of dopaminergic neurons from this nucleus is associated with Parkinson's disease

**Sudomotor** Affecting the activity of the sweat glands

**Supraspinal** Pertaining to the region above (rostral to) the spine

**Symmetrical waveform** Waveform with identical positive and negative phases

**Sympathetic block** Blocking of the sympathetic trunk (either side of the vertebral column) using paravertebral infiltration of an anaesthetic agent

**Sympathetic nervous system** Thoracolumbar division of the ANS, preparing the body for 'fight or flight'

**Sympatholytic** Sympathetic-calming

**Sympathotonic** Sympathetic-activating

**Synergistic** Acting together, (mutually) enhancing

**Systematic review** The process of conducting a comprehensive evidence synthesis from different studies, involving search strategy, evaluation of study quality and analysis

**Tail-flick latency** Pain threshold test, assessing response to noxious thermal or electric stimulus

**TDP far-infrared lamp** Gives out a radiation spectrum claimed to coincide with the 'bio-spectrum' of the human body, and a more deeply penetrating heat than standard heat lamps

**Tensegrity** Term coined by Buckminster Fuller, exemplified by James Oschman in the connective tissue matrix of the body, capable of converting one form of energy to another

**TENS-like EA (TLEA)** HF low intensity EA, with short pulse durations

**Tesla** Unit of magnetic flux density

**Tetanic** Smooth contraction of muscle above critical fusion frequency

**Thalamic syndrome** Contralateral hemianaesthesia, sometimes with severe chronic pain and other symptoms

**Thalamus** Part of the diencephalon in the brain, a relay between second order neurons from the dorsal horn and third order neurons to the cortex. The brain's principal pacemaker

**Theophylline** ▪ Compound found in tea leaves

**Thermography** ▪ Method of measuring temperature, either over large areas of the body or at individual points

**Theta (θ)** ▪ 3–7 Hz frequencies in the EEG

**Thoracic outlet syndrome** ▪ Any of a variety of neurovascular syndromes resulting from compression of the subclavian artery, brachial plexus nerve trunks, or axillary or subclavian vein

**Thrombolysis** ▪ Decomposition of a blood clot

**Thromboxane** ▪ Prostaglandin-related compound derived from arachidonic acid. Thromboxane $A_2$ induces platelet aggregation

**Tic douloureux** ▪ Trigeminal neuralgia

**Tolerance** ▪ Reduced response to a drug or other treatment following prolonged or repeated use

**Toxaemia** ▪ Any condition resulting from the spread of toxins in the blood, in pregnancy often associated with hypertension

**Train** ▪ A continuous series of pulses of limited duration

**Transcranial electrotherapy (TCET)** ▪ A form of CES using stronger intensities and sometimes higher frequencies, usually employed as a method of electroanalgesia or electroanaesthesia

**Transcutaneous electrical nerve stimulation (TENS)** ▪ Method of peripheral neuromodulation using surface electrodes

**Transcutaneous** ▪ Of electrodes, applied to the surface of the body

**Transcutaneous spinal electroanalgesia (TSE)** ▪ Method of treatment developed by the British medical acupuncturist Alexander Macdonald, using electrodes directly over the spine to obtain the effects of implanted spinal column stimulation but non-invasively

**Trigger point (TrP)** ▪ Tender point where sustained pressure reproduces pain in areas where it occurs spontaneously

**Trophic ulcer (or other disorder)** ▪ Ulcer (or other disorder) caused by poor nutrition of the affected area

**Type A (Aα, Aβ, Aγ and Aδ) and C nerve fibres** ▪ Types Aα, Aβ and Aγ are thick and myelinated, type Aδ are thin and myelinated, and type C are thin and unmyelinated

**Type I – IV muscle afferents** ▪ Afferent nerves from muscle, type I being the thickest, type IV the thinnest. Types I–II correspond roughly to Aα, Aβ and Aγ fibres, type III to Aδ, and type IV to C fibres

**Ultrasound** ▪ Vibration at a higher frequency than audible sound

**Ultraviolet (UV)** ▪ Electromagnetic radiation, with a higher frequency than visible light

**Unilateral** ▪ Pertaining to one side of the body

**Urge incontinence** ▪ Urge to urinate, followed within seconds or minutes by voiding, even though the individual attempts to delay it. Often associated with detrusor overactivity or instability

**Urolithiasis** ▪ Urinary stones

**Uroschesis** ▪ Urinary retention

**Uterine inertia** ▪ Uncoordinated or weak uterine contractions during labour

**Vagus nerve** ▪ Cranial nerve X (mixed), a key player in the ANS

**Vasoactive intestinal polypeptide (VIP)** ▪ A gut peptide

**Vasomotor** ▪ Affecting the diameter of a vessel

**Vasovagal** ▪ Usually evoked by anxiety or pain, a vasovagal attack is a transient reaction involving a rapid fall in blood pressure that can result in loss of consciousness. Preliminary signs include pallor, nausea, sweating and bradycardia

**Vegatest** ▪ 'Vegetative reflex test' devised by Helmut Schimmel as a simplified and less expensive method of meridian testing than EAV

**Version** ▪ Turning the baby

**Viscerotome** ▪ Viscera innervated from a single spinal segment. An alternative definition considers the viscerotome as the approximate superficial area to which pain is referred from a particular internal organ

**Visual analogue scale** ▪ Method of rating a response such as pain, using a vertical or horizontal line whose ends are labelled, for instance, 'no pain' and 'the worst pain imaginable'

**Volt** ▪ Unit of potential energy and potential difference

**Waveform** ▪ The shape of a wave

**Wavelength (λ)** ▪ The distance between successive wave crests

**Window** ▪ Narrow range of frequencies or amplitudes having a biological effect

**Xerophthalmia** ▪ Dry eyes, usually associated with night blindness

**Xerostomia** ▪ Dryness of the mouth due to salivary gland dysfunction

**β-endorphin (βEP)** ▪ Opioid peptide neurotransmitter (and neurohormone) considered responsible for many effects of EA

## RESOURCES USED IN COMPILING THIS GLOSSARY

The main source has been:

Anderson DM, Novak PD, Keith J, Elliott MA, 2000 (eds) Dorland's Illustrated Medical Dictionary. Saunders, Philadelphia, PA (30th edn)

# Index

Note: **bold type** signifies definitions; *italic type* signifies illustrations